Engineering and Characterisation of Novel Nanomedicine Formulations, 2nd Edition

Engineering and Characterisation of Novel Nanomedicine Formulations, 2nd Edition

Guest Editors

Ana Isabel Fraguas-Sánchez
Francisco Bolás-Fernández
Raquel Fernández García

MDPI

Basel • Beijing • Wuhan • Barcelona • Belgrade • Novi Sad • Cluj • Manchester

Guest Editors
Ana Isabel Fraguas-Sánchez
Department of Pharmaceutics and Food Technology
Complutense University of Madrid
Madrid
Spain

Francisco Bolás-Fernández
Departamento de Parasitología
Universidad Complutense de Madrid
Madrid
Spain

Raquel Fernández García
Department of Pharmaceutics and Food Technology
Complutense University of Madrid
Madrid
Spain

Editorial Office
MDPI AG
Grosspeteranlage 5
4052 Basel, Switzerland

This is a reprint of the Special Issue, published open access by the journal *Pharmaceutics* (ISSN 1999-4923), freely accessible at: https://www.mdpi.com/journal/pharmaceutics/special_issues/C2GH4Q0FJ7.

For citation purposes, cite each article independently as indicated on the article page online and as indicated below:

Lastname, A.A.; Lastname, B.B. Article Title. *Journal Name* **Year**, *Volume Number*, Page Range.

ISBN 978-3-7258-5281-9 (Hbk)
ISBN 978-3-7258-5282-6 (PDF)
https://doi.org/10.3390/books978-3-7258-5282-6

Contents

About the Editors

Ana Isabel Fraguas Sánchez

Ana Isabel Fraguas obtained her PhD in Pharmacy from Complutense University of Madrid in 2020, where she focused on the development of micro- and nanoparticles for the delivery of novel antineoplastics in breast and ovarian cancers. Her PhD thesis was awarded with the "Doctorate Extraordinary Award 2019" from the Faculty of Pharmacy of Complutense University and the "Juan Abello I" prize from the Doctor Academy of Spain. She also received "Juan Abello 2019 prize" of the Spanish Royal Academy of Pharmacy for her scientific research. She has participated in 22 research projects funded by Spanish and European institutions, and by pharmaceutical and related companies (7 of them as principal investigator). She is the author of 39 peer-reviewed articles and 6 book chapters and has participated in over 50 scientific conferences. She serves as an evaluator of research projects for institutions in Poland, Spain, and France, as well as a member of the board of directors of the Spanish Society of Industrial and Galenic Pharmacy. She has completed several predoctoral and postdoctoral research placements (Italy, Switzerland, Finland, and Greece). Currently, she is Assistant Professor of Pharmaceutics, Biopharmacy, and Pharmacokinetics at Complutense University of Madrid. Her research group is focused on the development, optimization, and preclinical evaluation of novel controlled drug delivery systems (with a special focus on implants, micro- and nanoparticles) for the treatment of cancer, inflammatory and infectious diseases.

Francisco Bolás Fernández

Francisco Bolás Fernández earned his PhD in Pharmacy from Complutense University of Madrid in 1981, where he focused on the anthelmintic activity of benzimidazole-carbamates in Trichinella spiralis. After his graduation, Francisco was awarded a Fleming Scholarship, which allowed him to continue his research career in the Department of Zoology at University of Nottingham, where he applied humoral and cellular immune responses to characterize antigens of Trichinella species from different geographical origin. This allowed him to return to Complutense University of Madrid as full-time professor, where he established his research group focused on the investigation of the immunological fundaments of the application of Trichuris and Trichinella sp. in the treatment of autoimmune diseases. Apart from that, he extended his research interest to the development of novel treatments for leishmaniasis. Francisco is the author of 130 publications and has been part of more than 150 scientific conferences. He has also been part of 33 research projects funded by public institutions and related companies.

Raquel Fernández García

Raquel Fernández García earned her PhD in Pharmacy from Complutense University of Madrid in 2020, where she focused in developing novel oral and topical treatments for infectious diseases. Her thesis was awarded an international distinction and the 'Folch Foundation award' in 2021. Later, she joined the School of Pharmacy at University of Nottingham as a postdoctoral research associate, where she worked in the optimization of stable formulations based on viral vectors for gene therapy and the use of nanotechnology in tree propagation. In 2025, she was appointed Assistant Professor of Pharmacy at Complutense University of Madrid. She has authored 17 articles and 1 book chapter and has collaborated with different academic institutions and industrial partners. She has recently established her independent research focusing on micro- and nanoparticles for the treatment of infectious diseases.

pharmaceutics

Editorial

Editorial for Special Issue 'Engineering and Characterisation of Novel Nanomedicine Formulations, 2nd Edition'

Raquel Fernández-García [1,*], Francisco Bolás-Fernández [2] and Ana Isabel Fraguas-Sánchez [3,4,*]

1 School of Pharmacy, University of Nottingham, University Park, Nottingham NG7 2RD, UK
2 Department of Microbiology and Parasitology, Faculty of Pharmacy, Complutense University, 28040 Madrid, Spain
3 Department of Pharmaceutics and Food Technology, Faculty of Pharmacy, Complutense University, 28040 Madrid, Spain
4 Institute of Industrial Pharmacy, Complutense University, 28040 Madrid, Spain
* Correspondence: raquel.fernandez-garcia@nottingham.ac.uk (R.F.-G.); aifraguas@ucm.es (A.I.F.-S.)

Nanomedicine applies nanotechnology to revolutionise healthcare through the development of systems at the nanoscale (below 1000 nm) to enhance drug delivery. These nanosystems are designed not only to optimise drug release profiles, but also to solve critical pharmaceutical challenges by encapsulating poorly soluble drugs and precisely targeting specific tissues, thus significantly reducing their adverse effects. Nanosystems can also protect drugs from degradation, proving especially valuable for sensitive therapeutic agents like proteins and RNA, thus unlocking new treatment possibilities.

This Special Issue, titled 'Engineering and Characterisation of Novel Nanomedicine Formulations, 2nd Edition', showcases cutting-edge developments in the nanomedicine field. The Special Issue consists of 11 research articles and 2 review articles that present diverse and significant advances in this rapidly evolving field. The articles cover multiple nanosystems, including inorganic and lipid nanoparticles, micelles, nanoemulsions, dendrimers and nanocrystals.

Mebeverine hydrochloride is an antispasmodic agent used to regulate bowel movements and relax intestinal smooth muscle; however, its application in clinical practice is limited due to its specific side effects [1]. Stoyanova et al. (contribution 1) developed silver nanoparticles loaded with this therapeutic agent to treat gastrointestinal spasmodic disorders [2]. These nanoparticles were synthesised using $AgNO_3$ under previously optimised conditions. This formulation proved promising compared to other commercially available drugs, although it showed a lower anti-inflammatory effect than free mebeverine hydrochloride.

As discussed by Fernández-García and Fraguas-Sánchez (contribution 2), pulmonary drug delivery has recently become a hot topic in pharmaceutical development to combat respiratory infections and lung cancer. One of the main challenges is successful drug deposition into the lungs, as the respiratory system tries to eliminate inhaled particles. In this context, nanomedicine has emerged as a useful strategy to engineer particles with prolonged pulmonary retention, as they can avoid clearance while reducing systemic drug distribution and, thus, adverse systemic effects. In this context Party et al. (contribution 3) developed a nanoparticle-based dry-powder inhaler as a strategy to enable ciprofloxacin to exert targeted antibacterial activity in the lungs. This system was characterised by large lung deposition and a suitable aerodynamic diameter, which allows for the potential treatment of patients with different respiratory infections. Khan et al. (contribution 4) explored the pulmonary delivery of nanostructured lipid carriers loaded with trans-resveratrol to treat lung cancer, which is the leading cause of cancer death worldwide [3]. They developed 24 formulations in which one solid lipid (Dynasan 116) was combined with four liquid lipids (Capryol 90, Lauroglycol 90, Miglyol 810 and Tributyrin) at different solid/liquid ratios and different drug concentrations. The optimised formulation was stable for six months and exhibited excellent aerosolisation performance when using an air-jet nebuliser. Encapsulating trans-resveratrol within lipid nanocarriers enabled sustained drug release, which was markedly visible after 3 h, where free-drug levels reached ~76% of the total drug concentration, while nanocarriers released ~37%.

Due to the recent global healthcare situation, lipid nanoparticles have been studied to determine their efficacy in combating severe acute respiratory syndrome coronavirus 2 (SARS-CoV-2), particularly in engineering vaccine platforms [4]. The manufacturing of lipid nanoparticles in SARS-CoV-2 mRNA vaccines has garnered attention, as these can preserve and deliver mRNA to specific cells with a low to moderate immunological response [5]. Their effectiveness has been confirmed, as multiple lipid-nanoparticle-based mRNA vaccines against SARS-CoV-2 have been approved by regulatory agencies. However, lipid nanoparticles tend to accumulate in the liver, meaning that only a fraction of each dose reaches the target, and their poor long-term storage stability remains an obstacle. Lipid nanoparticles primarily consist of lipid components, including ionisable lipids, helper lipids (phospholipids and cholesterol) and polyethylene glycol (PEG)-containing lipids. The latter has a significant effect on the physicochemical properties, stability and in vivo kinetics of the formulation [6]. In this context, Saraswat et al. (contribution 5) utilised polysorbate 80 as an alternative PEG-lipid to manufacture lipid nanoparticles for the SARS-CoV-2 vaccine. They prepared lipid nanoparticles with a lipid composition of (6Z,9Z,28Z,31Z)-heptatriacont-6,9,28,31-tetraene-19-yl 4-(dimethylamino)butanoate (DLin-MC3-DMA), distearoylphosphatidylcholine (DSPC), cholesterol and polysorbate 80. This formulation showed enhanced spleen tropism over liver accumulation, maintaining high mRNA encapsulation and activity after over six months of storage at −80 °C.

It is well known that using micelles is an excellent strategy to enhance the solubility of poorly soluble drugs [7]. D-α-tocopherol PEG 100 succinate (VitE-TPGS) is an amphiphilic molecule widely used in formulation, as it is capable of forming micelles in aqueous environments due to its low critical micelle concentration [8]. De Caro et al. (contribution 6) used VitE-TPGS to prepare micelles in the presence and absence of poorly soluble pharmaceutical compounds. These micelles were then investigated in terms of their morphology to assess their ability to solubilise poorly soluble pharmaceutical compounds. For this purpose, a novel theoretical approach to analysing the pair distribution function was developed. This model was able to estimate the relative fractions of drugs incorporated into the core and shell of the micelles.

Stankovic et al. (contribution 7) developed intravenous nanoemulsions with a pyrazoloquionline ligand to enhance drug delivery to the brain. This ligand showed a unique profile of selective binding to σ2 receptors; however, its poor solubility hampers its research and development. An in vitro blood–brain barrier study demonstrated that a substantial part of the ligand, when applied in a nanoemulsion, was able to permeate the barrier.

It should be noted that nanomedicine can also be useful in regenerative medicine and tissue engineering. Extracellular vesicles (EVs) are nanosized particles secreted by various cell types that mediate intercellular communication. Galbiati et al. (contribution 8) used fibroblast-derived EVs to functionalise hydrogels. These hydrogels consisted of gelatin methacrylate (GelMA), which is a widely used biomaterial with tuneable mechanical, chemical and biological properties that is also able to support wound healing. In a murine model, hydrogels loaded with fibroblast-derived EVs significantly accelerated wound healing. These hydrogels, containing trehalose and polyvinylpyrrolidone 40 (PVP40), maintained a uniform population of vesicles, making them essential for preserving the structural and functional characteristics of EVs during freeze-drying.

Strzelecka et al. (contribution 9) synthesised a novel poly(amidoamine) (PAMAM) dendrimer/camptothecin complex as a novel strategy for targeted cancer treatment. These complexes controlled the release of camptothecin over long periods of time (>400 h).

Nanocrystals can be used in pharmaceutical research as a drug delivery system to improve the oral bioavailability of Biopharmaceutics Classification System (BCS) class II and IV drugs. For example, Cheng et al. (contribution 10) developed curcumin nanocrystal liposomes to overcome the limited bioavailability of this drug. The encapsulation of nanocrystals within liposomes showed significantly slower dissolution rates in simulated intestinal fluid than the nanocrystal alone, showing that the lipid bilayer impeded rapid core nanocrystal dissolution while showing superior mucus-penetrating capabilities in cell uptakes studies.

Micro- and nanomotors are devices with the ability to generate autonomous movement through the conversion of several forms of stimulation [9]. Among these stimuli, chemical reagents, light, ultrasound frequencies and magnetic fields can be found. Their ability to exert continuous movement enhances their interaction with target molecules, thus facilitating drug delivery, improving the accumulation rate in complex biological environments and enabling their penetration into tissues. Donoso-González et al. (contribution 11) developed a novel core–shell micromotor that combined magnetic and photothermal properties. It was synthesised via the template-assisted electrodeposition of iron and reduced graphene oxide on a microtubular pore-shaped membrane. The resulting iron-reduced graphene oxide core–shell micromotors, loaded with doxorubicin, successfully released the drug upon near-infrared irradiation.

Hybrid lipid nanoparticles that combine proteins with lipids represent an emerging class of nanocarriers designed to leverage the advantages of both biological and synthetic components for drug delivery, gene therapy and vaccine applications [10]. Maeyouf et al. (contribution 12) developed novel hybrid lipid nanoparticles that contained zein and were conjugated to the cancer-targeting ligand transferrin. Specifically, these nanoparticles were designed to entrap the anticancer drug docetaxel and carry plasmid DNA. This formulation efficiently entrapped docetaxel, leading to its increased uptake by different cancer cell lines and enhancing its anti-proliferative efficacy. Furthermore, proficient DNA condensation was demonstrated, resulting in increased gene expression across all tested cell lines.

Finally, a review article by Malheiro et al. (contribution 13) discussed the emergence of Pharma 4.0 technologies, such as additive manufacturing, machine learning, in silico modelling and digital twins, and their application in the manufacturing of non-biological complex drugs.

Author Contributions: Conceptualisation, R.F.-G. and A.I.F.-S.; writing—original draft preparation, R.F.-G. and A.I.F.-S.; writing—review and editing, R.F.-G., F.B.-F. and A.I.F.-S. All authors have read and agreed to the published version of the manuscript.

Conflicts of Interest: The authors declare no conflicts of interest.

List of Contributions

1. Stoyanova, M.; Milusheva, M.; Gledacheva, V.; Todorova, M.; Kircheva, N.; Angelova, S.; Stefanova, I.; Pencheva, M.; Vasileva, B.; Hristova-Panusheva, K.; et al. Silver Nanoparticles with Mebeverine in IBS Treatment: DFT Analysis, Spasmolytic, and Anti-Inflammatory Effects. *Pharmaceutics* **2025**, *17*, 561. https://doi.org/10.3390/pharmaceutics17050561.

2. Fernández-García, R.; Fraguas-Sánchez, A.I. Nanomedicines for Pulmonary Drug Delivery: Overcoming Barriers in the Treatment of Respiratory Infections and Lung Cancer. *Pharmaceutics* **2024**, *16*, 1584. https://doi.org/10.3390/pharmaceutics16121584.
3. Party, P.; Klement, M.L.; Gaudio, B.M.; Sorrenti, M.; Ambrus, R. Nanoparticle-Based Dry Powder Inhaler Containing Ciprofloxacin for Enhanced Targeted Antibacterial Therapy. *Pharmaceutics* **2025**, *17*, 486. https://doi.org/10.3390/pharmaceutics17040486.
4. Khan, I.; Sunita, S.; Hussein, N.R.; Omer, H.K.; Elhissi, A.; Houacine, C.; Khan, W.; Yousaf, S.; Rathore, H.A. Development and Characterization of Novel Combinations and Compositions of Nanostructured Lipid Carrier Formulations Loaded with Trans-Resveratrol for Pulmonary Drug Delivery. *Pharmaceutics* **2024**, *16*, 1589. https://doi.org/10.3390/pharmaceutics16121589.
5. Saraswat, A.; Nomani, A.; Yong, L.-K.; Kuo, J.C.-T.; Brown, H.; Narayanareddygari, M.; Peace, A.; Fazily, R.; Blake, T.; Petro, C.D.; et al. A Polysorbate-Based Lipid Nanoparticle Vaccine Formulation Induces In Vivo Immune Response Against SARS-CoV-2. *Pharmaceutics* **2025**, *17*, 441. https://doi.org/10.3390/pharmaceutics17040441.
6. De Caro, L.; Stoll, T.; Grandeury, A.; Gozzo, F.; Giannini, C. Characterization of VitE-TPGS Micelles Linked to Poorly Soluble Pharmaceutical Compounds Exploiting Pair Distribution Function's Moments. *Pharmaceutics* **2025**, *17*, 431. https://doi.org/10.3390/pharmaceutics17040431.
7. Stanković, T.; Ilić, T.; Divović Matović, B.; Petkovic, M.; Dobričić, V.; Jančić, I.; Bufan, B.; Jezdić, K.; Đoković, J.; Pantelić, I.; et al. Intravenous Nanoemulsions Loaded with Phospholipid Complex of a Novel Pyrazoloquinolinone Ligand for Enhanced Brain Delivery. *Pharmaceutics* **2025**, *17*, 232. https://doi.org/10.3390/pharmaceutics17020232.
8. Galbiati, M.; Maiullari, F.; Ceraolo, M.G.; Bousselmi, S.; Fratini, N.; Gega, K.; Recchia, S.; Ferretti, A.M.; Scala, G.; Costantini, M.; et al. Bioactive Hydrogel Supplemented with Stromal Cell-Derived Extracellular Vesicles Enhance Wound Healing. *Pharmaceutics* **2025**, *17*, 162. https://doi.org/10.3390/pharmaceutics17020162.
9. Strzelecka, K.; Kasiński, A.; Biela, T.; Bocho-Janiszewska, A.; Laskowska, A.; Szeleszczuk, Ł.; Gawlak, M.; Sobczak, M.; Oledzka, E. Future-Oriented Nanosystems Composed of Polyamidoamine Dendrimer and Biodegradable Polymers as an Anticancer Drug Carrier for Potential Targeted Treatment. *Pharmaceutics* **2024**, *16*, 1482. https://doi.org/10.3390/pharmaceutics16111482.
10. Cheng, X.; Han, X.; Si, J.; Dong, C.; Ji, Z.; Zhao, S.; Wu, X.; Li, H.; Jin, X. Cationic Curcumin Nanocrystals Liposomes for Improved Oral Bioavailability: Formulation Development, Optimization, In Vitro and In Vivo Evaluation. *Pharmaceutics* **2024**, *16*, 1155. https://doi.org/10.3390/pharmaceutics16091155.
11. Donoso-González, O.; Riveros, A.L.; Marco, J.F.; Venegas-Yazigi, D.; Paredes-García, V.; Olguín, C.F.; Mayorga-Lobos, C.; Lobos-González, L.; Franco-Campos, F.; Wang, J.; et al. Iron-Reduced Graphene Oxide Core–Shell Micromotors Designed for Magnetic Guidance and Photothermal Therapy under Second Near-Infrared Light. *Pharmaceutics* **2024**, *16*, 856. https://doi.org/10.3390/pharmaceutics16070856.
12. Maeyouf, K.; Sakpakdeejaroen, I.; Somani, S.; Meewan, J.; Ali-Jerman, H.; Laskar, P.; Mullin, M.; MacKenzie, G.; Tate, R.J.; Dufès, C. Transferrin-Bearing, Zein-Based Hybrid Lipid Nanoparticles for Drug and Gene Delivery to Prostate Cancer Cells. *Pharmaceutics* **2023**, *15*, 2643. https://doi.org/10.3390/pharmaceutics15112643.

13. Malheiro, V.; Duarte, J.; Veiga, F.; Mascarenhas-Melo, F. Exploiting Pharma 4.0 Technologies in the Non-Biological Complex Drugs Manufacturing: Innovations and Implications. *Pharmaceutics* **2023**, *15*, 2545. https://doi.org/10.3390/pharmaceutics15112545.

References

1. Daniluk, J.; Malecka-Wojciesko, E.; Skrzydlo-Radomanska, B.; Rydzewska, G. The Efficacy of Mebeverine in the Treatment of Irritable Bowel Syndrome-A Systematic Review. *J. Clin. Med.* **2022**, *11*, 1044. [CrossRef] [PubMed]
2. Chakraborty, D.S.; Hazra, A.; Sil, A.; Pain, S. Will controlled release mebeverine be able to surpass placebo in treatment of diarrhoea predominant irritable bowel syndrome? *J. Fam. Med. Prim. Care* **2019**, *8*, 3173–3178. [CrossRef]
3. Bray, F.; Laversanne, M.; Sung, H.; Ferlay, J.; Siegel, R.L.; Soerjomataram, I.; Jemal, A. Global cancer statistics 2022: GLOBOCAN estimates of incidence and mortality worldwide for 36 cancers in 185 countries. *CA A Cancer J. Clin.* **2024**, *74*, 229–263. [CrossRef] [PubMed]
4. Wilson, B.; Geetha, K.M. Lipid nanoparticles in the development of mRNA vaccines for COVID-19. *J. Drug Deliv. Sci. Technol.* **2022**, *74*, 103553. [CrossRef] [PubMed]
5. Swetha, K.; Kotla, N.G.; Tunki, L.; Jayaraj, A.; Bhargava, S.K.; Hu, H.; Bonam, S.R.; Kurapati, R. Recent Advances in the Lipid Nanoparticle-Mediated Delivery of mRNA Vaccines. *Vaccines* **2023**, *11*, 658. [CrossRef] [PubMed]
6. Waggoner, L.E.; Miyasaki, K.F.; Kwon, E.J. Analysis of PEG-lipid anchor length on lipid nanoparticle pharmacokinetics and activity in a mouse model of traumatic brain injury. *Biomater. Sci.* **2023**, *11*, 4238–4253. [CrossRef] [PubMed]
7. Xu, W.; Ling, P.; Zhang, T. Polymeric Micelles, a Promising Drug Delivery System to Enhance Bioavailability of Poorly Water-Soluble Drugs. *J. Drug Deliv.* **2013**, *2013*, 340315. [CrossRef] [PubMed]
8. Shen, R.; Kim, J.J.; Yao, M.; Elbayoumi, T.A. Development and evaluation of vitamin E d-α-tocopheryl polyethylene glycol 1000 succinate-mixed polymeric phospholipid micelles of berberine as an anticancer nanopharmaceutical. *Int. J. Nanomed.* **2016**, *11*, 1687–1700. [CrossRef]
9. Zhou, H.; Mayorga-Martinez, C.C.; Pané, S.; Zhang, L.; Pumera, M. Magnetically Driven Micro and Nanorobots. *Chem. Rev.* **2021**, *121*, 4999–5041. [CrossRef] [PubMed]
10. Gaber, M.; Medhat, W.; Hany, M.; Saher, N.; Fang, J.Y.; Elzoghby, A. Protein-lipid nanohybrids as emerging platforms for drug and gene delivery: Challenges and outcomes. *J. Control. Release* **2017**, *254*, 75–91. [CrossRef] [PubMed]

pharmaceutics

MDPI

Article

Silver Nanoparticles with Mebeverine in IBS Treatment: DFT Analysis, Spasmolytic, and Anti-Inflammatory Effects

Mihaela Stoyanova [1], Miglena Milusheva [1,2], Vera Gledacheva [3], Mina Todorova [1], Nikoleta Kircheva [4], Silvia Angelova [4,5], Iliyana Stefanova [3], Mina Pencheva [3], Bela Vasileva [6], Kamelia Hristova-Panusheva [7], Natalia Krasteva [7], George Miloshev [6], Yulian Tumbarski [8], Milena Georgieva [6] and Stoyanka Nikolova [1,*]

[1] Department of Organic Chemistry, Faculty of Chemistry, University of Plovdiv, 4000 Plovdiv, Bulgaria; stoyanova@uni-plovdiv.bg (M.S.); miglena.milusheva@uni-plovdiv.bg or miglena.milusheva@mu-plovdiv.bg (M.M.); minatodorova@uni-plovdiv.bg (M.T.)

[2] Department of Bioorganic Chemistry, Faculty of Pharmacy, Medical University of Plovdiv, 4002 Plovdiv, Bulgaria

[3] Department of Medical Physics and Biophysics, Faculty of Pharmacy, Medical University of Plovdiv, 4002 Plovdiv, Bulgaria; vera.gledacheva@mu-plovdiv.bg (V.G.); iliyana.stefanova@mu-plovdiv.bg (I.S.); mina.pencheva@mu-plovdiv.bg (M.P.)

[4] Institute of Optical Materials and Technologies "Acad. J. Malinowski", Bulgarian Academy of Sciences, 1113 Sofia, Bulgaria; nkircheva@iomt.bas.bg (N.K.); sea@iomt.bas.bg (S.A.)

[5] University of Chemical Technology and Metallurgy, 1756 Sofia, Bulgaria

[6] Laboratory of Molecular Genetics, Epigenetics and Longevity, Institute of Molecular Biology "R. Tsanev", Bulgarian Academy of Sciences, 1113 Sofia, Bulgaria; byvasileva@gmail.com (B.V.); karamolbiol@gmail.com (G.M.); milenageorgy@gmail.com (M.G.)

[7] Institute of Biophysics and Biomedical Engineering, Bulgarian Academy of Sciences, 1113 Sofia, Bulgaria; kameliahristova@abv.bg (K.H.-P.); natalia.krasteva@yahoo.com (N.K.)

[8] Department of Microbiology and Biotechnology, Technological Faculty, University of Food Technologies, 4002 Plovdiv, Bulgaria; tumbarski@abv.bg

* Correspondence: tanya@uni-plovdiv.bg

Abstract: Background/Objectives: Mebeverine hydrochloride (MBH) is an antispasmodic agent used to regulate bowel movements and relax intestinal smooth muscle, but its application is limited by specific side effects; therefore, this study investigates the effects of previously synthesized MBH-loaded silver nanoparticles (AgNPs) on smooth muscle contractile activity and their anti-inflammatory potential as an alternative delivery system. **Methods:** The interactions of AgNPs with cholinergic inhibitors, selective antagonists, Ca^{2+} blockers, and key neurotransmitters were analyzed. In vitro, albumin denaturation suppression and ex vivo assays evaluated the anti-inflammatory effects of AgNPs-MBH, validated using a DFT in silico approach. To comprehensively assess the systemic impact and IBS treatment potential of AgNPs-MBH, we also examined in vitro their antimicrobial activity and hepatic cell responses, as the liver is a key organ in evaluating the overall safety and efficacy of nanoparticles. Additionally, the drug-release capabilities of Ag NPs were established. **Results**: Our findings indicate that AgNPs with MBH do not affect blocked cholinergic receptors, but their effects are more pronounced and distinct in amplitude and character than MBH. MBH-loaded AgNPs showed a lower anti-inflammatory effect than MBH but were still better than diclofenac. They also affected hepatic cell morphology and proliferation, suggesting potential for enhanced therapeutic efficacy. Drug-loaded AgNPs are considered not bactericidal. **Conclusions**: Based on our results, drug-loaded AgNPs might be a promising medication delivery system for MBH and a useful treatment option for IBS. Future in vivo and preclinical experiments will contribute to the establishment of drug-loaded AgNPs in IBS treatment.

Keywords: inflammatory bowel disease (IBD); gastrointestinal inflammation (GI); silver nanoparticles; drug delivery (DD); mebeverine hydrochloride (MBH); molecular docking; spasmolytic; anti-inflammatory activity; HepG2 cells

1. Introduction

Inflammatory bowel disease (IBD) is characterized by chronic gastrointestinal inflammation (GI) [1,2]. The condition affects between 5% and 10% of otherwise healthy individuals at any one point in time and, in most people, runs a relapsing and remitting course [3]. The occurrence of IBD in developing regions like Asia, Eastern Europe, and Africa has risen rapidly in recent years [4]. IBD is characterized as multifactorial, involving genetic susceptibility, immune dysfunction due to environmental factors (diet, chemicals, stress), and microbial exposure [5–8], with an imbalance in gut microbiota [6,9–11].

Although current treatments for IBD offer certain therapeutic benefits, their efficacy is often constrained by non-specific drug distribution, gastrointestinal metabolism, and notable side effects [12]. A well-designed drug delivery (DD) system can enhance therapeutic outcomes by employing controlled drug release, prodrugs, pH-responsive mechanisms, and micro- or nanoparticulate formulations [13,14]. Several pharmacological agents—including corticosteroids, antibiotics, and immunosuppressants—have recently demonstrated effectiveness in promoting mucosal healing. However, there remains a pressing need for innovative biomaterial-based platforms capable of delivering drugs more efficiently and with reduced adverse effects. Such platforms can serve as targeted DD systems, facilitating colon-specific delivery and ensuring sustained drug release at the injury site [15]. Although micro- and nanoscale DD strategies can potentially prolong colonic retention and offer additional therapeutic advantages for IBD, the accumulation of micro- and nanoparticles in inflamed intestinal tissues is size-dependent [16,17], underscoring their promise as leading candidates for regulated drug delivery.

Nanoparticles (NPs) of noble metals have gained considerable attention over the past few decades due to their expanding applications in pharmaceutical and biomedical fields, including DD, photothermal therapy, radiotherapy, and imaging [18]. Among these, gold and silver nanoparticles have been the most extensively synthesized, attributed to their remarkable biological activity and unique physicochemical properties [19–21]. A major challenge in utilizing silver nanoparticles (AgNPs) for DD—particularly in inflammatory bowel disease—is achieving precise, site-specific delivery to the colon [22,23].

The application of carbohydrates in NP synthesis has recently garnered significant interest. Various green synthesis approaches have been developed for producing nano-sized AgNPs, such as starch-mediated biosynthesis [24–26], and other methods employing polyoxometalates, polysaccharides, and classical chemical reactions like Tollens' and Fehling's [27–31]. A wide range of mono-, di-, and polysaccharides have been employed as reducing and capping agents in the synthesis of noble metal NPs, owing to their sustainability, availability, low cost, non-toxicity, renewability, biodegradability, and excellent biocompatibility [32–36].

Our recent work synthesized AgNPs functionalized with mebeverine hydrochloride (MBH) and assessed their cytotoxic and genotoxic properties [37]. To date, few strategies for MBH targeting have been reported, including MBH-loaded electrospun nanofibers [38], mucoadhesive buccal tablets for local anesthesia [39], and molecularly imprinted polymer-based electrochemical sensors for MBH detection [40]. MBH is an antispasmodic drug (Figure 1) that can potentially exert a local anesthetic effect via blocking voltage-gated Na^+ channels. As a musculotropic antispasmodic agent, MBH directly influences colonic muscle activity [41]. Due to its muscle-relaxing properties, MBH is widely used to treat GI spasmodic disorders such as abdominal pain, intestinal disturbances, and bowel discomfort [42].

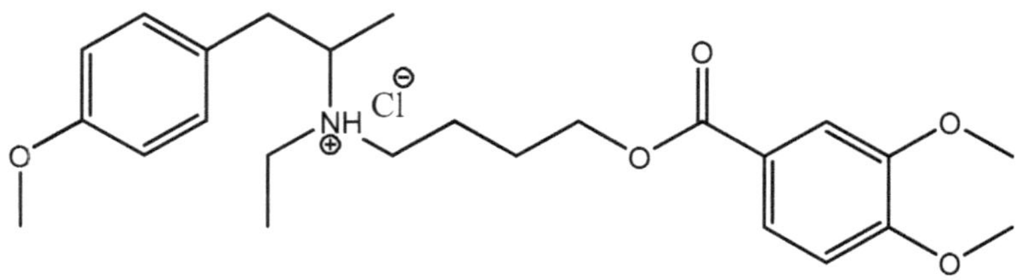

Figure 1. Chemical structure of mebeverine hydrochloride (MBH).

Unlike the mentioned and already reported molecules, when depositing MBH into NPs, a change in the spasmolytic activity of the drug-loaded AgNPs is expected, both in terms of the pharmacological profile and in terms of the speed of action and the duration of the effect [43–46]. Therefore, a plausible first step in the assessment of various characteristics that play a key role in the drug (ligand)/AgNP recognition process is calculations based on Density Functional Theory (DFT) [47–49]. These simulations provide valuable information about the electronic structure and physicochemical properties and the change of these properties when the drug is adsorbed on the nanoparticle's surface [50]. Integrating in silico calculations with experimental validation is crucial for retrieving solid evidence of the potential therapeutic application and probable mechanism of action. Advancements in computational and experimental methodologies will continue to enhance our understanding of AgNPs, paving the way for their safe and practical application in various fields.

The primary aim of this study is to investigate the specific effects of MBH-loaded silver nanoparticles (AgNPs) on smooth muscle (SM) contractility compared to the effects of free MBH. To achieve this, we explored the interactions of drug-loaded AgNPs with key regulators of SM function, including cholinergic inhibitors (atropine, ipratropium), selective muscarinic antagonists (pirenzepine, gallamine, 4-DAMP), calcium channel blockers (hexamethonium, decamethonium), and neurotransmitters (acetylcholine and 5-HT). These experiments were complemented by in silico modeling to validate the predicted antispasmodic properties of the conjugates. Additionally, we evaluated the anti-inflammatory potential of MBH-loaded AgNPs through albumin denaturation and ex vivo assays. We investigated their impact on hepatic cell morphology and proliferation to assess their safety and systemic effects. By integrating pharmacodynamic, anti-inflammatory, and cytotoxicity profiles, this study aims to comprehensively assess MBH-loaded AgNPs as a novel and targeted therapeutic strategy for irritable bowel syndrome (IBS).

2. Materials and Methods

2.1. Synthetic Protocol

MBH or 4-[ethyl-[1-(4-methoxyphenyl)propan-2-yl]amino]butyl 3,4-dimethoxybenzoate hydrochloride is a crystalline white powder with a molecular weight of 429.5 g/mol. The free base of mebeverine is essentially insoluble in water and ethanol, but its hydrochloride salt is very soluble in water and freely soluble in alcohol [51,52]. With a pKa of around 10 and a plasma half-life of 2.5 h, it requires frequent administration because of its short half-life [53]. MBH (Duspatalin) is marketed as a 200 mg extended-release capsule with a recommended dosage of two times per day. Its musculotropic antispasmodic activity, which directly affects the smooth muscles of the GI tract, is utilized. It is used effectively in treating IBS, a condition marked by abdominal pain and irregular bowel movements.

The NMR data was completely consistent with data reported in the literature [54]. HRMS electrospray ionization (ESI) m/z calcd. for $[M + H]^+$ $C_{25}H_{36}O_5N^+$ = 430.25880, found 430.25788 (mass error $\Delta m = -2.14$ ppm).

Drug-loaded AgNPs were synthesized according to previously reported methods [37]. Briefly, 1.25 g (0.007 mol) of fructose was dissolved in 25 mL of water and refluxed for 2 min; then, 0.63 mL of 0.01 M $AgNO_3$ solution was added. MBH was added to the solution at a concentration of 1 mg/mL. After roughly 5 min of reflux, the solution's color changed to a light yellow, signifying the formation of AgNPs. The synthesized AgNPs were characterized using different analytical techniques, such as UV-Vis, Transmission electron microscopy (TEM, Talos 1.15.3, Thermo Fisher Scientific, Waltham, MA, USA), dynamic light scattering (DLS, Brookhaven BI-200 goniometer, Brookhaven Instruments Corporation, Nashua, NH, USA), and the zeta potential (Brookhaven BI-200 goniometer, Brookhaven Instruments Corporation, Nashua, NH, USA). The TEM images confirmed the synthesis of smaller spherical particles up to 95 nm in size (Figure 2). The drug-loaded AgNPs were obtained with a controllable size due to carbohydrate assistance in the presence of $[Ag(NH_3)_2]^+$ [55]. The carbohydrate coating also decreases the agglomeration rate and size [56].

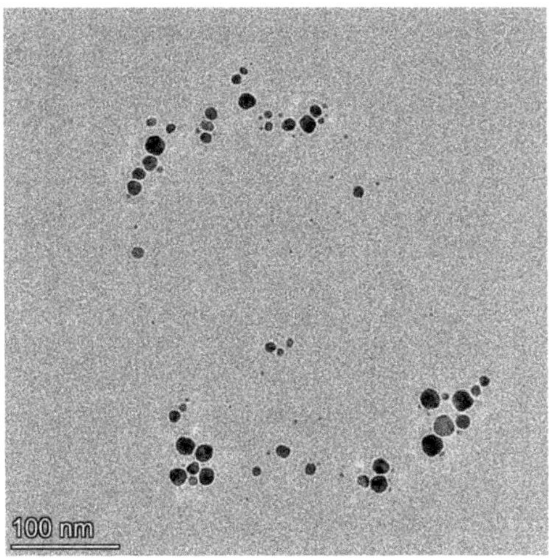

Figure 2. TEM visualization of drug-loaded silver nanoparticles with MBH.

The zeta potential of drug-loaded AgNPs was −19.19 mV. The negative charge of the zeta potential refers to the carboxylic groups of carboxylic acid obtained when Ag^+ is reduced to Ag°. Carboxylic acids, obtained in the oxidation of sugars, provide a negative surface charge density to counteract the van der Waals forces responsible for particle coalescence [30,31,57].

2.2. DFT Calculations

An initial step in the current research presents the theoretical assessment of the process of drug adsorption on the surface of AgNPs coated with carbohydrate molecules (e.g., fructose) and the further evaluation of the change of some specific physicochemical characteristics deriving from the HOMO-LUMO differences. For this purpose, the Density Functional Theory approach was utilized in the Gaussian 09 Suite of Programs [58]. The structures of the drug under study, MBH, in its two non-charged and cationic forms, and a simplified model for the carbohydrate surface comprising three fructose molecules, as well as the resulting complexes, were subjected to complete geometry optimization at the B3LYP level of theory in conjunction with the triple zeta 6-311++G(d,p) basis set in the gas phase found most suitable for the investigated systems in our previous research [59]. The lack of negative frequencies in the vibrational frequency analysis indicated a local minimum on the potential energy surface. Hence, following thermodynamics, ref. [60] the adsorption energy, ΔE_{ads}, can be found as follows:

$$\Delta E_{ads} = \Delta E_{ads}\ (\text{products}) - \Delta E_{ads}\ (\text{reactants}),$$

where the electronic energies obtained during optimization were implemented in the equation. For a more proper representation, thermal energies, including zero-point energy, Eth, were further retrieved and included in an equation for calculating the enthalpy, ΔH. The overall change in the enthalpy could then be computed as follows:

$$\Delta H = \Delta E_{ads} + \Delta E_{th}\ (\text{products}) - \Delta E_{th}\ (\text{reagents}) + P\Delta V,$$

where PΔV stands for a work term that accounts for the change in the number of molecules during a reaction; hence, a negative value of $\Delta E_{ads}/\Delta H$ indicates the successful adsorption of MBH on the carbohydrate layer, whereas a positive one suggests an improbable reaction.

2.3. *Cell Culturing Conditions and IC_{50} Determination for AgNPs with MBH Treatments*

HepG2 cells, originating from human liver carcinoma, were purchased from the European Collection of Authenticated Cell Cultures (ECACC) and maintained in Dulbecco's Modified Eagle Medium (DMEM) supplemented with 10% fetal bovine serum (FBS; Sigma-Aldrich, Darmstadt, Germany). The cells were incubated at 37 °C in a humidified atmosphere containing 5% CO_2. A solution of 0.05% trypsin and 0.02% EDTA (Sigma-Aldrich, Germany) was used to detach cells for subsequent experiments. HepG2 cells were seeded in 24-well plates at a density of 2.5×10^4 cells per well for cytotoxicity assessments, including cell viability. After an initial 24-h incubation period, the cells were exposed to AgNPs, MBH, and their combined nano-formulation for designated time points. Cell viability and metabolic activity were assessed using the WST-1 assay. After 24- and 72-h incubation periods with the tested compounds, the medium was removed, and the cells were rinsed with PBS. A fresh medium containing a WST-1 reagent (10% v/v) was added to each well, followed by a 1-h incubation in the dark. Absorbance was measured at 450 nm using a Thermo Scientific Multiskan Spectrum ELISA reader (Thermo Scientific, Tokyo, Japan). GraphPad software (GraphPad Prism, version 10.0.3; GraphPad Software, San Diego, CA, USA) calculated the half-maximal inhibitory concentrations (IC_{50}) based on dose-response curves.

2.4. *Fluorescence-Activated Cell Sorting (FACS) Analysis of HepG2 Cells*

Cell Cycle Analysis and Cellular Morphology

Flow cytometry (BD FACSCalibur™ Flow Cytometer; Becton Dickinson & Company, Franklin Lakes, NJ, USA) was used to assess cell cycle progression and morphological changes in HepG2 cells treated with MBH, AgNPs, and AgNPs with MBH at IC_{50} concentrations for 24 and 72 h. The cells were fixed in 76% cold ethanol and stored at −20 °C for 24 h. Following fixation, the cells were centrifuged, washed with PBS, and incubated with 100 µg/mL RNase A at 37 °C for 30 min. Propidium iodide (PI) staining was performed using a 50 µg/mL solution for 30 min in the dark. Fifty thousand events were recorded per sample using flow cytometry with the excitation at 488 nm, and the data were analyzed using FlowJo™ software (Version 10, Becton Dickinson, Franklin Lakes, NJ, USA).

2.5. Ex Vivo Spasmolytic Activity

The study was performed on the gastric SM of male Wistar rats weighing 270–290 g. Three or four muscle strips were taken from a rat's stomach. The number of muscle preparations used for each data point is indicated by n. The isolated SM preparation was placed upright in a thermostated vessel for isolated organs that was 15 mL in volume and oxygenated with physiological fluid at a temperature of 37 °C. The SM preparations consisted of circular dissections, 12–13 mm in length and 1.0–1.1 mm in width, which were used to record isometric contractile activity. All the transducers used in our experiments were made by the Tissue Organ Bath System (159920 Radnoti, Dublin, Ireland) according to a previously described procedure [59,61].

2.6. In Vitro Inhibition of Albumin's Denaturation

The denaturation inhibition was performed following Milusheva et al.'s method [61]. The reaction mixture contained 0.2 mL of the tested AgNPs in DMSO (0.5 mg/mL) and 0.5 mL of a 5% aqueous solution of human albumin (Albunorm 20, Octapharma (IP) SPRL, 1070 Anderlecht, Belgium). For 15 min, the samples were incubated at 37 °C. Subsequently, each tube was filled with 2.5 mL of phosphate-buffered saline (pH 6.3), and the samples were heated at 80 °C for 30 min before being cooled for 5 min. The turbidity was measured at 660 nm spectrophotometrically (Cary 60 UV-Vis, Agilent Technologies, Santa Clara, CA, USA). The percentage of the inhibition of protein denaturation was calculated as follows:

$$\text{percentage of inhibition of denaturation} = [(A_{\text{control}} - A_{\text{AgNPs}})/A_{\text{control}}] \times 100.$$

The control represents 100% protein denaturation. The commercially available anti-inflammatory drugs diclofenac and acetylsalicylic acid (ASA) were used for comparison. Additionally, MBH controls were made. Their anti-inflammatory effect was determined as a percentage of the inhibition of albumin denaturation, following the same protocol.

2.7. Immunohistochemistry

The sections (5 μm thick) obtained from rat stomachs were deparaffinized and subjected to the immunohistochemical analysis using the monoclonal antibody IL-1β (E-AB-52153) (Elabscience Biotechnology Inc., Houston, TX, USA) and the polyclonal antibody 5HT3, 1:300 (E-AB-32268), (Ellabscience Biotechnology Inc., Houston, TX, USA) [62].

All the microphotographs were taken using a Leica DM1000 LED microscope (Leica Microsystems, Wetzlar, Germany) and an ICC50W digital camera (Leica Microsystems, Wetzlar, Germany).

2.8. Morphometric Analysis

The immune response intensity in the SM cells was quantified in arbitrary units (AUs) on sections immunostained for IL-1β and 5HT3 receptors. The average pixel intensity was determined using specialized software, ranging from 0 (black) to 256 (white). Measurements were performed on microphotographs of the SM cells at ×200 magnification, with at least 50 points assessed per slice. A total of five slices were analyzed for each animal.

2.9. In Vitro Drug Release

In vitro drug release was evaluated using the dialysis bag approach. A dialysis membrane was hydrated in distilled water for 24 h (MWCO 12 kDa, Sigma-Aldrich, St. Louis, MO, USA). Drug-loaded Ag NPs were dispersed in 10 mL of phosphate-buffered saline (PBS), transferred to the dialysis bag, and closed with a plastic clamp. Each bag was placed into a beaker with 40 mL of PBS (dialysis medium, pH 7.4). Aliquots with 4 mL of each dialysis medium were taken for measurements, and then the fresh medium was added at specified intervals. The drug release experiment lasted 130 h. The mean results of triplicate measurements and standard deviations were reported. Additionally, drug-only controls were made.

2.10. Antimicrobial Assay

The agar diffusion method evaluated the antimicrobial activity of drug-loaded AgNPs against various microorganisms. The tested microorganisms included Gram-positive bacteria, such as *Enterococcus faecalis, Staphylococcus aureus, Listeria monocytogenes, Bacillus subtilis,* and *Bacillus amyloliquefaciens*; Gram-negative bacteria, including *Escherichia coli, Salmonella typhimurium, Pseudomonas aeruginosa, Proteus vulgaris* G, and *Klebsiella pneumoniae*; two yeasts, *Candida albicans* and *Saccharomyces cerevisiae*; and six fungi (*Aspergillus niger, Aspergillus flavus, Penicillium* sp., *Rhizopus* sp., *Mucor* sp. (plant isolate), and *Fusarium moniliforme*) from the collection of the Department of Microbiology at the University of Food Technologies—Plovdiv, Bulgaria.

The procedure involved spreading a suspension of each test microorganism (10^6 cfu/cm^3) onto specific nutrient agar media. Next, 6 mm diameter wells were created in the agar, and 60 µL of the tested substance solution (1 mg/cm^3) was added to each well. The Petri dishes were then incubated at appropriate temperatures (37 °C for bacteria and *C. albicans* and 30 °C for *S. cerevisiae*) for 24–48 h. The fungi *A. niger, A. flavus, Penicillium* sp., *Rhizopus* sp., *Mucor* sp., and *F. moniliforme* were grown on Malt Extract Agar at 30 °C for 7 days or until sporulation. After incubation, the inhibition zones around each well were measured, with zones more significant than 7 mm considered inhibition zones. Each test was performed in triplicate, and the results were reported as mean values of the inhibition zone diameters.

The antimicrobial activity was determined by measuring the diameter of the inhibition zones around the wells on the 24 h and 48 h of incubation. The tested microorganisms with inhibition zones of 18 mm or more were considered sensitive; those in which the zones were from 12 to 18 mm were considered moderately sensitive; and those in which the inhibition zones were up to 12 mm or completely missing were considered resistant [63].

2.11. Statistical Analysis

The SPSS 23.0 program (SPSS Inc., Chicago, IL, USA) was used for the statistical analysis. All the data are expressed as the mean ± SD (standard deviation). The number of tissue preparations used in each experiment is indicated by n. The statistical significance of the two independent groups was analyzed using an independent sample *t*-test. The level of statistical significance was considered as $p < 0.05$.

3. Results and Discussion

3.1. DFT Analysis in AgNP Evaluation

As the first step in the current research, an analysis of the most energetically favorable composition of the carbohydrate layer in the AgNPs was performed. A combination of three fructose molecules was modeled, as suggested in a previous study [59], following the computational restriction regarding the size of the studied system. Fructose is known to exist primarily in two forms: as a furanose (denoted as *f*) and a pyranose (denoted as *p*), with five- and six-membered rings, respectively [64]. Hence, six combinations between these forms were modeled, and their stability was assessed. The results obtained are presented in Figure 3.

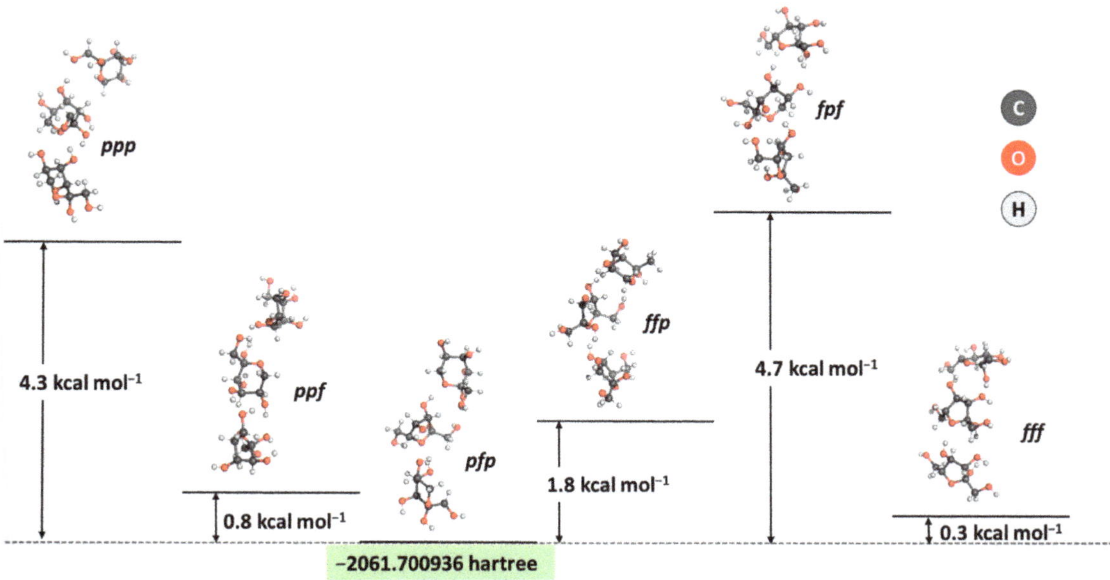

Figure 3. Optimized geometries and obtained energy differences between six combinations of the two most stable ring forms of fructose in solution (in kcal mol^{-1}). The five-membered cycle is denoted as *f*, whereas the six-membered ring is denoted as *p*.

The calculations prove the most thermodynamically favorable composition of three fructose molecules: the pyranose/furanose/pyranose combination appears to be the most stable configuration, closely followed by the trifuranose and pyranose/pyranose/furanose combinations, which differ by only 0.3 and 0.8 kcal mol^{-1} in stability, respectively. These results strongly correspond to experimental data claiming that fructose exists in a solution's 2:1 pyranose:furanose ratio [64]. Therefore, this particular composition for a simplified model of the carbohydrate outer layer in the nanoparticle was considered when further assessing the interaction with the MBH molecule. The energy and enthalpy for the absorption of MBH on the carbohydrate-coated surface of a silver nanoparticle were calculated and are depicted in Figure 4.

The performed computations indicate an energetically justified reaction of drug-loaded AgNP formation as the observed changes of ΔE_{ads} and enthalpy, ΔH, are strongly negative: $-6.2/-4.8$ and $-25.0/-23.3$ kcal mol^{-1} for the interaction between the carbohydrate layer and MBH in neutral/cationic form, respectively. Due to the positive charge of the ligand in the second reaction, however, the complexation appears much more favorable than a reaction for the neutral form, with an energy gain that is up to about 18 kcal mol^{-1} greater in the former case. This outcome could be explained by the stronger interaction between the charged amino group from the drug and the HO-groups from the fructose ring being ion–dipole in nature as opposed to the weaker dipole–dipole interaction in the case of a neutral MBH. Still, the calculations provide strong evidence for successful MBH adsorption on AgNPs regardless of the charge of the drug.

Further interpretation of the obtained results includes the frontier molecular orbitals energies, an indispensable parameter explaining the electronic behavior of the studied structures. Data regarding the energies of the highest occupied (HOMO)/lowest unoccupied (LUMO) molecular orbitals, along with the quantum chemical descriptors connected to them, are presented in Table 1.

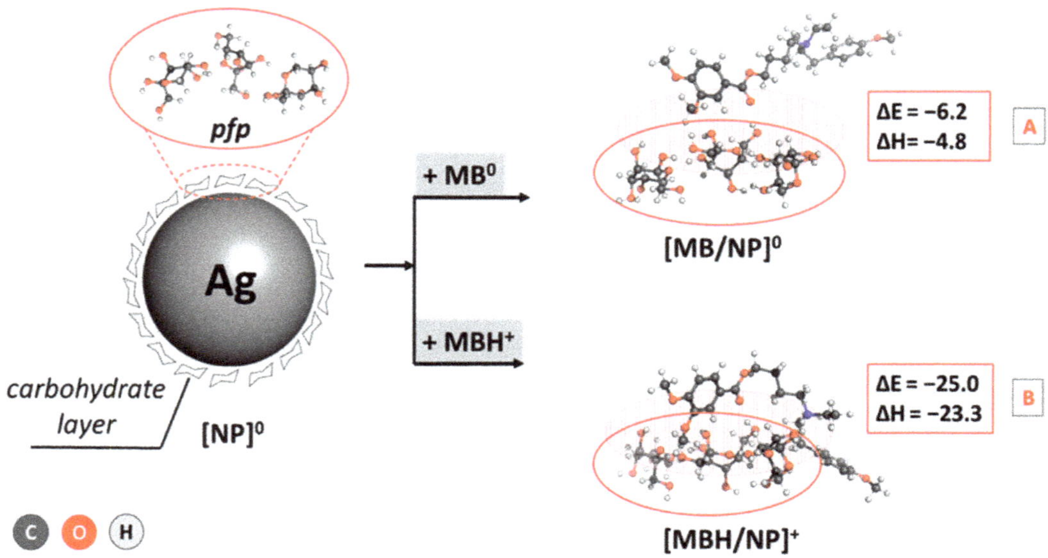

Figure 4. Adsorption energies and enthalpies of MBH/AgNP complex formation (in kcal mol^{-1}) for the drug in the [A] neutral form and the [B] cationic form. The structures are optimized at the B3LYP/6-311++G(d,p) level.

Table 1. Quantum chemical descriptors obtained through DFT calculation at the B3LYP/6-311++G(d,p) level of theory: E_{HOMO}, E_{LUMO}, $\Delta E = E_{LUMO} - E_{HOMO}$, $\chi = -(E_{HOMO} + E_{LUMO})/2$ (electronegativity), $Pi = -\chi$ (chemical potential), $\eta = (E_{LUMO} - E_{HOMO})/2$ (chemical hardness), $\sigma = 1/\eta$ (chemical softness), and $\omega = Pi^2/\eta$ (electrophilicity index). Data are presented in eV.

Compound	E_{HOMO}	E_{LUMO}	ÄE	÷	Pi	ç	6	ù
MBH^0	−5.71	−1.28	4.42	3.49	−3.49	2.21	0.45	5.52
MBH/AgNP^0	−5.66	−1.46	4.20	3.56	−3.56	2.10	0.48	6.05
MBH$^+$	−7.89	−3.70	4.19	5.80	−5.80	2.10	0.48	16.04
MBH/AgNP$^+$	−8.28	−3.46	4.82	5.87	−5.87	2.41	0.41	14.28

The energy gap, ΔE, accounts for a molecule's chemical reactivity and stability: the more significant the gap, the more reactive but less stable a compound is. Hence, the adsorption of MBH in its neutral form onto the surface of the carbohydrate layer promotes its reactivity but slightly lowers its stability. In contrast, this trend reverses in the case of a cation. Nevertheless, both the bare ligands and their complexes with fructose appear chemically stable and do not disintegrate to their primal elements, as evidenced by the negative value of the chemical potential Pi. Furthermore, the hard–soft–acid–base approximation states that soft compounds tend to interact with molecules of a biological origin more efficiently [65], which suggests that among the studied structures, drug-loaded AgNP^0 and MBH$^+$ would be more prone to interaction with proteins as their chemical softness, 6, is more significant compared to the rest of the compounds. The high electrophilicity index of MBH$^+$ outlines it as the best electron density acceptor with an estimated ù of 16.04 eV, which is an expected result when considering its positive charge. The adsorption on the fructose layer lowers this value to 14.28 eV for the drug-loaded AgNP$^+$ complex. This descriptor is much lower for the non-charged MBH and the corresponding drug-loaded AgNP^0 structure, estimated at 5.52/6.05 eV, suggesting that these compounds would be prone to supplying electrons. Overall, the provided DFT analysis of the structures under study draws a clear picture of the adsorption process of an MBH molecule (neutral and cationic) on the surface of a fructose-coated silver nanoparticle and is correlated with its physicochemical parameters of great significance and hence justifies further experiments. Note that the mechanism of therapeutic action of MBH corresponding to binding in the two active centers of albumin have already been subjected to investigation in our previous work [66] and will not be discussed any further.

3.2. Evaluation of Ex Vivo Spasmolytic Effect

It is common practice to investigate the drug concentration–response relationship using both in vitro and ex vivo models. The degree of influence can be ascertained by isometrically measuring concentration-dependent changes in the mechanokinetic parameters of spontaneous contractions after the tested chemical has been applied to the model system. To track target molecules' activating or inhibiting effects as modulators of muscle activity, we employed an isolated SM model from a rat's stomach in this investigation. After pretesting the isolated SM samples for viability with ACh, we determined the following details using the known cumulative dose-dependent effects of MBH and its deposition into AgNPs. MBH caused a sharp contractile reaction with dose-dependent changes in the tonic response and a statistically significant increase in the contraction amplitude (Figure 5a). AgNPs with MBH, on the other hand, exhibited mild tonic relaxation and a 50% reduction in the amplitude of spontaneous contraction. Neither substance induced statistically significant changes in the frequency of contractile activity (Figure 5b).

The observed differences point out different mechanisms of action on the cellular processes underlying SM's spontaneous reactions. At least three different mechanisms are involved in the polyvalent spasmolytic effects, which are known to be not specific to any one system. These mechanisms include competitive antimuscarinic activity, direct musculotropic action, including Ca^{2+} ion exchange, and local anesthetic action resulting from inhibiting norepinephrine uptake [67].

On the other hand, the single independent application of AgNPs does not alter the SM tonus in isolated SM from the trachea. However, the simultaneous application of AgNPs and ACh results in a slight increase in ACh-induced SM contractility, after which the muscle tone does not return to the baseline level. The authors of these reported findings attribute the observed effects to increased nitric oxide production [68].

To clarify the pathway of influence of the drug-loaded AgNPs in SM cellular mechanisms, we applied two of the primary neurotransmitters—ACh and 5HT [69,70]. After cholinergic or serotonergic stimulation, SM preparations respond with an initial sharp increase component (phasic contraction) due to the increased level of ionized cytosolic Ca^{2+}. This is followed by a stable tonic (sustained) contraction caused by extracellular Ca^{2+} influx into SM cells [71].

This contractile activity pathway appears unaffected by MBH-loaded AgNPs, as the pre-incubation of tissues does not significantly alter the responses to the two neurotransmitters. Interestingly, MBH itself causes a remarkable 98% reduction. The likely explanation is the presence of nanoparticles.

The ex vivo tissue bath model allows for the independent or combined exogenous application of these substances, monitoring and assessing changes in the electrical, pharmacological, or electro-pharmacological responses of treated tissue segments. Due to the potential differences in their mechanisms of action, which could result in either the contraction or the relaxation of the SM, we further investigated the changes in the contractile response strength of the SM under the influence of AgNPs with MBH at a volume of 20 μL in the presence of blockers and activators of spontaneous contractility (Table 2). We found that the effects of AgNPs and MBH are not significantly changed when mAChRs are blocked by the non-selective receptor antagonist atropine (10^{-6} M, n = 6).

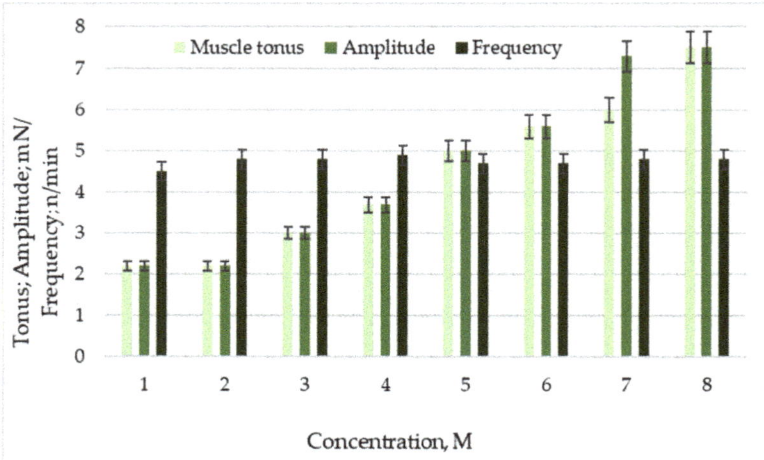

a

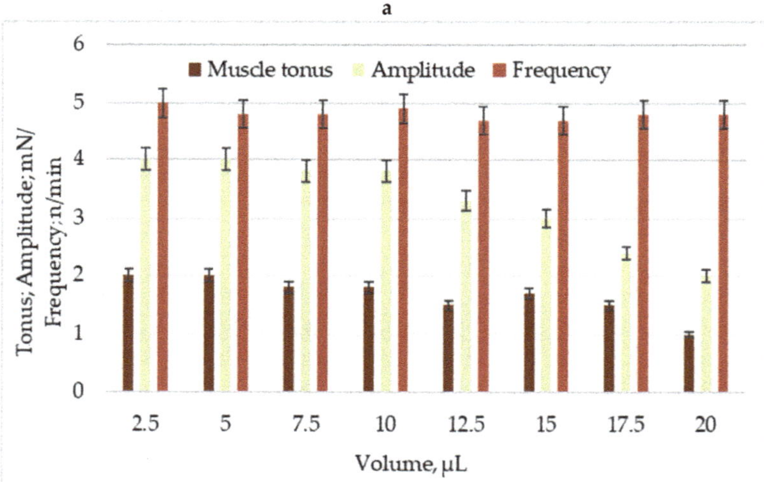

b

Figure 5. Changes in main parameters of spontaneous contractile activity: muscle tonus (mN), amplitude (mN), and frequency (n/min) under the influence of: (**a**) MBH; (**b**) AgNPs with MBH.

Table 2. Changes in the strength of the contractile response of SM under the influence of MBH and AgNPs with MBH in the presence of the main neurotransmitters (ACh and 5-HT) and atropine (non-selective mAChR antagonist).

Compound	Individual Application, mN	Strength of the Contractile Reaction in the Background, mN	
		AgNPs with MBH	MBH
ACh	5.70 ± 0.23	4.98 ± 0.36	0.10 * ± 0.02
5HT	6.33 ± 0.45	6.17 ± 0.41	4.25 * ± 0.33
atropine	2.00 ± 0.18	2.10 ± 0.21	1.87 ± 0.18

The comparison is between spontaneous effects on CA in Krebs solution before and after the application of testing substances. All the data were expressed as the mean values ± standard error of the mean (mean ± SEM); n = 9; * statistically significant differences ($p < 0.05$).

Additional research using specific and non-specific muscarinic and nicotinic acetylcholine receptor antagonists was conducted to better understand the mechanism of action of compounds encapsulated in Ag NPs. The responses to AgNPs with MBH were considerably changed by the use of specific antagonists, namely pirenzepine 10^{-5} M (M1 mAChR blocker), gallamine 10^{-5} M (M2 mAChR blocker), 4-DAMP 3×10^{-7} M (M3 mAChR blocker), hexamethonium 10^{-5} M (nAChR blocker), and decamethonium 10^{-5} M (nAChR blocker), to block muscarinic and nicotinic AChRs (Table 3).

Table 3. Changes in the strength of the contractile response of SM under the influence of AgNPs with MBH in the presence of a modulating agent of spontaneous contractility.

Compound	Individual Application	Strength of the Contractile Reaction in the Background of AgNPs with MBH, mN
Pirenzepine	1.16 ± 0.08	0.20 * ± 0.02
Gallamine	3.37 ± 0.21	1.22 * ± 0.12
4-DAMP	4.09 ± 0.40	1.08 * ± 0.07
Hexamethonium	3.78 ± 0.23	1.02 * ± 0.05
Decamethonium	2.55 ± 0.15	1.18 * ± 0.10

The comparison is between spontaneous effects on CA in Krebs solution before and after the application of testing substances. All the data were expressed as the mean values ± standard error of the mean (mean ± SEM); n = 6; * statistically significant differences ($p < 0.05$).

Through this particular cellular mechanism, we attribute the effects to the capacity of MBH and AgNPs with MBH to activate mAChRs and nAChRs on SM cells, thereby regulating the critical mechanokinetic parameters of spontaneous contractions. Our findings demonstrated that when Ag NPs with MBH interact with specifically blocked cholinergic receptors, their effects are more noticeable and different in amplitude and character, while MBH has no effect.

In summary, we suggest that the biological activity of drug-loaded AgNPs is due to an underlying mechanism that directly connects mAChR and nAChR activation.

3.3. *In Vitro Inhibition of Albumin Denaturation*

Steroidal and nonsteroidal anti-inflammatory drugs (NSAIDs) treat inflammation, fever, and pain. The indications, mode of action, administration, adverse effects, and monitoring of NSAIDs are essential for healthcare professionals [72,73]. Anti-inflammatory drugs can prevent thermally induced protein denaturation in a dose-dependent manner [66,74].

Our results for the in vitro anti-inflammatory activity of MBH and AgNPs with MBH were calculated as a percentage of the inhibition of albumin's thermal denaturation (Figure 6). We found that MBH-loaded AgNPs exhibit three times lower activity than MBH ($p < 0.05$). The anti-inflammatory effect of MBH could be explained by the potential for attaching the albumin molecule via its functional groups [66]. The lesser anti-inflammatory effect of MBH-loaded AgNPs is most likely due to the interaction of MBH's functional groups with the NPs.

We found that MBH and MBH-loaded AgNPs demonstrated 20-fold and 6-fold greater protection than diclofenac and 12-fold and 4-fold greater protection than ASA, respectively ($p < 0.05$) (Figure 7).

Further ex vivo experiments were carried out to verify these findings and assess the anti-inflammatory activity of AgNPs with MBH on nNOS and interleukin-1 (IL-1β) expression, compared to MBH.

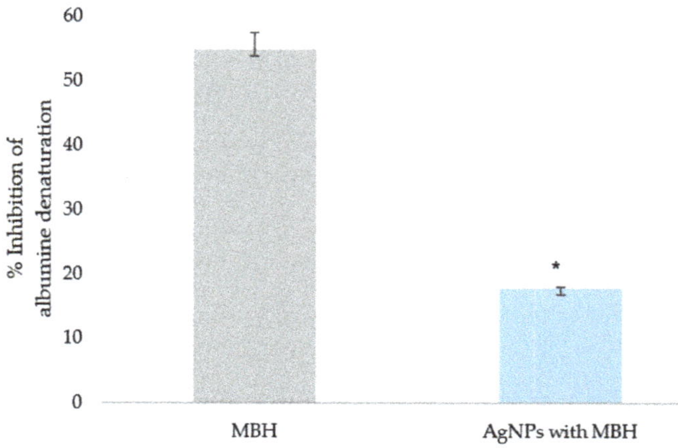

Figure 6. Inhibition of albumin's thermal denaturation by MBH and drug-loaded AgNPs (%); * $p < 0.05$.

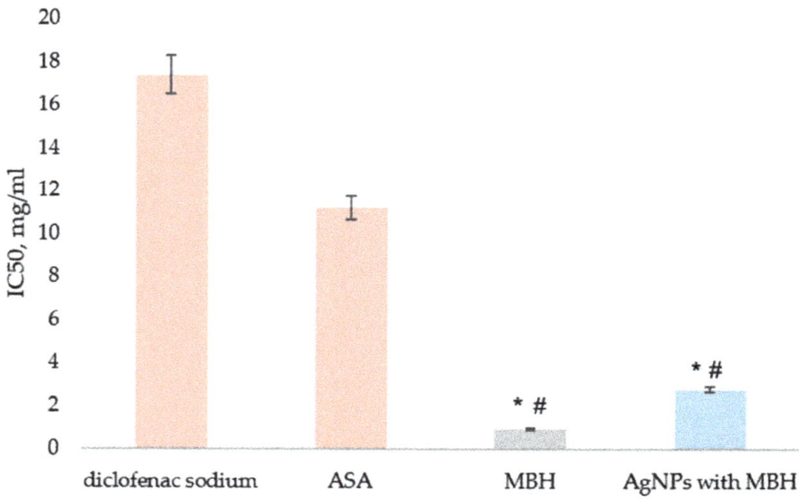

Figure 7. Inhibition of thermal denaturation of albumin by MBH (grey) and AgNPs with MBH (blue). The anti-inflammatory activity of the tested substances was compared to diclofenac's and acetylsalicylic acid (ASA)'s activity (orange). The results are expressed as IC_{50}, mg/mL. # $p < 0.05$ compared to diclofenac; * $p < 0.05$ compared to ASA.

3.4. *Ex Vivo Anti-Inflammatory Activity*

IBD and Crohn's disease are characterized by the increased production of inflammatory chemicals by immune cells [75]. Proinflammatory cytokines, including IL-1, IL-6, and IL-17, are released in response to many disease conditions, including IBD, and significantly trigger intestinal inflammation [76]. Drug-loaded AgNPs provide great promise for local delivery and fewer side effects when used to treat IBS. One of the goals of selective delivery is to use nanoparticles to deliver drugs and accumulate them at the site of inflammation through immune cell absorption [77–80].

In SM cells incubated with MBH, the measured intensity and density of IL-1β expression (160.1 ± 5.4 AU) were comparable to those incubated with the controls (169.7 ± 8.9 AU, $p < 0.001$, Figure 8A,C) (Figure 8B). In contrast, AgNPs with MBH (134.8 ± 3.2 AU) showed the lower expression of IL-1β (Figure 8B,E).

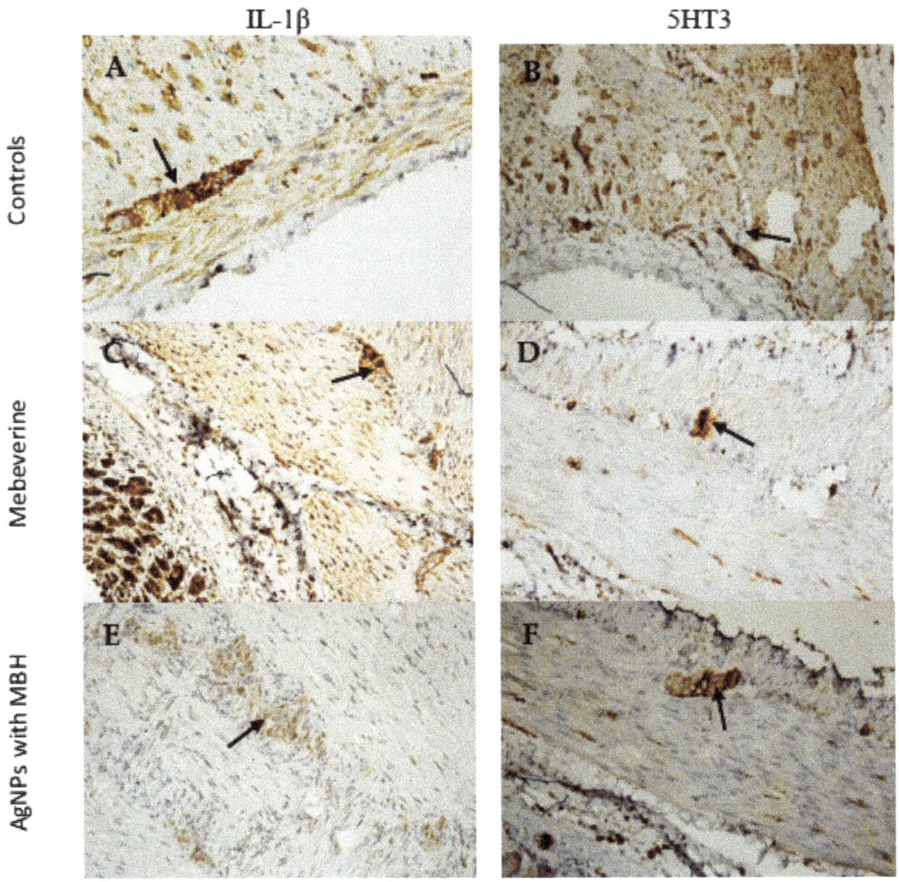

Figure 8. Microphotographs of SM preparations from the rat corpus incubated with MBH and MBH-loaded AgNPs for 1 h. (**A**) Control stained for IL-1β (black arrow), ×200. (**B**) Control stained for 5HT3 (black arrow), ×200. (**C**) SMs incubated with MBH showed the increased expression of IL-1β in the myenteric plexus (black arrow), ×200. (**E**) SMs incubated with AgNPs with MBH showed the weak expression of IL-1β in the myenteric plexus (black arrow), ×200. (**D**) SMs incubated with MBH, weakly stained cells in the myenteric plexus for 5HT3 (black arrow), ×200. (**F**) SMs incubated with AgNPs with MBH showed the weak expression of 5HT3 in the myenteric plexus (black arrow), ×200.

We found that the SMs incubated with MBH (155.5 ± 7.7 AU) had a lower intensity of expression than the control preparations (166.4 ± 6.6 AU, Figure 8B,D, $p < 0.001$) in the 5HT3 comparative analysis. In contrast, the SMs incubated with AgNPs with MBH (123.3 ± 6.9 AU) had a weaker expression of 5HT3 in the myenteric plexus (Figure 8A,F).

To confirm the in vitro anti-inflammatory effect of AgNPs with MBH, we also measured ex vivo IL-1β and 5HT3 expression. The data analysis revealed varying degrees of expression. Compared to the control SMs and MBH, AgNPs significantly decreased the intensity of IL-1β expression and suppressed 5HT3 expression. Our results demonstrated that AgNPs exhibited better anti-inflammatory effects in terms of IL-1β expression when compared to the control samples. Drug-loaded AgNPs also showed a superior inhibitory effect on the 5-HT3 channel receptor. Our results align with previous research demonstrating that 5-HT3 receptor antagonists, including ramosetron and ondansetron, reduce intestinal damage [81,82].

The obtained AgNPs are essential for testing anti-inflammatory properties and their effect on serotonin receptors, particularly the 5-HT3 channel receptor. The synthesized AgNPs can also be used in drug delivery and applying monoamine neurotransmitters [83].

3.5. Cytotoxicity Assessment of AgNPs with MBH in HepG2 Cells

To evaluate the cytotoxic effects of MBH, AgNPs, and their combined formulation drug-loaded AgNPs, IC_{50} values were determined at 24- and 72-h post-treatment in HepG2 cells. The results indicated a time-dependent increase in IC_{50} values for all the tested formulations (Table 4). At 24 h, the IC_{50} values were as follows: MBH—17.16 µg/mL, AgNPs—6.35 µg/mL, and AgNPs-MBH—14.16 µg/mL. After 72 h, the IC_{50} values increased to 27.50 µg/mL for MBH, 17.79 µg/mL for AgNPs, and 17.94 µg/mL for AgNPs with MBH.

Table 4. Cytotoxicity (IC_{50}) of MBH, AgNPs, and AgNPs-MBH in HepG2 cells at 24 and 72 h.

Samples	IC_{50} at 24 h [µg/mL]	IC_{50} at 72 h [µg/mL]
MBH	17.16	27.50
AgNPs	6.35	17.79
AgNPs-MBH	14.16	17.94

These findings suggest that AgNPs exhibited the highest cytotoxicity among the tested formulations, with the lowest IC_{50} values at both time points, which aligns with previous studies indicating the potent cytotoxic effects of AgNPs in hepatic cell lines [84]. The AgNPs-MBH combination demonstrated intermediate cytotoxicity, with slightly increased IC_{50} values at 72 h compared to 24 h, indicating potential cellular adaptation or reduced sensitivity over time. The observed increase in IC_{50} values over time for all compounds may indicate a cellular adaptation or reduced sensitivity to the treatments. This trend was noted in other studies where prolonged nanoparticle exposure resulted in increased IC_{50} values, possibly due to cellular defense mechanisms [85].

3.6. Fluorescence-Activated Cell Sorting (FACS) Analysis of HepG2 Cell Morphology and Granularity

The fluorescence-activated cell sorting (FACS) analysis revealed distinct effects of MBH, AgNPs, and their combination on HepG2 cell morphology over time (Figure 9).

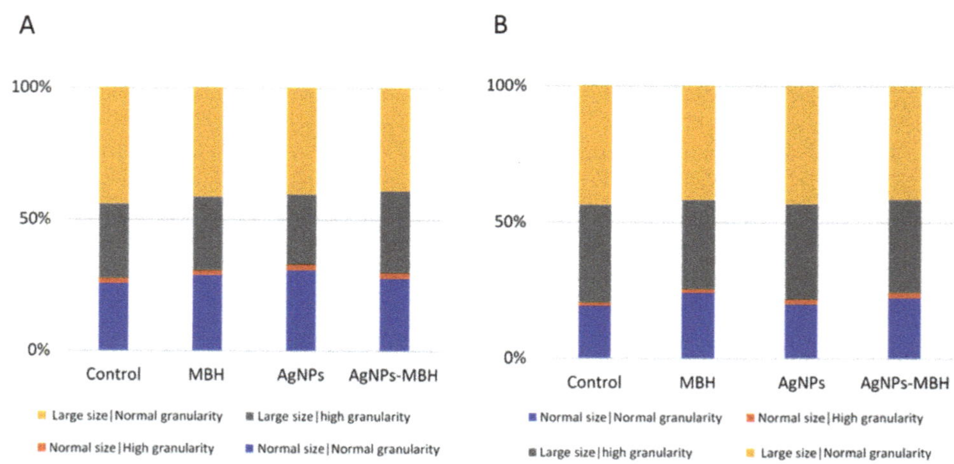

Figure 9. Effects of MBH, AgNPs, and their combination on HepG2 cell morphology and granularity at 24 h (**A**) and 72 h (**B**), assessed by FACS.

At 24 h, MBH, plain AgNPs and drug-loaded AgNPs increased the population of cells with standard size and granularity compared to the non-treated control cells. A minor rise in cells with high granularity was observed across all the treated groups. AgNPs reduced the proportion of larger cells with high granularity, whereas MBH and AgNPs with deposited MBH increased this population. The proportion of large cells with regular granularity remained relatively stable, with MBH slightly increasing and AgNPs reducing this population (Figure 9A). The relatively stable population of large cells with regular granularity under MBH treatment further supports its role in maintaining cellular integrity.

After 72 h, MBH maintained a higher number of normal-sized cells with regular granularity, and under AgNPs and drug-loaded AgNPs they were also increased (Figure 9B). The number of cells with high granularity was elevated under the AgNPs and AgNPs with MBH treatments compared to the control. Over time, AgNPs increased large cells with high granularity, while MBH and AgNPs-MBH led to a reduction, suggesting a potential cellular adaptation. In the population of large cells with regular granularity, AgNPs had the most pronounced increase, followed by MBH and drug-loaded AgNPs, indicating a time-dependent shift in cellular response.

These findings suggest that while MBH maintains a relatively stable cell distribution, AgNPs and their combination with MBH induce dynamic changes in cell size and granularity, possibly reflecting variations in cellular adaptation mechanisms.

3.7. The Fluorescence-Activated Cell Sorting (FACS) Analysis of the HepG2 Cell Cycle After 24 and 72 h of Treatment with MBH, AgNPs, and Their Combination

The fluorescence-activated cell sorting (FACS) analysis of the HepG2 cell cycle after 24 and 72 h of treatment revealed distinct effects of MBH, AgNPs, and their combination (Figure 10).

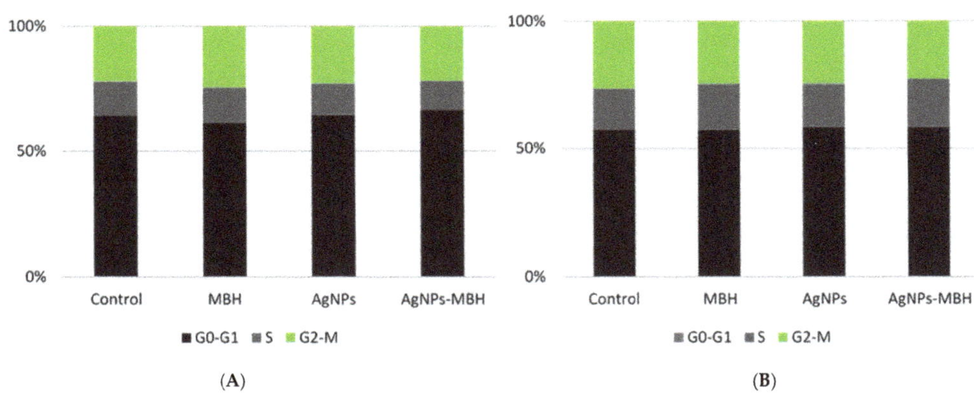

Figure 10. Effects of MBH, AgNPs, and their combination on HepG2 cell cycle at 24 h (**A**) and 72 h (**B**), assessed by FACS.

At 24 h, MBH slightly increased the proportion of cells in the G_0-G_1 phase compared to the control, suggesting a moderate delay in cell cycle progression. On the other hand, the AgNPs treatment led to a reduction in the G_0-G_1 phase, accompanied by decreases in both the S and G_2-M phases (Figure 10A). This pattern may reflect cytotoxic effects or potential cell cycle arrest induced by AgNPs, highlighting their impact on cellular proliferation and viability [86–88]. The drug-loaded AgNPs resulted in a significant increase in the G_0-G_1 population, with a slight decrease in the S phase and a moderate increase in the G_2-M phase. This indicates a potential synergistic effect, where the two agents together may promote a redistribution of cells across the different phases of the cell cycle.

At 72 h, the control cells showed a relatively stable distribution across all the phases. MBH treatment increased the proportion of cells in the S phase while slightly reducing G_2-M-phase cells, indicating possible interference with DNA synthesis (Figure 10B). The AgNPs treatment led to an accumulation of cells in the G_0-G_1 and S phases, with a minor reduction in G_2-M, suggesting a prolonged effect on cell cycle regulation. Interestingly, the drug-loaded AgNPs maintained a similar G_0-G_1-phase percentage to the control while increasing S-phase cells and decreasing G_2-M-phase cells, potentially indicating a shift in the balance of proliferation and arrest mechanisms. The results indicate that while MBH and AgNPs impact cell cycle dynamics individually, their combination exerts unique regulatory effects that may modulate HepG2 cell proliferation. Further studies are warranted to elucidate the underlying mechanisms driving these effects and their potential implications for cancer treatment protocols.

3.8. Antimicrobial Activity

The AgNPs exhibit excellent antimicrobial activity, and this property can be beneficial, especially against microorganisms resistant to conventional antimicrobials [27]. The antibacterial activity of AgNPs against various bacteria results in the diverse inhibitory zone diameters reported recently [89]. The potential use of the antispasmodic mebeverine against *Staphylococcus aureus* was recently examined [90,91]. The authors demonstrated that mebeverine was beneficial in lowering the dosage of antibiotics and reducing the need for subsequent antibiotic administration to patients with various problems, including infection, spasm difficulties, and gastrointestinal ulcers.

Since MBH is administered orally in clinical settings, we anticipated that the drug-loaded AgNPs would also be taken orally. Considering that AgNPs have antibacterial properties, our next aim was to evaluate the antimicrobial effects of drug-loaded AgNPs and to determine whether they could disturb the balance of intestinal flora. The inhibition zones of bacterial and fungal growth caused by MBH-loaded AgNPs are outlined in Table 5.

Table 5. Antimicrobial activity of drug-loaded AgNPs.

	Bacillus subtilis **ATCC 6633**	***Bacillus amyloliquefaciens*** **4BCL-YT**	***Staphylococcus aureus*** **ATCC 25923**	***Listeria monocytogenes*** **NBIMCC 8632**	***Enterococcus faecalis*** **ATCC 29212**	***Salmonella typhimurium*** **NBIMCC 1672**	***Escherichia coli*** **ATCC 25922**	***Pseudomonas aeruginosa*** **ATCC 9027**	***Aspergillus niger*** **ATCC 1015**	***Aspergillus flavus***	***Penicillium chrysogenum***	***Fusarium moniliforme*** **ATCC 38932**
Inhibition zone, mm	10 ± 0.0	10 ± 0.0	15 ± 0.2	15 ± 0.1	15 ± 0.5	12 ± 0.4	10 ± 0.1	12 ± 0.5	11 ± 0.0	8 ± 0.1	8 ± 0.0	11 ± 0.2

Our experiments used six Gram-positive bacteria, six Gram-negative bacteria, two yeasts, and six fungi. The obtained results confirmed previously published results that MBH is bacteriostatic on some Gram-negative bacteria [27], but it was highly bactericidal when tested against *S. aureus*. We found that drug-loaded AgNPs exerted only modest activity against Gram-positive bacteria, including *Staphylococcus aureus* ATCC 25923, *Listeria monocytogenes* NBIMCC 8632, and *Enterococcus faecalis* ATCC 29212. Therefore, we can conclude that drug-loaded AgNPs are not bactericidal. To further assess the stability of drug-loaded AgNPs, their in vitro drug release was evaluated.

3.9. Drug Release

DD systems enter the stomach and small intestine via the mouth and then reach the colon. The nature and pH of gastric secretion and mucus influence drug release and absorption. To reach the colon intact, the DD system should bypass the stomach and small intestine barriers. GI transit varies from 1–3 h depending upon fasting or non-fasting periods [92].

In general, the small intestinal transit is not influenced by the physical state, size of the dosage form, and presence of food in the stomach. The mean transit time required for the dosage form to reach the ileocaecal junction is 3–4 h, and the time is inconsistent. During transit, the dosage form is exposed to enzymes (such as esterase, amylase, lipase, protease, nuclease, glycosidase, disaccharidases, etc.) in the small intestine. The bioavailability of drugs can be highly influenced by the colonic transit time. Compared with the other regions of the GI tract, the movement of material through the colon is slow and influenced by various factors, such as diet, dietary fibers, mobility, stress, disease conditions, and drugs. The colonic transit time of a capsule in an adult is 20–35 h. The release and absorption of the drug from a dosage form are governed by an improved residence time with a longer transit time and the contact of the dosage form with microflora in the colon [92].

Drug-release profiles from dialysis-based assays determine NP formulations' in vivo–in vitro correlations and direct the development and quality control [93]. Under normal physiological conditions, the pH value from the stomach to the intestine showed an increasing trend, specifically, an acidic stomach (pH 1.5 to 3.5), duodenum (pH 6), terminal ileum (pH 7.4), terminal cecum (pH 6), and colon (pH 6.7) [94]. The drug-release study was carried out in a neutral medium (PBS, pH 7.4) to simulate the physiological conditions. A cellulose dialysis bag with a molecular weight cut-off of 12,400 Da was used to hold the solution of drug-containing Ag NPs. The pores in this cut-off were large enough to let the medication out of the dialysate while keeping the Ag NPs inside the membrane. Since the calibration curve for MBH was linear, it was possible to conduct the quantification tests.

The length of the intestine, the composition of the gut microbiota, individual variances in stomach and intestinal fluid, and peristalsis may all have a role in the transport time of the gastrointestinal system. There are considerable variations in gastrointestinal emptying periods, not just between healthy participants but also between IBD patients and healthy people, which may raise the uncertainty of when the medicine will reach the colon. Although the small intestine's average transport time is thought to be 4 h, individual differences often range from 2 to 6 h [94]. Therefore, determining the drug release at the first 6 h was crucial for our investigation.

During the initial 5 to 20 h of the drug release experiment, the absorbance intensity rose with time, indicating an increasing concentration of the MBH in the dialysate (Figure 11).

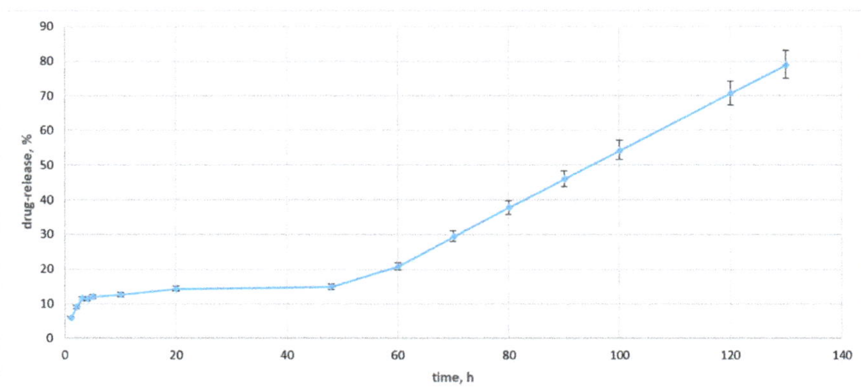

Figure 11. Drug-release concentrations for drug-loaded Ag NPs.

After the 48 h, the drug release pattern changed drastically, with the concentration of the released MBH in the dialysate increasing by 14%. Then, the concentration of the released drug rose, and at the 130 h, it indicated an 80% drug release. The observed drug release was slower than those previously measured [59]. We can explain this drug release with the carbohydrate coating. The fructose loads MBH more effectively and slows down the drug release.

According to these preliminary findings, Ag NPs might be a helpful medication delivery mechanism for MBH and a potent tool for treating inflammatory bowel disease. For this reason, additional research on long-acting delivery formulations and potential medical uses for drug-loaded Ag NPs will also be required to add to the benefits of this study.

4. Conclusions

Our results provide valuable insights into the biological activity of the drug-loaded AgNPs studied from a spasmolytic and anti-inflammatory point of view.

Drug-loaded AgNPs exhibited mild tonic relaxation and a 50% reduction in the amplitude of spontaneous contraction. At the same time, MBH caused a sharp contractile reaction with dose-dependent changes in the tonic response and a statistically significant increase in the contraction amplitude. When drug-loaded AgNPs interact with specifically blocked cholinergic receptors, their effects are more noticeable and different in amplitude and character, while MBH has no effect. Therefore, the biological activity of drug-loaded AgNPs is due to an underlying mechanism that directly connects mAChR and nAChR activation.

In vitro and ex vivo experiments were conducted to further investigate the anti-inflammatory effect of drug-loaded AgNPs. In vitro, the results showed that MBH and drug-loaded AgNPs demonstrated better protection in albumin denaturation than known NSAIDs. The ex vivo experiments confirmed these results, demonstrating that AgNPs exhibited better anti-inflammatory effects regarding IL-1β expression and a superior inhibitory effect on the 5-HT3 channel receptor.

The provided DFT analysis confirmed the adsorption process of an MBH molecule (neutral and cationic) on the surface of fructose-coated AgNPs. It correlated with its physicochemical parameters of great significance, which justifies experiments.

Drug-loaded AgNPs were identified as not being bactericidal. Additionally, their in vitro drug release was also assessed. We found that fructose loads MBH more effectively and slows down the drug release.

Future in vivo and preclinical experiments will contribute to the establishment of drug-loaded AgNPs as a potential antispasmodic against inflammatory diseases in the GI tract.

Cytotoxicity results showed that plain AgNPs exhibited the most potent cytotoxicity among the tested formulations (AgNPs, MBH, and drug-loaded AgNPs) in HepG2 cells, with the lowest IC_{50} values at 24 and 72 h. The drug-loaded AgNPs showed intermediate cytotoxicity, with a slight increase in IC_{50} values over time, which could indicate cellular adaptation or reduced sensitivity to the treatment. The overall trend of increasing IC_{50} values over time for all the compounds points to possible cellular defense mechanisms or adaptation to prolonged nanoparticle exposure.

Our results demonstrate the distinct effects of MBH and AgNPs on HepG2 cell morphology over time. MBH appears to support stable cell distribution and maintain normal morphology, whereas AgNPs and drug-loaded AgNPs induce dynamic alterations, suggesting varied cellular adaptation responses. These findings are essential for refining nanoparticle-based drug delivery strategies.

The flow cytometry analysis further showed that MBH and AgNPs individually influence the HepG2 cell cycle, while their combination produces unique regulatory effects that may impact cellular proliferation. Investigating these interactions is vital for developing more effective therapeutic approaches. Additional studies are needed to uncover the mechanisms underlying these observations and their potential relevance to cancer treatment.

Author Contributions: Conceptualization, S.N. and M.T.; methodology, M.S., M.M., V.G., M.T., M.P., K.H.-P., G.M., Y.T. and B.V.; investigation, contractile activity, V.G. and I.S.; anti-inflammatory activity, M.T., M.S., M.M., S.N. and M.P.; DFT and molecular docking, S.A. and N.K. (Nikoleta Kircheva); cytotoxicity: K.H.-P., B.V., G.M., N.K. (Natalia Krasteva) and M.G.; antimicrobial activity—Y.T., M.M. and M.S., software, S.A. and N.K. (Nikoleta Kircheva); writing—original draft preparation, S.N., V.G., N.K. (Nikoleta Kircheva), I.S., N.K. (Natalia Krasteva), M.G. and S.A.; writing—review and editing, S.N., V.G., N.K. (Natalia Krasteva), N.K. (Nikoleta Kircheva), Y.T. and M.G.; visualization, S.N., V.G., N.K. (Nikoleta Kircheva), N.K. (Natalia Krasteva), M.G. and S.A.; supervision, S.N., M.G., N.K. (Natalia Krasteva) and S.A.; project administration, S.N. All authors have read and agreed to the published version of the manuscript.

Funding: This research received no external funding.

Institutional Review Board Statement: Ethical Committee of the Bulgarian Food Agency with No 400/23.05.2024 approved the study protocol. All the studies were carried out according to the Institutional Animal Care guidelines and complied with the EU Directive 2010/63/EU. All the experiments were carried out according to the legislation on the Welfare and Protection of Animals Used for Experimental and Other Scientific Purposes. All efforts were made to minimize the number of used animals.

Informed Consent Statement: Not applicable.

Data Availability Statement: The original contributions presented in the study are included in the article; further inquiries can be directed to the corresponding author.

Acknowledgments: This study is part of Scientific Project 466 No KP-06-H73/11 of the National Fund for Scientific Research in Bulgaria, National Program for Basic Research Projects—2023.

Conflicts of Interest: The authors declare no conflicts of interest.

References

1. Kaplan, G.G. The Global Burden of IBD: From 2015 to 2025. *Nat. Rev. Gastroenterol. Hepatol.* **2015**, *12*, 720–727. [CrossRef] [PubMed]
2. Talaei, F.; Atyabi, F.; Azhdarzadeh, M.; Dinarvand, R.; Saadatzadeh, A. Overcoming Therapeutic Obstacles in Inflammatory Bowel Diseases: A Comprehensive Review on Novel Drug Delivery Strategies. *Eur. J. Pharm. Sci.* **2013**, *49*, 712–722. [CrossRef] [PubMed]
3. Ford, A.C.; Sperber, A.D.; Corsetti, M.; Camilleri, M. Irritable Bowel Syndrome. *Lancet* **2020**, *396*, 1675–1688. [CrossRef]
4. Zhang, Q.; Long, L.; Zhu, H.-L.; Peng, H.; Luo, X.-H.; Zhu, K.-S.; Wang, R.-P. Global Burden of Inflammatory Bowel Disease 1990-2019: A Systematic Examination of the Disease Burden and Twenty-Year Forecast. *World J. Gastroenterol.* **2023**, *29*, 5751–5767. [CrossRef]
5. Venkataraman, G.R.; Rivas, M.A. Rare and Common Variant Discovery in Complex Disease: The IBD Case Study. *Hum. Mol. Genet.* **2019**, *28*, R162–R169. [CrossRef]
6. Ananthakrishnan, A.N. Epidemiology and Risk Factors for IBD. *Nat. Rev. Gastroenterol. Hepatol.* **2015**, *12*, 205–217. [CrossRef]
7. Hammer, T.; Lophaven, S.N.; Nielsen, K.R.; Petersen, M.S.; Munkholm, P.; Weihe, P.; Burisch, J.; Lynge, E. Dietary Risk Factors for Inflammatory Bowel Diseases in a High-Risk Population: Results from the Faroese IBD Study. *United Eur. Gastroenterol. J.* **2019**, *7*, 924–932. [CrossRef]
8. Kaplan, G.G. Global Variations in Environmental Risk Factors for IBD. *Nat. Rev. Gastroenterol. Hepatol.* **2014**, *11*, 708–709. [CrossRef]
9. van der Sloot, K.W.J.; Weersma, R.K.; Dijkstra, G.; Alizadeh, B.Z. Development and Validation of a Web-Based Questionnaire to Identify Environmental Risk Factors for Inflammatory Bowel Disease: The Groningen IBD Environmental Questionnaire (GIEQ). *J. Gastroenterol.* **2018**, *54*, 238–248. [CrossRef]
10. Lim, J.S.; Lim, M.Y.; Choi, Y.; Ko, G. Modeling Environmental Risk Factors of Autism in Mice Induces IBD-Related Gut Microbial Dysbiosis and Hyperserotonemia. *Mol. Brain* **2017**, *10*, 14. [CrossRef]

11. Putignani, L.; Del Chierico, F.; Vernocchi, P.; Cicala, M.; Cucchiara, S.; Dallapiccola, B. Gut Microbiota Dysbiosis as Risk and Premorbid Factors of IBD and IBS along the Childhood–Adulthood Transition. *Inflamm. Bowel Dis.* **2016**, *22*, 487–504. [CrossRef] [PubMed]
12. Vong, L.; Mo, J.; Abrahamsson, B.; Nagasaki, Y. Specific accumulation of orally administered redox nanotherapeutics in the inflamed colon reducing inflammation with dose-response efficacy. *J. Control. Release* **2015**, *210*, 19–25. [CrossRef] [PubMed]
13. Tiwari, A.; Verma, A.; Kumar Panda, P.; Saraf, S.; Jain, A.; Jain, S.K. Stimuli-responsive polysaccharides for colon-targeted drug delivery. In *Biomaterials, Stimuli Responsive Polymeric Nanocarriers for Drug Delivery Applications*; Makhlouf, A.S.H., Abu-Thabit, N.Y., Eds.; Woodhead Publishing: Sawston, UK, 2019; pp. 547–566. [CrossRef]
14. Wang, C.-P.; Ji Byun, M.; Kim, S.-N.; Park, W.; Park, H.; Kim, T.-H.; Lee, J.; Park, C. Biomaterials as therapeutic drug carriers for inflammatory bowel disease treatment. *J. Control. Release* **2022**, *345*, 1–19. [CrossRef] [PubMed]
15. Collnot, E.-M.; Ali, H.; Lehr, C.-M. Nano- and microparticulate drug carriers for targeting of the inflamed intestinal mucosa. *J. Control. Release* **2012**, *161*, 235–246. [CrossRef]
16. Nidhi; Rashid, M.; Kaur, V.; Hallan, S.S.; Sharma, S.; Mishra, N. Microparticles as controlled drug delivery carrier for the treatment of ulcerative colitis: A brief review. *Saudi Pharm. J.* **2016**, *24*, 458–472. [CrossRef]
17. Katas, H.; Moden, N.Z.; Lim, C.S.; Celesistinus, T.; Chan, J.Y.; Ganasan, P.; Abdalla, S.S.I. Biosynthesis and potential applications of silver and gold nanoparticles and their chitosan-based nanocomposites in nanomedicine. *J. Nanotechnol.* **2018**, *2018*, 4290705. [CrossRef]
18. Jeevanandam, J.; Barhoum, A.; Chan, Y.; Dufresne, A.; Danquah, M. Review on nanoparticles and nanostructured materials: History, sources, toxicity and regulations. *Beilstein J. Nanotechnol.* **2018**, *9*, 1050–1074. [CrossRef]
19. Petros, R.; DeSimone, J. Strategies in the design of nanoparticles for therapeutic applications. *Nat. Rev. Drug Discov.* **2010**, *9*, 615–627. [CrossRef]
20. Virmani, I.; Sasi, C.; Priyadarshini, E.; Kumar, R.; Kumar Sharma, S.; Pratap Singh, G.; Babu Pachwarya, R.; Paulraj, R.; Barabadi, H.; Saravanan, M.; et al. Comparative Anticancer Potential of Biologically and Chemically Synthesized Gold Nanoparticles. *J. Clust. Sci.* **2020**, *31*, 867–876. [CrossRef]
21. Jain, A.; Pawar, P.; Sarkar, A.; Junnuthula, V.; Dyawanapelly, S. Bionanofactories for Green Synthesis of Silver Nano-particles: Toward Antimicrobial Applications. *Int. J. Mol. Sci.* **2021**, *22*, 11993. [CrossRef]
22. Rutgeerts, P.; Sandborn, W.J.; Feagan, B.G.; Reinisch, W.; Olson, A.; Johanns, J.; Travers, S.; Rachmilewitz, D.; Hanauer, S.B.; Lichtenstein, G.R.; et al. Infliximab for induction and mainte-nance therapy for ulcerative colitis. *N. Engl. J. Med.* **2005**, *353*, 2462–2476. [CrossRef] [PubMed]
23. Papadakis, K.A.; Shaye, O.A.; Vasiliauskas, E.A.; Ippoliti, A.; Dubinsky, M.C.; Birt, J.; Paavola, J.; Lee, S.K.; Price, J.; Targan, S.R.; et al. Safety and efficacy of adalimumab (D2E7) in Crohn's disease patients with an attenuated response to infliximab. *Am. J. Gastroenterol.* **2005**, *100*, 75–79. [CrossRef] [PubMed]
24. Chairam, S.; Poolperm, C.; Somsook, E. Starch vermicelli template-assisted synthesis of size/shape-controlled nanoparticles. *Carbohydr. Polym.* **2009**, *75*, 694–704. [CrossRef]
25. Kassaee, M.Z.; Akhavan, A.; Sheikh, N.; Beteshobabrud, R. γ-Ray synthesis of starch-stabilized silver nanoparticles with antibacterial activities. *Radiat. Phys. Chem.* **2008**, *77*, 1074–1078. [CrossRef]
26. Vigneshwaran, N.; Nachane, R.P.; Balasubramanya, R.H.; Varadarajan, P.V. A novel one-pot green synthesis of stable silver nanoparticles using soluble starch. *Carbohydr. Res.* **2006**, *341*, 2012–2018. [CrossRef]
27. Sharma, V.K.; Yngard, R.A.; Lin, Y. Silver nanoparticles: Green synthesis and their antimicrobial activities. *Adv. Colloid Interface Sci.* **2009**, *145*, 83–96. [CrossRef]
28. Panacek, A.; Kvítek, L.; Prucek, R.; Kolar, M.; Vecerova, R.; Pizúrova, N.; Sharma, V.; Nevecna, T.; Zboril, R. Silver colloid nanoparticles: Synthesis, characterization, and their antibacterial activity. *J. Phys. Chem. B* **2006**, *110*, 16248–16253. [CrossRef]
29. Kamble, S.; Bhosale, K.; Mohite, M.; Navale, S. Methods of Preparation of Nanoparticles. *Int. Adv. Res. Sci. Commun. Technol.* **2022**, *2*, 2581–9429. [CrossRef]
30. Filippo, E.; Manno, D.; Serra, A. Self assembly and branching of sucrose stabilized silver nanoparticles by microwave assisted synthesis: From nanoparticles to branched nanowires structures. *Colloids Surf. A Physicochem. Eng. Asp.* **2009**, *348*, 205–211. [CrossRef]
31. Filippo, E.; Serra, A.; Buccolieri, A.; Manno, D. Green synthesis of silver nanoparticles with sucrose and maltose: Morphological and structural characterization. *J. Non-Cryst. Solids* **2010**, *356*, 344–350. [CrossRef]
32. Caschera, D.; Toro, R.G.; Federici, F.; Montanari, R.; de Caro, T.; Al-Shemy, M.T.; Adel, A.M. Green Approach for the Fabrication of Silver-Oxidized Cellulose Nano-composite with Antibacterial Properties. *Cellulose* **2020**, *27*, 8059–8073. [CrossRef]
33. Garza-Cervantes, J.A.; Mendiola-Garza, G.; de Melo, E.M.; Dugmore, T.I.; Matharu, A.S.; Morones-Ramirez, J.R. An-timicrobial Activity of a Silver-Microfibrillated Cellulose Biocomposite against Susceptible and Resistant Bacteria. *Sci. Rep.* **2020**, *10*, 7281. [CrossRef] [PubMed]

34. Rather, R.A.; Sarwara, R.K.; Das, N.; Pal, B. Impact of Reducing and Capping Agents on Carbohydrates for the Growth of Ag and Cu Nanostructures and Their Antibacterial Activities. *Particuology* **2019**, *43*, 219–226. [CrossRef]
35. Shanmuganathan, R.; Edison, T.N.J.I.; LewisOscar, F.; Kumar, P.; Shanmugam, S.; Pugazhendhi, A. Chitosan Na-nopolymers: An Overview of Drug Delivery against Cancer. *Int. J. Biol. Macromol.* **2019**, *130*, 727–736. [CrossRef]
36. Maiti, P.K.; Ghosh, A.; Parveen, R.; Saha, A.; Choudhury, M.G. Preparation of Carboxy-Methyl Cellulose-Capped Na-nosilver Particles and Their Antimicrobial Evaluation by an Automated Device. *Appl. Nanosci.* **2019**, *9*, 105–111. [CrossRef]
37. Stoyanova, M.; Milusheva, M.; Georgieva, M.; Ivanov, P.; Miloshev, G.; Krasteva, N.; Hristova-Panusheva, K.; Feizi-Dehnayebi, M.; Mohammadi Ziarani, G.; Stojnova, K.; et al. Synthesis, Cytotoxic and Genotoxic Evaluation of Drug-Loaded Silver Nanoparticles with Mebeverine and Its Analog. *Pharmaceuticals* **2025**, *18*, 397. [CrossRef]
38. Illangakoon, U.E.; Nazir, T.; Williams, G.R.; Chatterton, N.P. Mebeverine-loaded electrospun nanofibers: Physicochemical characterization and dissolution studies. *J. Pharm. Sci.* **2014**, *103*, 283–292. [CrossRef]
39. Abdulhady, S.S.; Ibrahim, K.M.H. Preparation and evaluation of mebeverine hydrochloride as mucoadhesive buccal tablet for local anesthesia. *Trop. J. Pharm. Res.* **2017**, *16*, 1805–1812. [CrossRef]
40. Nezhadali, A.; Bonakdar, G.A. Multivariate optimization of mebeverine analysis using molecularly imprinted polymer electrochemical sensor based on silver nanoparticles. *J. Food Drug Anal.* **2019**, *27*, 305–314. [CrossRef]
41. Annaházi, A.; Róka, R.; Rosztóczy, A.; Wittmann, T. Role of Antispasmodics in the Treatment of Irritable Bowel Syndrome. *World J. Gastroenterol.* **2014**, *20*, 6031–6043. [CrossRef]
42. Sil, A.; Chakraborty, D.; Hazra, A.; Pain, S. Will Controlled Release Mebeverine Be Able to Surpass Placebo in Treatment of Diarrhoea Predominant Irritable Bowel Syndrome? *J. Fam. Med. Prim. Care* **2019**, *8*, 3173–3178. [CrossRef] [PubMed]
43. Touyz, R.M.; Alves-Lopes, R.; Rios, F.J.; Camargo, L.L.; Anagnostopoulou, A.; Arner, A.; Montezano, A.C. Vascular Smooth Muscle Contraction in Hypertension. *Cardiovasc. Res.* **2018**, *114*, 529–539. [CrossRef] [PubMed]
44. Ruggieri, M.R.; Braverman, A.S.; Vegesna, A.K.; Miller, L.S. Nicotinic Receptor Subtypes Mediating Relaxation of the Normal Human Clasp and Sling Fibers of the Upper Gastric Sphincter. *Neurogastroenterol. Motil.* **2014**, *26*, 1015–1025. [CrossRef]
45. Saab, H.; Aboeed, A.; Patel, P. Ipratropium. Available online: https://www.ncbi.nlm.nih.gov/books/NBK544261/ (accessed on 3 February 2025).
46. Di Natale, M.R.; Stebbing, M.J.; Furness, J.B. Autonomic Neuromuscular Junctions. *Auton. Neurosci.* **2021**, *234*, 102816. [CrossRef]
47. Biswas, N.; Thomas, S.; Sarkar, A.; Mukherjee, T.; Kapoor, S. Adsorption of Methimazole on Silver Nanoparticles: FTIR, Raman, and Surface-Enhanced Raman Scattering Study Aided by Density Functional Theory. *J. Phys. Chem. C* **2009**, *113*, 7091–7100. [CrossRef]
48. Arroyave, J.M.; Ambrusi, R.E.; Pronsato, M.E.; Juan, A.; Pistonesi, M.F.; Centurión, M.E. Experimental and DFT Studies of Hybrid Silver/Cdots Nanoparticles. *J. Phys. Chem. B* **2020**, *124*, 2425–2435. [CrossRef]
49. Makkar, P.; Ghosh, N.N. A Review on the Use of DFT for the Prediction of the Properties of Nanomaterials. *RSC Adv.* **2021**, *11*, 27897–27924. [CrossRef]
50. Kanagamani, K.; Muthukrishnan, P.; Ilayaraja, M.; Shankar, K.; Kathiresan, A. Synthesis, Characterisation and DFT Studies of Stigmasterol Mediated Silver Nanoparticles and Their Anticancer Activity. *J. Inorg. Organomet. Polym. Mater.* **2017**, *28*, 702–710. [CrossRef]
51. Radwan, M.A.; Foda, N.H.; Al Deeb, O.A. Mebeverine Hydrochloride. In *Analytical Profiles of Drug Substances and Excipients*; Brittain, H.G., Ed.; Academic Press: San Diego, CA, USA, 1998; Volume 25, pp. 165–207, ISBN 978-0-12-260825-4, ISSN 1075-6280. [CrossRef]
52. Brittain, H.G. *Analytical Profiles of Drug Substances and Excipients*, 1st ed.; Academic Press: San Diego, CA, USA, 2001; Volume 28, ISBN 978-0-12-260828-5.
53. Abdullah, G.Z.; Abdulkarim, M.F.; Chitneni, M.; Mutee, A.F.; Ameer, O.Z.; Salman, I.M.; Noor, A.M. Preparation and in vitro evaluation of mebeverine HCl colon-targeted drug delivery system. *Pharm. Dev. Technol.* **2011**, *16*, 331–342. [CrossRef]
54. Blagbrough, I.S.; Elmasry, M.S.; Woodman, T.J.; Saleh, H.M.; Aboul Kheir, A. Quantitative determination of mebeverine HCl by NMR chemical shift migration. *Tetrahedron* **2009**, *65*, 4930–4936. [CrossRef]
55. Iravani, S.; Korbekandi, H.; Mirmohammadi, S.; Zolfaghari, B. Synthesis of Silver Nanoparticles: Chemical, Physical, and Biological Methods. *Res. Pharm. Sci.* **2014**, *9*, 385–406. [PubMed]
56. Younas, M.; Ahmad, M.A.; Jannat, F.T.; Ashfaq, T.; Ahmad, A. 18—Role of Silver Nanoparticles in Multifunctional Drug Delivery. In *Micro and Nano Technologies, Nanomedicine Manufacturing and Applications*; Verpoort, F., Ahmad, I., Ahmad, A., Khan, A., Chee, C.Y., Eds.; Elsevier: Orlando, FL, USA, 2021; pp. 297–319.
57. Mulvaney, P.; Liz-Marzan, L.; Giersig, M.; Ung, T.J. Silica encapsulation of quantum dots and metal clusters. *J. Mater. Chem.* **2000**, *10*, 1259–1270. [CrossRef]
58. Frisch, M.; Trucks, G.; Schlegel, H.B.; Scuseria, G.E.; Robb, M.A.; Cheeseman, J.R.; Scalmani, G.; Barone, V.; Mennucci, B.; Petersson, G. *Gaussian 09*; Revision d. 01; Gaussian, Inc.: Wallingford, CT, USA, 2009; p. 201.

59. Nikolova, S.; Milusheva, M.; Gledacheva, V.; Feizi-Dehnayebi, M.; Kaynarova, L.; Georgieva, D.; Delchev, V.B.; Stefanova, I.; Tumbarski, Y.; Mihaylova, R.; et al. Drug-Delivery Silver Nanoparticles: A New Perspective for Phenindione as an Anticoagulant. *Biomedicines* **2023**, *11*, 2201. [CrossRef] [PubMed]
60. Cox, H.; Macquarrie, D.A.; Simon, J.D. *Physical Chemistry: A Molecular Approach Problems and Solutions to Accompany McQuarrie and Simon: Physical Chemistry*; University Science Books: Sausalito, CA, USA, 1997; ISBN 9780935702439.
61. Milusheva, M.; Gledacheva, V.; Stefanova, I.; Feizi-Dehnayebi, M.; Mihaylova, R.; Nedialkov, P.; Cherneva, E.; Tumbarski, Y.; Tsoneva, S.; Todorova, M.; et al. Synthesis, Molecular Docking, and Biological Evaluation of Novel Anthranilic Acid Hybrid and Its Diamides as Antispasmodics. *Int. J. Mol. Sci.* **2023**, *24*, 13855. [CrossRef]
62. Khan, H.A.; Ibrahim, K.E.; Khan, A.; Alrokayan, S.H.; Alhomida, A.S. Immunostaining of Proinflammatory Cytokines in Renal Cortex and Medulla of Rats Exposed to Gold Nanoparticles. *Histol. Histopathol.* **2017**, *32*, 597–607. [CrossRef]
63. Tumbarski, Y.; Deseva, I.; Mihaylova, D.; Stoyanova, M.; Krastev, L.; Nikolova, R.; Yanakieva, V.; Ivanov, I. Isolation, Characterization and Amino Acid Composition of a Bacteriocin Produced by Bacillus methylotrophicus Strain BM47. *Food Technol. Biotechnol.* **2018**, *56*, 546–552. [CrossRef]
64. Barclay, T.; Ginic-Markovic, M.; Cooper, P.D.; Petrovsky, N. The Chemistry and Sources of Fructose and Their Effect on Functionality and Health Implications. *J. Excip. Food Chem.* **2012**, *3*, 67.
65. Ismael, M.; Abdel-Mawgoud, A.M.; Rabia, M.K.; Abdou, A. Ni(II) Mixed-Ligand Chelates Based on 2-Hydroxy-1-Naphthaldehyde as Antimicrobial Agents: Synthesis, Characterization, and Molecular Modeling. *J. Mol. Liq.* **2019**, *330*, 115611. [CrossRef]
66. Stoyanova, M.; Milusheva, M.; Gledacheva, V.; Stefanova, I.; Todorova, M.; Kircheva, N.; Angelova, S.; Pencheva, M.; Stojnova, K.; Tsoneva, S.; et al. Spasmolytic Activity and Anti-Inflammatory Effect of Novel Mebeverine Derivatives. *Biomedicines* **2024**, *12*, 2321. [CrossRef]
67. Daniluk, J.; Malecka-Wojciesko, E.; Skrzydlo-Radomanska, B.; Rydzewska, G. The Efficacy of Mebeverine in the Treatment of Irritable Bowel Syndrome—A Systematic Review. *J. Clin. Med.* **2022**, *11*, 1044. [CrossRef]
68. González, C.; Salazar-García, S.; Palestino, G.; Martínez-Cuevas, P.P.; Ramírez-Lee, M.A.; Jurado-Manzano, B.B.; Rosas-Hernández, H.; Gaytán-Pacheco, N.; Martel, G.; Espinosa-Tanguma, R.; et al. Effect of 45 Nm Silver Nanoparticles (AgNPs) upon the Smooth Muscle of Rat Trachea: Role of Nitric Oxide. *Toxicol. Lett.* **2011**, *207*, 306–313. [CrossRef] [PubMed]
69. Zholos, A.V.; Bolton, T.B.; Dresvyannikov, A.V.; Kustov, M.V.; Tsvilovskii, V.V.; Shuba, M.F. Cholinergic Excitation of Smooth Muscles: Multiple Signaling Pathways Linking M2 and M3 Muscarinic Receptors to Cationic Channels. *Neurophysiology* **2004**, *36*, 398–406. [CrossRef]
70. Janssen, P.; Prins, N.H.; Meulemans, A.L.; Lefebvre, R.A. Smooth Muscle 5-HT2A Receptors Mediating Contraction of Porcine Isolated Proximal Stomach Strips. *Br. J. Pharmacol.* **2002**, *137*, 1217–1224. [CrossRef] [PubMed]
71. Perez, J.F.; Sanderson, M.J. The Frequency of Calcium Oscillations Induced by 5-HT, ACH, and KCl Determine the Contraction of Smooth Muscle Cells of Intrapulmonary Bronchioles. *J. Gen. Physiol.* **2005**, *125*, 535–553. [CrossRef]
72. Harirforoosh, S.; Asghar, W.; Jamali, F. Adverse Effects of Nonsteroidal Anti-inflammatory Drugs: An Update of Gastrointestinal, Cardiovascular and Renal Complications. *J. Pharm. Pharm. Sci.* **2014**, *16*, 821–847. [CrossRef]
73. Yasir, M.; Sonthalia, S.; Goyal, A. *Corticosteroid Adverse Effects*; StatPearls Publishing: Treasure Island, FL, USA, 2023. Available online: https://www.ncbi.nlm.nih.gov/books/NBK531462/ (accessed on 10 March 2025).
74. Jayashree, V.; Bagyalakshmi, S.; Manjula Devi, K.; Richard, D.D. In Vitro Anti-Inflammatory Activity of 4-Benzylpiperidine. *Asian J. Pharm. Clin. Res.* **2016**, *9*, 108–110. [CrossRef]
75. Stack, W.; Mann, S.; Roy, A.; Heath, P.; Sopwith, M.; Freeman, J.; Holmes, G.; Long, R.; Forbes, A.; Kamm, M.; et al. Randomised Controlled Trial of CDP571 Antibody to Tumour Necrosis Factor-α in Crohn's Disease. *Lancet* **1997**, *349*, 521–524. [CrossRef]
76. Elson, C.O.; Sartor, R.B.; Tennyson, G.S.; Riddell, R.H. Experimental Models of Inflammatory Bowel Disease. *Gastroenterology* **1995**, *109*, 1344–1367. [CrossRef]
77. Traverso, G.; Schoellhammer, C.M.; Schroeder, A.; Maa, R.; Lauwers, G.Y.; Polat, B.; Anderson, D.G.; Blankschtein, D.; Langer, R. Microneedles for Drug Delivery via the Gastrointestinal Tract. *J. Pharm. Sci.* **2015**, *104*, 362–367. [CrossRef]
78. Patra, J.K.; Das, G.; Fraceto, L.F.; Campos, E.V.R.; Rodriguez-Torres, M.d.P.; Acosta-Torres, L.S.; Diaz-Torres, L.A.; Grillo, R.; Swamy, M.K.; Sharma, S.; et al. Nano Based Drug Delivery Systems: Recent Developments and Future Prospects. *J. Nanobiotechnol.* **2018**, *16*, 71. [CrossRef]
79. Yusuf, A.; Almotairy, A.R.Z.; Henidi, H.; Alshehri, O.Y.; Aldughaim, M.S. Nanoparticles as Drug Delivery Systems: A Review of the Implication of Nanoparticles' Physicochemical Properties on Responses in Biological Systems. *Polymers* **2023**, *15*, 1596. [CrossRef] [PubMed]
80. Hsu, C.-Y.; Rheima, A.M.; Kadhim, M.M.; Ahmed, N.; Mohammed, S.H.; Abbas, F.H.; Abed, Z.T.; Mahdi, Z.M.; Abbas, Z.S.; Hachim, S.K.; et al. An Overview of Nanoparticles in Drug Delivery: Properties and Applications. *S. Afr. J. Chem. Eng.* **2023**, *46*, 233–270. [CrossRef]
81. Kato, S. Role of Serotonin 5-HT$_3$ Receptors in Intestinal Inflammation. *Biol. Pharm. Bull.* **2013**, *36*, 1406–1409. [CrossRef]

82. Yasuda, H.; Park, E.; Yun, C.-H.; Sng, N.J.; Lucena-Araujo, A.R.; Yeo, W.-L.; Huberman, M.S.; Cohen, D.W.; Nakayama, S.; Ishioka, K.; et al. Structural, Biochemical and Clinical Characterization of Epidermal Growth Factor Receptor (EGFR) Exon 20 Insertion Mutations in Lung Cancer. *Sci. Transl. Med.* **2013**, *5*, 216ra177. [CrossRef]
83. Jiang, Y.; Zou, D.; Li, Y.; Gu, S.; Dong, J.; Ma, X.; Xu, S.; Wang, F.; Huang, J.H. Monoamine Neurotransmitters Control Basic Emotions and Affect Major Depressive Disorders. *Pharmaceuticals* **2022**, *15*, 1203. [CrossRef]
84. Xue, Y.; Huang, Y.; Gong, F.; Zhang, T.; Tang, M. Cytotoxicity of Silver Nanoparticles Was Influenced by Dispersion Media in HepG2 Cells. In Proceedings of the 6th International Conference on Biomedical Engineering and Informatics, Hangzhou, China, 16–18 December 2013; pp. 358–362. [CrossRef]
85. Tabbasam, R.; Khursid, S.; Ishaq, Y.; Farrukh, S.Y. Synergistic Cytotoxic Effects of Doxorubicin Loaded Silver, Gold and Zinc Oxide Nanoparticles in HepG2 Liver Cancer Cells. *BioNanoScience* **2024**, *15*, 105. [CrossRef]
86. Pozarowski, P.; Darzynkiewicz, Z. Analysis of Cell Cycle by Flow Cytometry. *Methods Mol. Biol.* **2004**, *281*, 301–311. [CrossRef]
87. Darzynkiewicz, Z.; Zhao, H. *Encyclopedia of Life Sciences*; John Wiley & Sons: London, UK; New York, NY, USA, 2005; Volume 4, pp. 26–30, ISBN 9780470016176.
88. Wang, F.; Chen, Z.; Wang, Y.; Ma, C.; Bi, L.; Song, M.; Jiang, G. Silver Nanoparticles Induce Apoptosis in HepG2 Cells through Particle-Specific Effects on Mitochondria. *Environ. Sci. Technol.* **2022**, *56*, 5706–5713. [CrossRef]
89. Said, A.; Abu-Elghait, M.; Atta, H.M.; Salem, S.S. Antibacterial activity of green synthesized silver nanoparticles using *Lawsonia inermis* against common pathogens from urinary tract infection. *Appl. Biochem. Biotechnol.* **2024**, *196*, 85–98. [CrossRef]
90. Akilandeswari, A.; Ruckmani, K. Antibacterial potentiality of antiulcer and antispasmodic drugs with selected antibiotics against methicillin resistant Staphylococcus aureus: In vitro and in silico studies. *Bangladesh J. Pharmacol.* **2015**, *10*, 875–883. [CrossRef]
91. Nandini, P.; Deepnandan, D. Synthetic Process Study and Pharmacological Evaluation of Antispasmodic Drug as Potential Antimicrobial Agent. *Asian J. Res. Chem.* **2009**, *2*, 494–500.
92. Sowmya, C.; Reddy, C.S.; Priya, N.V.; Sandhya, R.; Keerthi, K. Colon specific drug delivery systems: A review on phar-maceutical approaches with current trends. *Int. Res. J. Pharm.* **2012**, *3*, 45–55.
93. Kumar, B.; Jalodia, K.; Kumar, P.; Gautam, H.K. Recent Advances in Nanoparticle-Mediated Drug Delivery. *J. Drug Deliv. Sci. Technol.* **2017**, *41*, 260–268. [CrossRef]
94. Cui, M.; Zhang, M.; Liu, K. Colon-targeted drug delivery of polysaccharide-based nanocarriers for synergistic treatment of inflammatory bowel disease: A review. *Carbohydr. Polym.* **2021**, *272*, 118530. [CrossRef] [PubMed]

pharmaceutics

MDPI

Review

Nanomedicines for Pulmonary Drug Delivery: Overcoming Barriers in the Treatment of Respiratory Infections and Lung Cancer

Raquel Fernández-García [1,*] and Ana I. Fraguas-Sánchez [2,3,*]

1 School of Pharmacy, University of Nottingham, University Park, Nottingham NG7 2RD, UK
2 Department of Pharmaceutics and Food Technology, School of Pharmacy, Complutense University, 28040 Madrid, Spain
3 Institute of Industrial Pharmacy, Complutense University, 28040 Madrid, Spain
* Correspondence: raquel.fernandezgarcia@nottingham.ac.uk (R.F.-G.); aifraguas@ucm.es (A.I.F.-S.)

Abstract: The pulmonary route for drug administration has garnered a great deal of attention in therapeutics for treating respiratory disorders. It allows for the delivery of drugs directly to the lungs and, consequently, the maintenance of high concentrations at the action site and a reduction in systemic adverse effects compared to other routes, such as oral or intravenous. Nevertheless, the pulmonary administration of drugs is challenging, as the respiratory system tries to eliminate inhaled particles, being the main responsible mucociliary escalator. Nanomedicines represent a primary strategy to overcome the limitations of this route as they can be engineered to prolong pulmonary retention and avoid their clearance while reducing drug systemic distribution and, consequently, systemic adverse effects. This review analyses the use of pulmonary-administered nanomedicines to treat infectious diseases affecting the respiratory system and lung carcinoma, two pathologies that represent major health threats.

Keywords: pulmonary delivery; nanomedicine; infectious diseases; tuberculosis; cancer; dry powder inhalers; inhalable nanoparticles

1. Introduction

The pulmonary route for drug administration has garnered a great deal of attention in therapeutics for both local drug action and systemic effect. This route is considered non-invasive, making its administration more comfortable for patients and improving treatment adherence [1–3]. On the one hand, the pulmonary route allows for the delivery of drugs directly to the lungs and, consequently, the maintenance of high concentrations at the action site and a reduction in systemic adverse effects compared to other routes, such as oral or intravenous. This is the preferred route for treating respiratory diseases such as asthma, chronic obstructive pulmonary disease (COPD), and idiopathic pulmonary fibrosis. In recent years, there has also been an increased interest in treating other pathologies affecting the respiratory system, such as pulmonary infections or lung carcinomas [4–6]. On the other hand, this route is also useful for systemic effects. The lungs have a large surface area (in the range of 70–140 m^2 in adult humans) and a high vascularisation, which provides fast absorption and availability in the bloodstream and allows for a rapid onset of action. Moreover, it has a minimal metabolism compared with oral and other administration routes as it bypasses the hepatic first-pass effect [7,8].

Nevertheless, the pulmonary administration of drugs is challenging. The respiratory system tries to maintain exogenous substances out of the lungs, removing or inactivating therapeutics after deposition. The conducting airways of the lungs are mainly layered by the mucociliary escalator, consisting of cilia embedded in a mucous layer [9–11]. The mucus is mainly secreted by goblet cells and consists of mucin, which is the principal structural and functional constituent, other smaller proteins, salt, and water [12,13]. The mucociliary escalator is one of the most important mechanisms responsible for removing inhaled substances. Mucins are glycoproteins with a high molecular weight crosslinked with cysteine residues [14]. They create a physical barrier that captures inhaled particles that are then removed by cilia and expelled from the respiratory system (Figure 1). The clearance of these particles occurs within 15 min to 2 h after inhalation, showing in healthy adults a mucociliary clearance in the range of 4–20 mm/min [15].

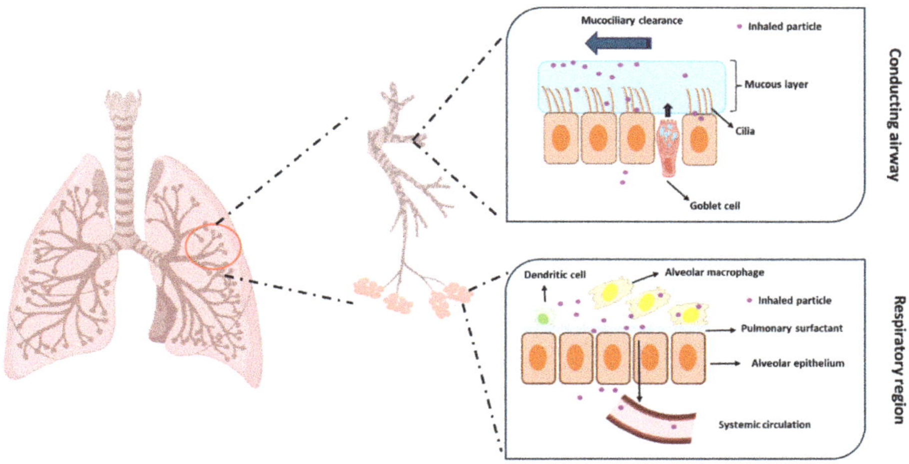

Figure 1. Schematic representation of the clearance of inhaled particles by the mucociliary escalator.

The immune system of the respiratory tract also plays an essential role in host defence and the removal of foreign particles. Alveolar macrophages are the most abundant cell type, accounting for more than 90% of the cells of this immune system. Inhaled foreign particles can be internalised by alveolar macrophages, transported to phagosomes, and degraded [16,17]. It should be mentioned that the alveolar space is covered by a layer of pulmonary surfactant comprising lipids and proteins that can interact with inhaled particles and facilitate their internalisation by alveolar macrophages and, consequently, their elimination [18].

Diverse physicochemical properties of the inhaled particles, such as particle size, surface charge and hygroscopicity, among others, condition the clearance and, consequently, the efficacy of this route [19]. It has been reported that particles above 1000 nm are easily entrapped in the mucous layer [11]. Particles with a positive surface charge are also quickly immobilised as mucus is negatively charged [20]. In this context, nanomedicines represent a promising strategy to overcome the limitations of the pulmonary route and improve its efficacy. Nanomedicines can be engineered to prolong pulmonary retention and avoid their clearance. They represent an excellent tool to improve the stability of drugs, protecting them from degradation (this is of particular interest for the delivery of proteins or nucleic acids); to release the drugs gradually, offering sustained therapeutic levels and reducing the frequency of administration; to access deeper regions of the respiratory system, as, due to their small particle size, they can penetrate deeper into the lungs; and to deliver drugs to specific cells of regions within the lung, among other advantages (Figure 2). Moreover, nanomedicines can be administered using inhalers and nebulisers [21–23]. This review analyses the use of pulmonary-administered nanomedicines to treat infectious diseases affecting the respiratory system and lung carcinoma. These are disorders where nanomedicines and the pulmonary route show a high utility.

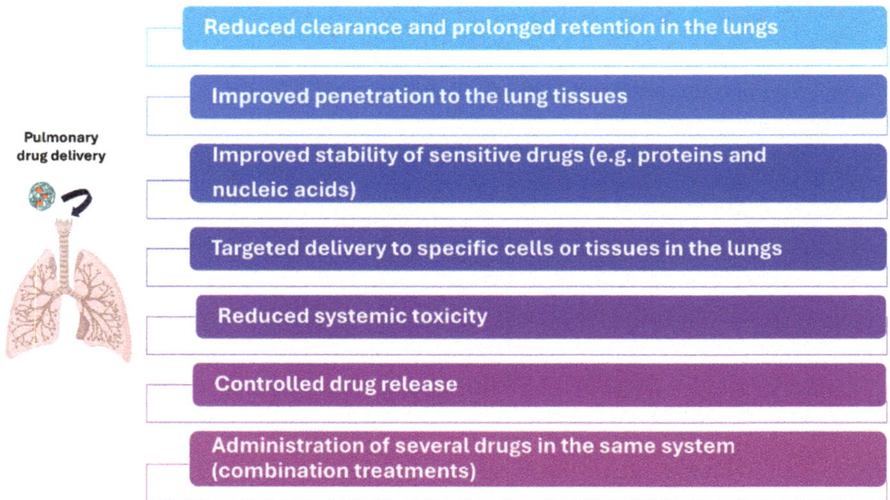

Figure 2. Advantages of nanomedicines over conventional formulations for pulmonary drug delivery.

2. Nanomedicine in Pulmonary Drug Delivery

2.1. Types of Nanocarriers

Nanotechnology represents an excellent strategy for improving the efficacy and decreasing the toxicity of antimicrobials and antineoplastics [24–26]. Nanomedicines are also useful for overcoming the resistances developed by microorganisms and tumoral cells. These systems can evade efflux pumps, which actively expel conventional drugs from cells, reducing their effectiveness. Moreover, nanoparticles protect against enzymatic degradation, which can deactivate drugs. This latter mechanism is particularly important in microorganisms [27,28]. Nevertheless, it should be mentioned that pathogens, and cancer cells, can develop resistances to nanomedicines. For example, it has been demonstrated that bacteria induce the production of proteins like flagellin that trigger particle aggregation and make their internalisation difficult [29].

In general, nanoparticles can be divided into organic (including lipid, polymeric, and protein nanocarriers) and inorganic nanocarriers [30]. Among lipid nanocarriers, liposomes are particularly noteworthy [31]. They are spherical lipid nanovesicles consisting of an aqueous inner core surrounded by one or more bilayers of phospholipids. They are considered the most exploited nanocarrier for the delivery of both hydrophobic and hydrophilic molecules [32,33] due to several factors, including their high biocompatibility and easier manufacturing process at the industrial level compared to other types of nanomedicines [34,35] (Figure 3). Several liposomal formulations are currently approved for the delivery of antifungals (e.g., AmBisome® or Arikayce®) and antineoplastics (e.g., Doxil®, Depocyt®, Mepact® or Lipusu®), among other therapeutics [36]. Similarly to liposomes, niosomes have demonstrated a potential utility in drug delivery. They are self-assembled nanovesicles with an inner aqueous phase surrounded by a lipid bilayer composed of non-ionic surfactants, often combined with cholesterol [37,38]. Apart from liposome-type systems, solid lipid nanoparticles have also emerged as promising lipid drug delivery systems in the last decade due to their high biocompatibility, low toxicity, and industrially scalable manufacturing [39,40] (Figure 3). They are particularly interesting for the delivery of nucleic acids [41].

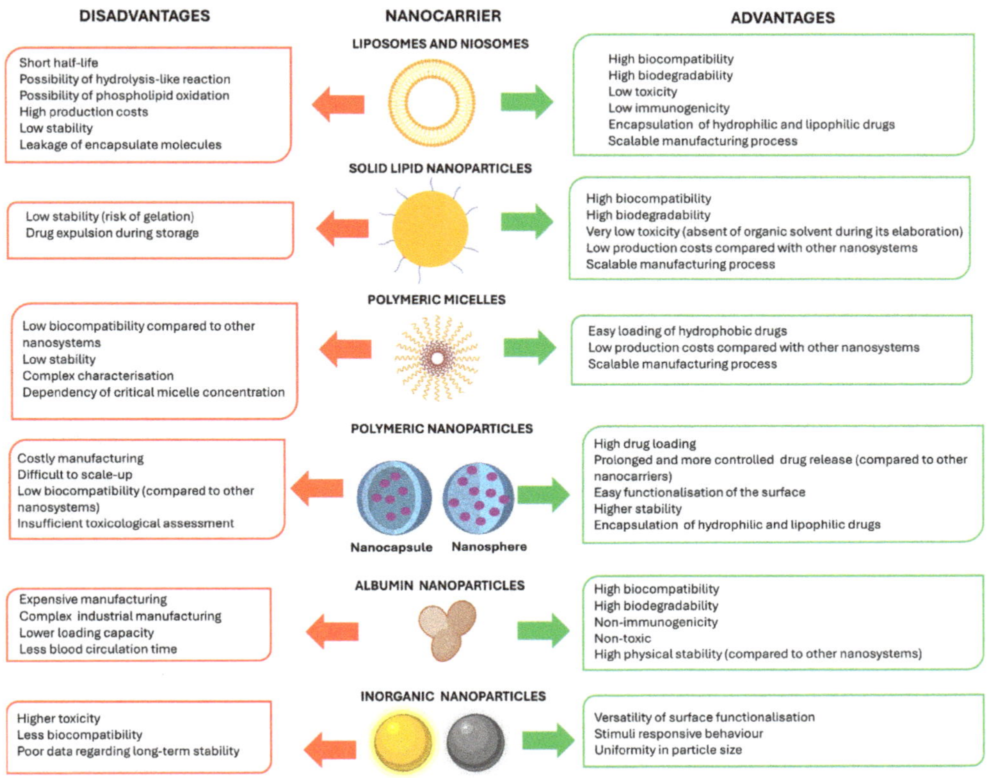

Figure 3. Advantages and disadvantages of each type of nanocarrier.

Polymeric nanocarriers are also valuable systems. Micelles are self-assembled nanoparticles of amphiphilic polymers with a hydrophobic core and a hydrophilic corona that have been widely investigated for the delivery of antineoplastics [42,43], with several formulations approved in the market (e.g., Genexol® or Paclical®, both encapsulating paclitaxel) [44,45]. Polymeric nanoparticles offer different advantages, such as controlled drug release over extended periods, high versatility due to easily modifiable surfaces for controlling drug biodistribution, and superior drug encapsulation efficiency compared to other systems (Figure 3). They can be divided into nanocapsules (reservoir-type system), consisting of an inner core where the drug is usually dissolved surrounded by the polymeric layer, and nanospheres (matrix type system) composed of a continuous polymeric network in which the drug is entrapped. The latter are more commonly developed systems [46,47].

Albumin is a water-soluble globular protein that can bind many drugs by either covalent or non-covalent linkage, becoming an attractive carrier for drug delivery. It is a biocompatible, safe, and non-antigenic carrier, and albumin nanoparticles can be developed at the industrial level [48,49] (Figure 3). They are particularly interesting for administering antineoplastics as they tend to accumulate in the tumour area. Albumin nanoparticles bind to glycoprotein 60 receptors expressed on vascular endothelial cells of the tumours. Through these receptors, albumin nanoparticles are internalised to the tumour interstitium, where they bind to secreted acidic proteins rich in cysteine (SPARC) that are overexpressed in many tumours, such as lung, breast, and pancreatic carcinomas [50,51]. Abraxane® and Fyaro® are two formulations of albumin nanoparticles encapsulating paclitaxel and sirolimus, respectively, currently approved for treating several carcinomas [52].

Finally, inorganic nanoparticles such as gold nanoparticles, iron oxide nanoparticles and mesoporous silica nanoparticles have also emerged as promising nanoplatforms. They have shown great potential in diagnosis (with some formulations approved in the market for this purpose) and in drug delivery. Compared to organic nanosystems, inorganic nanoparticles exhibited a higher stability and ease surface of functionalisation, but a lower biodegradability and biocompatibility [53–55] (Figure 3).

2.2. *Impact of Physicochemical Properties of Nanoparticles on Pulmonary Drug Delivery*

Despite the considerable potential of the pulmonary administration route for treating respiratory diseases, the effective delivery of drugs by this route is challenged. Maintaining an aerodynamic particle size below 5 μm is essential for particles to effectively reach the mid and deep lung parenchyma. In this context, the use of nanocarriers is more than worthwhile. However, it should also be considered that particles smaller than 0.5 μm are usually prone to rapid exhalation [56], and consequently, developing pulmonary administered nanoformulations that can avoid rapid lung clearance is not easy. Particle size, particle morphology, surface charge, and hydrophobicity are critical parameters affecting the fate of pulmonary administered nanoparticles (Figure 4).

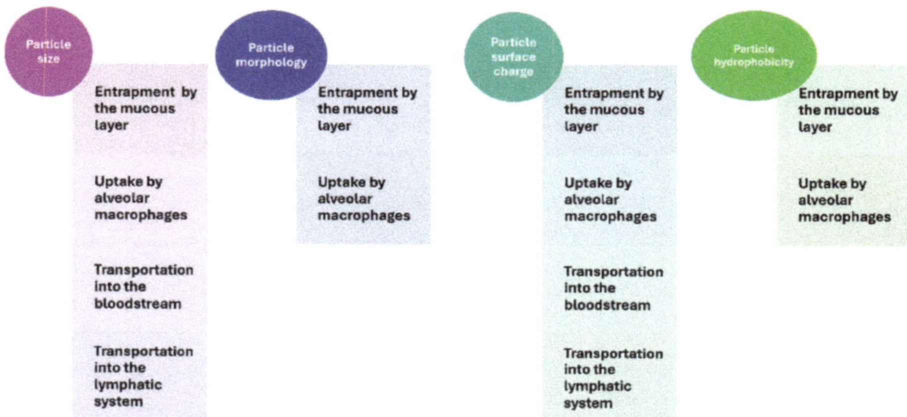

Figure 4. Impact of physicochemical properties of nanoparticles on pulmonary drug delivery.

To optimise pulmonary drug delivery, innovative nanocarrier strategies, specifically 'Trojan Horse microparticles' or nano-in-microparticle, drug delivery systems have been developed. These advanced systems ingeniously integrate porous nanoparticles within microparticulate structures, typically ranging from 2 to 5 μm in diameter. By combining the targeted drug delivery capabilities of nanoparticles with the superior aerodynamic properties of microparticles, these hybrid systems offer a sophisticated approach to improving therapeutic effectiveness. The fabrication of these systems has been successfully achieved using different strategies, including the spray drying of supercritical CO_2 [56].

2.2.1. Influence of Particle Size

As aforementioned, the mucous layer of conducting airways offers a physical barrier that entraps inhaled particles as mucin glycoproteins create a crosslinked network acting like a filter. It has been reported that the upper airway region filters around 90% of inhaled particles [57]. Aerodynamic particle size is a critical parameter determining the retention of nanoparticles in the mucous layer and their mucociliary clearance. The larger the particle size, the higher the retention in the mucous layer. Schuster and collaborators demonstrated that polystyrene nanoparticles coated with polyethylene glycol (PEG) of 100 and 200 nm were not retained in the mucus. In comparison, particles of around 500 nm could not penetrate this layer efficiently, being entrapped [58]. Similar results were also found by Schenieider et al., who also reported that at least 70% of the administered dose of PEG-coated-polystyrene nanoparticles with a particle size around 300 nm were retained in the lung parenchyma 2 h after the administration [59]. The remaining 30% of the dose was removed from the respiratory tract. Finally, almost 90% of the administered 200 nm gold nanoparticles remain in the lung 2 h after their pulmonary administration [60].

Alveolar macrophages also play a significant role in the clearance of inhaled particles, phagocyting and degrading them, and particle size strongly influences macrophage phagocytosis. Macrophage uptake increases as particle size increases. Nanoparticles usually escape from alveolar macrophages due to their small particle size. Nevertheless, Chono and coworkers demonstrated that particle size was an influencing factor for liposome uptake. The phagocytosis of liposomal particles of 400 nm was two-fold higher than the uptake of liposomes of 100 nm [61].

Another aspect to be considered after the pulmonary administration of nanomedicines for treating respiratory disorders is the possible translocation of nanoparticles from the lungs into the circulatory or lymphatic systems. Very low amounts of intact nanoparticles can generally access the bloodstream or extrapulmonary organs after their pulmonary administration. However, some authors have reported this fact. For example, the capacity of PEG-poly(lactic-co-glycolic) acid (PLGA) micelles with a small particle size of around 28 nm to access the brain when administered intratracheally has been demonstrated in rats [62]. Kreling and collaborators demonstrated that particle size is a critical factor affecting nanoparticle transportation to the bloodstream. The translocation of 15 nm iridium nanoparticles was 1.5-fold higher than the transportation of 80 nm nanoparticles [63]. However, the amount of gold nanoparticles with a particle size of 20 and 200 nm was similar [60]. This suggests the influence of other properties of the formulations.

Smaller nanoparticles are generally more easily transported to the lymphatic system by both cellular and non-cellular pathways. Choi et al. found that polystyrene nanoparticles with a particle size below 34 nm were rapidly transported from the alveolar luminal surface into the septal interstitium and then to the regional lymph nodes [64]. Similar results were also reported by Mohammad et al., who demonstrated that polystyrene nanoparticles of 50 nm had a higher overall lymph deposition ($\approx$21%) compared to 100 and 250 nm nanoparticles ($\approx$15 and 12.5%) 5 h after their administration [65].

Therefore, particle size is a critical parameter that conditions the efficacy of pulmonary-administered nanomedicines, as it influences their ability to access the mid-deep parenchyma and their ability to be retained in this region. Nanomedicines must be small enough to pass through the mucous layer of the respiratory conducting airways, penetrate the lung parenchyma, and avoid phagocytosis by the alveolar macrophages, but large enough to avoid rapid exhalation and translocation to the lymphatic and circulatory systems.

2.2.2. Influence of Particle Morphology

Particle shape may also affect the fate of pulmonary administered nanoparticles, as it influences the uptake of alveolar macrophages. In general, it has been reported that this uptake is superior in spherical particles [66]. This aspect has been widely investigated and demonstrated in pulmonary administered microparticles [67,68], but less researched in nanoparticles. Several researchers have demonstrated that non-spherical (rod-shaped or pollen-shaped) microparticles show better flowability, aerosolisation, and deposition properties than spherical microparticles [68,69]. In this context, shifting from spherical to non-spherical nanoparticles may be a good technological strategy to decrease the macrophage clearance of inhaled particles.

2.2.3. Influence of the Surface Charge

The surface charge of nanoparticles is another crucial factor that conditions the efficacy of pulmonary-administered nanoparticles. As aforementioned, the mucous layer is negatively charged due to the carboxyl and sulphate groups of the oligosaccharide chains [20], and positively charged nanoparticles are entrapped in this layer through electrostatic interactions, which may hinder their diffusion through the mucous layer and penetration to the lung parenchyma [70]. By contrast, neutral and negatively charged nanoparticles penetrate the mucous layer easily [11,71]. Dawson and collaborators found that neutral-charged polystyrene nanoparticles showed the highest mucus permeability [72]. In this context, coating nanoparticles with compounds that provide a neutral charge could be a good strategy to facilitate mucus penetration. For example, the coating of nanoparticles with dense PEG can bring the surface of the charge to neutral [68] and improve mucus penetration. Polystyrene nanoparticles coated with PEG exhibited superior mucus penetration. This penetration was 15- and 35-fold higher in 100 nm and 200 nm nanoparticles, respectively, compared to non-pegylated nanoparticles [58]. As positively charged inhaled nanoparticles are retained in the mucus, their mucociliary clearance is lower compared to non-positive nanoparticles. This could be useful when it is required to increase retention in the respiratory system.

The surface charge of nanoparticles is also crucial for macrophage phagocytosis. It has been reported that positively charged nanoparticles are generally more easily phagocyted by macrophages due to their interaction with the negatively charged sialic acid of these cells [11]. Seydoux and collaborators reported that phagocytosis by alveolar macrophages of positively charged-polyvinyl alcohol (PVA)-gold nanoparticles was higher than negatively charged-PVA-gold particles [73]. Similar results were found in negatively and positively charged PLGA nanoparticles [74].

As positively charged nanoparticles tend to be retained in the mucous layer, the possibility of their translocation to the bloodstream is extremely low compared to negatively charged formulations. Kreyling et al. showed that around 5% of positively charged gold nanoparticles ($\approx$3 nm) were detected in extrapulmonary organs 24 h after their intratracheal instillation, while negatively charged nanoparticles showed significantly lower translocation percentages ($\approx$1%) [75]. Similar results were found in metallic oxide nanoparticles with negative and positive surface charges [76].

Surface charge can also influence the translocation of nanoparticles to the lymphatic system. Choi and collaborators demonstrated that it is critical in lymph translocation via the non-cellular pathway in particles below 34 nm. In this case, nanoparticles with a neutral or negative surface charge rapidly translocated from the lung to the mediastinal lymph nodes, while in positive nanoparticles, this translocation was inhibited [64]. The surface charge of nanoparticles did not seem to influence nanoparticles translocated via cellular pathways [77].

Therefore, the surface charge of nanoparticles is another key factor influencing the fate of pulmonary administered nanoparticles. Neutral and negatively charged nanoparticles show a lower interaction with the mucous layer and a higher penetration than positive nanoparticles, especially net-neutral formulation. Non-positive nanoparticles also demonstrated a lower uptake by alveolar macrophages and a lower translocation from the lungs to the blood circulation.

2.2.4. Influence of Surface Hydrophobicity

The surface hydrophobicity of the nanoparticles is another factor influencing the penetration of particles through the mucous layer. Large amounts of lipids can be absorbed or bound to the mucous, specifically to the mucin network of non-PTS (proline, threonine, and serine) regions. These lipids can interact with hydrophobic nanoparticles, favouring their retention. Hydrophilic nanoparticles can penetrate the mucous layer better, accessing the lung parenchyma. This also explains why coating the surface of the nanoparticles with PEG (a hydrophilic polymer) is a good strategy to improve their penetration [78]. However, not all PEG polymers are helpful for promoting penetration through the mucous layer. Wang and collaborators reported that the chain of PEG with high molecular weight can entangle with mucins and hamper nanoparticle penetration. However, low-molecular-weight PEG polymers avoid this problem [79]. In general, PEG polymers with a molecular weight in the range of 2 to 5 kDa are adequate to improve the penetration of inhaled nanoparticles through the mucous layer of conducting airways [80].

Incorporating PEG and other hydrophilic polymers on the surface of the particles also decreases their macrophage-mediated phagocytosis. For example, Murata and collaborators reported that incorporating PVA (PVA also provides a hydrophilic surface) to the surface of liposomes also decreases recognition and uptake by alveolar macrophages [81].

2.3. *Impact of Patient-Specific Factors*

Another key point to consider in the design of pulmonary administration medications is that respiratory function, as well as the mechanisms (e.g., mucociliary escalator, alveolar macrophage phagocytosis, and lung surfactant interaction) involved in the removal of inhaled particles, vary significantly across different patients, such as smokers or individuals with chronic lung diseases, affecting the success of inhaled therapies.

2.3.1. Smoking

Smoking significantly alters the respiratory system of patients, which in turn affects the outcome of inhaled medications [82]. One of the main consequences is a reduction in lung capacity and ventilation, which reduces the ability of the patient to inhale deeply. As a result, lower doses reach the lungs and the efficacy is reduced. Moreover, smoking leads to changes in the mucociliary escalator. Smoking reduces ciliary function and produces an exacerbation of mucus production [83]. The excess of mucus can retain more nanoparticles and hinder their diffusion to the lungs, decreasing their efficacy. Moreover, microorganisms can also be retained, increasing the risk of developing infections.

2.3.2. Chronic Obstructive Pulmonary Disease

Chronic Obstructive Pulmonary Disease (COPD) is characterised by a progressive reduction in lung function due to persistent airflow obstruction [84], which can influences the outcome of inhaled medications, including nanomedicines. In these patients, the secretion of mucus is exacerbated, producing a more viscous and harder-to-clear mucous layer that retains inhaled particles [85]. Moreover, the chronic inflammation of COPD increases the activity of alveolar macrophages, which can trigger an enhanced phagocytosis and reduces the dose that reaches the lungs.

2.3.3. Cystic Fibrosis

In patients with cystic fibrosis, a similar situation occurs. This disease also involves a chronic inflammation of the conducting airways, a decline in lung function and an excessive production of sticky mucus. Patients with cystic fibrosis experience multiple bacterial infections, and inhaled antibiotics represent a good treatment approach [86], including the administration of nanomedicines. However, it should be considered that this mucus is not only more viscous, but also enriched with DNA, proteins, and cellular debris, and creates a dense barrier that significantly hinders the penetration and distribution of nanoparticles to deeper areas of the respiratory system.

2.3.4. Asthma

Asthma is a prevalent condition characterised by the intermittent and reversible obstruction of respiratory airways, heightened sensitivity, and chronic inflammation of the respiratory system [87]. The pulmonary administration route is widely used for the treatment of asthma, providing effective and rapid relief by delivering therapeutic agents directly to the lungs. However, it is important to consider that the pathological damage associated with asthma, particularly chronic inflammation, can influence the accessibility and efficacy of inhaled formulations. Persistent airway inflammation leads to a thickening of the airway walls, increased mucus production, and altered epithelial permeability that may hinder the access of nanoparticles.

2.3.5. Lung Cancer

Inhaled nanomedicine holds significant potential for the delivery of anticancer drugs in lung cancer. However, this pathology induces changes in the respiratory system that can affect the efficacy of inhaled nanoformulations [88]. Firstly, the lung capacity of these patients may be reduced, which impacts the effectiveness of this therapy, as proper inhalation technique and adequate pulmonary function are essential. Moreover, tumours often induce chronic inflammation, leading to increased mucus production that retains nanoparticles and hinders their access to cancer cells.

3. Pulmonary-Administered Nanomedicines to Combat Respiratory Tract Infections

A wide variety of bacteria, viruses, and fungi are the causative agents of respiratory infections. Respiratory tract infections occur in both the upper and lower regions of the respiratory system [89]. Upper respiratory tract infections are usually defined as self-limited irritation and inflammation of the upper conducting airways without evidence of pneumonia, and their complications are rare [90]. Nevertheless, lower respiratory infections are usually more severe and difficult to handle [91,92].

Lower respiratory infections are a major health problem. According to the World Health Organization (WHO), they represented the fifth leading cause of death globally in 2021 and the first cause in low-income countries. There are countless therapeutic options for their treatment, and in clinical practice, an empirical regimen of oral or parenteral antimicrobials is followed [93]. Nevertheless, systemic side effects and drug resistance remain considerable limitations in treating respiratory infections [94]. The administration of antimicrobials by the pulmonary route can overcome these challenges. Compared to oral or parenteral routes, pulmonary administration delivers drugs directly into the lungs, allowing for high therapeutic concentrations at the action site with lower doses and reducing the systemic exposure of antimicrobials and, consequently, systemic adverse effects [21,95]. In fact, due to the advantages of the pulmonary route in clinical practice, some intravenous formulations are repurposed for nebulisation [96]. Table 1 displays the available pulmonary formulations for treating bacterial and fungal infections.

Table 1. Inhaled formulations available for treating pulmonary infections.

Formulation	Drug	Pharmaceutical Dosage Form	Indication
Tobi® *	Tobramycin	Solution for inhalation	Cystic fibrosis patients infected with *Pseudomonas aeruginosa*
Betkis® *	Tobramycin	Solution for inhalation	Cystic fibrosis patients infected with *P. aeruginosa*
Cayston® *	Aztreonam	Solution for inhalation	Cystic fibrosis patients infected with *P. aeruginosa*
Tobi® Podhaler *	Tobramycin	Dry powder inhaler	Cystic fibrosis patients infected with *P. aeruginosa*
Kitabis® Pak *	Tobramycin	Solution for inhalation	Cystic fibrosis patients infected with *P. aeruginosa*
Arikayce® *	Amikacin	Liposomal inhalation suspension	Nontuberculous mycobacterial lung disease
Opelconazole	Opelconazole	Dry powder inhaler	Aspergillosis
PUR1900	Itraconazole	Dry powder inhaler	Fungal pulmonary infections
Voriconazole	Voriconazole	Dry powder inhaler	Fungal pulmonary infections
Apulmiq	Ciprofloxacin	Liposomal inhalation suspension	Chronic lung infections with *P. aeruginosa*
MRT5005	Ciprofloxacin	Lipid nanoparticles	Cystic fibrosis

* Approved formulations.

Nevertheless, pulmonary drug delivery is challenging. Using nanocarriers may overcome the limitations of this route [97]. Moreover, nanoparticles can be engineered to overcome drug resistance. In fact, a liposomal formulation of amikacin for pulmonary administration (Arikayce®) is currently approved for treating nontuberculous mycobacterial lung disease in adults (Table 1) [98,99].

3.1. Bacterial Infections

Bacteria are the dominant causative agents of pulmonary infectious diseases [100]. They usually occur as a consequence of another respiratory condition, including viral infections, COPD, and cystic fibrosis [93]. These infections might be caused by different types of bacteria, including *Streptococcus pneumoniae*, *Legionella pneumophila*, *Mycoplasma pneumoniae*, *Chlamydia pneumoniae*, *Haemophilus influenzae*, and *Mycobacterium tuberculosis* [101]. Table 2 shows a summary of novel nanotechnology-based antibacterial therapy approaches.

3.1.1. Tuberculosis

M. tuberculosis is the causative agent of tuberculosis (TB) [102]. While it is a preventable and treatable condition, TB continues to pose a significant global health challenge [103]. Each year, over 10 million individuals are diagnosed with the disease, predominantly in low-income nations [104]. Despite a substantial decline in TB-related mortality over the past three decades, it remains one of the leading causes of death worldwide, accounting for 1.6 million fatalities in 2021 [105,106].

The pharmacotherapy of TB has faced challenges due to the absence of an optimal treatment with favourable safety and pharmacokinetic profiles, despite the availability of these drugs for nearly 80 years. Additionally, drug-resistant TB is a major complication, contributing to over 10% of TB-related deaths [107,108]. The four cornerstone drugs used in anti-TB treatment (rifampicin, isoniazid, pyrazinamide, and ethambutol) exhibit diverse mechanisms of action and are administered in combination to prevent the development of resistance [109,110]. Alternative antibiotics, such as ciprofloxacin, levofloxacin, rifabutin, and linezolid can be employed as second- and third-line treatments [111].

Although TB primarily affects the lungs, current therapeutic options predominantly involve the systemic oral administration of antibiotics. This method may be nonspecific, potentially targeting other tissues and causing toxicity while also achieving inadequate drug concentrations in the lung [93]. Such issues can promote the emergence of resistance. Furthermore, TB treatment regimens are lengthy, typically lasting 6 to 9 months [112], which can lead to poor patient adherence, premature treatment discontinuation, relapse, and resistance development [95]. It is also important to note that *M. tuberculosis* is particularly challenging to eradicate. Alveolar macrophages play a crucial role as the first line of defence in the innate immune response against pulmonary infections; they phagocytise and destroy inhaled pathogens. However, *M. tuberculosis* evades macrophage responses by inhibiting phagosome maturation and preventing lysosome fusion, thereby transforming the hostile macrophage environment into one conducive to its survival and replication [113,114].

In this context, there is an urgent need for novel anti-TB therapies that enhance the tolerability and biodistribution of antimicrobials, promote efficacy with lower doses, increase patient adherence by shortening treatment durations, and reduce resistance emergence. The pulmonary route has yet to be fully utilised in clinical anti-TB therapies, but it offers potential advantages over systemic drugs, such as minimising systemic side effects and toxicity while achieving therapeutic concentrations at the target site with lower doses [115]. Nanomedicine has emerged as a promising approach for TB treatment, as it can be engineered to specifically target infected macrophages [116,117].

Various nanomedicine formulations have been developed to encapsulate anti-TB drugs, including liposomes, nanoparticles, polymeric micelles, and niosomes (Table 2) [107]. For instance, Ma et al. created mannose-modified solid lipid nanoparticles carrying a pH-sensitive isoniazid prodrug for pulmonary administration. The surface modification enhanced macrophage uptake significantly, achieving 97.2% compared to 42.4% for unmodified nanoparticles [118]. Viswanathan et al. developed inhalable liposomes containing liquorice extract, intended as a potential standalone treatment for TB or as an adjuvant to existing therapies. Their in vitro studies indicated favourable flow properties for inhalation, while in vivo studies showed that 46% of the administered drug reached the lungs, with 16% retained 24 h post-administration [119]. Silva et al. explored the use of antimicrobial peptides (AMPs), specifically LLKKK18, which has demonstrated effectiveness against *M. tuberculosis* and *Mycobacterium avium*. This AMP was encapsulated in self-assembling hyaluronic acid nanogels, enhancing stability, reducing cytotoxicity, and improving targeting to infection sites. In vivo studies indicated significantly reduced infection levels after just five doses [120]. Wu et al. introduced lung-targeted nanogel particles composed of genipin-crosslinked deacetylated chitosan loaded with isoniazid and rifampicin. These particles exhibited extended antibacterial activity due to sustained drug release, with a single pulmonary dose maintaining therapeutic concentrations of 40–60% in the lungs for 24 h while keeping levels in other organs below 5% [121]. Lastly, Scolari et al. designed nanoparticles made of sodium alginate coated with chitosan and Tween® 80, encapsulating rifampicin and ascorbic acid, utilising a design-of-experiments approach to optimise the formulation. The addition of ascorbic acid, shown to enhance the efficacy of anti-TB drugs like isoniazid and rifampicin [122], resulted in improved activity against nine clinical strains of *M. tuberculosis*. The formulation also included sucrose or mannitol to facilitate easy redispersion and prevent particle aggregation during lyophilisation [123].

3.1.2. Bacterial Pneumonia

Beyond TB, lower respiratory tract infections caused by other bacterial pathogens are also a significant issue, particularly in developing countries, which account for over 95% of global cases. It is estimated that around 4 million deaths occur annually due to these infections [124]. Bacterial pneumonia can be categorised into community-acquired pneumonia, primarily caused by *S. pneumoniae*, *M. pneumoniae*, *H. influenzae*, *C. pneumoniae*, and *L. pneumophila* (listed in order of frequency), and hospital-acquired pneumonia, which has a high mortality rate and is mainly associated with *Pseudomonas aeruginosa*, *Enterobacteriaceae*, and *Staphylococcus aureus* [125,126].

Timely administration of antibiotics is crucial to alleviate symptoms and reduced mortality associated with bacterial pneumonia. The choice of antibiotic depends on the causative agents and the severity of the illness. Commonly used classes of antibiotics include macrolides, doxycycline, β-lactams, aminoglycosides, fluoroquinolones, and carbapenems. In cases where the causative agent cannot be identified, empirical treatment with broad-spectrum antibiotics may be necessary, which can contribute to the development of resistant bacterial strains [95].

Inhaled therapies have also shown promise in treating bacterial pneumonia, and several nanoformulations for pulmonary drug delivery have been developed. For example, Arikayce® is a liposomal formulation of amikacin approved for treating lung infections caused by the *M. avium* complex (Table 1). However, it is important to note that the excessive mucus production and inflammatory response in pneumonia patients can hinder the effectiveness of inhaled therapies [70].

Additionally, there are ongoing studies investigating nanomedicine-based treatments for the pulmonary administration of other bacterial infections (Table 2). One approach involves developing poly(2-ethyl-2-oxazoline) (PEtOx) nanoparticles designed to encapsulate ciprofloxacin, enhancing in vivo solubility and optimising lung delivery. These nanoparticles demonstrated sustained release for up to 7 days, indicating their potential as an alternative therapeutic option for lower respiratory tract infections [127]. AMPs have also gained attention as alternatives to traditional antibiotics for pulmonary infections [93]. One specific AMP, SET-M33, was incorporated into dextran-based nanoparticles targeting *P. aeruginosa* infections, resulting in significantly prolonged lung residence time (approximately 12-fold greater than the free peptide) while maintaining acceptable toxicity levels. This was achieved through non-covalent interactions under suitable pH conditions [128].

Derbali et al. compared poly(lactic) (PLA)-grafted-PEG nanoparticles with anionic and cationic liposomes to encapsulate levofloxacin, ultimately identifying anionic liposomes as the most promising formulation. These anionic liposomes exhibited a sustained release of levofloxacin over 72 h while preserving antibacterial activity against five strains of *P. aeruginosa*. Notably, despite their negative charge, the liposomes effectively interacted with *P. aeruginosa* membranes in a dose-dependent manner, demonstrating a favourable safety profile on A549 epithelial cells, even at high concentrations [129]. Another study investigated a liposomal formulation combining levofloxacin and lysozyme formulation for pulmonary delivery. This formulation was developed using a pH gradient method and spray dried with a lysozyme-containing solution. Efficacy against *S. aureus* was tested in rats, where the liposomes containing both levofloxacin and lysozyme significantly reduced microbial burden in the lungs, bronchoalveolar lavage fluid, and nasal fluid, with acute toxicity studies confirming the safety of the formulation [130]. Lastly, an innovative approach utilised liposomes containing colistin for treating *P. aeruginosa* infections. These liposomes were designed with sodium cholesteryl sulphate to enhance electrostatic interactions between the drug and lipids. In vivo studies demonstrated prolonged retention of colistin in the lungs while minimising transfer to the bloodstream and kidneys, leading to improved therapeutic efficacy in a murine model of pulmonary *P. aeruginosa* infection [131].

3.2. Fungal Infections

Respiratory fungal infections, similar to bacterial lung infections, pose a serious global health threat, causing approximately 1.5 million deaths annually [132]. Over recent decades, the incidence of these infections has risen, likely due to the growing population of immune-compromised individuals, resulting from factors such as organ transplants, cancer treatments, autoimmune diseases, acquired immunodeficiency syndrome (AIDS), and corticosteroid therapies, among others [133]. The primary pathogens behind fungal lung infections include *Aspergillus*, *Cryptococcus*, *Pneumocystis*, and *Candida albicans*, which account for over 90% of fungal infection-related deaths. Treatment strategies typically involve either oral or parenteral administration of broad-spectrum azoles (e.g., voriconazole or posaconazole) or the parenteral administration of amphotericin B or echinocandins (e.g., anidulafungin or caspofungin) [134,135]. Although amphotericin B is a key treatment for fungal infections, its parenteral application is often problematic for lung infections due to severe side effects, including kidney and liver toxicity [136,137]. Pulmonary drug delivery offers a promising alternative by reducing systemic exposure and toxicity. In some cases, intravenous formulations of antifungal are adapted for inhalation to take advantage of the localised effects of pulmonary delivery [96].

Nanotechnology has recently been explored to enhance the treatment of respiratory fungal infections through pulmonary delivery systems. Table 3 provides an overview of recent nanotechnology-based approaches. A novel approach by Kaur et al. involved using chitosan nanoparticles loaded with voriconazole, which were aerosolised into microdroplets for pulmonary administration. These nanoparticles showed effectiveness against *Aspergillus* species and improved lung retention in pharmacokinetic studies [138]. Another study by Ali et al. evaluated silver nanoparticles with *Artemisia sieberi* leaf extract in a mouse model of invasive pulmonary aspergillosis (IPA), which significantly reduced lung tissue damage by inhibiting fungal growth and biofilm formation, while also increasing antioxidant enzyme activity [139].

Further advancements include the development of a pulmonary dapsone delivery system to prevent *Pneumocystis carinii* pneumonia in immunocompromised patients. Dapsone was encapsulated in liposomes and formulated into a dry powder inhaler (DPI) with hydrolysed gelatin-based carriers for sustained release up to 16 h, following Higuchi's release model [140]. Chitosan-stearic acid nanomicelles encapsulating amphotericin B have also been developed, showing enhanced antifungal activity and stability post-nebulisation [141]. Additionally, Nasr et al. reported that nebulised nanoemulsions successfully delivered amphotericin B to the peripheral respiratory airways. Formulations prepared with Clinoleic®

(an emulsion elaborated with olive oil, sodium oleate, egg phospholipids, soybean oil, and glycerol) showed a better performance than nanoemulsions based on Intralipid® (fat emulsion prepared from egg phospholipids, soybean oil, and glycerol) with deposition percentages of around 80 and 57%, respectively [142]. Another study utilised ligand-coated liposomal aerosols with alveolar macrophage-targeting ligands for amphotericin B, which demonstrated efficient lung accumulation and prolonged retention in macrophages [143]. Finally, nanostructured aggregates containing mannitol and lecithin were created using ultra-rapid freezing for itraconazole delivery. This formulation displayed favourable aerodynamic properties, reaching the deepest lung regions and achieving systemic levels in mice [144].

Table 2. Novel formulations to treat bacterial pulmonary infections.

Formulation	Drugs	Mechanism of Action	Disease	Excipients	Comments	Reference
Solid lipid nanoparticles	Isoniazid	Inhibition of the synthesis of mycolic acid	TB	PP SA Poloxamer 188 Mannose Leucine	pH-sensitive response achieved by adding isoniazid as a prodrug	[118]
Liposomes	Liquorice extract (glycyrrhizin)	Membrane disruption	TB	Lipoid® 100 Cholesterol	In total, 46% of the drug reached the lungs, with 16% remaining in the lungs 24 h post-administration	[119]
Nanogels	LLKKK18	Membrane disruption	TB	HA	Infection levels significantly reduced after just five to ten doses	[120]
Nanogels	Isoniazid Rifampicin	Inhibition of the synthesis of mycolic acid (isoniazid) + inhibition of RNA synthesis (rifampicin)	TB	Carboxymethyl chitosan Genipin	Selective targeting of lungs, maintaining drug concentrations of 40–60% after 24 h	[121]
Polymeric nanoparticles	Rifampicin Ascorbic acid	Inhibition of RNA synthesis (rifampicin) + adjuvant (ascorbic acid)	TB	Sodium alginate Tween® 80 Sucrose Mannitol	Demonstrated activity against nine clinical strains of *M. tuberculosis*	[123]
Polymeric nanoparticles	Ciprofloxacin	Inhibition of type IV topoisomerase	Lower respiratory tract infections—unspecified	PEtOx Tannic acid	Sustained release over the course of 7 days	[127]

Table 2. *Cont.*

Formulation	Drugs	Mechanism of Action	Disease	Excipients	Comments	Reference
Polymeric nanoparticles	SET-M33	Binding to LPS	Infection caused by *P. aeruginosa*	Dextran	Prolonged residence time (12-fold higher) compared to free peptide; demonstrated efficacy and safety in vivo	[128]
Anionic liposomes	Levofloxacin	Inhibition of type IV topoisomerase	Infection caused by *P. aeruginosa* in cystic fibrosis patients	DSPC Cholesterol DSPE-PEG 2000	Sustained release over 72 h and demonstrated activity against five strains of *P. aeruginosa*	[129]
Liposomes	Levofloxacin Lysozyme	Inhibition of type IV topoisomerase (levofloxacin) + hydrolysis of peptidoglycan in bacterial cell wall (lysozyme)	Infection caused by *S. aureus*	Phospholipon® 90G Phospholipon® 90H Cholesterol Lactose	Demonstrated decrease in microbial burden in lungs, bronchoalveolar lavage fluid, and nasal fluid	[130]
Liposomes	Colistin	Displacement of magnesium and calcium in LPS	Infection caused by *P. aeruginosa*	Sodium cholesteryl sulphate Lipoid® S75	Prolonged drug retention in the lung and enhanced in vivo efficacy	[131]

Key: tuberculosis (TB); palmityl palmitate (PP); stearyl amine (SA); hyaluronic acid (HA); poly(2-ethyl-2-oxazoline) (PEtOx); lipopolysaccharide (LPS); 1,2-distearoyl-sn-glycero-3-phosphocholine (DSPC); 1,2-distearoyl-sn-glycero-3-phosphoethanolamine-N-(polyethylene-glycol)-2000.

Table 3. Novel formulations to treat fungal pulmonary infections.

Formulation	Drugs	Mechanism of Action	Excipients	Comments	Reference
Polymeric nanoparticles	Voriconazole	Inhibition of ergosterol demethylation	Chitosan	Enhanced lung deposition and demonstrated in vitro efficacy against *Aspergillus*	[138]
Inorganic nanoparticles	Leaf extract of *Artemisia sieberi*	Not reported	Silver ($AgNO_3$)	Demonstrated efficacy against *Aspergillus*, reducing lung tissue damage, and reduced oxidative stress	[139]
Liposomes	Dapsone	Inhibition of synthesis of dihydrofolic acid	DPPC Cholesterol	Prolonged in vitro release up to 16 h	[140]

Table 3. *Cont.*

Formulation	Drugs	Mechanism of Action	Excipients	Comments	Reference
Micelles	Amphotericin B	Membrane disruption	Chitosan Stearic acid	Aerosolisation of amphotericin B with improved activity compared to the free drug	[141]
Liposomes	Amphotericin B	Membrane disruption	Egg PC Cholesterol OPM OPP	Improved in vivo airway penetration in rats and accumulation in lung tissue for over 24 h	[143]
Nanostructured aggregates	Itraconazole	Inhibition of ergosterol demethylation	Mannitol Lecithin	Achieved lung deposition and systemic levels in mice	[144]

Key: 1,2-dipalmitoyl-*sn*-glycero-3-phosphocholine (DPPC), phosphatidylcholine (PC), O-palmitoylated mannan (OPM), O-palmitoylated pullulan (OPP).

3.3. *Viral Infections*

Respiratory infections caused by viruses typically impact the upper airways and are often self-limiting. However, certain infections can spread to the lower respiratory tract, developing into severe diseases, especially among children and the elderly in low- and middle-income countries [145]. Influenza and respiratory syncytial virus (RSV) are common viral agents responsible for significant morbidity in older adults. Recently, severe acute respiratory syndrome coronavirus 2 (SARS-CoV-2) had an unparalleled impact on healthcare systems and society.

Nanotechnology has emerged as a promising area for enhancing viral infection treatments [146] since nanocarriers can be engineered to target viruses at various stages of infection [147]. In particular, pulmonary-administered nanoformulations offer potential advantages for treating lung-related illnesses. Some examples of pulmonary formulations for viral infections are shown in Table 4.

3.3.1. SARS-CoV-2

The virus responsible for coronavirus disease 2019 (COVID-19), SARS-CoV-2, was initially identified in Wuhan (China) in December 2019 and rapidly became a global pandemic [148,149]. COVID-19 has led to over 6 million deaths [150], with elderly individuals showing higher mortality rates [151]. To improve COVID-19 treatments, various pulmonary nanomedicines have been developed [152].

During the pandemic, remdesivir, a prodrug metabolically converted into a nucleoside triphosphate, received authorisation for emergency use from the U.S. Food and Drug Administration (FDA) for hospitalised patients with severe COVID-19 [153]. Remdesivir was among the first drugs to demonstrate improved patient outcomes; however, its use is limited due to its physicochemical properties and pharmacokinetics, including metabolism by both CYP and non-CYP enzymes and its incompatibility with oral administration. Additionally, it has systemic side effects, such as hepatotoxicity [154]. Pulmonary administration has been explored as a way to address these issues and enhance the efficacy of remdesivir.

Sanna and colleagues designed inhalable polymeric nanoparticles loaded with remdesivir to target the human angiotensin-converting enzyme 2 (ACE2), which SARS-CoV-2 utilises to infect host cells [155]. This formulation exhibited increased antiviral activity compared to free remdesivir [156]. Meng et al. demonstrated that dexamethasone-loaded nanoparticles, created with neutrophil-derived nanovesicles and cholesterol, reduced lung inflammation and injury in rhesus macaques infected with SARS-CoV-2. Notably, inhalation was more effective than intravenous administration, as the pulmonary delivery of 10 μg/kg dexamethasone outperformed intravenous administration of 100 μg/kg due to greater accumulation in inflamed lungs, as these nanovesicles showed improved targeting to macrophages, inhibiting the inflammatory response of a broad range of cytokines [157].

Fouad et al. developed an inhalable nanosuspension of remdesivir with polycaprolactone (PCL) and Pluronic® F127, which was transformed into inhalable microparticles with hyaluronic acid and mannitol. This formulation showed improved drug release over free remdesivir, with a 1.5- and 1.9-fold increases at 24 and 48 h, respectively, along with an enhanced safety profile [158]. Halevas et al. created a nano-based delivery system using 2,2,-bis(hydroxymethyl)propionic acid (bis-MPA) dendritic nanocarriers to improve the solubility of remdesivir. Release studies indicated complete drug release within 24 h, following first-order kinetics. Toxicity tests on lung fibroblasts and alveolar macrophages confirmed non-toxic profiles similar to free remdesivir [159].

Ali et al. developed nanostructured lipid carriers for the pulmonary delivery of hydroxychloroquine, a repurposed drug during COVID-19. This drug presented a few limitations, including reduced efficacy and cardiac toxicity. The nanoformulation provided full drug release within 24 h and demonstrated effectiveness in reducing lung inflammation and injury in an acute lung injury mouse model. However, the cardiac toxicity of the formulation still needs to be assessed [160].

3.3.2. Other Viral Infections

Nanomedicine-based approaches for viral infections extend beyond SARS-CoV-2. While the COVID-19 pandemic heightened focus on this virus, research has also targeted other respiratory viruses, including RSV and influenza [161]. Chang et al. developed resveratrol nanoparticles via sonication-assisted self-assembly, enhancing solubility and dissolution rates. Nebulised resveratrol nanoparticles improved pharmacological effects by inhibiting RSV replication and reducing pro-inflammatory cytokine production. RSV-infected mice treated with these nanoparticles showed reduced viral loads and improved lung microenvironment [161]. Peng et al. designed a chitosan-coated liposome delivery system for oxymatrine, a herbal compound with antiviral activity against RSV. Encapsulation within chitosan-coated liposomes enhanced lung tissue retention and improved therapeutic effects in RSV-infected mice by overcoming the mucous barrier [162].

Gil et al. created interferon-λ (IFN-λ)-loaded nanoparticles combined with pulmonary surfactants for inhalation against influenza A. This formulation notably restricted viral replication from day three post-infection and fully improved lung pathology, surpassing recombinant IFN-λ in effectiveness and immunological response, evidenced by increased monocyte frequency and restored T and B cell profiles [163].

Table 4. Novel formulations to treat viral pulmonary infections.

Formulation	Drugs	Mechanism of Action	Disease	Excipients	Comments	Reference
Polymeric nanoparticles	Remdesivir	Inhibition of RNA polymerase	COVID-19	PLGA PCL	Selective targeting to ACE2 membrane receptor and enhanced antiviral effect compared to free drug	[156]

Table 4. *Cont.*

Formulation	Drugs	Mechanism of Action	Disease	Excipients	Comments	Reference
Nanovesicles	Dexamethasone	Agonist of the glucocorticoid receptor	COVID-19	Nanovesicles were obtained from neutrophils from bone marrow of mice or rhesus macaques	Better outcome when the formulation was inhaled instead of injected. Improved targeting to macrophages.	[157]
Nanosuspension	Remdesivir	Inhibition of RNA polymerase	COVID-19	PCL Pluronic® F127 HA Mannitol	Enhanced drug release compared to free drug (1.5-fold increase at 24 h and 1.9-fold increase at 48 h) and better safety index (1.3-fold higher).	[158]
Dendritic nanocarriers	Remdesivir	Inhibition of RNA polymerase	COVID-19	Hyperbranched G4-PEG6k-OH	First-order release kinetics with total release of remdesivir after 24 h and similar toxicity profile than free drug.	[159]
Nanostructured lipid carriers	Hydroxychloro-quine	Inhibition of TLR9	COVID-19	Sweet almond oil Glyceryl behenate PC Gelucire®	Improved lung tissue targeting of hydroxychloro-quine, but further investigation needed to confirm its potential for COVID-19 treatment	[160]
Nanoparticles	Resveratrol	Activation of Sirt-1	Infection caused by RSV	Unspecified	In vivo models demonstrated extended lung residence and reduced viral load compared to free drug	[161]
Liposomes	Oxymatrine	Antiviral activity induced by promoting difference cytokines	Infection caused by RSV	DPPC HSPC DPPG Cholesterol DSPE-PEG Chitosan	Selective distribution and improved retention in lung tissue compared to the free drug	[162]

Table 4. *Cont.*

Formulation	Drugs	Mechanism of Action	Disease	Excipients	Comments	Reference
Lipid nanoparticles	IFN-λ	Recruitment of neutrophils and NK cells	Influenza	Protamine Unspecified lipids Unspecified proteins	Improved delivery of IFN-λ to lungs and superior efficacy compared to recombinant IFN	[163]

Key: coronavirus disease 2019 (COVID-19); poly(lactic-co-glycolic) acid (PLGA); polycaprolactone (PCL); angiotensin-converting enzyme 2 (ACE2); hyaluronic acid (HA); toll-like receptor (TLR); phosphatidylcholine (PC); sirtuin-1 (Sirt-1); respiratory syncytial virus (RSV); interferon-λ (IFN-λ); natural killer cells (NK); dipalmitoylphosphatidylcholine (DPPC); hydrogenated soybean phosphatidylcoline (HSPC); dipalmitoylphosphatidylglycerol (DPPG); 1,2-distearoyl-*sn*-glycero-3phosphoethanolamine-*N*-[amino(polyethylene glycol)] (DSPE-PEG).

4. Nanovaccines

Nanostructures used in vaccine formulations can serve multiple purposes: they can act as adjuvants to enhance vaccine effectiveness, function as antigen delivery systems, or improve antigen presentation to the immune system or even serve as the primary component to the vaccine. The role of nanotechnology in vaccine development has a long history; for instance, two nanovaccines, Epaxal® and Inflexal®, were approved in the 1990s for hepatitis A and influenza prevention, respectively [164]. These vaccines use virosomes (liposome-like particles embedded with viral proteins) as carriers [165]. Epaxal® virosomes contain formalin-deactivated hepatitis A antigen within a phospholipid bilayer, facilitating absorption into immunocompetent cells [166,167], while Inflexal® contains virosomal particles from three influenza strains, selected following WHO guidelines, that express hemagglutinin and neuraminidase glycoproteins [168].

The COVID-19 pandemic renewed interest in nanovaccine technology, with years of research enabling clinical trials to start rapidly after the genome of the virus became available [169]. Among approved COVID-19 vaccines, Spikevax (Moderna™) and Comirnaty (Pfizer Ltd./BioNTech SE) use lipid nanoparticles to stabilise mRNA and facilitate cellular uptake [169]. Spikevax includes lipids such as SM-102 (heptadecane-9-yl 8-((2-hydroxyethyl) [6-oxo-6-(undecyloxy)hexyl]amino)octanoate), 1,2-distearoyl-*sn*-glycero-3-phosphocholine (DSPC), cholesterol, and 1,2-dimyristoyl-rac-glycero-3-methoxypolyethylene glycol-2000 (PEG2000-DMG), while the lipid structure of Comirnaty incorporates ((4-hydroxybutyl)azanediyl)bis(hexane-6,1-diyl)bis(2-hexyldecanoate) (ALC-0315) and 2-[(polyethylene glycol)-2000]-*N*,*N*-ditetradecylacetamide (ALC-0159) for mRNA electrochemical interaction, with cholesterol and DSPC added to enhance stability [170,171]. Ultimately, PEG-modified lipids are incorporated to enhance the solubility of the lipid nanoparticles [172]. These PEGylated lipids, lacking an ionic charge, contribute to the colloidal stability of the lipid nanoparticles. Furthermore, the PEGylated lipids confer the ability for the vaccine to evade phagocytosis by the mononuclear phagocyte system [173].

Beyond the commonly used subcutaneous and intramuscular administration, the pulmonary delivery of nanovaccines has gained attention, especially for respiratory infections. This route is crucial for establishing mucosal immunity, which can prevent pathogen transmission by inducing tissue resident memory T cells and immunoglobulin A antibodies [174,175]. Subcutaneous or intramuscular administered vaccines promote systemic immunity but do not offer mucosal immunity. The vaccines must be administered by the nasal or pulmonary administration routes to develop robust mucosal immunity in the respiratory tract [176,177]. Nanocarriers explored for pulmonary delivery include liposomes, polymeric nanoparticles, lipid–polymer hybrids, and virus-like particles (VLPs). Several nanovaccines for respiratory diseases like COVID-19 and influenza have shown promise in this approach. A few examples of these nanovaccines for pulmonary delivery have been summarised in Table 5.

For example, Wang et al. developed a hybrid nanovaccine by combining nanovesicles expressing the receptor-binding domain (RBD) with pulmonary surfactant-mimicking liposomes containing monophosphoryl-lipid-A (MPLA). This nanovaccine provided notable advantages over traditional subcutaneous vaccination, including efficient targeting and activation of alveolar macrophages via the toll-like receptor 4/nuclear factor κ-light-chain-enhancer of activated B cells (TLR4/NF-κB) pathway. This process induced strong T and B responses, yielding high levels of RBD-specific IgG and secretory IgA antibodies. Additionally, it demonstrated broad neutralising activity against several SARS-CoV-2 variants (wild type, delta, and omicron pseudoviruses) while showing reduced side effects, with this inhalable delivery system particularly enhancing mucosal immunity [178].

Zheng et al. designed a bionic-virus nanovaccine comprising polyionisic–polycytidylic acid (poly(I:C)) as an adjuvant, biomimetic pulmonary surfactant liposomes as a virus-like capsid, and SARS-CoV-2 RBDs as the spike protein. This nanovaccine, designed for intranasal or inhalable administration, closely mimicked natural SARS-CoV-2 infection and elicited stronger mucosal immunity than conventional intramuscular or subcutaneous vaccines. This was demonstrated by elevated SARS-CoV-2-specific secretory IgA levels in respiratory secretions, effectively neutralising the virus [179].

Lokugamage et al. applied a systematic cluster-based approach to develop lipid nanoparticles comprising various lipids, either neutral or cationic helper lipids, and PEG. They discovered that the PEG molar ratio and the type of helper lipid were critical factors: lower PEG ratios performed best with neutral helper lipids, while higher ratios suited cationic lipids. This optimised nanoparticle design effectively delivered mRNA encoding antibodies against influenza H1N1, protecting mice from lethal infection and performing better than previous lipid nanoparticle systems intended for systemic delivery [180].

Lopez et al. designed a polyanhydride nanoparticle-based vaccine platform aimed at broad protection against influenza A virus. Several H3N2-based nanovaccine versions were tested, which induced robust systemic and mucosal antibody responses along with enhanced lung-resident and systemic cellular immunity. These immune responses were correlated with protection against both homologous and heterosubtypic infections [181].

Table 5. Nanovaccine formulations for pulmonary administration.

Formulation	Infection	Excipients	Comments	Reference
Nanovesicles + liposomes	COVID-19	DPPC, DPPE, DPPG, Cholesterol	Demonstrated neutralisation of multiple coronavirus variants and effective at generating mucosal immunity	[178]
Liposomes	COVID-19	DPPC, DPPG, DPPE-PEG-COOH	Elicited stronger mucosal protective immunity compared to intramuscular or subcutaneous vaccination	[179]
Lipid nanoparticles	Influenza A	DMPE, DPSE, Cholesterol, DOPE, DSPC, DOTAP, DOTMA, DODA	All the mentioned lipids were tested, but the composition of the optimised composition is unspecified. Successfully delivered mRNA encoding antibodies against influenza A	[180]

Table 5. *Cont.*

Formulation	Infection	Excipients	Comments	Reference
Polymeric nanoparticles	Influenza A	CPTEG, CPH	Elicited robust systemic and mucosal humoral immune responses and enhanced systemic and lung-resident cellular immunity	[181]

Key: coronavirus disease 2019 (COVID-19); dipalmitoylphosphatidylcholine (DPPC); 1,2-bis(disphenylphosphino)ethane (DPPE); dipalmitoylphosphatidylglycerol (DPPG); polyethylene glycol (PEG); 1,2-dimyristoyl-sn-glycero-3-phosphoethanolamine-N-[methoxy(polyethyleneglycol)-2000] (DMPE); 1,2-distearoyl-sn-glycero-3-phosphoethanolamine-N-[methoxy(polyethyleneglycol)-2000] (DPSE); 1,2-dioleyl-sn-glycero-3-phosphoethanolamine (DOPE); 1,2-dioleyl-3-trimethylammonium-propane (DOTAP); 1,2-di-O-octadecenyl-3-trimethylammonium propane (DOTMA); dimethyldioctadecylammonium (DODA); 1,8-bis(p-carboxyphenoxy)-3,6-dioxoctane (CPTEG); 1,6-bis(p-carboxyphenoxy)hexane (CPH).

5. Pulmonary-Administered Nanomedicines to Combat Lung Cancer

Lung cancer is the most diagnosed carcinoma and the main leading cause of cancer-related death, with more than 2 million new cases and nearly 1.9 million deaths worldwide in 2022 [182]. This neoplasm can be classified into small-cell lung cancer (SCLC) and non-small-cell lung cancer (NSCLC). This latter represents about 85% of all lung carcinomas and can be subdivided into different histological subtypes, including adenocarcinoma, adenosquamous carcinoma, squamous cell carcinoma, and large-cell carcinoma. Adenocarcinoma is the most common subtype, accounting for 50% of NSCLCs, and represents a significant health problem, as the 5-year survival rate is low (≈15%) [183].

Different treatment strategies are currently available for patients with lung cancer, including surgery, radiotherapy, immunotherapy, and chemotherapy. Tumour resection in combination with radiotherapy, is the preferable treatment option. However, most patients are not suitable for surgery due to local invasion or distant metastases. In these patients, systemic therapies, chemotherapy, and immunotherapy are the primary treatment strategies [184]. Delivering these drugs by the pulmonary route offers certain advantages (Figure 2) for treating lung carcinoma [185]. In fact, several clinical trials have evaluated the efficacy of inhalable chemotherapy (Table 6). Lemarie and collaborators demonstrated that the pulmonary administration of gemcitabine was safe and exhibited minimal signs of systemic toxicity, as very low plasma gemcitabine levels were detected. Around 42% of the administered dose remained in the lungs. Regarding anticancer activity, a minor overall response was detected in one patient and stable disease was detected in four patients. A total of 11 patients were enrolled in this study [186]. Similar results in terms of toxicity were also appreciated in patients treated with inhaled doxorubicin or 5-fluorouracil; meagre amounts of these antineoplastics were detected in the bloodstream [187,188]. In terms of efficacy, it should be noted that the administration of 5-fluorouracil was effective. A satisfactory anticancer effect was detected in 60% of treated patients [188].

Table 6. Inhaled antineoplastics evaluated in clinics.

Drug	Dose	Cancer Type	Reference
Gemcitabine	1–4 mg/kg	NSCLC	[186]
Doxorrubicin	0.4–9.4 mg/m^2	Primary and metastases in the lungs	[187]
5-Fluorouracil	250 mg	NSCLC	[188]
Carboplatin (iv or inhaled) +Docetaxel (iv)	Docetaxel: 100 mg/m^2 Carboplatin: AUC 5.5	NSCLC	[189]
Liposomal cisplatin	1.5–48 mg/m^2	NSCLC	[190]
Liposomal 9-Nitrocamptothecin	6.7–26.6 µg/kg/day	Primary lung cancer Metastases in the lungs	[191]

Key: non-small cell lung cancer (NSCLC); intravenous (iv); area under the curve (AUC).

Interestingly, Zarogoudilis and collaborators compared the efficacy of intravenous and inhaled carboplatin in NSCLC patients. They demonstrated that the pulmonary administration of carboplatin was more effective than its intravenous administration. The patients receiving inhaled carboplatin showed a higher, although non-significant, survival rate (benefit of 25 days). Nevertheless, these patients exhibited a lower lung function measured as forced expiratory volume in one second [189].

The studies mentioned above indicate that the pulmonary administration of antineoplastics allows for its localisation in the respiratory system; a meagre amount of antineoplastics reaches the bloodstream, reducing the systemic toxicity of these drugs. However, patients may experience an impairment in pulmonary function related to the local toxicity of these drugs that must be evaluated. In this context, administering antineoplastics encapsulated into nanocarriers may decrease their local toxicity and increase their anticancer activity, as these systems can be engineered to deliver drugs selectively at the tumour site [192].

Currently, there are two nanoformulations approved for lung cancer treatment: (i) Genexol-PM, polymeric micelles encapsulating paclitaxel, approved for the treatment of NSCLC and breast cancer in Korea, and (ii) Abraxane®, albumin nanoparticles containing paclitaxel approved by FDA and EMA for the treatment of advanced NSCLC and metastatic breast and pancreatic carcinomas. EMA recently authorised a bioequivalent formulation of Abraxane®, known as Pazenir® [193,194]. It should be noted that these formulations are approved for intravenous administration. However, the efficacy of some inhalable nanoparticles encapsulating anticancer agents has also been tested in lung cancer patients. For example, Wittgen and colleagues evaluated the efficacy of inhaled liposomes encapsulating cisplatin in NSCLC patients. This formulation was, in general, safe without detecting dose-limiting toxicity. Signs of haematologic toxicity, nephrotoxicity, ototoxicity, or neurotoxicity (effects commonly associated with this antineoplastic) were not detected. The most common adverse effects were gastrointestinal (nausea and vomiting) and pulmonary (dyspnoea, fatigue, and hoarseness) toxicities. More than 40% of the patients exhibited these adverse effects. Regarding efficacy, tumour regression was not appreciated in any patient, but around 70% exhibited a stable disease [190]. Pulmonary-administered 9-nitrocamptothecin-loaded-liposomes were also safe at doses lower than 26.6 μg/kg/day. In this case, the most common adverse effects were nausea, vomiting, cough, bronchial irritation, and fatigue. However, higher levels of antineoplastics were absorbed systemically compared to the other formulations. Finally, in terms of efficacy, stable disease was detected in three patients with primary lung cancer [191].

In addition to these clinically tested formulations, many other pulmonary delivery nanosystems have been designed and evaluated at the preclinical level for lung cancer treatment (Table 7). Curcumin, a phenolic constituent in Curcuma longa L., attains significant interest in treating cancer, including lung carcinoma [195]. Zhang and collaborators developed curcumin-loaded liposomes of around 95 nm intended for pulmonary administration using a dry powder inhaler. This formulation demonstrated a higher lung deposition than free curcumin and a selective cytotoxic effect against lung cancer cells. Moreover, studies in rats also demonstrated higher anticancer activity. Tumour nodes and lung bleeding decreased in liposome-treated rats compared to the free-curcumin-treated group [196].

Similar results were also found with paclitaxel-loaded liposomes. The intratracheal administration of this formulation showed a 26-fold higher lung accumulation of paclitaxel compared to the intravenous injection in the tail vein. These liposomes also reduced tumour growth in the lungs and prolonged the survival rate of the mice [197]. The delivery of paclitaxel via other lipid nanoparticles (specifically nanostructured lipid carriers) was also effective. Pulmonary administration of these nanomedicines allowed for the accumulation of paclitaxel in the lungs, limiting systemic exposure and reducing systemic toxicity [198]. Moreover, a higher anticancer effect than free paclitaxel was obtained [199].

Erlotinib is a tyrosine kinase inhibitor approved for treating NSCLC overexpressing epidermal growth factor receptors [200]. Szabová et al. developed pegylated liposomes loaded for the pulmonary administration of this drug. These liposomes were able to penetrate the lungs. While air jet nebulisers led to deeper penetration, vibrating mesh nebulisers showed a lower leakage of the administered dose, as around 98% of the encapsulated dose was effectively delivered into the lungs [201]. The good penetration of this liposomal formulation through the respiratory system can be attributed, among other aspects, to PEG coating. As aforementioned, the presence of PEG on the surface of nanoparticles improves their penetration through the mucous layer and their access to deep lung regions. The anticancer efficacy of this formulation was not evaluated. However, it is expected to show an increased anticancer effect compared to free erlotinib due to its local delivery into the lungs.

Hu and colleagues developed solid lipid nanoparticles of around 225 nm for the pulmonary administration of doxorubicin. This inhalable formulation allows for the delivery of higher doses of doxorubicin within the lungs than the pulmonary administration of free doxorubicin. Doxorubicin-loaded solid lipid nanoparticles exhibited a respirable fraction of around 79%, and non-encapsulated doxorubicin showed a significantly lower value of around 60%. Moreover, the encapsulated drug was able to reach deeper regions of the lungs. Higher plasmatic levels ($\approx$2-fold higher plasma area under the curve values) were observed in rats treated with nanoparticles compared to animals receiving the free drug [202].

Apart from lipid nanoparticles, inhalable polymeric nanosystems have also been designed. Sorafenib-loaded inhalable PLGA nanoparticles showed suitable aerosolization properties and promising in vivo anticancer activity in an NSCLC tumour model [203]. Quinacrine, also known as mepacrine, is an antimalarial drug that recently demonstrated anticancer properties [204]. PLGA nanoparticles loaded with this agent and coated with albumin were also developed. It showed excellent aerosolization properties and an improved in vitro anticancer activity in NSCLC compared to the free drug. A higher apoptosis induction was also detected [205]. It should be noted that this superior efficacy can be attributed not only to the higher accumulation of quinacrine in the lung due to its pulmonary administration but also to the incorporation of albumin on the surface of quinacrine-loaded nanoparticles. As described above, albumin nanoparticles tend to accumulate in NSCLC due to the presence of GP-60 receptors in tumoral blood vessels and the overexpression of SPARC proteins in the tumour.

One advantage of nanomedicines is the possibility of co-encapsulating several compounds simultaneously, allowing for simultaneous release into the tumour environment. For example, Kaur and colleagues developed lipid nanoparticles containing paclitaxel and doxorubicin. The studies reported that this inhalable nanoformulation showed superior in vitro anticancer activity against A549 cells and higher drug distribution in the lungs compared to non-encapsulated antineoplastics [206]. Saimi and collaborators developed niosomes containing gemcitabine and cisplatin. They showed excellent aerosolization properties (aerosol output was 96.22%). This formulation exhibited significantly lower toxicity against healthy lung cells (MRC5 cell line). While the combination of free gemcitabine and free cisplatin was very toxic ($IC_{50} < 1.6$ µg/mL), the niosomal formulation containing both drugs was weakly toxic ($IC_{50} = 280$ µg/mL). This is interesting, as a lower toxicity in the lung tissue could be expected with this nanoformulation. However, regarding efficacy, a cytotoxic effect was also appreciated in lung cancer cells. In A549 cells, the administration of free drugs showed an $IC_{50} < 1.6$ µg/mL and for niosomes an IC_{50} of around 46 µg/mL. This lower antiproliferative effect could be related to the controlled release of these drugs [207].

Table 7. Inhalable nanomedicines developed at the preclinical level for treating lung carcinoma.

Nanocarrier	Drug	Observations	Reference
Liposomes	Curcumin	Better aerosolization properties. Selective cytotoxicity against lung cancer cells compared to healthy lung cells. Higher in vivo anticancer activity.	[196]
	Pirfenidone	Good aerosolization performance More cytotoxic effect against A549 cells than non-encapsulated drug.	[208]
	Paclitaxel	Higher lung accumulation of paclitaxel compared to i.v. administration. Tumour reduction compared to non-treated animals. Higher survival rate compared to non-treated animals.	[197]
	Erlotinib	Good aerosolization performance using vibrating mesh nebulisers.	[201]
Niosomes	Gemcitabine and paclitaxel	Aerosol output of 96.2%. Lower toxicity in healthy lung cells (MRC5) compared to free drugs (IC_{50} = 280 µg/mL vs IC_{50} < 1.6 µg/mL). Lower cytotoxic activity in lung cancer (A529 cells) compared to free drugs (IC_{50} = 46 µg/mL vs IC_{50} < 1.6 µg/mL).	[207]
Nanostructured lipid particles	Paclitaxel	Higher distribution in the lungs of the pulmonary route compared to intravenous injection. No signs of systemic toxicity after pulmonary administration.	[198]
	Paclitaxel	Better lung accumulation compared to free paclitaxel. Higher anticancer activity than free paclitaxel.	[199]
	Paclitaxel and Doxorrubicin	Higher antiproliferative effect in A549 cells. Higher distribution in the lungs compared to non-encapsulated drugs.	[206]
Solid lipid nanoparticles	Doxorubicin	Higher deposition of administered doses compared to inhaled free doxorubicin. Reach deeper regions in the lungs. Higher plasmatic level of doxorubicin compared to the administration of inhaled free doxorubicin.	[202]
Polymeric nanoparticles	Quinacrine (mepacrine)	Nanoparticles incorporating albumin on their surface. Good aerosolization properties. Improved in vitro anticancer activity in NSCLC compared to the free drug. Higher apoptosis induction.	[205]
	Sorafenib	Appropriate aerosolization properties. Higher in vivo anticancer activity in NSCLC	[203]

Key: intravenous (iv); non-small cell lung cancer (NSCLC).

6. Challenges in Clinical Translation

Despite substantial progress in developing nanomedicines for pulmonary administration, a significant gap remains between preclinical research and clinical translation [209]. Cost presents a critical barrier to nanomedicine development. Manufacturing these advanced medicines is substantially more expensive than traditional pharmaceutical approaches, resulting in significantly higher selling prices and acquisition costs for healthcare institutions [210]. The commercialisation landscape is predominantly shaped by small and medium-sized enterprises, who bear the burden of navigating extensive and expensive validation processes and clinical trial requirements, while larger pharmaceutical companies maintain a 'low profile', showing low interest in these emerging technologies [210]. This economic challenge particularly impacts affordability in middle- and low-income countries, effectively limiting potential market implementation [211].

Regulatory frameworks struggle to keep pace with rapid technological advancements, creating a complex approval environment [212]. The absence of standardised protocols for characterising nanomedicine formulations further complicates research efforts, as different research groups employ varying analytical tools and testing methods. This inconsistency makes comprehensive comparative assessments difficult [213].

While the scientific literature often emphasises successful experimental outcomes and promising results, this approach can inadvertently introduce publication bias. By underreporting failures, setbacks, and null results, researchers risk presenting an incomplete and potentially overly optimistic view of the current state of nanomedicine.

Additional developmental challenges include scaling production from laboratory to industrial levels, ensuring formulation stability and appropriate shelf life, addressing potential nanomaterial toxicity and achieving consistent drug loading and release profiles. Complex interactions with biological systems, potential long-term tissue accumulation effects, immune system responses, and environmental implications of nanomaterials further complicate research and development efforts.

7. Conclusions

The pulmonary route of administration is of interest in treating respiratory infections and lung cancer, as it would allow for the localisation of drugs in the lungs (action site) and a reduction in their systemic exposure. Nevertheless, the efficient pulmonary delivery of drugs is challenged, as the respiratory system (mainly through mucociliary escalator) tends to eliminate inhaled particles. Moreover, the lungs have a large surface area, and drugs can be rapidly translocated into the bloodstream and distributed to other organs. Certainly, nanomedicine holds the potential to overcome the limitations of the pulmonary route. Of all the types of nanosystems, lipid nanocarriers, particularly liposomes, are the most investigated nanomedicines. To date, one formulation, Arikayce®, consisting of liposomes of amikacin, is currently approved. It should be noted that although, commonly, drugs administered via the pulmonary route show less toxicity than drugs administered through other systemic routes, like intravenous administration, severe toxicity can occur at the pulmonary level and impair the respiratory function of patients. This aspect is especially problematic in the case of the administration of antineoplastics, which show high toxicity. The administration of nanomedicines is safer than the administration of non-encapsulated drugs. However, they are not devoid of causing severe lung damage and must be deeply investigated. Inhalable nanovaccines have the potential to revolutionise the prophylaxis and therapy of respiratory infections and lung cancer due to the improved mucosal immunity achieved through this route, although investigation in this field is still limited. To sum up, inhalable nanomedicines show great potential for administering antimicrobials and antineoplastics in patients suffering respiratory tract infections and lung carcinoma and for immunising against microorganisms entering by this route.

Author Contributions: Conceptualization, A.I.F.-S. and R.F.-G.; methodology, A.I.F.-S. and R.F.-G.; software, A.I.F.-S. and R.F.-G., writing—original draft preparation, A.I.F.-S. and R.F.-G.; writing—review and editing, A.I.F.-S. and R.F.-G. Funding acquisition, A.I.F.-S. All authors have read and agreed to the published version of the manuscript.

Funding: This research was partially funded by UCM-Research group "Formulation and Bioavailability of new medicines" (Ref: 910939).

Conflicts of Interest: The authors declare no conflicts of interest.

References

1. Mansour, H.M.; Rhee, Y.S.; Wu, X. Nanomedicine in pulmonary delivery. *Int. J. Nanomed.* **2009**, *4*, 299–319. [CrossRef] [PubMed]
2. Dames, P.; Gleich, B.; Flemmer, A.; Hajek, K.; Seidl, N.; Wiekhorst, F.; Eberbeck, D.; Bittmann, I.; Bergemann, C.; Weyh, T.; et al. Targeted delivery of magnetic aerosol droplets to the lung. *Nat. Nanotechnol.* **2007**, *2*, 495–499. [CrossRef] [PubMed]
3. Seresirikachorn, B.; Ghadiri, M. Chapter 7—Absorption enhancement of macromolecule-administered intrapulmonary. In *Targeting Chronic Inflammatory Lung Diseases Using Advanced Drug Delivery Systems*; Dua, K., Ed.; Academic Press: Cambridge, MA, USA, 2020; pp. 147–161.
4. Lam, J.K.W.; Zhou, Q. Advances in Pulmonary Drug Delivery Systems and Inhalation Formulations. *Pharm. Res.* **2023**, *40*, 1013–1014. [CrossRef] [PubMed]
5. Jain, H.; Bairagi, A.; Srivastava, S.; Singh, S.B.; Mehra, N.K. Recent advances in the development of microparticles for pulmonary administration. *Drug Discov. Today* **2020**, *25*, 1865–1872. [CrossRef]
6. Anaya, B.J.; D'Angelo, D.; Bettini, R.; Molina, G.; Sanz-Perez, A.; Dea-Ayuela, M.A.; Galiana, C.; Rodríguez, C.; Tirado, D.F.; Lalatsa, A.; et al. Heparin-azithromycin microparticles show anti-inflammatory effects and inhibit SARS-CoV-2 and bacterial pathogens associated to lung infections. *Carbohydr. Polym.* **2025**, *348*, 122930. [CrossRef]
7. Torres-Suárez, A.I.; Martín-Sabroso, C.; Fraguas-Sánchez, A.I.; Rojo, M.Á.; Garrosa, M.; Fernández-Carballido, A. Chapter 7—Design of dosage forms: Influences of anatomy and administration routes. In *Dosage Forms, Formulation Developments and Regulations*; Nayak, A.K., Sen, K.K., Eds.; Academic Press: Cambridge, MA, USA, 2024; pp. 183–221. [CrossRef]
8. He, S.; Gui, J.; Xiong, K.; Chen, M.; Gao, H.; Fu, Y. A roadmap to pulmonary delivery strategies for the treatment of infectious lung diseases. *J. Nanobiotechnology* **2022**, *20*, 101. [CrossRef]
9. Stannard, W.; O'Callaghan, C. Ciliary function and the role of cilia in clearance. *J. Aerosol Med.* **2006**, *19*, 110–115. [CrossRef]
10. Araujo, F.; Martins, C.; Azevedo, C.; Sarmento, B. Chemical modification of drug molecules as strategy to reduce interactions with mucus. *Adv. Drug Deliv. Rev.* **2018**, *124*, 98–106. [CrossRef]
11. Liu, Q.; Guan, J.; Qin, L.; Zhang, X.; Mao, S. Physicochemical properties affecting the fate of nanoparticles in pulmonary drug delivery. *Drug Discov Today* **2020**, *25*, 150–159. [CrossRef]
12. Bansil, R.; Turner, B.S. The biology of mucus: Composition, synthesis and organization. *Adv. Drug Deliv. Rev.* **2018**, *124*, 3–15. [CrossRef]
13. Hill, D.B.; Button, B.; Rubinstein, M.; Boucher, R.C. Physiology and pathophysiology of human airway mucus. *Physiol. Rev.* **2022**, *102*, 1757–1836. [CrossRef] [PubMed]
14. Wang, W.; Huang, Z.; Huang, Y.; Zhang, X.; Huang, J.; Cui, Y.; Yue, X.; Ma, C.; Fu, F.; Wang, W.; et al. Pulmonary delivery nanomedicines towards circumventing physiological barriers: Strategies and characterization approaches. *Adv. Drug Deliv. Rev.* **2022**, *185*, 114309. [CrossRef] [PubMed]
15. Taherali, F.; Varum, F.; Basit, A.W. A slippery slope: On the origin, role and physiology of mucus. *Adv. Drug Deliv. Rev.* **2018**, *124*, 16–33. [CrossRef] [PubMed]
16. Hetzel, M.; Ackermann, M.; Lachmann, N. Beyond "Big Eaters": The Versatile Role of Alveolar Macrophages in Health and Disease. *Int. J. Mol. Sci.* **2021**, *22*, 3308. [CrossRef]
17. Patel, B.; Gupta, N.; Ahsan, F. Particle engineering to enhance or lessen particle uptake by alveolar macrophages and to influence the therapeutic outcome. *Eur. J. Pharm. Biopharm.* **2015**, *89*, 163–174. [CrossRef]
18. Hidalgo, A.; Cruz, A.; Pérez-Gil, J. Barrier or carrier? Pulmonary surfactant and drug delivery. *Eur. J. Pharm. Biopharm.* **2015**, *95*, 117–127. [CrossRef]
19. Newman, S.P. Drug delivery to the lungs: Challenges and opportunities. *Ther. Deliv.* **2017**, *8*, 647–661. [CrossRef]
20. García-Díaz, M.; Birch, D.; Wan, F.; Nielsen, H.M. The role of mucus as an invisible cloak to transepithelial drug delivery by nanoparticles. *Adv. Drug Deliv. Rev.* **2018**, *124*, 107–124. [CrossRef]
21. Kole, E.; Jadhav, K.; Shirsath, N.; Dudhe, P.; Verma, R.K.; Chatterjee, A.; Naik, J. Nanotherapeutics for pulmonary drug delivery: An emerging approach to overcome respiratory diseases. *J. Drug Deliv. Sci. Technol.* **2023**, *81*, 104261. [CrossRef]
22. García-Fernández, A.; Sancenón, F.; Martínez-Máñez, R. Mesoporous silica nanoparticles for pulmonary drug delivery. *Adv. Drug Deliv. Rev.* **2021**, *177*, 113953. [CrossRef]
23. Kumar, M.; Hilles, A.R.; Almurisi, S.H.; Bhatia, A.; Mahmood, S. Micro and nano-carriers-based pulmonary drug delivery system: Their current updates, challenges, and limitations—A review. *JCIS Open* **2023**, *12*, 100095. [CrossRef]
24. Fraguas-Sánchez, A.I.; Martín-Sabroso, C.; Lozza, I.; Torres-Suárez, A.I. Nanomedicine Applications in Cancer Treatment. In *Handbook of Cancer and Immunology*; Rezaei, N., Ed.; Springer International Publishing: Cham, Switzerland, 2022; pp. 1–37. [CrossRef]
25. Rubey, K.M.; Brenner, J.S. Nanomedicine to fight infectious disease. *Adv. Drug Deliv. Rev.* **2021**, *179*, 113996. [CrossRef]
26. Khan, A.; Alsahli, M.A.; Aljasir, M.A.; Maswadeh, H.; Mobark, M.A.; Azam, F.; Allemailem, K.S.; Alrumaihi, F.; Alhumaydhi, F.A.; Alwashmi, A.S.S.; et al. Safety, Stability, and Therapeutic Efficacy of Long-Circulating TQ-Incorporated Liposomes: Implication in the Treatment of Lung Cancer. *Pharmaceutics* **2022**, *14*, 153. [CrossRef]
27. Hu, T.; Gong, H.; Xu, J.; Huang, Y.; Wu, F.; He, Z. Nanomedicines for Overcoming Cancer Drug Resistance. *Pharmaceutics* **2022**, *14*, 1606. [CrossRef] [PubMed]

28. Yang, X.; Ye, W.; Qi, Y.; Ying, Y.; Xia, Z. Overcoming Multidrug Resistance in Bacteria Through Antibiotics Delivery in Surface-Engineered Nano-Cargos: Recent Developments for Future Nano-Antibiotics. *Front. Bioeng. Biotechnol.* **2021**, *9*, 696514. [CrossRef] [PubMed]
29. Kamat, S.; Kumari, M. Emergence of microbial resistance against nanoparticles: Mechanisms and strategies. *Front Microbiol* **2023**, *14*, 1102615. [CrossRef] [PubMed]
30. Serrano, D.R.; Kara, A.; Yuste, I.; Luciano, F.C.; Ongoren, B.; Anaya, B.J.; Molina, G.; Diez, L.; Ramirez, B.I.; Ramirez, I.O.; et al. 3D Printing Technologies in Personalized Medicine, Nanomedicines, and Biopharmaceuticals. *Pharmaceutics* **2023**, *15*, 313. [CrossRef]
31. Osouli-Bostanabad, K.; Puliga, S.; Serrano, D.R.; Bucchi, A.; Halbert, G.; Lalatsa, A. Microfluidic Manufacture of Lipid-Based Nanomedicines. *Pharmaceutics* **2022**, *14*, 1940. [CrossRef]
32. Nsairat, H.; Khater, D.; Sayed, U.; Odeh, F.; Al Bawab, A.; Alshaer, W. Liposomes: Structure, composition, types, and clinical applications. *Heliyon* **2022**, *8*, e09394. [CrossRef]
33. He, K.; Tang, M. Safety of novel liposomal drugs for cancer treatment: Advances and prospects. *Chem.-Biol. Interact.* **2018**, *295*, 13–19. [CrossRef]
34. Fraguas-Sánchez, A.I.; Lozza, I.; Torres-Suárez, A.I. Actively Targeted Nanomedicines in Breast Cancer: From Pre-Clinal Investigation to Clinic. *Cancers* **2022**, *14*, 1198. [CrossRef] [PubMed]
35. Fraguas-Sánchez, A.I.; Martín-Sabroso, C.; Fernández-Carballido, A.; Torres-Suárez, A.I. Current status of nanomedicine in the chemotherapy of breast cancer. In *Cancer Chemotherapy and Pharmacology*; Springer: Berlin/Heidelberg, Germany, 2019; Volume 84, pp. 689–706.
36. Bulbake, U.; Doppalapudi, S.; Kommineni, N.; Khan, W. Liposomal Formulations in Clinical Use: An Updated Review. *Pharmaceutics* **2017**, *9*, 12. [CrossRef] [PubMed]
37. Izhar, M.P.; Hafeez, A.; Kushwaha, P.; Simrah. Drug Delivery Through Niosomes: A Comprehensive Review with Therapeutic Applications. *J. Clust. Sci.* **2023**, *34*, 2257–2273. [CrossRef]
38. Moammeri, A.; Chegeni, M.M.; Sahrayi, H.; Ghafelehbashi, R.; Memarzadeh, F.; Mansouri, A.; Akbarzadeh, I.; Abtahi, M.S.; Hejabi, F.; Ren, Q. Current advances in niosomes applications for drug delivery and cancer treatment. *Mater. Today Bio* **2023**, *23*, 100837. [CrossRef]
39. Duan, Y.; Dhar, A.; Patel, C.; Khimani, M.; Neogi, S.; Sharma, P.; Kumar, N.S.; Vekariya, R.L. A brief review on solid lipid nanoparticles: Part and parcel of contemporary drug delivery systems. *RSC Adv.* **2020**, *10*, 26777–26791. [CrossRef]
40. Scioli Montoto, S.; Muraca, G.; Ruiz, M.E. Solid lipid nanoparticles for drug delivery: Pharmacological and biopharmaceutical aspects. *Front. Mol. Biosci.* **2020**, *7*, 587997. [CrossRef] [PubMed]
41. Liu, G.W.; Guzman, E.B.; Menon, N.; Langer, R.S. Lipid nanoparticles for nucleic acid delivery to endothelial cells. *Pharm. Res.* **2023**, *40*, 3–25. [CrossRef] [PubMed]
42. Perumal, S.; Atchudan, R.; Lee, W. A Review of Polymeric Micelles and Their Applications. *Polymers* **2022**, *14*, 2510. [CrossRef]
43. Ghezzi, M.; Pescina, S.; Padula, C.; Santi, P.; Del Favero, E.; Cantù, L.; Nicoli, S. Polymeric micelles in drug delivery: An insight of the techniques for their characterization and assessment in biorelevant conditions. *J. Control. Release* **2021**, *332*, 312–336. [CrossRef]
44. Miguel, R.D.A.; Hirata, A.S.; Jimenez, P.C.; Lopes, L.B.; Costa-Lotufo, L.V. Beyond Formulation: Contributions of Nanotechnology for Translation of Anticancer Natural Products into New Drugs. *Pharmaceutics* **2022**, *14*, 1722. [CrossRef]
45. Hwang, D.; Ramsey, J.D.; Kabanov, A.V. Polymeric micelles for the delivery of poorly soluble drugs: From nanoformulation to clinical approval. *Adv. Drug Deliv. Rev.* **2020**, *156*, 80–118. [CrossRef] [PubMed]
46. Beach, M.A.; Nayanathara, U.; Gao, Y.; Zhang, C.; Xiong, Y.; Wang, Y.; Such, G.K. Polymeric Nanoparticles for Drug Delivery. *Chem. Rev.* **2024**, *124*, 5505–5616. [CrossRef] [PubMed]
47. Zielińska, A.; Carreiró, F.; Oliveira, A.M.; Neves, A.; Pires, B.; Venkatesh, D.N.; Durazzo, A.; Lucarini, M.; Eder, P.; Silva, A.M.; et al. Polymeric Nanoparticles: Production, Characterization, Toxicology and Ecotoxicology. *Molecules* **2020**, *25*, 3731. [CrossRef] [PubMed]
48. Zwain, T.; Taneja, N.; Zwayen, S.; Shidhaye, A.; Palshetkar, A.; Singh, K.K. Chapter 9—Albumin nanoparticles—A versatile and a safe platform for drug delivery applications. In *Nanoparticle Therapeutics*; Kesharwani, P., Singh, K.K., Eds.; Academic Press: Cambridge, MA, USA, 2022; pp. 327–358. [CrossRef]
49. Spada, A.; Emami, J.; Tuszynski, J.A.; Lavasanifar, A. The Uniqueness of Albumin as a Carrier in Nanodrug Delivery. *Mol. Pharm.* **2021**, *18*, 1862–1894. [CrossRef]
50. Ji, Q.; Zhu, H.; Qin, Y.; Zhang, R.; Wang, L.; Zhang, E.; Zhou, X.; Meng, R. GP60 and SPARC as albumin receptors: Key targeted sites for the delivery of antitumor drugs. *Front. Pharmacol.* **2024**, *15*, 1329636. [CrossRef]
51. Hartley, C.; Rowan, D.; Chen, X.; Gomez-Arellano, L.; West, A.M.; Oshima, K.; Mackinnon, A.C. Increased SPARC expression is associated with neoadjuvant therapy in resectable pancreatic ductal adenocarcinoma. *Pract. Lab. Med.* **2020**, *21*, e00171. [CrossRef]
52. Qu, N.; Song, K.; Ji, Y.; Liu, M.; Chen, L.; Lee, R.J.; Teng, L. Albumin Nanoparticle-Based Drug Delivery Systems. *Int. J. Nanomed.* **2024**, *19*, 6945–6980. [CrossRef]
53. Unnikrishnan, G.; Joy, A.; Megha, M.; Kolanthai, E.; Senthilkumar, M. Exploration of inorganic nanoparticles for revolutionary drug delivery applications: A critical review. *Discov. Nano* **2023**, *18*, 157. [CrossRef]
54. Mitchell, M.J.; Billingsley, M.M.; Haley, R.M.; Wechsler, M.E.; Peppas, N.A.; Langer, R. Engineering precision nanoparticles for drug delivery. *Nat. Rev. Drug Discov.* **2021**, *20*, 101–124. [CrossRef]

55. Morillas-Becerill, L.; De Cola, L.; Zuidema, J.M. Inorganic nanoparticle empowered biomaterial hybrids: Engineered payload release. *Front. Nanotechnol.* **2022**, *4*, 999923. [CrossRef]
56. de Pablo, E.; Fernández-García, R.; Ballesteros, M.P.; Torrado, J.J.; Serrano, D.R. Nebulised antibiotherapy: Conventional versus nanotechnology-based approaches, is targeting at a nano scale a difficult subject? *Ann. Transl. Med.* **2017**, *5*, 448. [CrossRef] [PubMed]
57. Patil, J.S.; Sarasija, S. Pulmonary drug delivery strategies: A concise, systematic review. *Lung India* **2012**, *29*, 44–49. [PubMed]
58. Schuster, B.S.; Suk, J.S.; Woodworth, G.F.; Hanes, J. Nanoparticle diffusion in respiratory mucus from humans without lung disease. *Biomaterials* **2013**, *34*, 3439–3446. [CrossRef] [PubMed]
59. Schneider, C.S.; Xu, Q.; Boylan, N.J.; Chisholm, J.; Tang, B.C.; Schuster, B.S.; Henning, A.; Ensign, L.M.; Lee, E.; Adstamongkonkul, P.; et al. Nanoparticles that do not adhere to mucus provide uniform and long-lasting drug delivery to airways following inhalation. *Sci. Adv.* **2017**, *3*, e1601556. [CrossRef] [PubMed]
60. Furuyama, A.; Kanno, S.; Kobayashi, T.; Hirano, S. Extrapulmonary translocation of intratracheally instilled fine and ultrafine particles via direct and alveolar macrophage-associated routes. *Arch. Toxicol.* **2009**, *83*, 429–437. [CrossRef]
61. Chono, S.; Tanino, T.; Seki, T.; Morimoto, K. Influence of particle size on drug delivery to rat alveolar macrophages following pulmonary administration of ciprofloxacin incorporated into liposomes. *J. Drug Target.* **2006**, *14*, 557–566. [CrossRef]
62. Hu, X.; Yang, F.-F.; Quan, L.-H.; Liu, C.-Y.; Liu, X.-M.; Ehrhardt, C.; Liao, Y.-H. Pulmonary delivered polymeric micelles—Pharmacokinetic evaluation and biodistribution studies. *Eur. J. Pharm. Biopharm.* **2014**, *88*, 1064–1075. [CrossRef]
63. Kreyling, W.G.; Semmler, M.; Erbe, F.; Mayer, P.; Takenaka, S.; Schulz, H.; Oberdörster, G.; Ziesenis, A. Translocation of ultrafine insoluble iridium particles from lung epithelium to extrapulmonary organs is size dependent but very low. *J. Toxicol. Environ. Health—Part A* **2002**, *65*, 1513–1530. [CrossRef]
64. Choi, H.S.; Ashitate, Y.; Lee, J.H.; Kim, S.H.; Matsui, A.; Insin, N.; Bawendi, M.G.; Semmler-Behnke, M.; Frangioni, J.V.; Tsuda, A. Rapid translocation of nanoparticles from the lung airspaces to the body. *Nat. Biotechnol.* **2010**, *28*, 1300–1303. [CrossRef]
65. Mohammad, A.K.; Amayreh, L.K.; Mazzara, J.M.; Reineke, J.J. Rapid Lymph Accumulation of Polystyrene Nanoparticles Following Pulmonary Administration. *Pharm. Res.* **2013**, *30*, 424–434. [CrossRef]
66. Garapaty, A.; Champion, J.A. Tunable particles alter macrophage uptake based on combinatorial effects of physical properties. *Bioeng. Transl. Med.* **2017**, *2*, 92–101. [CrossRef] [PubMed]
67. Zellnitz, S.; Zellnitz, L.; Müller, M.T.; Meindl, C.; Schröttner, H.; Fröhlich, E. Impact of drug particle shape on permeability and cellular uptake in the lung. *Eur. J. Pharm. Sci.* **2019**, *139*, 105065. [CrossRef] [PubMed]
68. Hassan, M.S.; Lau, R.W.M. Effect of Particle Shape on Dry Particle Inhalation: Study of Flowability, Aerosolization, and Deposition Properties. *AAPS PharmSciTech* **2009**, *10*, 1252–1262. [CrossRef] [PubMed]
69. Shukla, S.K.; Sarode, A.; Kanabar, D.D.; Muth, A.; Kunda, N.K.; Mitragotri, S.; Gupta, V. Bioinspired particle engineering for non-invasive inhaled drug delivery to the lungs. *Mater. Sci. Eng. C* **2021**, *128*, 112324. [CrossRef] [PubMed]
70. Huang, Z.; Kłodzińska, S.N.; Wan, F.; Nielsen, H.M. Nanoparticle-mediated pulmonary drug delivery: State of the art towards efficient treatment of recalcitrant respiratory tract bacterial infections. *Drug Deliv. Transl. Res.* **2021**, *11*, 1634–1654. [CrossRef]
71. Murgia, X.; Loretz, B.; Hartwig, O.; Hittinger, M.; Lehr, C.-M. The role of mucus on drug transport and its potential to affect therapeutic outcomes. *Adv. Drug Deliv. Rev.* **2018**, *124*, 82–97. [CrossRef]
72. Dawson, M.; Wirtz, D.; Hanes, J. Enhanced Viscoelasticity of Human Cystic Fibrotic Sputum Correlates with Increasing Microheterogeneity in Particle Transport. *J. Biol. Chem.* **2003**, *278*, 50393–50401. [CrossRef]
73. Seydoux, E.; Rodriguez-Lorenzo, L.; Blom, R.A.M.; Stumbles, P.A.; Petri-Fink, A.; Rothen-Rutishauser, B.M.; Blank, F.; von Garnier, C. Pulmonary delivery of cationic gold nanoparticles boost antigen-specific CD4+ T Cell Proliferation. *Nanomed. Nanotechnol. Biol. Med.* **2016**, *12*, 1815–1826. [CrossRef]
74. Areny-Balagueró, A.; Mekseriwattana, W.; Camprubí-Rimblas, M.; Stephany, A.; Roldan, A.; Solé-Porta, A.; Artigas, A.; Closa, D.; Roig, A. Fluorescent PLGA Nanocarriers for Pulmonary Administration: Influence of the Surface Charge. *Pharmaceutics* **2022**, *14*, 1447. [CrossRef]
75. Kreyling, W.G.; Hirn, S.; Möller, W.; Schleh, C.; Wenk, A.; Celik, G.; Lipka, J.; Schäffler, M.; Haberl, N.; Johnston, B.D.; et al. Air–Blood Barrier Translocation of Tracheally Instilled Gold Nanoparticles Inversely Depends on Particle Size. *ACS Nano* **2014**, *8*, 222–233. [CrossRef]
76. George, I.; Naudin, G.; Boland, S.; Mornet, S.; Contremoulins, V.; Beugnon, K.; Martinon, L.; Lambert, O.; Baeza-Squiban, A. Metallic oxide nanoparticle translocation across the human bronchial epithelial barrier. *Nanoscale* **2015**, *7*, 4529–4544. [CrossRef] [PubMed]
77. Fromen, C.A.; Rahhal, T.B.; Robbins, G.R.; Kai, M.P.; Shen, T.W.; Luft, J.C.; DeSimone, J.M. Nanoparticle surface charge impacts distribution, uptake and lymph node trafficking by pulmonary antigen-presenting cells. *Nanomed. Nanotechnol. Biol. Med.* **2016**, *12*, 677–687. [CrossRef] [PubMed]
78. Witten, J.; Samad, T.; Ribbeck, K. Selective permeability of mucus barriers. *Curr. Opin. Biotechnol.* **2018**, *52*, 124–133. [CrossRef] [PubMed]
79. Wang, Y.-Y.; Lai, S.K.; Suk, J.S.; Pace, A.; Cone, R.; Hanes, J. Addressing the PEG Mucoadhesivity Paradox to Engineer Nanoparticles that "Slip" through the Human Mucus Barrier. *Angew. Chem. Int. Ed.* **2008**, *47*, 9726–9729. [CrossRef]
80. Huang, X.; Chisholm, J.; Zhuang, J.; Xiao, Y.; Duncan, G.; Chen, X.; Suk, J.S.; Hanes, J. Protein nanocages that penetrate airway mucus and tumor tissue. *Proc. Natl. Acad. Sci. USA* **2017**, *114*, E6595–E6602. [CrossRef]

81. Murata, M.; Tahara, K.; Takeuchi, H. Real-time in vivo imaging of surface-modified liposomes to evaluate their behavior after pulmonary administration. *Eur. J. Pharm. Biopharm.* **2014**, *86*, 115–119. [CrossRef]
82. Weers, J.; Clark, A. The Impact of Inspiratory Flow Rate on Drug Delivery to the Lungs with Dry Powder Inhalers. *Pharm. Res.* **2017**, *34*, 507–528. [CrossRef]
83. Ahmadi, K.; Gharibi, Z.; Davoodian, P.; Gouklani, H.; Hassaniazad, M.; Ahmadi, N. The Effect of Smoking on the Increase of Infectious Diseases. *Tob. Health* **2022**, *1*, 100–106. [CrossRef]
84. Jo, Y.S. Long-Term Outcome of Chronic Obstructive Pulmonary Disease: A Review. *Tuberc. Respir. Dis.* **2022**, *85*, 289–301. [CrossRef]
85. Shah, B.K.; Singh, B.; Wang, Y.; Xie, S.; Wang, C. Mucus Hypersecretion in Chronic Obstructive Pulmonary Disease and Its Treatment. *Mediat. Inflamm.* **2023**, *2023*, 8840594. [CrossRef]
86. Taccetti, G.; Francalanci, M.; Pizzamiglio, G.; Messore, B.; Carnovale, V.; Cimino, G.; Cipolli, M. Cystic Fibrosis: Recent Insights into Inhaled Antibiotic Treatment and Future Perspectives. *Antibiotics* **2021**, *10*, 338. [CrossRef] [PubMed]
87. Papi, A.; Blasi, F.; Canonica, G.W.; Morandi, L.; Richeldi, L.; Rossi, A. Treatment strategies for asthma: Reshaping the concept of asthma management. *Allergy Asthma Clin. Immunol.* **2020**, *16*, 75. [CrossRef] [PubMed]
88. Kumbhar, P.; Manjappa, A.; Shah, R.; Jha, N.K.; Singh, S.K.; Dua, K.; Disouza, J.; Patravale, V. Inhalation delivery of repurposed drugs for lung cancer: Approaches, benefits and challenges. *J. Control. Release* **2022**, *341*, 1–15. [CrossRef] [PubMed]
89. Elahe, D.-N. An Overview of Bacterial Respiratory Tract Infections and their Etiologies. *J. Med. Bacteriol.* **2023**, *11*, 36–46. [CrossRef]
90. Thomas, M.; Bomar, P.A. Upper Respiratory Tract Infection. In *StatPearls*; StatPearls Publishing LLC.: Treasure Island, FL, USA, 2024.
91. Mariyam, N.; Reji, S.; Saijan, S.; George, S.; Subscription, C. Assessment of Antibiotic Sensitivity Pattern in RTI Patients in a Secondary Care Hospital. *J. Pharma Innov.* **2020**, *1*, 41–47.
92. Troeger, C.; Blacker, B.; Khalil, I.A.; Rao, P.C.; Cao, J.; Zimsen, S.R.; Albertson, S.B.; Deshpande, A.; Farag, T.; Abebe, Z.; et al. Estimates of the global, regional, and national morbidity, mortality, and aetiologies of lower respiratory infections in 195 countries, 1990–2016: A systematic analysis for the Global Burden of Disease Study 2016. *Lancet Infect. Dis.* **2018**, *18*, 1191–1210. [CrossRef]
93. Chee, E.; García, A.J. Biomaterial therapeutic strategies for treatment of bacterial lung infections. *Biofilm* **2023**, *5*, 100111. [CrossRef]
94. Cantón, R.; Gottlieb, T.; Coombs, G.W.; Woo, P.C.Y.; Korman, T.M.; Garcia-Castillo, M.; Daley, D.; Bauer, K.A.; Wong, M.; Wolf, D.J.; et al. Antimicrobial surveillance: A 20-year history of the SMART approach to addressing global antimicrobial resistance into the future. *Int. J. Antimicrob. Agents* **2023**, *62*, 107014. [CrossRef]
95. Li, J.; Zheng, H.; Leung, S.S.Y. Pulmonary Delivery of Emerging Antibacterials for Bacterial Lung Infections Treatment. *Pharm. Res.* **2023**, *40*, 1057–1072. [CrossRef]
96. Muthu, V.; Sehgal, I.S.; Agarwal, R. Aerosolized Antifungals for the Treatment of Pulmonary Fungal Diseases. *Curr. Fungal Infect. Rep.* **2024**, *18*, 154–162. [CrossRef]
97. Feng, X.; Shi, Y.; Zhang, Y.; Lei, F.; Ren, R.; Tang, X. Opportunities and Challenges for Inhalable Nanomedicine Formulations in Respiratory Diseases: A Review. *Int. J. Nanomed.* **2024**, *19*, 1509–1538. [CrossRef] [PubMed]
98. Khan, O.; Chaudary, N. The Use of Amikacin Liposome Inhalation Suspension (Arikayce) in the Treatment of Refractory Nontuberculous Mycobacterial Lung Disease in Adults. *Drug Des. Dev. Ther.* **2020**, *14*, 2287–2294. [CrossRef] [PubMed]
99. Shirley, M. Amikacin Liposome Inhalation Suspension: A Review in Mycobacterium avium Complex Lung Disease. *Drugs* **2019**, *79*, 555–562. [CrossRef] [PubMed]
100. Murray, C.J.L.; Aravkin, A.Y.; Zheng, P.; Abbafati, C.; Abbas, K.M.; Abbasi-Kangevari, M.; Abd-Allah, F.; Abdelalim, A.; Abdollahi, M.; Abdollahpour, I.; et al. Global burden of 87 risk factors in 204 countries and territories, 1990–2019: A systematic analysis for the Global Burden of Disease Study 2019. *Lancet* **2020**, *396*, 1223–1249. [CrossRef]
101. Pneumonia. 2022. Available online: https://medlineplus.gov/spanish/pneumonia.html (accessed on 25 April 2023).
102. Lawn, S.D.; Zumla, A.I. Tuberculosis. *Lancet* **2011**, *378*, 57–72. [CrossRef]
103. Villar-Hernández, R.; Ghodousi, A.; Konstantynovska, O.; Duarte, R.; Lange, C.; Raviglione, M. Tuberculosis: Current challenges and beyond. *Breathe* **2023**, *19*, 220166. [CrossRef]
104. WHO. *Global Tuberculosis Report 2023*; World Health Organization: Geneva, Switzerland, 2023.
105. Tuberculosis. 2022. Available online: https://www.who.int/news-room/fact-sheets/detail/tuberculosis (accessed on 21 November 2022).
106. Chakaya, J.; Khan, M.; Ntoumi, F.; Aklillu, E.; Fatima, R.; Mwaba, P.; Kapata, N.; Mfinanga, S.; Hasnain, S.E.; Katoto, P.D.M.C.; et al. Global Tuberculosis Report 2020—Reflections on the Global TB burden, treatment and prevention efforts. *Int. J. Infect. Dis.* **2021**, *113*, S7–S12. [CrossRef]
107. Grotz, E.; Tateosian, N.; Amiano, N.; Cagel, M.; Bernabeu, E.; Chiappetta, D.A.; Moretton, M.A. Nanotechnology in Tuberculosis: State of the Art and the Challenges Ahead. *Pharm. Res.* **2018**, *35*, 213. [CrossRef]
108. Eldholm, V.; Balloux, F. Antimicrobial Resistance in Mycobacterium tuberculosis: The Odd One Out. *Trends Microbiol.* **2016**, *24*, 637–648. [CrossRef]
109. Grange, J.M.; Zumla, A. The global emergency of tuberculosis: What is the cause? *J. R. Soc. Promot. Health* **2002**, *122*, 78–81. [CrossRef]

110. Garcia-Prats, A.J.; Willemse, M.; Seifart, H.I.; Jordaan, A.M.; Werely, C.J.; Donald, P.R.; Schaaf, H.S. Acquired drug resistance during inadequate therapy in a young child with tuberculosis. *Pediatr. Infect. Dis. J.* **2014**, *33*, 883–885. [CrossRef] [PubMed]
111. Nasiruddin, M.; Neyaz, M.K.; Das, S. Nanotechnology-Based Approach in Tuberculosis Treatment. *Tuberc. Res. Treat.* **2017**, *2017*, 4920209. [CrossRef] [PubMed]
112. Singh, V.K.; Chau, E.; Mishra, A.; DeAnda, A.; Hegde, V.L.; Sastry, J.K.; Haviland, D.; Jagannath, C.; Godin, B.; Khan, A. CD44 receptor targeted nanoparticles augment immunity against tuberculosis in mice. *J. Control. Release* **2022**, *349*, 796–811. [CrossRef] [PubMed]
113. Cirillo, J.D.; Kong, Y. *Tuberculosis Host-Pathogen Interactions*; Springer: Berlin/Heidelberg, Germany, 2019.
114. Chai, Q.; Zhang, Y.; Liu, C.H. Mycobacterium tuberculosis: An adaptable pathogen associated with multiple human diseases. *Front. Cell. Infect. Microbiol.* **2018**, *8*, 158. [CrossRef]
115. Grotz, E.; Tateosian, N.L.; Salgueiro, J.; Bernabeu, E.; Gonzalez, L.; Manca, M.L.; Amiano, N.; Valenti, D.; Manconi, M.; García, V.; et al. Pulmonary delivery of rifampicin-loaded soluplus micelles against Mycobacterium tuberculosis. *J. Drug Deliv. Sci. Technol.* **2019**, *53*, 101170. [CrossRef]
116. Chae, J.; Choi, Y.; Tanaka, M.; Choi, J. Inhalable nanoparticles delivery targeting alveolar macrophages for the treatment of pulmonary tuberculosis. *J. Biosci. Bioeng.* **2021**, *132*, 543–551. [CrossRef]
117. Baranyai, Z.; Soria-Carrera, H.; Alleva, M.; Millán-Placer, A.C.; Lucía, A.; Martín-Rapún, R.; Aínsa, J.A.; de la Fuente, J.M. Nanotechnology-Based Targeted Drug Delivery: An Emerging Tool to Overcome Tuberculosis. *Adv. Ther.* **2021**, *4*, 2000113. [CrossRef]
118. Ma, C.; Wu, M.; Ye, W.; Huang, Z.; Ma, X.; Wang, W.; Wang, W.; Huang, Y.; Pan, X.; Wu, C. Inhalable solid lipid nanoparticles for intracellular tuberculosis infection therapy: Macrophage-targeting and pH-sensitive properties. *Drug Deliv. Transl. Res.* **2021**, *11*, 1218–1235. [CrossRef]
119. Viswanathan, V.; Pharande, R.; Bannalikar, A.; Gupta, P.; Gupta, U.; Mukne, A. Inhalable liposomes of Glycyrrhiza glabra extract for use in tuberculosis: Formulation, in vitro characterization, in vivo lung deposition, and in vivo pharmacodynamic studies. *Drug Dev. Ind. Pharm.* **2019**, *45*, 11–20. [CrossRef]
120. Silva, J.P.; Gonçalves, C.; Costa, C.; Sousa, J.; Silva-Gomes, R.; Castro, A.G.; Pedrosa, J.; Appelberg, R.; Gama, F.M. Delivery of LLKKK18 loaded into self-assembling hyaluronic acid nanogel for tuberculosis treatment. *J. Control. Release* **2016**, *235*, 112–124. [CrossRef]
121. Wu, T.; Liao, W.; Wang, W.; Zhou, J.; Tan, W.; Xiang, W.; Zhang, J.; Guo, L.; Chen, T.; Ma, D.; et al. Genipin-crosslinked carboxymethyl chitosan nanogel for lung-targeted delivery of isoniazid and rifampin. *Carbohydr. Polym.* **2018**, *197*, 403–413. [CrossRef] [PubMed]
122. Vilchèze, C.; Kim, J.; Jacobs, W.R., Jr. Vitamin C Potentiates the Killing of Mycobacterium tuberculosis by the First-Line Tuberculosis Drugs Isoniazid and Rifampin in Mice. *Antimicrob. Agents Chemother.* **2018**, *62*, 10-1128. [CrossRef] [PubMed]
123. Scolari, I.R.; Páez, P.L.; Sánchez-Borzone, M.E.; Granero, G.E. Promising Chitosan-Coated Alginate-Tween 80 Nanoparticles as Rifampicin Coadministered Ascorbic Acid Delivery Carrier Against Mycobacterium tuberculosis. *AAPS PharmSciTech* **2019**, *20*, 67. [CrossRef] [PubMed]
124. Sattar, S.B.A.; Nguyen, A.D.; Sharma, S. Bacterial Pneumonia. In *StatPearls*; StatPearls Publishing LLC.: Treasure Island, FL, USA, 2024.
125. Garg, M.; Prabhakar, N.; Gulati, A.; Agarwal, R.; Dhooria, S. Spectrum of imaging findings in pulmonary infections. Part 1: Bacterial and viral. *Pol. J. Radiol.* **2019**, *84*, e205. [CrossRef]
126. Eshwara, V.K.; Mukhopadhyay, C.; Rello, J. Community-acquired bacterial pneumonia in adults: An update. *Indian J. Med. Res.* **2020**, *151*, 287–302. [CrossRef]
127. Sabuj, M.Z.R.; Dargaville, T.R.; Nissen, L.; Islam, N. Inhaled ciprofloxacin-loaded poly(2-ethyl-2-oxazoline) nanoparticles from dry powder inhaler formulation for the potential treatment of lower respiratory tract infections. *PLoS ONE* **2021**, *16*, e0261720. [CrossRef]
128. Falciani, C.; Zevolini, F.; Brunetti, J.; Riolo, G.; Gracia, R.; Marradi, M.; Loinaz, I.; Ziemann, C.; Cossío, U.; Llop, J.; et al. Antimicrobial Peptide-Loaded Nanoparticles as Inhalation Therapy for Pseudomonas aeruginosa Infections. *Int. J. Nanomed.* **2020**, *15*, 1117–1128. [CrossRef]
129. Derbali, R.M.; Aoun, V.; Moussa, G.; Frei, G.; Tehrani, S.F.; Del'Orto, J.C.; Hildgen, P.; Roullin, V.G.; Chain, J.L. Tailored Nanocarriers for the Pulmonary Delivery of Levofloxacin against Pseudomonas aeruginosa: A Comparative Study. *Mol. Pharm.* **2019**, *16*, 1906–1916. [CrossRef]
130. Gupta, P.V.; Nirwane, A.M.; Nagarsenker, M.S. Inhalable Levofloxacin Liposomes Complemented with Lysozyme for Treatment of Pulmonary Infection in Rats: Effective Antimicrobial and Antibiofilm Strategy. *AAPS PharmSciTech* **2018**, *19*, 1454–1467. [CrossRef]
131. Li, Y.; Tang, C.; Zhang, E.; Yang, L. Electrostatically entrapped colistin liposomes for the treatment of Pseudomonas aeruginosa infection. *Pharm. Dev. Technol.* **2017**, *22*, 436–444. [CrossRef]
132. Palmieri, F.; Koutsokera, A.; Bernasconi, E.; Junier, P.; von Garnier, C.; Ubags, N. Recent Advances in Fungal Infections: From Lung Ecology to Therapeutic Strategies with a Focus on *Aspergillus* spp. *Front. Med.* **2022**, *9*, 832510. [CrossRef] [PubMed]
133. Bongomin, F.; Gago, S.; Oladele, R.O.; Denning, D.W. Global and multi-national prevalence of fungal diseases—Estimate precision. *J. Fungi* **2017**, *3*, 57. [CrossRef] [PubMed]

134. Ben-Ami, R. Systemic Antifungal Therapy for Invasive Pulmonary Infections. *J. Fungi* **2023**, *9*, 144. [CrossRef] [PubMed]
135. McKeny, P.T.; Nessel, T.A.; Zito, P.M. Antifungal Antibiotics. In *StatPearls*; StatPearls Publishing LLC.: Treasure Island, FL, USA, 2024.
136. Jenks, J.D.; Hoenigl, M. Treatment of Aspergillosis. *J. Fungi* **2018**, *4*, 98. [CrossRef] [PubMed]
137. Fernández-García, R.; de Pablo, E.; Ballesteros, M.P.; Serrano, D.R. Unmet clinical needs in the treatment of systemic fungal infections: The role of amphotericin B and drug targeting. *Int. J. Pharm.* **2017**, *525*, 139–148. [CrossRef] [PubMed]
138. Kaur, R.; Dennison, S.R.; Burrow, A.J.; Rudramurthy, S.M.; Swami, R.; Gorki, V.; Katare, O.P.; Kaushik, A.; Singh, B.; Singh, K.K. Nebulised surface-active hybrid nanoparticles of voriconazole for pulmonary Aspergillosis demonstrate clathrin-mediated cellular uptake, improved antifungal efficacy and lung retention. *J. Nanobiotechnology* **2021**, *19*, 19. [CrossRef]
139. Ali, E.M.; Abdallah, B.M. Effective Inhibition of Invasive Pulmonary Aspergillosis by Silver Nanoparticles Biosynthesized with Artemisia sieberi Leaf Extract. *Nanomaterials* **2021**, *12*, 51. [CrossRef]
140. Chougule, M.; Padhi, B.; Misra, A. Development of Spray Dried Liposomal Dry Powder Inhaler of Dapsone. *AAPS PharmSciTech* **2008**, *9*, 47–53. [CrossRef]
141. Gilani, K.; Moazeni, E.; Ramezanli, T.; Amini, M.; Fazeli, M.R.; Jamalifar, H. Development of Respirable Nanomicelle Carriers for Delivery of Amphotericin B by Jet Nebulization. *J. Pharm. Sci.* **2011**, *100*, 252–259. [CrossRef]
142. Nasr, M.; Nawaz, S.; Elhissi, A. Amphotericin B lipid nanoemulsion aerosols for targeting peripheral respiratory airways via nebulization. *Int. J. Pharm.* **2012**, *436*, 611–616. [CrossRef]
143. Vyas, S.P.; Quraishi, S.; Gupta, S.; Jaganathan, K.S. Aerosolized liposome-based delivery of amphotericin B to alveolar macrophages. *Int. J. Pharm.* **2005**, *296*, 12–25. [CrossRef] [PubMed]
144. Yang, W.; Tam, J.; Miller, D.A.; Zhou, J.; McConville, J.T.; Johnston, K.P.; Williams, R.O. High bioavailability from nebulized itraconazole nanoparticle dispersions with biocompatible stabilizers. *Int. J. Pharm.* **2008**, *361*, 177–188. [CrossRef] [PubMed]
145. van Doorn, H.R.; Yu, H. Viral Respiratory Infections. In *Hunter's Tropical Medicine and Emerging Infectious Diseases*; Elservier: Amsterdam, The Netherlands, 2020; pp. 284–288. [CrossRef]
146. Zhou, J.; Krishnan, N.; Jiang, Y.; Fang, R.H.; Zhang, L. Nanotechnology for virus treatment. *Nano Today* **2021**, *36*, 101031. [CrossRef] [PubMed]
147. Rao, L.; Tian, R.; Chen, X. Cell-membrane-mimicking nanodecoys against infectious diseases. *ACS Nano* **2020**, *14*, 2569–2574. [CrossRef]
148. Symptoms of COVID-19. 2022. Available online: https://www.mayoclinic.org/diseases-conditions/coronavirus/symptoms-causes/syc-20479963 (accessed on 24 April 2023).
149. McKinnon, T.; Watson, A.; Richards, L.; Sears, J.; Brookes, M.J.; Green, C.A. The Volunteers in Research Programme: Supporting COVID-19 research and improving medical training in parallel. *Clin. Med.* **2021**, *21*, 182–188. [CrossRef]
150. Cascella, M.; Rajnik, M.; Aleem, A.; Dulebohn, S.C.; Di Napoli, R. Features, Evaluation, and Treatment of Coronavirus (COVID-19). In *StatPearls*; StatPearls Publishing LLC.: Treasure Island, FL, USA, 2024.
151. Docherty, A.B.; Harrison, E.M.; Green, C.A.; Hardwick, H.E.; Pius, R.; Norman, L.; Holden, K.A.; Read, J.M.; Dondelinger, F.; Carson, G. Features of 20 133 UK patients in hospital with COVID-19 using the ISARIC WHO Clinical Characterisation Protocol: Prospective observational cohort study. *Bmj* **2020**, *369*, m1985. [CrossRef]
152. Abdellatif, A.A.H.; Tawfeek, H.M.; Abdelfattah, A.; El-Saber Batiha, G.; Hetta, H.F. Recent updates in COVID-19 with emphasis on inhalation therapeutics: Nanostructured and targeting systems. *J. Drug Deliv. Sci. Technol.* **2021**, *63*, 102435. [CrossRef]
153. Grein, J.; Ohmagari, N.; Shin, D.; Diaz, G.; Asperges, E.; Castagna, A.; Feldt, T.; Green, G.; Green, M.L.; Lescure, F.-X.; et al. Compassionate Use of Remdesivir for Patients with Severe COVID-19. *N. Engl. J. Med.* **2020**, *382*, 2327–2336. [CrossRef]
154. Deb, S.; Reeves, A.A.; Hopefl, R.; Bejusca, R. ADME and Pharmacokinetic Properties of Remdesivir: Its Drug Interaction Potential. *Pharmaceuticals* **2021**, *14*, 655. [CrossRef]
155. Lan, J.; Ge, J.; Yu, J.; Shan, S.; Zhou, H.; Fan, S.; Zhang, Q.; Shi, X.; Wang, Q.; Zhang, L. Structure of the SARS-CoV-2 spike receptor-binding domain bound to the ACE2 receptor. *Nature* **2020**, *581*, 215–220. [CrossRef]
156. Sanna, V.; Satta, S.; Hsiai, T.; Sechi, M. Development of targeted nanoparticles loaded with antiviral drugs for SARS-CoV-2 inhibition. *Eur. J. Med. Chem.* **2022**, *231*, 114121. [CrossRef]
157. Meng, Q.-F.; Tai, W.; Tian, M.; Zhuang, X.; Pan, Y.; Lai, J.; Xu, Y.; Xu, Z.; Li, M.; Zhao, G.; et al. Inhalation delivery of dexamethasone with iSEND nanoparticles attenuates the COVID-19 cytokine storm in mice and nonhuman primates. *Sci. Adv.* **2023**, *9*, eadg3277. [CrossRef]
158. Fouad, S.A.; Malaak, F.A.; Teaima, M.H.; Omar, S.; Kutkat, O.; Elhabal, S.F.; El-Nabarawi, M. Novel inhalable nano-based/microparticles for enhanced sustained pulmonary delivery of remdesivir—A patient malleable treatment for coronaviruses infection: In vitro aerosolization, cytotoxicity assays and antiviral activity studies. *J. Drug Deliv. Sci. Technol.* **2024**, *101*, 106196. [CrossRef]
159. Halevas, E.; Mavroidi, B.; Kokotidou, C.; Moschona, A.; Sagnou, M.; Mitraki, A.; Litsardakis, G.; Pelecanou, M. Remdesivir-loaded bis-MPA hyperbranched dendritic nanocarriers for pulmonary delivery. *J. Drug Deliv. Sci. Technol.* **2022**, *75*, 103625. [CrossRef]
160. Ali, A.S.; Alrashedi, M.G.; Ahmed, O.A.; Ibrahim, I.M. Pulmonary Delivery of Hydroxychloroquine Nanostructured Lipid Carrier as a Potential Treatment of COVID-19. *Polymers* **2022**, *14*, 2616. [CrossRef]

161. Chang, C.; Lu, C.; Zheng, Y.; Ji, J.; Lin, L.; Chen, L.; Chen, Z.; Chen, R. Sonication-Assisted Self-Assembled Resveratrol Nanoparticles with Enhanced Antiviral and Anti-inflammatory Activity against Respiratory Syncytial Virus-Induced Pneumonia. *ACS Appl. Mater. Interfaces* **2024**, *16*, 50442–50458. [CrossRef]
162. Peng, J.; Wang, Q.; Guo, M.; Liu, C.; Chen, X.; Tao, L.; Zhang, K.; Shen, X. Development of Inhalable Chitosan-Coated Oxymatrine Liposomes to Alleviate RSV-Infected Mice. *Int. J. Mol. Sci.* **2022**, *23*, 15909. [CrossRef]
163. Gil, C.H.; Oh, C.; Lee, J.; Jang, M.; Han, J.; Cho, S.-D.; Park, S.-H.; Park, J.-H.; Kim, H.J. Inhalation Delivery of Interferon-λ-Loaded Pulmonary Surfactant Nanoparticles Induces Rapid Antiviral Immune Responses in the Lung. *ACS Appl. Mater. Interfaces* **2024**, *16*, 11147–11158. [CrossRef]
164. Cojocaru, F.-D.; Botezat, D.; Gardikiotis, I.; Uritu, C.-M.; Dodi, G.; Trandafir, L.; Rezus, C.; Rezus, E.; Tamba, B.-I.; Mihai, C.-T. Nanomaterials Designed for Antiviral Drug Delivery Transport across Biological Barriers. *Pharmaceutics* **2020**, *12*, 171. [CrossRef]
165. Chapter 14—Vaccination. In *Primer to the Immune Response*, 2nd ed.; Mak, T.W., Saunders, M.E., Jett, B.D., Eds.; Academic Cell: Boston, MA, USA, 2014; pp. 333–375. [CrossRef]
166. Gholizadeh, O.; Akbarzadeh, S.; Ghazanfari Hashemi, M.; Gholami, M.; Amini, P.; Yekanipour, Z.; Tabatabaie, R.; Yasamineh, S.; Hosseini, P.; Poortahmasebi, V. Hepatitis A: Viral Structure, Classification, Life Cycle, Clinical Symptoms, Diagnosis Error, and Vaccination. *Can. J. Infect. Dis. Med. Microbiol.* **2023**, *2023*, 4263309. [CrossRef]
167. Poon, C.; Patel, A.A. Organic and inorganic nanoparticle vaccines for prevention of infectious diseases. *Nano Express* **2020**, *1*, 012001. [CrossRef]
168. Shichinohe, S.; Watanabe, T. Advances in Adjuvanted Influenza Vaccines. *Vaccines* **2023**, *11*, 1391. [CrossRef] [PubMed]
169. Vu, M.N.; Kelly, H.G.; Kent, S.J.; Wheatley, A.K. Current and future nanoparticle vaccines for COVID-19. *eBioMedicine* **2021**, *74*, 103699. [CrossRef] [PubMed]
170. Spikevax, Data Sheet. 2022. Available online: https://www.ema.europa.eu/en/documents/product-information/spikevax-previously-covid-19-vaccine-moderna-epar-product-information_en.pdf (accessed on 24 April 2023).
171. Comirnaty, Data Sheet. 2022. Available online: https://www.ema.europa.eu/en/documents/product-information/comirnaty-epar-product-information_en.pdf (accessed on 24 April 2023).
172. Klimek, L.; Novak, N.; Hamelmann, E.; Werfel, T.; Wagenmann, M.; Taube, C.; Bauer, A.; Merk, H.; Rabe, U.; Jung, K.; et al. Severe allergic reactions after COVID-19 vaccination with the Pfizer/BioNTech vaccine in Great Britain and USA: Position statement of the German Allergy Societies: Medical Association of German Allergologists (AeDA), German Society for Allergology and Clinical Immunology (DGAKI) and Society for Pediatric Allergology and Environmental Medicine (GPA). *Allergo J. Int.* **2021**, *30*, 51–55. [CrossRef]
173. Hatziantoniou, S.; Maltezou, H.C.; Tsakris, A.; Poland, G.A.; Anastassopoulou, C. Anaphylactic reactions to mRNA COVID-19 vaccines: A call for further study. *Vaccine* **2021**, *39*, 2605–2607. [CrossRef]
174. Lavelle, E.C.; Ward, R.W. Mucosal vaccines—Fortifying the frontiers. *Nat. Rev. Immunol.* **2022**, *22*, 236–250. [CrossRef]
175. Tang, W.; Zhang, Y.; Zhu, G. Pulmonary delivery of mucosal nanovaccines. *Nanoscale* **2022**, *14*, 263–276. [CrossRef]
176. Al-Halifa, S.; Gauthier, L.; Arpin, D.; Bourgault, S.; Archambault, D. Nanoparticle-Based Vaccines Against Respiratory Viruses. *Front. Immunol.* **2019**, *10*, 22. [CrossRef]
177. Wei, C.-J.; Crank, M.C.; Shiver, J.; Graham, B.S.; Mascola, J.R.; Nabel, G.J. Next-generation influenza vaccines: Opportunities and challenges. *Nat. Rev. Drug Discov.* **2020**, *19*, 239–252. [CrossRef]
178. Wang, S.; Ding, P.; Shen, L.; Fan, D.; Cheng, H.; Huo, J.; Wei, X.; He, H.; Zhang, G. Inhalable hybrid nanovaccines with virus-biomimetic structure boost protective immune responses against SARS-CoV-2 variants. *J. Nanobiotechnology* **2024**, *22*, 76. [CrossRef]
179. Zheng, B.; Peng, W.; Guo, M.; Huang, M.; Gu, Y.; Wang, T.; Ni, G.; Ming, D. Inhalable nanovaccine with biomimetic coronavirus structure to trigger mucosal immunity of respiratory tract against COVID-19. *Chem. Eng. J.* **2021**, *418*, 129392. [CrossRef] [PubMed]
180. Lokugamage, M.P.; Vanover, D.; Beyersdorf, J.; Hatit, M.Z.C.; Rotolo, L.; Echeverri, E.S.; Peck, H.E.; Ni, H.; Yoon, J.-K.; Kim, Y.; et al. Optimization of lipid nanoparticles for the delivery of nebulized therapeutic mRNA to the lungs. *Nat. Biomed. Eng.* **2021**, *5*, 1059–1068. [CrossRef] [PubMed]
181. Lopez, C.E.; Zacharias, Z.R.; Ross, K.A.; Narasimhan, B.; Waldschmidt, T.J.; Legge, K.L. Polyanhydride nanovaccine against H3N2 influenza A virus generates mucosal resident and systemic immunity promoting protection. *Npj Vaccines* **2024**, *9*, 96. [CrossRef] [PubMed]
182. Bray, F.; Laversanne, M.; Sung, H.; Ferlay, J.; Siegel, R.L.; Soerjomataram, I.; Jemal, A. Global cancer statistics 2022: GLOBOCAN estimates of incidence and mortality worldwide for 36 cancers in 185 countries. *CA Cancer J. Clin.* **2024**, *74*, 229–263. [CrossRef]
183. Seguin, L.; Durandy, M.; Feral, C.C. Lung Adenocarcinoma Tumor Origin: A Guide for Personalized Medicine. *Cancers* **2022**, *14*, 1759. [CrossRef]
184. Alexander, M.; Kim, S.Y.; Cheng, H. Update 2020: Management of Non-Small Cell Lung Cancer. *Lung* **2020**, *198*, 897–907. [CrossRef]
185. Sardeli, C.; Zarogoulidis, P.; Kosmidis, C.; Amaniti, A.; Katsaounis, A.; Giannakidis, D.; Koulouris, C.; Hohenforst-Schmidt, W.; Huang, H.; Bai, C.; et al. Inhaled chemotherapy adverse effects: Mechanisms and protection methods. *Lung Cancer Manag.* **2020**, *8*, Lmt19. [CrossRef]

186. Lemarie, E.; Vecellio, L.; Hureaux, J.; Prunier, C.; Valat, C.; Grimbert, D.; Boidron-Celle, M.; Giraudeau, B.; le Pape, A.; Pichon, E.; et al. Aerosolized Gemcitabine in Patients with Carcinoma of the Lung: Feasibility and Safety Study. *J. Aerosol Med. Pulm. Drug Deliv.* **2011**, *24*, 261–270. [CrossRef]
187. Otterson, G.A.; Villalona-Calero, M.A.; Sharma, S.; Kris, M.G.; Imondi, A.; Gerber, M.; White, D.A.; Ratain, M.J.; Schiller, J.H.; Sandler, A.; et al. Phase I study of inhaled Doxorubicin for patients with metastatic tumors to the lungs. *Clin Cancer Res* **2007**, *13*, 1246–1252. [CrossRef]
188. Tatsumura, T.; Koyama, S.; Tsujimoto, M.; Kitagawa, M.; Kagamimori, S. Further study of nebulisation chemotherapy, a new chemotherapeutic method in the treatment of lung carcinomas: Fundamental and clinical. *Br. J. Cancer* **1993**, *68*, 1146–1149. [CrossRef]
189. Zarogoulidis, P.; Eleftheriadou, E.; Sapardanis, I.; Zarogoulidou, V.; Lithoxopoulou, H.; Kontakiotis, T.; Karamanos, N.; Zachariadis, G.; Mabroudi, M.; Zisimopoulos, A.; et al. Feasibility and effectiveness of inhaled carboplatin in NSCLC patients. *Investig. New Drugs* **2012**, *30*, 1628–1640. [CrossRef] [PubMed]
190. Wittgen, B.P.; Kunst, P.W.; van der Born, K.; van Wijk, A.W.; Perkins, W.; Pilkiewicz, F.G.; Perez-Soler, R.; Nicholson, S.; Peters, G.J.; Postmus, P.E. Phase I study of aerosolized SLIT cisplatin in the treatment of patients with carcinoma of the lung. *Clin. Cancer Res.* **2007**, *13*, 2414–2421. [CrossRef] [PubMed]
191. Verschraegen, C.F.; Gilbert, B.E.; Loyer, E.; Huaringa, A.; Walsh, G.; Newman, R.A.; Knight, V. Clinical Evaluation of the Delivery and Safety of Aerosolized Liposomal 9-Nitro-20(S)-Camptothecin in Patients with Advanced Pulmonary Malignancies. *Clin. Cancer Res.* **2004**, *10*, 2319–2326. [CrossRef] [PubMed]
192. Zhang, S.; Li, R.; Jiang, T.; Gao, Y.; Zhong, K.; Cheng, H.; Chen, X.; Li, S. Inhalable nanomedicine for lung cancer treatment. *Smart Mater. Med.* **2024**, *5*, 261–280. [CrossRef]
193. Rodríguez, F.; Caruana, P.; De la Fuente, N.; Español, P.; Gámez, M.; Balart, J.; Llurba, E.; Rovira, R.; Ruiz, R.; Martín-Lorente, C.; et al. Nano-Based Approved Pharmaceuticals for Cancer Treatment: Present and Future Challenges. *Biomolecules* **2022**, *12*, 784. [CrossRef]
194. Zheng, X.; Song, X.; Zhu, G.; Pan, D.; Li, H.; Hu, J.; Xiao, K.; Gong, Q.; Gu, Z.; Luo, K.; et al. Nanomedicine Combats Drug Resistance in Lung Cancer. *Adv. Mater.* **2024**, *36*, 2308977. [CrossRef]
195. Kaur, G.; Bose, S.; Kataria, T.; Tyagi, A.; Singla, K.; Sharma, S.; Ghosh, S.; Jha, C.B. Curcumin as a Potential Phytoconstituent used for Cancer Treatment: An Overview. *Nat. Prod. J.* **2024**, *14*, 1–13. [CrossRef]
196. Zhang, T.; Chen, Y.; Ge, Y.; Hu, Y.; Li, M.; Jin, Y. Inhalation treatment of primary lung cancer using liposomal curcumin dry powder inhalers. *Acta Pharm. Sin. B* **2018**, *8*, 440–448. [CrossRef]
197. Koshkina, N.V.; Waldrep, J.C.; Roberts, L.E.; Golunski, E.; Melton, S.; Knight, V. Paclitaxel Liposome Aerosol Treatment Induces Inhibition of Pulmonary Metastases in Murine Renal Carcinoma Model1. *Clin. Cancer Res.* **2001**, *7*, 3258–3262.
198. Garbuzenko, O.B.; Kuzmov, A.; Taratula, O.; Pine, S.R.; Minko, T. Strategy to enhance lung cancer treatment by five essential elements: Inhalation delivery, nanotechnology, tumor-receptor targeting, chemo- and gene therapy. *Theranostics* **2019**, *9*, 8362–8376. [CrossRef]
199. Kaur, P.; Garg, T.; Rath, G.; Murthy, R.S.; Goyal, A.K. Development, optimization and evaluation of surfactant-based pulmonary nanolipid carrier system of paclitaxel for the management of drug resistance lung cancer using Box-Behnken design. *Drug Deliv.* **2016**, *23*, 1912–1925. [CrossRef] [PubMed]
200. Abdelgalil, A.A.; Al-Kahtani, H.M.; Al-Jenoobi, F.I. Chapter Four—Erlotinib. In *Profiles of Drug Substances, Excipients and Related Methodology*; Brittain, H.G., Ed.; Academic Press: Cambridge, MA, USA, 2020; Volume 45, pp. 93–117.
201. Szabová, J.; Mišík, O.; Fučík, J.; Mrázová, K.; Mravcová, L.; Elcner, J.; Lízal, F.; Krzyžánek, V.; Mravec, F. Liposomal form of erlotinib for local inhalation administration and efficiency of its transport to the lungs. *Int. J. Pharm.* **2023**, *634*, 122695. [CrossRef] [PubMed]
202. Hu, L.; Jia, Y.; Wen, D. Preparation and characterization of solid lipid nanoparticles loaded with epirubicin for pulmonary delivery. *Pharmazie* **2010**, *65*, 585–587. [PubMed]
203. Shukla, S.K.; Kulkarni, N.S.; Farrales, P.; Kanabar, D.D.; Parvathaneni, V.; Kunda, N.K.; Muth, A.; Gupta, V. Sorafenib Loaded Inhalable Polymeric Nanocarriers against Non-Small Cell Lung Cancer. *Pharm. Res.* **2020**, *37*, 67. [CrossRef]
204. Oien, D.B.; Pathoulas, C.L.; Ray, U.; Thirusangu, P.; Kalogera, E.; Shridhar, V. Repurposing quinacrine for treatment-refractory cancer. *Semin Cancer Biol.* **2021**, *68*, 21–30. [CrossRef]
205. Vaidya, B.; Kulkarni, N.S.; Shukla, S.K.; Parvathaneni, V.; Chauhan, G.; Damon, J.K.; Sarode, A.; Garcia, J.V.; Kunda, N.; Mitragotri, S.; et al. Development of inhalable quinacrine loaded bovine serum albumin modified cationic nanoparticles: Repurposing quinacrine for lung cancer therapeutics. *Int. J. Pharm.* **2020**, *577*, 118995. [CrossRef]
206. Kaur, P.; Mishra, V.; Shunmugaperumal, T.; Goyal, A.K.; Ghosh, G.; Rath, G. Inhalable spray dried lipidnanoparticles for the co-delivery of paclitaxel and doxorubicin in lung cancer. *J. Drug Deliv. Sci. Technol.* **2020**, *56*, 101502. [CrossRef]
207. Mohamad Saimi, N.I.; Salim, N.; Ahmad, N.; Abdulmalek, E.; Abdul Rahman, M.B. Aerosolized Niosome Formulation Containing Gemcitabine and Cisplatin for Lung Cancer Treatment: Optimization, Characterization and In Vitro Evaluation. *Pharmaceutics* **2021**, *13*, 59. [CrossRef]
208. Parvathaneni, V.; Kulkarni, N.S.; Shukla, S.K.; Farrales, P.T.; Kunda, N.K.; Muth, A.; Gupta, V. Systematic development and optimization of inhalable pirfenidone liposomes for non-small cell lung cancer treatment. *Pharmaceutics* **2020**, *12*, 206. [CrossRef]

209. Wang, W.; Zhong, Z.; Huang, Z.; Hiew, T.N.; Huang, Y.; Wu, C.; Pan, X. Nanomedicines for targeted pulmonary delivery: Receptor-mediated strategy and alternatives. *Nanoscale* **2024**, *16*, 2820–2833. [CrossRef]
210. Bosetti, R.; Jones, S.L. Cost–Effectiveness of Nanomedicine: Estimating the Real Size of Nano-Costs. *Nanomedicine* **2019**, *14*, 1367–1370. [CrossRef] [PubMed]
211. Uskoković, V. Nanomedicine for the poor: A lost cause or an idea whose time has yet to come? *Nanomedicine* **2021**, *16*, 1203–1218. [CrossRef] [PubMed]
212. Kendal, E. Ethical, Legal and Social Implications of Emerging Technology (ELSIET) Symposium. *J. Bioethical Inq.* **2022**, *19*, 363–370. [CrossRef] [PubMed]
213. McClements, J.; McClements, D.J. Standardization of Nanoparticle Characterization: Methods for Testing Properties, Stability, and Functionality of Edible Nanoparticles. *Crit. Rev. Food Sci. Nutr.* **2016**, *56*, 1334–1362. [CrossRef]

pharmaceutics

Article

Nanoparticle-Based Dry Powder Inhaler Containing Ciprofloxacin for Enhanced Targeted Antibacterial Therapy

Petra Party [1], Márk László Klement [1], Bianca Maria Gaudio [2], Milena Sorrenti [2] and Rita Ambrus [1,*]

[1] Institute of Pharmaceutical Technology and Regulatory Affairs, University of Szeged, 6720 Szeged, Hungary; party.petra@szte.hu (P.P.); klementmark@outlook.com (M.L.K.)
[2] Department of Drug Sciences, University of Pavia, 27100 Pavia, Italy; bianca.gaudio@gmail.com (B.M.G.); milena.sorrenti@unipv.it (M.S.)
* Correspondence: ambrus.rita@szte.hu; Tel.: +36-62-545-572

Abstract: Background: Ciprofloxacin (CIP) is a poorly water-soluble fluoroquinolone-type antibiotic that can be useful in the treatment of lung infections. When the drugs are delivered directly to the lungs, a smaller dosage is needed to achieve the desired effect compared to the oral administration. Moreover, the application of nanoparticles potentially enhances the effectiveness of the treatments while lowering the possible side effects. Therefore, we aimed to develop a "nano-in-micro" structured dry powder inhaler formulation containing CIP. **Methods**: A two-step preparation method was used. Firstly, a nanosuspension was first prepared using a high-performance planetary mill by wet milling. After the addition of different additives (leucine and mannitol), the solid formulations were created by spray drying. The prepared DPI samples were analyzed by using laser diffraction, nanoparticle tracking analysis, scanning electron microscopy, X-ray powder diffraction, and differential scanning calorimetry. The solubility and in vitro dissolution tests in artificial lung fluid and in vitro aerodynamic investigations (Spraytec® device, Andersen Cascade Impactor) were carried out. **Results**: The nanosuspension (D50: 140.0 ± 12.8 nm) was successfully prepared by the particle size reduction method. The DPIs were suitable for inhalation based on the particle diameter and their spherical shape. Improved surface area and amorphization after the preparation processes led to faster drug release. The excipient-containing systems were characterized by large lung deposition (fine particle fraction around 40%) and suitable aerodynamic diameter (between 3 and 4 μm). **Conclusions**: We have successfully formulated a nanosized antibiotic-containing formulation for pulmonary delivery, which could provide a potential treatment for patients with different respiratory infections.

Keywords: ciprofloxacin; nanosuspension; dry powder inhaler; wet milling; spray drying; aerodynamic characterization

1. Introduction

One of the major issues affecting the new drugs under development is the solubility aspect, which affects around 90% of newly developed medications, drugs falling into BCS classes II and IV. There are many approaches to increasing the rate of dissolution, but over the decades, the consistent strategy of interest has been concerned with the reduction in particle size, which can be achieved through nanonization. Drug nanocrystals were introduced in the early 1990s, and the commercialization of the first products started in the early 2000s [1]. Nowadays, the global nanotechnology drug delivery market is at USD 105.95 billion in 2025 and is expected to double by 2034. In this field, the most representative technology segments concern nanoparticles and nanocrystals, and, secondly, liposomes,

 https://doi.org/10.3390/pharmaceutics17040486

micelles, and nanotubes, in various branches of medicine such as neurology, oncology, cardiovascular/physiology, anti-inflammatory/immunology, and anti-infective [2].

Nanosuspensions (NS) consist of pure drugs and a minimal proportion of surfactants or polymers to generate a carrier-free colloidal system in a size range between 10 and 1000 nm. The definition of nanomaterials according to the European Union (EU) requires the particle size to be under 100 nm [3]. Pharmaceutical nanoparticles are defined as individual particles with a size below 1 μm. This met the definition of products prepared by nanotechnology according to the U.S. Food and Drug Administration (FDA) [4], which is relevant for bioavailability [5]. Due to their nearly 100% drug load, nanocrystals require fewer excipients, which may be hazardous, and have a higher concentration of active ingredients at the site of action. However, the application of stabilizing agents is indispensable to avoid the aggregation of colloidal particles and thus improve stability. Preparation of NSs is a promising strategy for the efficient delivery of hydrophobic drugs and poorly soluble actives. They have a great potential for the selective and controlled delivery of drugs to target cells and organs [6,7].

For nanocrystal products, oral medication administration is the most popular method. They are available as solid oral dosage forms made from NSs, like tablets, using techniques like lyophilization, or as liquid oral dosage forms, such as suspensions. Another appealing option is parenteral delivery, which requires sterility but has high active loading. Research has also focused on nanocarrier-based active delivery systems for ocular drug delivery, as they are able to overcome many of the biological barriers of the eye and thus improve the ocular bioavailability of drugs used for eye infections and glaucoma. Dermal administration of nanocrystals is also a promising route. The favorable characteristics of these systems can ensure a greater concentration gradient so that a sufficiently large area of direct surface contact of the crystals with the superficial layers of the skin is achieved. Regarding drug delivery to the lungs, drug absorption, and local bioavailability are two aspects that depend on the fraction of drug deposited and dissolved in lung fluids. Mucociliary clearance and drug absorption are two competitive mechanisms that influence drug fate. Since nano-systems are characterized by a high dissolution rate as shown above, they may be particularly efficient when administered by inhalation [8,9]. Due to the large surface area of the lungs, dissolution and penetration are exceptionally fast. Because of their size, nanoparticles can easily enter through the mucus, eliminating the mechanism of mucociliary clearance. The systems could prolong the retention time of inhaled nanoparticles, providing sufficient duration of time for drug release, leading to improved bioavailability. The liberated nanosized drug can effectively reach the epithelium because they are not eliminated by the size-dependent uptake of the alveolar macrophages [10–12]. Nanoparticles have advantages in moving through biological barriers and can improve drug uptake into cells through various endocytosis-based pathways as well [13–15]. In general, the required dosage can be reduced due to enhanced drug transport [16]. However, the prolonged residence of the particles in the lung may lead to cellular injury, biological responses, and undesired effects. The impacts (e.g., increased reactivity, oxidative stress, cellular injury, and interruption of cellular processes) of nanocrystals are significantly influenced by their properties. Therefore, to characterize nanoparticles for toxicological investigations, a number of nanomaterial characteristics must be considered, including size distribution, surface area, morphology, solubility, chemical composition, and particle agglomeration [17–19].

Ciprofloxacin (CIP) is a second-generation fluoroquinolone, patented in 1983 and marketed since 1987 by Bayer, included in the World Health Organization's list of essential antibiotics. CIP is effective in a wide range of infections, including those that are difficult to treat. Due to its broad-spectrum bactericidal activity, oral efficacy, and good tolerability, it is widely used for the blind therapy of urinary tract infections, acute uncomplicated cystitis, chronic bacterial prostatitis, lower respiratory tract infections, skin infections, typhoid fever, bone (osteochondritis) and joint infections, as well as pyelonephritis. It has been recognized as a second-line agent for the treatment of cholera and tuberculosis in cases of resistance or non-response to first-line anti-tuberculotic drugs. It can be administered orally, intravenously, or through pulmonary delivery for the treatment of chronic Pseudomonas aeruginosa infections in patients with cystic fibrosis [20–23]. At the physiological pH of the lungs, CIP exists as a zwitterion, with a net neutral charge. The molecule is close to its isoelectric point and, therefore, is very poorly soluble, but it a has slower dissolution rate, providing an extended residence time in the lungs [24,25]. The zwitterionic form has a prolonged terminal elimination half-life when instilled intratracheally as compared with oral delivery [26]. Nanoparticles are often stabilized through electrostatic repulsion. If the active ingredient is neutral, it does not contribute to surface charge, which can increase the likelihood of aggregation. However, adding steric stabilizers or surfactants can improve the stability of the nanoparticles [27].

A potentially interesting field of application of CIP nanocrystals is the preparation of dry powders for pulmonary administration through inhalation. Pulmonary formulations can be liquid preparations that are dispersed in nebulizers or soft mist inhalers. An intermediate between liquid and dry formulation is pressurized metered dose inhaler preparations. Dry powder inhalers (DPIs) are propellant-free systems, so they have lower greenhouse gas emission potential [28]. DPIs are considered the most stable but are the most challenging due to the detrimental characteristics of micronized materials: they come along with high surface energy, which renders them very cohesive, resulting in poor flowability. Thus, DPI formulations need much engineering on the particle level to balance interparticulate forces in the dry powder bulk and ensure sufficient stability during processing and storage, as well as optimal dispersion and fine particle generation during inhalation. In this context, particles with a mean particle diameter between 200 nm and a few micrometers are used because of various aspects in order to obtain the highest dose fraction deposition in the lower airways: they may incorporate and protect the active pharmaceutical ingredient (API) and are suitable for controlled and sustained drug release; and they are considered to overcome biological barriers, such as epi- or endothelial barriers, via various transport mechanisms and are most promising for effective cell uptake. The usage of nanopharmaceuticals for pulmonary delivery allows us to combine the advantages of nanomaterials and the lung as a target [29–31].

The emergence of inhaled CIP shows promise for effectively managing chronic lower respiratory tract infections. Inhaled CIP treatment demonstrated superior efficacy in several phases of clinical trials and in preclinical settings [32]. Moreover, the exploration of nanomaterials for respiratory infections is an area of research that is full of potential and has the fastest clinical application [33]. Our research group previously worked with CIP for pulmonary delivery; however, none of the research work was related to nanoparticles [34,35]. In addition, the team worked on nanoparticle-based non-steroidal anti-inflammatory drug-containing formulations [36,37]. In the literature, the following nano-in-micro structured CIP-containing DPIs can be found. There are CIP nanocrystals prepared by anti-solvent precipitation [38], which was followed by spray or freeze drying as solidification methods [39–42]. Another previously used method is the combination of sonication and lyophilization [43,44]. There is only one wet milling and spray-drying-based CIP-containing article in the literature [45]. We aimed to develop a nanoparticle-based CIP-containing dry powder inhaler for enhanced targeted antibacterial therapy. We applied more efficient wet milling for the preparation of the NS, thereby achieving a high drug loading in the final DPI formulation without the application of an organic solvent. Therefore, the preparation process used and the final inhaled form are also environmentally friendly.

2. Materials and Methods

2.1. Materials

Ciprofloxacin (CIP) was used as the active pharmaceutical ingredient (Sigma-Aldrich Chemie GmbH, Darmstadt, Germany). Poly-vinyl-alcohol 4–98 (PVA) was used (Sigma Aldrich Chemie GmbH, Darmstadt, Germany), which can promote stable suspension formation due to the steric or electrosteric stabilization of solid particles [46]. The coating effect of PVA prevents nanoparticles from aggregating and ensures a uniform particle size distribution [47]. The application of PVA would minimize the nanoparticle fusions during drying as well as milling. Its decreasing effect on surface tension could result in smaller particles. PVA produces particles with low moisture content, despite its high hydrophilicity [48]. It can be non-toxic when used at the right concentration of PVA, which makes it appropriate for pulmonary applications [36,49]. L-leucine (LEU) (AppliChem GmbH, Darmstadt, Germany) has a low surface energy and forms a hydrophobic shell around drug particles, minimizing cohesion and adhesion between the particles and the attachment to the capsule. This enhances powder flowability and dispersion upon inhalation. Moreover, LEU tends to form wrinkled surfaces when spray-dried, reducing particle density and increasing deep lung deposition by reducing particles [50–52]. The application of LEU can lead to moisture protection, therefore improving the product's physical storage stability [53]. LEU is commonly used in the development of DPIs, and it is well tolerated in pulmonary applications, making it a safe excipient for inhalable formulations [54]. D-mannitol (MAN) (Molar Chemicals Kft, Halásztelek, Hungary) was a matrix former in the spray-dried formulations. It promotes proper, spherical shape and reduces interparticle cohesion, leading to improved aerosol performance. MAN is less hygroscopic than some of the other sugars, e.g., lactose, which is beneficial in terms of better physical and chemical stability of the DPI formulation [55,56]. Additionally, MAN is an FDA-approved excipient for pulmonary delivery and is non-irritant to the lungs [57,58].

2.2. Production of the NS by Wet Milling

A high-performance planetary ball mill (Fritsch GmbH Planetary Micro Mill Pulverisette 7, Fritsch, Idar-Oberstein, Germany) was used to reduce the particle size of the CIP. The following material composition was used: 2.00 g of CIP, 18.0 g of 5% (*w*/*w*%) PVA solution, and 20.00 g of ZrO_2 beads (d = 0.3 mm). The PVA concentration and the ratio of the suspension and the beads were chosen based on a previous work of our team, where a different API and a planetary ball were used [59]. The milling parameters were also optimized previously using factorial design to reduce milling time by increasing the speed of the rotation using the high-performance ball mill. The final milling time was 30 min with a rotational speed of 800 rpm. After milling, the suspension was diluted by adding 180 g of purified water.

2.3. DPI Formulations by Spray Drying

Three spray-dried (SPD) compositions were prepared by adding different amounts of LEU and MAN to the NS (Table 1). Inhalable microparticles were produced using a spray dryer equipped with a two-fluid nozzle of 0.7 mm (Büchi Mini Spray Dryer B-191, Büchi, Flawil, Switzerland). The spray-drying properties were as follows: inlet temperature, 130 °C; outlet temperature, 70 °C; aspirator capacity, 75%; airflow rate, 500 L/h; and feed pump rate, 5%. The parameters were based on a previously published work [60] and preliminary experiments, where the particle size, particle size distribution, and the morphology of the dried particles were observed. The properties of the CIP allow the application of high temperatures, which can decrease the humidity in the final product and improve the yield. The applied aspirator capacity also helped the mentioned properties. The final particle size was influenced by the feed rate used as well [61].

Table 1. Composition and API content of the SPD samples and the PMs.

Sample Name	CIP (g)	PVA (g)	LEU (g)	MAN (g)	API Content (%)
nanoCIP_SPD	2.00	0.90	0.00	0.00	66.04 ± 4.37
nanoCIP_LEU_SPD	2.00	0.90	0.40	0.00	40.11 ± 5.85
nanoCIP_LEU_MAN_SPD	2.00	0.90	0.40	0.25	31.94 ± 1.73
CIP_PM	2.00	0.90	0.00	0.00	68.97
CIP_LEU_PM	2.00	0.90	0.40	0.00	60.61
CIP_LEU_MAN_PM	2.00	0.90	0.40	0.25	56.34

2.4. Preparation of the Physical Mixtures

Physical mixtures (PM) were prepared from the raw materials to observe the effect of the excipients. The compositions of the PMs were similar to the SPD samples (Table 1). During the experiments, the different qualities of the SPD samples were compared to the PM.

2.5. Determination of the Drug Content

The API contents of the different DPIs were determined by dissolving 1.0 mg of powder in 25 mL of methanol and pH 7.4 phosphate buffer (60 + 40 *V*/*V*%). The solutions were filtered (pore size = 0.45 μm and 0.10 μm, Millex-HV filter unit, Millipore Corporation, Bedford, MS, USA) and analyzed by UV/Vis spectrophotometry (ATI-Unicam, Cambridge, UK) at a wavelength of 271 nm. The measurement was carried out three times.

2.6. Laser Diffraction-Based Particle Size Measurement

The particle size, particle size distribution (PSD), and specific surface area (SSA) of the NS were determined by laser diffraction (Mastersizer Scirocco 2000, Malvern Instruments Ltd., Worcestershire, UK). The wet dispersion unit was used. The refractive index (RI) of the CIP was adjusted to 1.50. The suspension was measured three times in purified water with stirring at 2000 rpm. Laser diffraction was also applied to determine the particle size, PSD, and SSA of the SPD samples. In this case, the dry dispersion unit was used. The dispersion air pressure was set to 3.0 bar and a vibration feed was applied. Each sample was measured three times. PSD was characterized by the values of D10 (10% of the volume distribution is below this value), D50 (50% of the volume distribution is below this value), and D90 (90% of the volume distribution is below this value) (Equation (1)). The SSA was calculated from the PSD data under the assumption of spherical particles.

$$\text{Span} = (\text{D90} - \text{D10})/(\text{D50}) \quad (1)$$

2.7. Nanoparticle Tracking Analysis of the NS

The NanoSight NS 3000 device (Malvern Instruments, Worcestershire, UK) for nanoparticle tracking analysis (NTA) was used to obtain high-resolution particle size information about the NS. The instrument was equipped with a 565 nm laser, a high-sensitivity sCMOS camera, and a syringe pump. The CIP suspension was diluted and loaded into the device using a syringe pump speed of 50. The experiment videos were analyzed using NTA 3.4 Build 3.4.4 after being captured in script control mode (3 videos of 30 s per measurement). A total of 1500 frames per sample were examined.

2.8. Investigation of the Morphology of the Nanocrystals and the DPIs

The shape of the particles was analyzed using scanning electron microscopy (SEM, Hitachi S4700; Hitachi Ltd., Tokyo, Japan). The investigation conditions were the following: 10 kV high voltage, 10 mA amperage, and 1.3–13.1 mPa air pressure. A high vacuum evaporator and argon atmosphere were applied to make the sputter-coated samples conductive with gold–palladium (Bio-Rad SC 502; VG Microtech, Uckfield, UK). For the implementation of the particle diameter investigation, ImageJ, a public domain image analyzer software, was used (ImageJ 1.53e, https://imagej.net/ij/, accessed on 20 January 2025).

2.9. Analysis of the Crystalline Structure

The crystalline structure was investigated using X-ray powder diffraction (XRPD). The Bruker D8 advance diffractometer and the VANTEC-1 detector (Bruker AXS GmbH, Karlsruhe, Germany) were used with Cu KλI radiation. The powders were placed on a flat quartz glass with an etched square. Scanning was performed at a uniform voltage of 40 kV and a current of 40 mA from 3° to 40°, the scanning time constant was 0.1°/min, and the angular step was 0.01°. The DIFFRACplus EVA program was used for the evaluation.

2.10. Thermoanalytical Measurement

Differential scanning calorimetry (DSC) measurements were performed with a Mettler Toledo DSC 821e system with the STARe thermal analysis program V9.1 (Mettler Inc., Schwerzenbach, Switzerland). The samples (from 3 to 5 mg) were heated to temperatures between 25 and 300 °C at a rate of 10 °C/min while maintaining a steady flow of argon at a rate of 10 L/h.

2.11. Fourier-Transform Infrared Spectroscopy Investigation

The interactions between CIP and the excipients were investigated by Fourier-transform Infrared Spectroscopy (FT-IR), using the AVATAR 330 FT–IR spectrometer (Thermo Nicolet, Thermo Fisher Scientific Inc., Waltham, MA, USA). The samples were homogenized with 150 mg of KBr in an achate mortar, and the mixtures were pressed to prepare pastilles using a Specac® hydraulic press (Specac, Inc., Orpington, UK) with a 10-ton pressing force. The spectra were recorded from 4000 to 400 cm^{-1} at an optical resolution of 4 cm^{-1}.

2.12. Solubility Test

The apparent solubility tests of the SPD products were implemented in 3 mL of artificial lung fluid (0.68 g/L NaCl, 2.27 g/L $NaHCO_3$, 0.02 g/L $CaCl_2$, 0.1391 g/L NaH_2PO_4, 0.37 g/L glycine and 5.56 mL/L 0.1 M H_2SO_4) [62]. The pH of the medium was 7.4 ± 0.1. The samples were stirred with a magnetic stirrer at 25 °C for 24 h, filtered (pore size = 0.45 μm, and 0.1 μm, Millex-HV filter unit, Millipore Corporation, Bedford, MS, USA), and then the drug content was analyzed using a UV/VIS spectrophotometer (ATI-Unicam, Cambridge, UK) at a wavelength of 271 nm. The samples were measured in triplicate.

2.13. In Vitro Dissolution Test of the DPIs

A modified paddle method (Hanson SR8 Plus, Teledyne Hanson Research, Chatsworth, CA, USA) of the European Pharmacopeia was used to define the release of CIP from the dosage form [63]. At the present time, there are no regulatory requirements for the in vitro dissolution testing of inhaled products. The estimated value of the lung lining fluid is between 10 and 70 mL [64]; therefore, 50 mL of the previously mentioned simulated lung medium was applied. The samples contained 3.25 mg of CIP, which is a tenth of the estimated dose for pulmonary delivery [26]; therefore, the test was carried out in sink conditions. The samples were introduced to the vessel in a powder form. The paddle was rotated at 100 rpm and the measurement was performed up to 60 min at 37 °C. Samples of 5 mL were taken after 5, 10, 15, 30, and 60 min. The medium was replenished in all cases. After filtration (pore size: 0.45 μm, Millex-HV syringe-driven filter unit, Millipore Corporation, Bedford, MA, USA), the dissolved quantity of CIP was determined spectrophotometrically at a wavelength of 271 nm. The measurement was performed three times.

2.14. In Vitro Aerodynamic Characterization

The aerosolization properties of the SPD formulations were evaluated in vitro, using an Andersen cascade impactor (ACI, Apparatus D, Copley Scientific Ltd., Nottingham, UK) [65]. The inhalation flow rate was set at 60 L/min (High-capacity Pump model HCP5, Critical Flow Controller model TPK, Copley Scientific Ltd., Nottingham, UK). The actual airflow through the impactor was measured by a mass flow meter (Flow Meter model DFM 2000, Copley Scientific Ltd., Nottingham, UK). The inhalation time was 4 s. The Breezhaler® single-dose device (Novartis International AG, Basel, Switzerland) was applied, which is classified as a low-resistance inhaler. Transparent size 3 Ezeeflo™ hydroxypropyl methylcellulose capsules (ACG—Associated Capsules Pvt. Ltd., Mumbai, India) were filled with the powders. Measurements were carried out in triplicate. To simulate the pulmonary adhesive conditions, the collection plates were coated with a mixture of Span 85 and cyclohexane (1 + 99 *w*/*w*%). After the measurement, the device, capsules, induction port, plates, and filter (A/E glass fiber filter, Pall Corporation, NY, USA) were washed with methanol and pH 7.4 phosphate buffer (60 + 40 *V*/*V*%) to dissolve the deposited amount of MX. The API was quantified by UV/Vis spectrophotometry at a wavelength of 271 nm. Aerodynamic properties were evaluated using Inhalytix™ software (Copley Scientific Ltd., Nottingham, UK). The fine particle fraction (FPF) and mass median aerodynamic diameter (MMAD) values were determined. FPF is defined as the percentage of mass of the particles consisting of API with an MMAD of less than 5 μm divided by the emitted dose of the formulations. The emitted fraction (EF) was also calculated, which is the released fraction from the DPI device. The geometric standard deviation (GSD) was employed to characterize the aerodynamic diameter distribution.

2.15. Aerodynamic Particle Size Analysis Using the Spraytec® Device

The aerodynamic diameter was determined using a Spraytec® laser diffractometer equipped with an inhalation cell (Malvern Instruments Ltd., Worcestershire, UK) and ACI. The investigation accounts for the EF of the DPI formulation and measures PSD directly from the inhalation device. SPD formulations were aerosolized from a size 3 HPMC capsule inserted into a Breezhaler® device connected to an induction port of the inhalation cell. The assembly was attached to an ACI, which created a closed system that allowed measurement of the size under controlled circumstances [66]. The inhalation flow rate was set at 60 L/min. The inhalation time was 4 s. Measurements were made in triplicate.

3. Results

3.1. Characterization of the NS

3.1.1. Results of the Laser Diffraction-Based Particle Size Distribution of the NS

The initial diameter of the API was in the micrometric size range (D50 = 5.98 μm SSA = 1.33 m^2/g) and the PSD was heterodisperse (Span = 38.70). The particle size of CIP was successfully reduced by wet milling to the nano range (D10 = 120 ± 7.9 nm, D50 = 189.3 ± 11.6 nm, 257.67 ± 14.47 nm) with a Span of 0.727 ± 0.02. PVA coated the CIP particles during milling, which inhibited particle aggregation [47]. SSA significantly increased (34.93 ± 2.23 m^2/g), which predicts a higher rate of dissolution compared to the raw CIP [67]. The technique can obtain NS in 30 min of milling, increasing the cost-effectiveness of the preparation.

3.1.2. Outcomes of the Nanoparticle Tracking Analysis of the NS

NTA was used to determine the size distribution of the sample using nanoparticle light scattering and Brownian motion. NTA simultaneously detects large and small particles, resulting in a precise particle distribution [68,69]. According to NTA, the D50 of the CIP NS was 140.0 ± 12.8 nm and the PSD was monodisperse (Span = 1.59 ± 0.43) (Figure 1), which met the results of the laser diffraction-based particle size analysis.

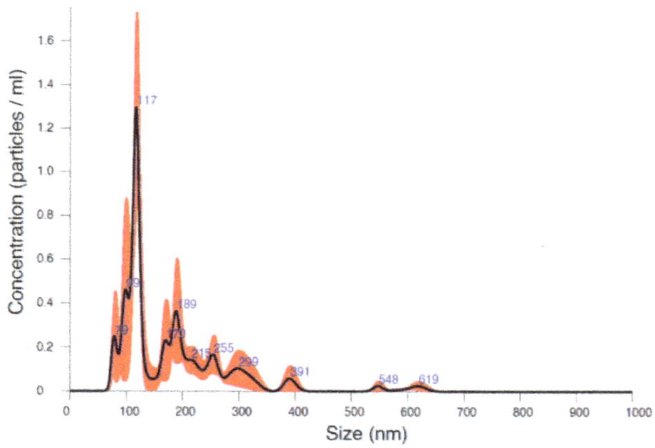

Figure 1. The particle size result of the suspension according to the NTA.

3.1.3. Morphology Results of the Dried NS

The prepared NS was dried and investigated by SEM. The solvent was evaporated at 40 °C in a vacuum drying chamber (Binder VD53, BINDER GmbH, Tuttlingen, Germany). In the images (Figure 2), the nanosized API particles were observed on the PVA matrix. The particle size was determined by the ImageJ program and the diameter of the particles (65.60 nm ± 22.70) was smaller in comparison to the results of wet investigation methods.

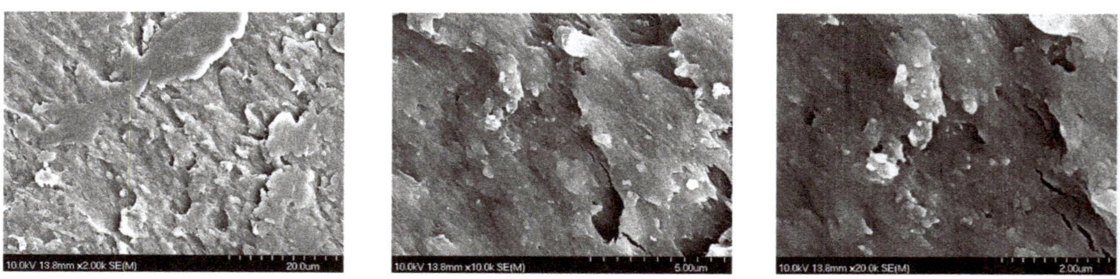

(a) (b) (c)

Figure 2. SEM pictures of the dried NS at a magnification of 2000-fold (**a**), 10,000-fold (**b**), and 20,000-fold (**c**).

3.2. Characterization of the Dry Powder Inhaler Formulation

3.2.1. Outcomes of the Laser Diffraction-Based Particle Size Measurement

The size of the SPD particles was applicable for pulmonary delivery since the D50 values were in the 1–5 μm range in the case of the nanoCIP_LEU_SPD and nanoCIP_LEU_MAN_SPD (Table 2). The geometric diameter of the LEU- and MAN-free samples was above 5 µm. Moreover, its PSD was heterodisperse (Span > 2.0), given that the higher the Span value, the broader the distribution. PSD was monodisperse in the case of LEU- and MAN-containing products, which is important for targeting the lungs and for the application of standard drug doses [70].

Table 2. The particle size, Span, and SSA values of the DPIs. Data are means ± S.D. (n = 3 measurements).

Sample Name	D10 (µm)	D50 (µm)	D90 (µm)	Span	SSA (m^2/g)
nanoCIP_SPD	2.63 ± 0.20	5.66 ± 0.31	15.46 ± 0.50	2.27 ± 0.07	1.23 ± 0.03
nanoCIP_LEU_SPD	2.50 ± 0.05	4.86 ± 0.17	9.41 ± 0.64	1.42 ± 0.08	1.40 ± 0.04
nanoCIP_LEU_MAN_SPD	2.25 ± 0.12	4.59 ± 0.09	9.18 ± 0.44	1.51 ± 0.10	1.52 ± 0.06

3.2.2. Findings of the Morphology Investigation

On the SEM images (Figure 3) of the DPIs, the effects of the additives were noticeable. The nanoCIP_SPD showed elongated needle-like particles associated with agglomerates. The size of this sample evaluated by ImageJ did not correspond with the findings of the particle size analysis. The average size of the particles was 3.65 ± 1.11 µm for nanoCIP_SPD because the particles tend to be more easily aggregated without LEU and MAN. Based on the picture, the PSD was not monodisperse and the shape of the particles is not preferable. However, a nearly spherical shape was observed in the case of the other two samples, which was the result of the combination of the excipients and the optimized spray-drying method. The spherical form met the requirements of DPIs [71]. Smooth surfaces are not preferred for pulmonary delivery because they tend to increase the interaction between particles, while rough surfaces enhance aerosolization efficiency, which effect was promoted by LEU. Applying MAN, the spherical morphology shifted to a donut-shaped appearance. The internal hollows, reflecting a low density, can lead to improved aerodynamic properties [51]. The diameters of the particles were the following: 3, 4.29 ± 1.14 µm for nanoCIP_LEU_SPD and 4.12 ± 0.95 µm for nanoCIP_LEU_MAN_SPD. The data are the means ± S.D. (n = 100 independent measurements), which was similar to the results of the laser diffraction-based measurement. Therefore, particles containing LEU predicted a proper drug delivery to the bronchial and acinar regions as well [72].

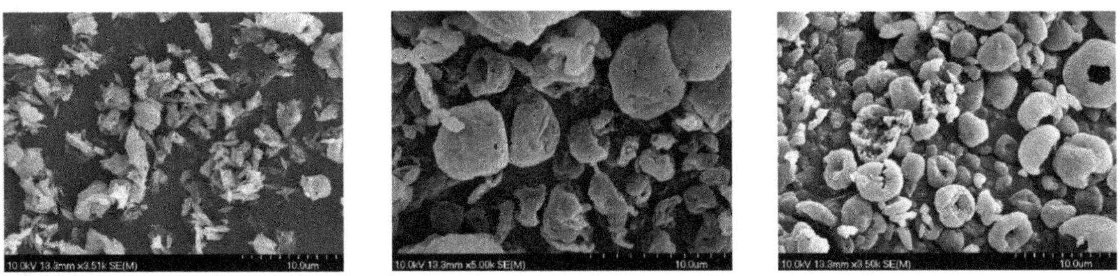

(a) (b) (c)

Figure 3. SEM pictures of the SPD samples: (**a**) nanoCIP_SPD; (**b**) nanoCIP_LEU_SPD; (**c**) nanoCIP_LEU_MAN_SPD.

3.2.3. Characteristics of the Crystalline Structure

The XRPD was used to characterize the crystalline state of CIP before and after the preparation process in the case of the pulmonary preferable samples. The XRPD pattern of the raw material and the PMs demonstrated the crystalline structure of CIP (Figure 4). In the PMs containing PVA, the three main peaks of CIP are also observable; however, they are of lower intensity at 14.5, 20.5, and 25°. Moreover, between 18 and 20° theta, there is an overlap of the peaks in the sample due to the presence of amorphous PVA in the sample. In the case of the products, the intensities of the characteristic peaks decreased due to the effects of milling and spray drying on the crystallinity of the API. Considering the sample consisting of only CIP and PVA, it can be observed that all the peaks inherent in the crystalline CIP are no longer present in the product. Referring to the nanoCIP_LEU_SPD sample preparation method resulted in a markedly amorphous product: the only peaks that can be distinguished in this case are those of LEU at about 2.5° and the one at 19.5°. A similar conclusion can be drawn for the last sample: the degree of crystallinity of the LEU and MAN also decreased during solidification. The amorphization can lead to faster dissolution of the CIP in comparison to the crystalline drug. Moreover, it can also affect the stability of the final product, which requires further investigation. However, based on the literature, recrystallization does not significantly happen over 1 year in the case of similar "nano-in-micro" systems. In the case of CIP-containing DPIs, the recrystallization did not influence the particle size distribution and aerodynamic performance [28,60,73].

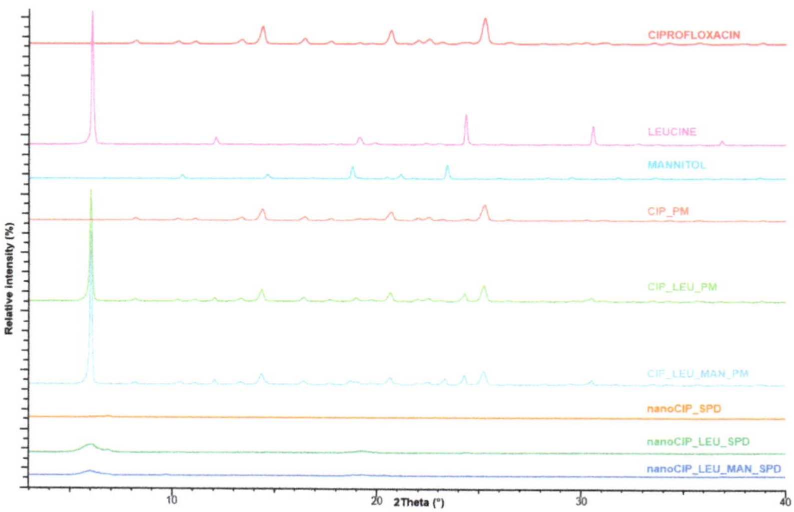

Figure 4. XRPD curves of the initial materials, PMs, and SPD samples.

3.2.4. Results of the Thermoanalytical Measurement

The DSC was employed to investigate the CIP melting process in the case of the raw form, PMs, and SPD products (Figure 5). The raw CIP showed a sharp endothermic peak at 271.61 °C, reflecting its melting point and crystallinity. Based on the DSC curves, the amorphization of the CIP is possible. The melting point in the case of CIP_PM indicated the crystallinity of CIP. However, on the curve of CIP_LEU_PM, the starting point around 255 °C detected the melting of LEU not to the CIP. Since there was no observable peak at 260 °C in the case of nanoCIP_SPD, LEU and CIP were solved in the melted MAN. Due to the smaller particle size, a small amount of the remaining CIP crystals in the nanoCIP_SPD melted at a lower temperature than the raw CIP. It is not feasible to determine whether the curves with melting points of 250–260 °C in the case of LEU-containing products relate to CIP or LEU. But, according to the XRPD spectra, the API in the spray-dried samples was in an amorphous state.

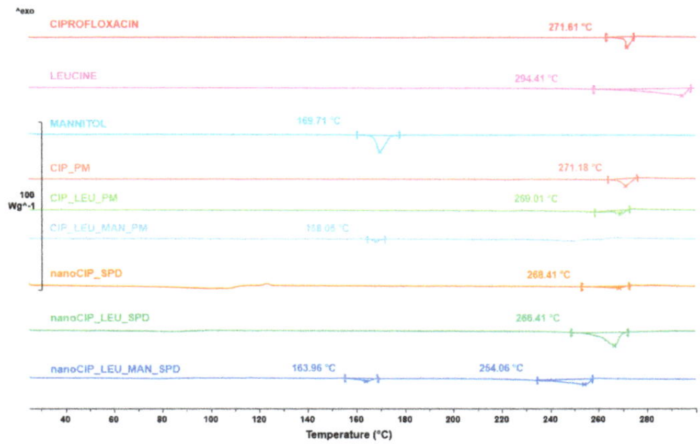

Figure 5. DSC curves of the initial materials, PMs, and SPD samples.

3.2.5. Results of the FTIR Analysis

FT-IR spectral analysis was performed to study the possibility of molecular interactions between CIP and the excipients (PVA, MAN, LEU). To identify the changes occurring during nanonization and spray drying, the initial materials, FT-IR spectra of the physical mixtures, and the spray-dried formulations were compared (Figure 6). CIP has characteristic peaks at 1616, 1498, 1285, and 1035 cm^{-1}. All the mentioned peaks of CIP were detected in the spray-dried samples, indicating that the preparation process did not cause any structural changes. The peaks related to PVA (3367 and 2943 cm^{-1}) were observed in the nanoCIP_PVA, with a shift to 3392 cm^{-1} due to hydrogen bonding interactions between PVA and CIP. The peaks of LEU (2957, 2871 cm^{-1}) did not change during the preparation method. The presence of MAN caused a slight shift in the O-H stretching peak (from 3324 to 3287 cm^{-1}), indicating that MAN forms hydrogen bonds with PVA. The findings of the FTIR analysis can affect the dissolution and stability as well.

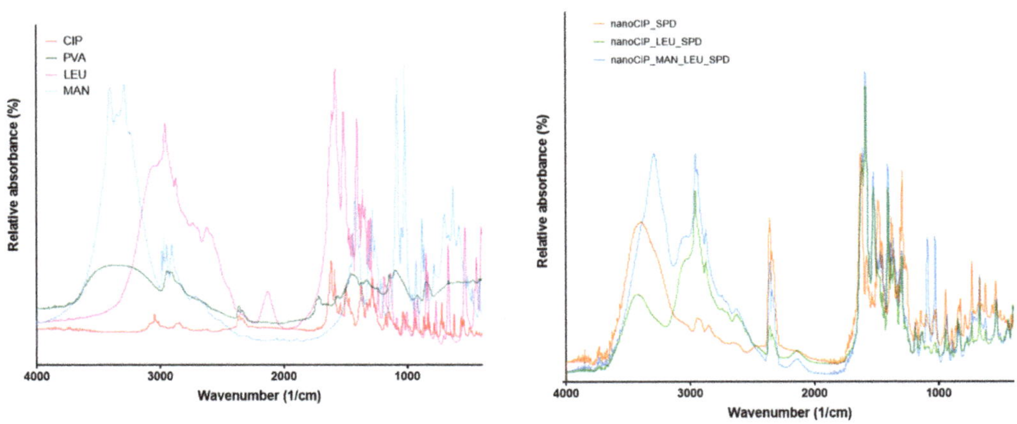

(**a**) (**b**)

Figure 6. FTIR spectra of the initial materials (**a**) and SPD samples (**b**).

3.2.6. Effects of the Formulation on the Solubility

The initial solubility of the raw CIP was 0.021 ± 0.002 mg/mL in artificial lung medium. As a result of the increased surface area of CIP, the solubility of the SPD samples improved in both cases: 0.061 ± 0.010 mg/mL of nanoCIP_LEU_SPD, 0.056 ± 0.012 mg/mL of nanoCIP_LEU_MAN_SPD. The reduction in drug particle size in the nano-range led to an increased surface area, which promoted the increase in solubility [74]. The improved solubility exceeds the minimum inhibitory concentration of different pathogens, such as *Pseudomonas aeruginosa*, which is a common cause of bacterial infection in cystic fibrosis [75,76]. Higher concentrations were previously achieved in the sputum of patients with cystic fibrosis, but this could be related to the different composition of the media [77].

3.2.7. Results of the In Vitro Dissolution Test

During the in vitro drug release test, the amount of CIP was the lowest for samples containing raw materials (Figure 7). Approximately 20% of the drug was released from the SPD samples within the first 5 min. These improvements are related to the higher specific surface area, enhanced solubility, and amorphization of the CIP in both cases. Hydrophilic PVA inhibited aggregation and increased polarity, LEU reduced the cohesion between the particles; therefore, a larger amount of CIP was liberated. In all cases, the water-soluble MAN improved the drug dissolution. Additionally, faster drug release could be achieved in the presence of the used excipients due to their combined effect increasing the drug–solvent interactions [78]. The outcomes demonstrated that the nanosized CIP dissolved better than the PMs. Nevertheless, the time was insufficient for the complete drug dose release, which should be taken into consideration when determining the final drug dosage.

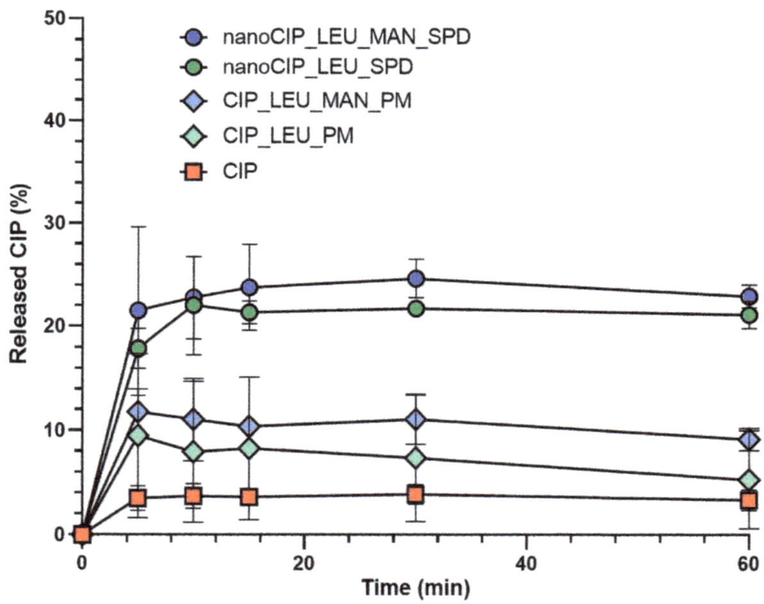

Figure 7. In vitro dissolution results of the DPIs. Data are means ± S.D. (n = 3 measurements).

3.2.8. Outcomes of the In Vitro Aerodynamic Characterization

The in vitro aerodynamic investigation was carried out by ACI. The distribution of CIP-containing powders on the plates of the stages is shown in Figure 8. It can be concluded that the performance of nanoCIP_LEU_SPD and nanoCIP_LEU_MAN_SPD was quite similar. The application of MAN decreased the deposited amount of powder in the first five stages, which is preferable for lung targeting.

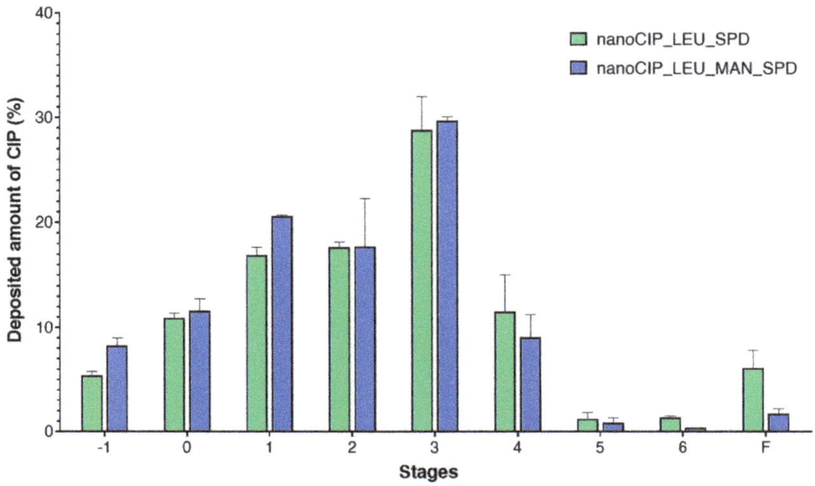

Figure 8. Distribution of the DPIs at a flow rate of 60 L/min. Data are means ± S.D. (*n* = 3 measurements).

The in vitro aerodynamic results evaluated by the Inhalytix^{TM} software are presented in Table 3. The MMAD results showed the different behavior of the particles during aerosolization. Now, the size of the MAN-containing powder was larger. However, thanks to its hollow structure, the FPF and EF values were more promising in comparison to nanoCIP_LEU_SPD. The FPF values were higher than the commercially available DPI formulations in the Breezhaler® device [79]. Due to the appropriate excipients being employed, the particle was attached neither to the capsule nor the device, and the EF values exceeded 80%. The GSD values were calculated to be less than 2, indicating that the aerodynamic diameter distribution of nanoaggregate microparticles was narrow [80].

Table 3. MMAD, FPF, and EF of the DPIs. Data are means ± S.D. (*n* = 3 independent measurements).

Sample Name	MMAD (µm)	FPF by Size (%)	FPF by Stage (%)	EF (%)	GSD
nanoCIP_LEU_SPD	3.25 ± 0.11	36.49 ± 4.89	41.85 ± 5.96	83.55 ± 0.01	1.99 ± 0.03
nanoCIP_LEU_MAN_SPD	3.71 ± 0.03	41.43 ± 2.88	49.56 ± 3.11	86.65 ± 0.08	1.78 ± 0.08

3.2.9. Findings of the Aerodynamic Particle Size Analysis Using the Spraytec® Device

According to the Spraytec® test, the D50 values of the samples were between 4.91 and 5.22 µm and showed a narrow PSD (Table 4). The values were similar to the laser diffraction results in Section 3.2.1. The pulmonary applicability in terms of particle size was proved again. However, the increased particle size by MAN was observable, like in the case of the MMAD results of ACI.

Table 4. The particle size, Span, and SSA values of the DPIs according to Spraytec® measurement Data are means ± S.D. (*n* = 3 measurements).

Sample Name	D10 (µm)	D50 (µm)	D90 (µm)	Span	SSA (m^2/g)
nanoCIP_LEU_SPD	2.59 ± 0.05	4.91 ± 0.03	9.06 ± 0.06	1.32 ± 0.03	1.38 ± 0.01
nanoCIP_LEU_MAN_SPD	2.59 ± 0.04	5.22 ± 0.16	10.39 ± 0.56	1.49 ± 0.05	1.32 ± 0.04

4. Discussion

Compared to conventional oral and intravenous antibiotic therapies, direct pulmonary delivery offers the advantage of localized drug action, reducing systemic exposure and associated side effects. Additionally, the nanosized drug particles enhance dissolution and absorption in the lungs, which could lead to faster therapeutic onset and improved efficacy, particularly in patients with chronic or resistant bacterial infections.

We have successfully developed nanosized CIP-containing DPI products combining LEU and MAN for the treatment of respiratory infections. To produce the NS, which was only 30 min long, a particle size reduction technique without the use of organic solvents was employed. To combine the advantages of nanoparticles and pulmonary delivery, the NS was solidified by spray drying using LEU and MAN. A comprehensive physicochemical and dosage form investigation was executed. We managed to adjust the particle size of the SPD formulation under 5 µm to target the appropriate regions of the lung. The LEU-containing formulation showed a spherical form, and the LEU- and MAN-containing formulations appeared to have a donut-like form. The dissolution profile of the nanosized CIP-containing samples was improved in comparison to the initial drug, which was promoted by the reduced size and the partial amorphization of the drug. Moreover, the aerodynamic properties also proved to be adequate, the MMAD results were also in the pulmonary adequate range and the FPF values were around 40%. The measurements with the ACI and Spraytec® device clarified that the behavior of the particles changes during aerosolization.

To contextualize our formulation within the existing literature, we compared its performance to previously published formulations. Spray-dried micelles exhibited a slightly higher FPF while maintaining comparable drug dissolution within the first hour [81]. Several studies utilizing spray drying from organic solvent-based nanosuspension technology did not include an aerodynamic performance evaluation [39,82]. Other nanoparticle formulations prepared using organic solvent-based techniques, followed by freeze-drying, demonstrated similar or improved drug release profiles, when aerodynamic investigations were assessed, performance was either slightly inferior or exceeded our findings. Spray-dried formulations containing sugars displayed comparable aerodynamic characteristics [83,84]. Regarding milling techniques, micronized ciprofloxacin (CIP) obtained by spray drying with isopropyl alcohol exhibited a higher FPF but a lower EF [85]. In conclusion, while numerous studies have employed organic solvents in formulation development, our approach offers a safer and more environmentally friendly alternative.

Despite the promising findings, several challenges must be addressed to facilitate the translation of this technology into clinical practice. One major concern is the scalability of the production process. While wet milling and spray drying are well-established techniques, maintaining batch-to-batch consistency in nanoparticle size, crystallinity, and aerodynamic properties during large-scale manufacturing requires further optimization. Process parameters such as milling time, spray-drying conditions, and excipient ratios must be carefully controlled to ensure reproducibility and long-term stability of the formulation. Furthermore, it is important to note the limitations of the work. Our study provides comprehensive in vitro characterization; however, in vivo validation is essential to confirm the efficacy and safety of our formulation. Moreover, the amorphous formulations may present stability challenges, such as recrystallization and moisture absorption; therefore, the stability of the product should be tested. While our work focused on the development and characterization of a novel DPI formulation, direct comparisons with a currently commercially available DPI product could be informative to observe the potential benefits and limitations of our formulation in relation to existing options. Therefore, future directions are the mentioned limitations, such as in vivo animal study in rats to determine the lung concentration of the drug and long-term stability investigation. We plan to conduct comparative tests with different marketed products, ensuring the clinical relevance of the formulations.

5. Conclusions

To conclude, the preparation of the "nano-in-micro" structured DPIs containing CIP was carried out using LEU and MAN, offering an environmentally friendly alternative. The formulation can provide the possibility to deliver the antibiotic directly to the lungs, a viable treatment option for respiratory infections, potentially offering a more effective and patient-friendly alternative to existing antibiotic therapies.

Author Contributions: Conceptualization and Methodology, P.P. and R.A.; Investigation, P.P., M.L.K. and B.M.G.; Evaluation, P.P.; Writing—Original Draft, P.P.; Writing—Review and Editing, M.S. and R.A.; Supervision, M.S. and R.A. All authors have read and agreed to the published version of the manuscript.

Funding: This research was funded by the University of Szeged Open Access Fund, grant number 7567.

Institutional Review Board Statement: Not applicable.

Informed Consent Statement: Not applicable.

Data Availability Statement: The original contributions presented in the study are included in the article, and further inquiries can be directed to the corresponding author.

Acknowledgments: This research was supported by the National Research, Development and Innovation Office, NKFIH OTKA K_146148. Project no TKP2021-EGA-32 has been implemented with the support provided by the Ministry of Culture and Innovation of Hungary from the National Research, Development and Innovation Fund, financed under the TKP2021-EGA funding scheme.

Conflicts of Interest: The authors declare no conflicts of interest.

References

1. Gigliobianco, M.R.; Casadidio, C.; Censi, R.; Di Martino, P. Nanocrystals of Poorly Soluble Drugs: Drug Bioavailability and Physicochemical Stability. *Pharmaceutics* **2018**, *10*, 134. [CrossRef] [PubMed]
2. Gokhale, S. Nanotechnology Drug Delivery Market Size, Share, and Trends 2025 to 2034. Available online: https://www.precedenceresearch.com/nanotechnology-drug-delivery-market (accessed on 1 February 2025).
3. Potočnik, J. Comission Recommendation of 18 October 2011 on the Definition of Nanomaterial. *Off. J. Eur. Union* **2011**.
4. U.S. Food and Drug Administration Guidance for Industry Considering Whether an FDA-Regulated Product Involves the Application of Nanotechnology. Available online: https://www.fda.gov/media/88423/download (accessed on 10 January 2025).
5. Merisko-Liversidge, E.; Liversidge, G.G. Nanosizing for Oral and Parenteral Drug Delivery: A Perspective on Formulating Poorly-Water Soluble Compounds Using Wet Media Milling Technology. *Adv. Drug Deliv. Rev.* **2011**, *63*, 427–440. [CrossRef] [PubMed]
6. Dahan, A.; Miller, J.M.; Amidon, G.L. Prediction of Solubility and Permeability Class Membership: Provisional BCS Classification of the World ' s Top Oral Drugs. *AAPS J.* **2009**, *11*, 740–746. [CrossRef]
7. Singhal, M.; Baumgartner, A.; Turunen, E.; van Veen, B.; Hirvonen, J.; Peltonen, L. Nanosuspensions of a Poorly Soluble Investigational Molecule ODM-106: Impact of Milling Bead Diameter and Stabilizer Concentration. *Int. J. Pharm.* **2020**, *587*, 119636. [CrossRef]
8. Malamatari, M.; Taylor, K.M.G.; Malamataris, S.; Douroumis, D.; Kachrimanis, K. Pharmaceutical Nanocrystals: Production by Wet Milling and Applications. *Drug Discov. Today* **2018**, *23*, 534–547. [CrossRef]
9. Fernández-García, R.; Fraguas-Sánchez, A.I. Nanomedicines for Pulmonary Drug Delivery: Overcoming Barriers in the Treatment of Respiratory Infections and Lung Cancer. *Pharmaceutics* **2024**, *16*, 1584. [CrossRef] [PubMed]
10. Liu, Q.; Guan, J.; Qin, L.; Zhang, X.; Mao, S. Physicochemical Properties Affecting the Fate of Nanoparticles in Pulmonary Drug Delivery. *Drug Discov. Today* **2020**, *25*, 150–159. [CrossRef]
11. Thorley, A.J.; Tetley, T.D. New Perspectives in Nanomedicine. *Pharmacol. Ther.* **2013**, *140*, 176–185. [CrossRef]
12. Ruge, C.C.; Kirch, J.; Lehr, C.M. Pulmonary Drug Delivery: From Generating Aerosols to Overcoming Biological Barriers-Therapeutic Possibilities and Technological Challenges. *Lancet Respir. Med.* **2013**, *1*, 402–413. [CrossRef]
13. Malamatari, M.; Charisi, A.; Malamataris, S.; Kachrimanis, K.; Nikolakakis, I. Spray Drying for the Preparation of Nanoparticle-Based Drug Formulations as Dry Powders for Inhalation. *Processes* **2020**, *8*, 788. [CrossRef]
14. Wang, W.; Huang, Z.; Huang, Y.; Zhang, X.; Huang, J.; Cui, Y.; Yue, X.; Ma, C.; Fu, F.; Wang, W.; et al. Pulmonary Delivery Nanomedicines towards Circumventing Physiological Barriers: Strategies and Characterization Approaches. *Adv. Drug Deliv. Rev.* **2022**, *185*, 114309. [CrossRef]

15. Donahue, N.D.; Acar, H.; Wilhelm, S. Concepts of Nanoparticle Cellular Uptake, Intracellular Trafficking, and Kinetics in Nanomedicine. *Adv. Drug Deliv. Rev.* **2019**, *143*, 68–96. [CrossRef]
16. Torge, A.; Grützmacher, P.; Mücklich, F.; Schneider, M. The Influence of Mannitol on Morphology and Disintegration of Spray-Dried Nano-Embedded Microparticles. *Eur. J. Pharm. Sci.* **2017**, *104*, 171–179. [CrossRef]
17. Bakand, S.; Hayes, A. Toxicological Considerations, Toxicity Assessment, and Risk Management of Inhaled Nanoparticles. *Int. J. Mol. Sci.* **2016**, *17*, 929. [CrossRef] [PubMed]
18. Hayes, A.J.; Bakand, S. Toxicological Perspectives of Inhaled Therapeutics and Nanoparticles. *Expert Opin. Drug Metab. Toxicol.* **2014**, *10*, 933–947. [CrossRef] [PubMed]
19. Kole, E.; Jadhav, K.; Shirsath, N.; Dudhe, P.; Verma, R.K.; Chatterjee, A.; Naik, J. Nanotherapeutics for Pulmonary Drug Delivery: An Emerging Approach to Overcome Respiratory Diseases. *J. Drug Deliv. Sci. Technol.* **2023**, *81*, 104261. [CrossRef]
20. Rusch, M.; Spielmeyer, A.; Zorn, H.; Hamscher, G. Biotransformation of Ciprofloxacin by Xylaria Longipes: Structure Elucidation and Residual Antibacterial Activity of Metabolites. *Appl. Microbiol. Biotechnol.* **2018**, *102*, 8573–8584. [CrossRef]
21. Bush, N.G.; Diez-santos, I.; Abbott, L.R.; Maxwell, A. Quinolones: Mechanism, Lethality and Their Contributions to Antibiotic Resistance. *Molecules* **2020**, *25*, 5662. [CrossRef]
22. Sharma, P.C.; Jain, A.; Jain, S.; Pahwa, R.; Yar, M.S. Ciprofloxacin: Review on Developments in Synthetic, Analytical, and Medicinal Aspects. *J. Enzyme Inhib. Med. Chem.* **2010**, *25*, 577–589. [CrossRef]
23. Stass, H.; Weimann, B.; Nagelschmitz, J.; Rolinck-Werninghaus, C.; Staab, D. Tolerability and Pharmacokinetic Properties of Ciprofloxacin Dry Powder for Inhalation in Patients with Cystic Fibrosis: A Phase I, Randomized, Dose-Escalation Study. *Clin. Ther.* **2013**, *35*, 1571–1581. [CrossRef] [PubMed]
24. Olivera, M.E.; Manzo, R.H.; Junginger, H.E.; Midha, K.K.; Shah, V.P.; Stavchansky, S.; Dressman, J.B. Biowaiver Monographs for Immediate Release Solid Oral Dosage Forms: Ciprofloxacin Hydrochloride. *J. Pharm. Sci.* **2011**, *100*, 22–33. [CrossRef] [PubMed]
25. Mcshane, P.J.; Weers, G.; Tarara, T.E.; Haynes, A.; Durbha, P.; Miller, D.P.; Mundry, T.; Operschall, E.; Elborn, J.S. Pulmonary Pharmacology & Therapeutics Cipro Fl Oxacin Dry Powder for Inhalation (Ciprofloxacin DPI): Technical Design and Features of an e Ffi Cient Drug—Device Combination. *Pulm. Pharmacol. Ther.* **2018**, *50*, 72–79. [CrossRef]
26. Stass, H.; Nagelschmitz, J.; Willmann, S.; Delesen, H.; Gupta, A.; Baumann, S. Inhalation of a Dry Powder Ciprofloxacin Formulation in Healthy Subjects: A Phase I Study. *Clin. Drug Investig.* **2013**, *33*, 419–427. [CrossRef]
27. Chin, W.W.L.; Parmentier, J.; Widzinski, M.; Tan, E.N.H.; Gokhale, R. A Brief Literature and Patent Review of Nanosuspensions to a Final Drug Product. *J. Pharm. Sci.* **2014**, *103*, 2980–2999. [CrossRef] [PubMed]
28. Party, P.; Ambrus, R. Investigation of Physico-Chemical Stability and Aerodynamic Properties of Novel "Nano-in-Micro" Structured Dry Powder Inhaler System. *Micromachines* **2023**, *14*, 1348. [CrossRef]
29. Scherließ, R.; Bock, S.; Bungert, N.; Neustock, A.; Valentin, L. Particle Engineering in Dry Powders for Inhalation. *Eur. J. Pharm. Sci.* **2022**, *172*, 106158. [CrossRef]
30. Lechanteur, A.; Evrard, B. Influence of Composition and Spray-Drying Process Parameters on Carrier-Free DPI Properties and Behaviors in the Lung: A Review. *Pharmaceutics* **2020**, *12*, 55. [CrossRef]
31. Cao, J.; Xu, Y.; Zhang, J.; Fang, T.; Wu, F.; Zhen, Y.; Yu, X.; Liu, Y.; Li, J.; Wang, D. "Nano-in-Micro" Structured Dry Powder Inhalers for Pulmonary Delivery: Advances and Challenges. *J. Drug Deliv. Sci. Technol.* **2024**, *96*, 105648. [CrossRef]
32. Panthi, V.K.; Fairfull-smith, K.E.; Islam, N. Ciprofloxacin-Loaded Inhalable Formulations against Lower Respiratory Tract Infections: Challenges, Recent Advances, and Future Perspectives. *Pharmaceutics* **2024**, *16*, 648. [CrossRef]
33. Feng, X.; Shi, Y.; Zhang, Y.; Lei, F.; Ren, R.; Tang, X. Opportunities and Challenges for Inhalable Nanomedicine Formulations in Respiratory Diseases: A Review. *Int. J. Nanomed.* **2024**, *19*, 1509–1538.
34. Karimi, K.; Pallagi, E.; Szabó-Révész, P.; Csóka, I.; Ambrus, R. Development of a Microparticle-Based Dry Powder Inhalation Formulation of Ciprofloxacin Hydrochloride Applying the Quality by Design Approach. *Drug Des. Dev. Ther.* **2016**, *10*, 3331–3343. [CrossRef]
35. Benke, E.; Winter, C.; Szabó-Révész, P.; Roblegg, E.; Ambrus, R. The Effect of Ethanol on the Habit and in Vitro Aerodynamic Results of Dry Powder Inhalation Formulations Containing Ciprofloxacin Hydrochloride. *Asian J. Pharm. Sci.* **2021**, *16*, 471–482. [CrossRef]
36. Party, P.; Kókai, D.; Burián, K.; Nagy, A.; Hopp, B.; Ambrus, R. Development of Extra-Fine Particles Containing Nanosized Meloxicam for Deep Pulmonary Delivery: In Vitro Aerodynamic and Cell Line Measurements. *Eur. J. Pharm. Sci.* **2022**, *176*, 106247. [CrossRef] [PubMed]
37. Party, P.; Klement, M.L.; Révész, P.S.; Ambrus, R. Preparation and Characterization of Ibuprofen Containing Nano—Embedded—Microparticles for Pulmonary Delivery. *Pharmaceutics* **2023**, *15*, 545. [CrossRef]
38. Türeli, N.G.; Torge, A.; Juntke, J.; Schwarz, B.C.; Türeli, A.E.; Lehr, C.; Schneider, M. Ciprofloxacin-Loaded PLGA Nanoparticles against Cystic Fibrosis P. Aeruginosa Lung Infections. *Eur. J. Pharm. Biopharm.* **2017**, *117*, 363–371. [CrossRef]
39. Ma, Y.; Cong, Z.; Wang, Y.; Gao, P. A Novel Multi-Drugs Ciprofloxacin-Curcumin-N-Acetylcysteine Co-Delivery System Based on Hybrid Nanocrystals for Dry Powder Inhalations. *Next Nanotechnol.* **2024**, *6*, 100084. [CrossRef]

40. Guan, W.; Liu, Y.; Ding, S.; Wang, Y. Ciprofloxacin Nanocrystals and N—Acetylcysteine Co—Solidified Powders for Pulmonary Drug Delivery: Development and in Vitro and in Vivo Characterization. *J. Nanoparticle Res.* **2022**, *24*, 41. [CrossRef]
41. Liu, Y.; Ma, Y.; Xue, L.; Guan, W.; Wang, Y. Pulmonary Multidrug Codelivery of Curcumin Nanosuspensions and Ciprofloxacin with N-Acetylcysteine for Lung Infection Therapy. *J. Drug Deliv. Sci. Technol.* **2023**, *84*, 104474. [CrossRef]
42. Dillen, K.; Vandervoort, J.; Van Den Mooter, G.; Ludwig, A. Evaluation of Ciprofloxacin-Loaded Eudragit® RS100 or RL100/PLGA Nanoparticles. *Int. J. Pharm.* **2006**, *314*, 72–82. [CrossRef]
43. El-Gendy, N.; Desai, V.; Berkland, C. Agglomerates of Ciprofloxacin Nanoparticles Yield Fine Dry Powder Aerosols. *J. Pharm. Innov.* **2010**, *5*, 79–87. [CrossRef]
44. Arnold, M.M.; Gorman, E.M.; Schieber, L.J.; Munson, E.J.; Berkland, C. NanoCipro Encapsulation in Monodisperse Large Porous PLGA Microparticles. *J. Control Release* **2007**, *121*, 100–109. [CrossRef] [PubMed]
45. Xu, Z.; Bera, H.; Wang, H.; Cun, D.; Feng, Y. Inhalable Ciprofloxacin/Polymyxin B Dry Powders in Respiratory Infection Therapy Inhalable Ciprofloxacin/Polymyxin B Dry Powders in Respiratory Infection Therapy. *Acta Mater. Medica* **2023**, *2*, 142–156. [CrossRef]
46. Małgorzata, W.; Ostolska, I.; Szewczuk-Karpisz, K.; Chibowski, S.; Terpiłowski, K.; Gun'ko, V.I.; Zarko, V.I. Investigation of the Polyvinyl Alcohol Stabilization Mechanism and Adsorption Properties on the Surface. *J. Nanoparticle Res.* **2015**, *17*, 12. [CrossRef]
47. Bartos, C.; Jójárt-Laczkovich, O.; Katona, G.; Budai-Szűcs, M.; Ambrus, R.; Bocsik, A.; Gróf, I.; Deli, M.A.; Szabó-Révész, P. Optimization of a Combined Wet Milling Process in Order to Produce Poly(Vinyl Alcohol) Stabilized Nanosuspension. *Drug Des. Dev. Ther.* **2018**, *12*, 1567–1580. [CrossRef]
48. Wang, Y.; Kho, K.; Cheow, W.S.; Hadinoto, K. A Comparison between Spray Drying and Spray Freeze Drying for Dry Powder Inhaler Formulation of Drug-Loaded Lipid-Polymer Hybrid Nanoparticles. *Int. J. Pharm.* **2012**, *424*, 98–106. [CrossRef]
49. Chvatal, A.; Alzhrani, R.; Tiwari, A.K.; Ambrus, R.; Szabó-Révész, P.; Boddu, S.H.S. Cytotoxicity of Inhalable Dry Powders in A549 Human Lung Cancer Cell Line. *Farmacia* **2018**, *66*, 172–175.
50. Yue-xing, C.; Fei-fei, Y.; Han, W.; Tao-tao, F.; Chun-yu, L.; Li-hui, Q.; Yong-hong, L. The Effect of L-Leucine on the Stabilization and Inhalability of Spray-Dried Solid Lipid Nanoparticles. *J. Drug Deliv. Sci. Technol.* **2018**, *46*, 474–481. [CrossRef]
51. Chvatal, A.; Ambrus, R.; Party, P.; Katona, G.; Jójárt-Laczkovich, O.; Szabó-Révész, P.; Fattal, E.; Tsapis, N. Formulation and Comparison of Spray Dried Non-Porous and Large Porous Particles Containing Meloxicam for Pulmonary Drug Delivery. *Int. J. Pharm.* **2019**, *559*, 68–75. [CrossRef]
52. Ordoubadi, M.; Shepard, K.B.; Wang, H.; Wang, Z.; Pluntze, A.M.; Churchman, J.P.; Vehring, R. On the Physical Stability of Leucine-Containing Spray-Dried Powders for Respiratory Drug Delivery. *Pharmaceutics* **2023**, *15*, 435. [CrossRef]
53. Sibum, I.; Hagedoorn, P.; Kluitman, M.P.G.; Kloezen, M.; Frijlink, H.W.; Grasmeijer, F. Dispersibility and Storage Stability Optimization of High Dose Isoniazid Dry Powder Inhalation Formulations with L-Leucine or Trileucine. *Pharmaceutics* **2020**, *12*, 24. [CrossRef] [PubMed]
54. Ke, W.; Yoon, R.; Chang, K.; Chan, H. Engineering the Right Formulation for Enhanced Drug Delivery. *Adv. Drug Deliv. Rev.* **2022**, *191*, 114561. [CrossRef] [PubMed]
55. Party, P.; Piszman, Z.I.; Farkas, Á.; Ambrus, R. Comprehensive In Vitro and In Silico Aerodynamic Analysis of High-Dose Ibuprofen- and Mannitol-Containing Dry Powder Inhalers for the Treatment of Cystic Fibrosis. *Pharmaceutics* **2024**, *16*, 1465. [CrossRef]
56. Hertel, N.; Birk, G.; Scherließ, R. Performance Tuning of Particle Engineered Mannitol in Dry Powder Inhalation Formulations. *Int. J. Pharm.* **2020**, *586*, 119592. [CrossRef] [PubMed]
57. Bronchitol. Available online: https://www.ema.europa.eu/en/medicines/human/EPAR/bronchitol (accessed on 10 February 2025).
58. Shetty, N.; Cipolla, D.; Park, H.; Zhou, Q.T. Physical Stability of Dry Powder Inhaler Formulations. *Expert Opin. Drug Deliv.* **2020**, *17*, 77–96. [CrossRef]
59. Bartos, C. Optimization of a Combined Wet Milling Process to Produce Nanosuspension and Its Transformation into Surfactant-Free Solid Compositions to Increase the Product Stability and Drug Bioavailability. Ph.D. Thesis, University of Szeged, Szeged, Hungary, 2019.
60. Benke, E.; Farkas, Á.; Balásházy, I.; Szabó-Révész, P.; Ambrus, R. Stability Test of Novel Combined Formulated Dry Powder Inhalation System Containing Antibiotic: Physical Characterization and In Vitro–In Silico Lung Deposition Results. *Drug Dev. Ind. Pharm.* **2019**, *45*, 1369–1378. [CrossRef]
61. Vehring, R. Pharmaceutical Particle Engineering via Spray Drying. *Pharm. Res.* **2008**, *25*, 999–1022. [CrossRef]
62. Parlati, C. Respirable Microparticles of Aminoglycoside Antibiotics for Pulmonary Administration. Ph.D. Thesis, University of Parma, Parma, Italy, 2008.
63. 2.9.3. Dissolution Test for Solid Dosage Forms. In *European Pharmacopoeia 11.0*; European Directorate for the Quality of Medicines & HealthCare: Strasbourg, France, 2024; pp. 348–355.
64. Fröhlich, E.; Mercuri, A.; Wu, S.; Salar-Behzadi, S. Measurements of Deposition, Lung Surface Area and Lung Fluid for Simulation of Inhaled Compounds. *Front. Pharmacol.* **2016**, *7*, 1–10. [CrossRef]

65. 2.9.18. Preparation for Inhalation: Aerodynamic Assessment of Fine Particles. In *European Pharmacopoeia 11.0*; European Directorate for the Quality of Medicines & HealthCare: Strasbourg, France, 2024; pp. 369–382.
66. Levet, V.; Rosière, R.; Merlos, R.; Fusaro, L.; Berger, G.; Amighi, K.; Wauthoz, N. Development of Controlled-Release Cisplatin Dry Powders for Inhalation against Lung Cancers. *Int. J. Pharm.* **2016**, *515*, 209–220. [CrossRef]
67. Dubey, R. Impact of Nanosuspension Technology on Drug Discovery and Development. *Drug Deliv. Technol.* **2006**, *5*, 67–71.
68. Hou, J.; Ci, H.; Wang, P.; Wang, C.; Lv, B.; Miao, L.; You, G. Nanoparticle Tracking Analysis versus Dynamic Light Scattering: Case Study on the Effect of Ca^{2+} and Alginate on the Aggregation of Cerium Oxide Nanoparticles. *J. Hazard. Mater.* **2018**, *360*, 319–328. [CrossRef]
69. Maguire, C.M.; Sillence, K.; Roesslein, M.; Hannell, C.; Suarez, G.; Sauvain, J.J.; Capracotta, S.; Contal, S.; Cambier, S.; El Yamani, N.; et al. Benchmark of Nanoparticle Tracking Analysis on Measuring Nanoparticle Sizing and Concentration. *J. Micro Nano-Manuf.* **2017**, *5*, 041002. [CrossRef]
70. Chvatal, A.; Farkas, Á.; Balásházy, I.; Szabó-Révész, P.; Ambrus, R. Aerodynamic Properties and in Silico Deposition of Meloxicam Potassium Incorporated in a Carrier-Free DPI Pulmonary System. *Int. J. Pharm.* **2017**, *520*, 70–78. [CrossRef] [PubMed]
71. Pallagi, E.; Karimi, K.; Ambrus, R.; Szabó-Révész, P.; Csóka, I. New Aspects of Developing a Dry Powder Inhalation Formulation Applying the Quality-by-Design Approach. *Int. J. Pharm.* **2016**, *511*, 151–160. [CrossRef] [PubMed]
72. Das, S.C.; Khadka, P.; Shah, R.; McGill, S.; Smyth, H.D.C. *Nanomedicine in Pulmonary Delivery*; Elsevier Inc.: Amsterdam, The Netherlands, 2021; ISBN 9780128204665.
73. Karimi, K.; Katona, G.; Csóka, I.; Ambrus, R. Physicochemical Stability and Aerosolization Performance of Dry Powder Inhalation System Containing Ciprofloxacin Hydrochloride. *J. Pharm. Biomed. Anal.* **2018**, *148*, 73–79. [CrossRef]
74. Böhm, B.H.L.; Müller, R.H. Lab-Scale Production Unit Design for Nanosuspensions of Sparingly Soluble Cytotoxic Drugs. *Pharm. Sci. Technol. Today* **1999**, *2*, 336–339. [CrossRef] [PubMed]
75. Cirz, R.T.; Neill, B.M.O.; Hammond, J.A.; Head, S.R.; Romesberg, F.E. Defining the Pseudomonas Aeruginosa SOS Response and Its Role in the Global Response to the Antibiotic Ciprofloxacin. *J. Bacteriol.* **2006**, *188*, 7101–7110. [CrossRef]
76. Chalkley, L.J.; Koornhof, H.J. Antimicrobial Activity of Ciprofloxacin against Pseudomonas Aeruginosa, Escherichia Coli, and Staphylococcus Aureus Determined by the Killing Curve Method: Antibiotic Comparisons and Synergistic Interactions. *Antimicrob. Agents Chemother.* **1985**, *28*, 331–342.
77. Phase, A.I.; Stass, H.; Staab, D. Safety and Pharmacokinetics of Ciprofloxacin Dry Powder for Inhalation in Cystic Fibrosis: A Phase I, Randomized, Single-Dose, Dose-Escalation Study Heino. *J. Aerosol Med. Pulm. Drug Deliv.* **2014**, *27*, 1–10. [CrossRef]
78. Sharif, S.; Muneer, S.; Izake, E.L.; Islam, N. Impact of Leucine and Magnesium Stearate on the Physicochemical Properties and Aerosolization Behavior of Wet Milled Inhalable Ibuprofen Microparticles for Developing Dry Powder Inhaler Formulation. *Pharmaceutics* **2023**, *15*, 674. [CrossRef]
79. Chapman, K.R.; Fogarty, C.M.; Peckitt, C.; Lassen, C. Delivery Characteristics and Patients ' Handling of Two Single-Dose Dry-Powder Inhalers Used in COPD. *Int. J. COPD* **2011**, *6*, 353–363.
80. Huang, Y.; Tang, H.; Meng, X.; Liu, D.; Liu, Y.; Chen, B. Highly Drug-Loaded Nanoaggregate Microparticles for Pulmonary Delivery of Cyclosporin A Highly Drug-Loaded Nanoaggregate Microparticles for Pulmonary Delivery of Cyclosporin A. *Int. J. Nanomed.* **2024**, *19*, 7529–7546. [CrossRef] [PubMed]
81. Farhangi, M.; Mahboubi, A.; Kobarfard, F.; Vatanara, A.; Mortazavi, S.A. Optimization of a Dry Powder Inhaler of Ciprofloxacin-Loaded Polymeric Nanomicelles by Spray Drying Process. *Pharm. Dev. Technol.* **2019**, *24*, 584–592. [CrossRef]
82. Sabuj, M.Z.R.; Rashid, M.A.; Dargaville, T.R.; Islam, N. Stability of Inhaled Ciprofloxacin-Loaded Poly(2-Ethyl-2-Oxazoline) Nanoparticle Dry Powder Inhaler Formulation in High Stressed Conditions. *Pharmaceuticals* **2022**, *15*, 1223. [CrossRef] [PubMed]
83. Adi, H.; Young, P.M.; Chan, H.K.; Agus, H.; Traini, D. Co-Spray-Dried Mannitol-Ciprofloxacin Dry Powder Inhaler Formulation for Cystic Fibrosis and Chronic Obstructive Pulmonary Disease. *Eur. J. Pharm. Sci.* **2010**, *40*, 239–247. [CrossRef]
84. Razuc, M.; Piña, J.; Ramírez-Rigo, M.V. Optimization of Ciprofloxacin Hydrochloride Spray-Dried Microparticles for Pulmonary Delivery Using Design of Experiments. *AAPS PharmSciTech* **2018**, *19*, 3085–3096. [CrossRef]
85. Cayli, Y.A.; Sahin, S.; Buttini, F.; Balducci, A.G.; Montanari, S.; Vural, I.; Oner, L.; Akdag, Y.; Sahin, S.; Buttini, F.; et al. Dry Powders for the Inhalation of Ciprofloxacin or Levofloxacin Combined with a Mucolytic Agent for Cystic Fibrosis Patients. *Drug Dev. Ind. Pharm.* **2017**, *43*, 1378–1389. [CrossRef]

pharmaceutics MDPI

Article

Development and Characterization of Novel Combinations and Compositions of Nanostructured Lipid Carrier Formulations Loaded with Trans-Resveratrol for Pulmonary Drug Delivery

Iftikhar Khan [1,*], Sunita Sunita [1], Nozad R. Hussein [2], Huner K. Omer [2], Abdelbary Elhissi [3], Chahinez Houacine [4], Wasiq Khan [5], Sakib Yousaf [1] and Hassaan A. Rathore [3,*]

[1] School of Pharmacy and Biomolecular Sciences, Liverpool John Moores University, Liverpool L3 3AF, UK; gradsunita@outlook.com (S.S.); s.s.yousaf@ljmu.ac.uk (S.Y.)
[2] College of Pharmacy, Hawler Medical University, Erbil 44001, Iraq; nozad.hussein@hmu.edu.krd (N.R.H.); huner.omer@hmu.edu.krd (H.K.O.)
[3] Department of Pharmaceutical Sciences, College of Pharmacy, QU Health Sector, Qatar University, Doha 2713, Qatar; aelhissi@qu.edu.qa
[4] School of Pharmacy and Biomedical Sciences, University of Central Lancashire, Preston PR1 2HE, UK; chahinez.houacine1@gmail.com
[5] Faculty of Engineering and Technology, Liverpool John Moores University, Liverpool L3 3AF, UK; w.khan@ljmu.ac.uk
* Correspondence: i.khan@ljmu.ac.uk (I.K.); hrathore@qu.edu.qa (H.A.R.)

Abstract: Background/Objectives: This study aimed to fabricate, optimize, and characterize nanostructured lipid carriers (NLCs) loaded with trans-resveratrol (TRES) as an anti-cancer drug for pulmonary drug delivery using medical nebulizers. Methods: Novel TRES-NLC formulations (F1–F24) were prepared via hot, high-pressure homogenization. One solid lipid (Dynasan 116) was combined with four liquid lipids (Capryol 90, Lauroglycol 90, Miglyol 810, and Tributyrin) in three different ratios (10:90, 50:50, and 90:10 *w*/*w*), with a surfactant (Tween 80) in two different concentrations (0.5 and 1.5%), and a co-surfactant, soya phosphatidylcholine (SPC S-75; 50 mg). Results: Amongst the analyzed 24 TR-NLC formulations, F8, F14, and F22 were selected based on their physicochemical stability when freshly prepared and following storage (4 weeks 25 °C), as well as in terms of particle size (<145 nm), polydispersity index (PDI; <0.21) and entrapment efficiency (>96%). Furthermore, F14 showed greater stability at 4 and 25 °C for six months and exhibited enhanced aerosolization performance, demonstrating the greater deposition of TRES in the later stages of the next-generation impactor (NGI) when using an air-jet nebulizer than when using an ultrasonic nebulizer. The F14 formulation exhibited greater stability and release in acetate buffer (pH 5.4), with a cumulative release of 95%. Conclusions: Overall, formulation F14 in combination with an air-jet nebulizer was identified as a superior combination, demonstrating higher emitted dose (ED; 80%), fine particle dose (FPD; 1150 µg), fine particle fraction (FPF; 24%), and respirable fraction (RF; 94%). These findings are promising in the optimization and development of NLC formulations, highlighting their versatility and targeting the pulmonary system via nebulization.

Keywords: nanostructured lipid carriers; cancer; anti-cancer; pulmonary system; aerosolization

1. Introduction

Advancements in inhalational drug delivery systems have resulted in successful applications in the prophylaxis and treatment of localized lung diseases (e.g., asthma, chronic obstructive pulmonary disease, cystic fibrosis, pulmonary hypertension, and cancer) [1]. However, due to the added advantage of bypassing first-pass metabolism, this route has started to attract growing interest for the treatment/management of systemic diseases [2,3]. The lung is distinguished by its large contact surface area (~100 m^2), thin epithelium (i.e., 0.1–0.2 µm), and rich blood supply. Drug bioavailability following inhalation can further be promoted by low enzymatic degradation, high membrane permeability, and rapid onset of action [1,4,5]. For these reasons, the development of advanced delivery systems, particularly for those that use nanotechnology, has seen a surge in interest to exploit this non-invasive route of administration [6,7]. Specifically, nanoparticles are known to offer a large surface to volume ratio, high drug encapsulation, higher biodistribution, controlled and site-specific drug release [8,9], potentially low systemic toxicity [10,11], and better formulation stability during nebulization [12].

Lipid nanoparticle drug delivery systems provide considerable benefits, including easy preparation, high biodegradability, scale-up feasibility, reduced toxicity, and targeted delivery [12,13]. Various types of lipid-based formulations have achieved the successful delivery of both hydrophilic and hydrophobic compounds [14]. There are several types of lipid nanoparticles including liposomes [14,15]. Prominent examples of liposome products include Doxil®, which is a doxorubicin-loaded PEGylated liposome formulation designed for the treatment of breast and ovarian cancer [14,16]. Other lipid nanoparticle formulations include niosomes [17,18], transfersomes [1], ethosomes, and surfactosmes [19].

Advancements in technology have led to the development of second-generation lipid nanoparticles, which started with solid lipid nanocarriers (SLNs), followed by third-generation nanocarriers, referred to as nanostructured lipid carriers (NLCs). SLNs have been vastly explored for delivering various types of agents (e.g., iron oxide, tachnitium-99, and insulin) [20, 21]. SLNs are biocompatible delivery systems having low toxicity and a smaller size (50–1000 nm) and can be easily manufactured on a large scale [22]. Despite these advantages, SLNs have shortcomings such as poor drug loading capacity (attributed to the crystalline nature of the solid lipid), drug leakage (following polymorphic transition), lipid particle growth, as well as particle aggregation and solidification. Consequently, NLCs were introduced to improve drug loading, stability, and compatibility. NLCs are combinations of solid and liquid lipids and hence possess a less crystalline matrix and imperfect solidified core, which prevent the leakage of the drug [23].

TRES, a natural polyphenol (chemically known as 3,4′,5-trans-trihydroxystilbene), is a biologically active compound and possesses multiple biological activities (i.e., anti-inflammatory, anti-oxidant, anti-tumor, as well as neuro- and cardioprotective effects) [11,24–26]. Despite the promising biological effects, it has low systematic availability due to rapid clearance, limiting its clinical application [27]. Moreover, TRES is hydrophobic molecule with slow dissolution and low oral bioavailability [28]. NLC formulations can improve absorption and protect against the rapid metabolism of drugs. The success of pulmonary therapy is not only dependent on the pharmacology of the inhaled drug but also on the site and extent of drug deposition in the respiratory tract [29]. Thus, for pulmonary targeting using lipid-based formulations, these must possess optimum aerodynamic properties such as aerosol median aerodynamic diameter and polydispersity, which determine the fine particle dose (FPD), and fine particle fraction (FPF) of the inhaled aerosol. Nebulizers are highly recommended for the delivery of liquid formulations (i.e., solutions or suspension) into the pulmonary system. The in vitro assessment of the aerodynamic diameter of aerosol particles released from nebulizers can be analyzed via a next-generation impactor (NGI) [30].

The present study aimed to formulate, optimize, and characterize TRES-NLC formulations for their deposition in an NGI. TRES-NLC formulations were studied based on their novel combination and composition ratios of different types of solid lipid, liquid lipid, surfactant, and co-surfactant ingredients. These were assessed in terms of particle size, PDI, zeta potential, drug entrapment efficiency, and percentage recovery. The formulations were stored at 4 and 25 °C for six months to analyze their stability at different temperatures. Based on their physicochemical properties and the stability studies, the optimum TRES-NLC formulation was selected for an aerosolization study using air-jet and ultrasonic nebulizers. Additionally, in vitro release was studied to determine the effect of two media with different pH values at 37 °C on the release profile of TRES.

2. Materials and Methods

2.1. Materials

HPLC-grade acetonitrile, formic acid, absolute ethanol, tetrahydrofuran and ammonium molybdate were purchased from Fischer Scientific Ltd., Loughborough, UK. Trans-resveratrol ($C_{14}H_{12}O_3$) was procured from Manchester Organics (Runcorn, UK). Tripalmitin (Dynasan 116; $C_{51}H_{98}O_6$) and caprylic triglyceride (Miglyol 810; $C_{21}H_{40}O_5$) were gifted by IOI Oleochemical GmbH (Witten, Germany). Propylene glycol monocaprylate type II (Capryol 90; $C_{11}H_{22}O_3$) and propylene glycol monolaurate (Lauroglycol 90; $C_{15}H_{30}O_3$) were provided by Gattefose (Ascot, Berkshire, UK). Tributyrin ($C_{15}H_{26}O_6$) was bought from Across Organics (New Jersey, NJ, USA). Tween 80 ($C_{64}H_{124}O_{26}$) was purchased from Sigma Aldrich, Gillingham, UK. Soya phosphatidylcholine S-75 grade (SPC; $C_{42}H_{80}NO_{26}P$) was gifted by Lipoid GmbH, Ludwigshafen, Germany.

2.2. Preparation and Optimization of Nanostructured Lipid Carriers (NLCs)

Combinations of one solid lipid and four different types of liquid lipids were used at three different ratios (10:90, 50:50, and 90:10 *w*/*w*) to form the lipid phase. Each combination of lipid phase was then formulated with two different percentages of the surfactant Tween 80 (i.e., 0.5 and 1.5%) to prepare 24 different TRES-NLC formulations via hot, high-pressure homogenization. Dynasan 116 was used as the solid lipid, whereas the four liquid lipids employed included Capryol 90, Lauroglycol 90, Miglyol 810, and Tributyrin. Tween 80 and SPC S-75 were employed as the surfactant and co-surfactant in all formulations. Each TRES-NLC formulation was prepared using three different phases, i.e., liquid phase, aqueous phase, and drug phase (Table 1).

Table 1. Composition of TRES-NLC formulations consisting of one solid lipid (Dynasan 116) and four liquid lipids (Capryol 90, Lauroglycol 90, Miglyol 810, and Tributyrin) in three different weight ratios, 10:90 (200 mg:1800 mg), 50:50 (1000 mg:1000 mg), or 90:10 (1800 mg:200 mg), where Tween 80 was used in two concentration (0.5% (250 mg) or 1.5% (750 mg)) as a surfactant and SPC-75 (50 mg) as a co-surfactant, and trans-resveratrol (TRES) (50 mg) was employed as the drug to prepare 24 TRES-NLC formulations.

Formulation	Solid Lipid (mg)	Liquid Lipid (mg)	Solid Lipid: Liquid Lipid (*w*/*w*)	Tween-80 (%)	Co-Surfactant (mg)	TRES (mg)
F1	Dynasan 116	Capryol 90	10:90	0.5	50	50
F2	Dynasan 116	Capryol 90	10:90	1.5	50	50
F3	Dynasan 116	Capryol 90	50:50	0.5	50	50
F4	Dynasan 116	Capryol 90	50:50	1.5	50	50
F5	Dynasan 116	Capryol 90	90:10	0.5	50	50
F6	Dynasan 116	Capryol 90	90:10	1.5	50	50
F7	Dynasan 116	Lauroglycol 90	10:90	0.5	50	50
F8	Dynasan 116	Lauroglycol 90	10:90	1.5	50	50
F9	Dynasan 116	Lauroglycol 90	50:50	0.5	50	50
F10	Dynasan 116	Lauroglycol 90	50:50	1.5	50	50
F11	Dynasan 116	Lauroglycol 90	90:10	0.5	50	50
F12	Dynasan 116	Lauroglycol 90	90:10	1.5	50	50
F13	Dynasan 116	Miglyol 810	10:90	0.5	50	50
F14	Dynasan 116	Miglyol 810	10:90	1.5	50	50
F15	Dynasan 116	Miglyol 810	50:50	0.5	50	50
F16	Dynasan 116	Miglyol 810	50:50	1.5	50	50
F17	Dynasan 116	Miglyol 810	90:10	0.5	50	50
F18	Dynasan 116	Miglyol 810	90:10	1.5	50	50
F19	Dynasan 116	Tributyrin	10:90	0.5	50	50
F20	Dynasan 116	Tributyrin	10:90	1.5	50	50
F21	Dynasan 116	Tributyrin	50:50	0.5	50	50
F22	Dynasan 116	Tributyrin	50:50	1.5	50	50
F23	Dynasan 116	Tributyrin	90:10	0.5	50	50
F24	Dynasan 116	Tributyrin	90:10	1.5	50	50

The lipid phase (4% of total formulation) was prepared by heating a solid lipid (Dynasan 116) and one of the liquid lipids (Capryol 90, Lauroglycol 90, Miglyol 810, or Tributyrin) in a ratio of 10:90 (200 mg:1800 mg) and melted at 70 °C (~10 °C above the phase transition temperature of the solid lipid) using digital hotplate magnetic stirrer (ADS-HP-NT, Asynt, IKA laboratories equipment, Germany). Similarly, other combinations of solid lipid and liquid lipids i.e., 50:50 *w/w* (1000 mg:1000 mg) and 90:10 *w/w* (1800 mg:200 mg), were used to prepare separate lipid phases. The aqueous phase was prepared separately by preheating deionized water at 70 °C (sufficient to prepare 50 mL of formulation), using Tween 80 at two different concentrations (0.5% (250 mg) and 1.5% (750 mg)), which were combined using a digital hotplate magnetic stirrer. The drug phase was prepared by dissolving 500 mg of TRES and 500 mg of SPC-S75 in 10 mL of ethanol. Subsequently, 1 mL (containing 50 mg of TRES and 50 mg of SPC-S75) of this phase was transferred into the preheated molten lipid phase. This was followed by the addition of the preheated aqueous phase into the lipid phase using continuous stirring (1250 rpm) for 15 min in order to prepare a dispersion system (i.e., microemulsion). For uniform homogenization, the obtained dispersion was subjected to homogenization (T18 Ultra-Turarax; IKA, Königswinter, Germany.) for 3 min at 10,000 rpm. The resultant uniform microemulsion was homogenized to a nano size by probe-sonication (Qsonica Probe Sonicator, Newtown, CT, USA) for 5 min using an amplitude intensity of 60%. TRES-NLC formulations were successfully obtained following cooling of the solid lipid to room temperature (25 °C).

2.3. Particle Size and Zeta Potential Analysis

For the calculation of size and zeta potential, 0.5 mL of TRES-NLC formulation was diluted with 10 mL of water. Particle size and polydispersity index (PDI) of TRES-NLC formulations were measured by dynamic light scattering (DLS) using a Zetasizer (Malvern Zetasizer Nano series, Malvern, Worcestershire, UK) at 25 °C. Moreover, after aerosolization, TRES-NLC formulations deposited in various stages of the NGI were washed with water and subjected to vortex-mixing for 1 min (Labnet International, Edison, NJ, USA), followed by particle size analysis. A Zetasizer was also employed to determine the zeta potential of the TRES-NLC particles using laser doppler velocimetry (LDV).

2.4. Determination of Entrapment Efficiency of Drug

The entrapment efficiency of the TRES-NLC formulations were determined via Millipore filters (3 kDa; Fisher Scientific, Loughborough, UK). To determine the unentrapped or free drug (TRES), 0.5 mL of TRES-NLC formulation was pipetted into a Millipore centrifuge filter that was fitted into an Eppendorf tube. Bench centrifugation (Spectrafuge 24D, Labnet International, Edison, NJ, USA) was then conducted at 5900 rcf for 15 min. The clear filtrate at the bottom of the Eppendorf tube was collected (centrifuge filters allowed the free drug to pass through their pores, while retaining the TRES entrapped in the NLCs) and concentration of free TRES was determined using high-performance liquid chromatography (HPLC) (Agilent 1200 Series Instrument, Waldborn, Germany). To quantify the total drug, 1 mL of TRES-NLC formulation was diluted with tetrahydrofuran, followed by running through HPLC. An HPLC instrument was used at 25 °C at a wavelength of 239 nm. A reverse-phase Luna C-18 column (Phenomenex, Torrance, CA, USA) with a 5 µm particle size, 4.6 mm internal diameter, and 250 mm length was used as the stationary phase. The flow rate was set t 1 mL/min with an injection volume of 20 µL. HPLC analysis was performed using a mobile phase (comprised of 0.1% formic acid and acetonitrile).

The entrapment efficiency of TRES was calculated using Equation (1), and percentage recovery was calculated using Equation (2).

$$\text{Entrapment efficiency } (\%) = \frac{\text{Totaldrug} - \text{Unentrappeddrug}}{\text{Total drug}} \times 100 \tag{1}$$

$$\text{Recovery}(\%) = \frac{\text{Practical amount of drug obtained from HPLC calibration curve}}{\text{Theoretical amount (amount of drug added during preparation)}} \times 100 \tag{2}$$

2.5. TRES-NLCs Formulation Stability Study

The initial stability studies of the TRES-NLC formulations were conducted for particle size, PDI, zeta potential, and entrapment efficiency in order to compare the physicochemical properties between the freshly prepared formulations as well as following storage at 25 °C for four weeks. All formulations were kept in an amber-colored glass bottles (25 mL), and the temperature was maintained throughout this study. Particle size analysis and zeta potential measurements were conducted as described in Section 2.3 and entrapment efficiency as described in Section 2.4.

Based on the stability study of the F1–F24 formulations, only selected TRES-NLC formulations were used for subsequent studies. These selected formulations were then characterized (particle size, PDI, zeta potential, entrapment efficiency, and drug recovery) over a period of six months under two different temperatures (4 and 25 °C).

2.6. Morphology Study via Transmission Electron Microscopy (TEM)

One drop of the TRES-NLC formulation and two drops of a negative stain ammonium molybdate were mixed and transferred onto a carbon-coated copper grid (400 mesh) (TAAB Laboratories Equipment Ltd., Aldermaston, UK) and then allowed to dry for 1 h. Samples were then placed in the TEM instrument (Morgagni 268D, EFI, MegaView, Brno, Czech Republic), and the morphology of the TRES-NLC formulations was observed.

2.7. Aerosolization Study of TRES-NLC Formulation Using Next-Generation Impactor (NGI)

The NGI (Copley Scientific, Nottingham, UK) was operated with a critical airflow controller (Copley TPK 2000, Copley Scientific, UK) and vacuum pump (Copley flow HCP5, Copley Scientific, UK). The airflow was adjusted to 15 L/min (European Pharmacopeia general chapter 2.9.44) for the aerodynamic assessment of nebulized aerosols.

Before aerosolization, the NGI and its collecting compartments were all kept in a fridge for 90 min at 5 °C. Two nebulizers were used: an air-jet (PARI GmbH Tourboboy 5 air-jet, Starnberg, Germany) and an ultrasonic nebulizer (Rechargeable Ultrasonic Inhaler MY-520B, China). All empty collection trays, induction port (mouthpiece), and nebulizers were weighed separately prior to starting nebulization. TRES-NLC formulations (5 mL) were pipetted into the nebulizer and weighed. The nebulizer was positioned in front of the induction port before starting nebulization. After completed nebulization (i.e., when the nebulizer stopped producing aerosols), the nebulization time (continuous formation of aerosols) and sputtering time (the intermittent formation of aerosols until no further aerosol formation) were recorded. The mass output (Equation (3)) and mass output rate (Equation (4)) were calculated. Moreover, the quantity of formulation deposited into each stage was determined via HPLC analysis.

$$\text{Mass output}(\%) = \frac{\text{Weight of nebulized formulation}}{\text{Weight of formulation present in nebulizer before nebulization}} \times 100 \quad (3)$$

$$\text{Mass output rate}\left(\frac{\text{mg}}{\text{min}}\right) = \frac{\text{Weight of nebulized formulation}}{\text{Complete nebulization time}} \quad (4)$$

The emitted dose (ED) was the total amount TRES in the formulation emitted from the nebulizer. The fine particle dose (FPD) was the mass of particles less than 5 μm in diameter of the total ED. The fine particle fraction (FPF) was the fraction of particles (i.e., less than 5 μm in diameter) correlated to the emitted mass, and the respirable fraction (RF) represented the fraction of particles entering stages 2–7. ED (Equation (5)), RF (Equation (6)), FPD (Equation (7)) and FPF (Equation (8)) were calculated using the following equations:

$$\text{ED}(\%) = \frac{\text{Initial mass in nebulizer} - \text{Final mass remaining in nebulizer}}{\text{Initial mass in nebulizer}} \times 100 \quad (5)$$

$$\text{RF}(\%) = \frac{\text{Fine particle dose}}{\text{Total particle mass on all stages}} \times 100 \quad (6)$$

$$\text{FPD} = \text{Mass of drug deposited on stage 2 through 7} \quad (7)$$

$$\text{FPF}(\%) = \frac{\text{Fine particle dose}}{\text{Initial particle mass loaded in nebulizer}} \times 100 \quad (8)$$

2.8. Study of TRES Released from NLC Formulations

The release profile of TRES from the NLCs (1 mg/1 mL) was studied using dialysis tubing (a cut-off MWCO; 3500 Daltons) placed in the dissolution apparatus II USP (Varion Instrument, Cary, NC, USA). The dialysis bag was selected based on its pore size, which should ideally be 5–10 times larger than the molecular weight of TRES (i.e., 228 Daltons) [7]. This allowed the TRES molecules only to pass through the dialysis bag, while retaining the NLC particles due to their large size. TRES-NLC formulations (5 mL) were sealed in the dialysis bag and placed in release media (900 mL), and the rotation speed of the paddles was adjusted to 100 rpm at 37 °C. The time-dependent release of the drug was investigated in two different media: acetate buffer (pH 5) and deionized water (pH 7). Samples (1 mL) were withdrawn from each media at specific time intervals (0.5, 1, 2, 3, 4, 5, and 24 h) and replaced each time with the same volume of drug-free media. TRES alone (5 mg/5 mL) was also employed as a control for comparison. The amounts of TRES released were estimated using HPLC (Section 2.4).

2.9. Statistical Analysis

Analysis of variance (ANOVA) and Student's *t*-tests were performed using SPSS software (IBM SPSS Statistics 28.0) in order to determine whether the difference was significant between the groups. A p value lower than 0.05 indicated the difference was statistically significant. All experiments were conducted in triplicate using three different batches.

3. Results and Discussion

3.1. Initial Investigation and Selection of TRES-NLC Formulations

The initial selection of TRES-NLC formulations was conducted based on particle size, PDI, zeta potential, and entrapment efficiency. Comparisons were made between freshly prepared formulations and formulations stored at 25 °C for four weeks.

In the TRES-NLC formulations prepared using Capryol 90 as a liquid lipid, larger particles were observed, attributed to particle aggregation; thus, a significant difference ($p < 0.05$) was noted in particle size between the freshly prepared TRES-NLCs and the TRES-NLCs stored at 25 °C for four weeks. This may have been related to the higher viscosity of Capryol 90, which may have prevented oil droplet emulsification, resulting in larger nanoparticles [31]. Lauroglycol 90 is a medium-chain mono-glyceride, and Miglyol 810 and Tributyrin are medium- to short-chain triglycerides; when medium- to shorter-chain glycerides were employed in the formulations, enhanced stability in terms of particle size was observed, linked to the lower viscosity of the employed glycerides (Table 2) [32]. Moreover, upon comparing the particle size and PDI of the freshly prepared TRES-NLC formulations, it was observed that the formulations containing higher liquid lipid (i.e., 10:90, solid to liquid lipid w/w ratio) and surfactant concentrations (i.e., 1.5%) had smaller particle size and PDI when compared to the formulations with low concentrations of liquid lipid and surfactant (produced large particles and a broader PDI) (Table 2). F22 showed greater potential based on its stability, particularly in terms of particle size and growth of the NLCs. In contrast, F20 exhibited a higher tendency for aggregation and sedimentation during storage, which could lead to stability issues upon long-term storage.

Table 2. Particle size, polydispersity index (PDI), zeta potential, and drug entrapment efficiency of the freshly prepared TRES-NLC formulations and those stored at 25 °C for four weeks. The molar ratios (drug to solid and liquid lipids) remained the same for freshly prepared TRES-NLC formulations and for those stored at 25 °C for four weeks. Data are reported as mean ± SD, n = 3.

Formulations	Size (nm)		PDI		Zeta Potential (mV)		Entrapment Efficiency (%)		Molar Ratios (Drug:Lipids)
	After Preparation	After Four Weeks	After Preparation	After Four Weeks	After Preparation	After Four Weeks	After Preparation	After Four Weeks	After Preparation and After Four Weeks
F1	245.46 ± 7.68	514.47 ± 8.75	0.25 ± 0.03	0.77 ± 0.18	−26.75 ± 4.77	−28.27 ± 5.12	97.15 ± 9.54	95.92 ± 7.82	0.02:1
F2	202.68 ± 8.52	258.72 ± 8.49	0.24 ± 0.08	0.31 ± 0.11	−26.35 ± 4.98	−30.85 ± 5.44	96.46 ± 7.25	95.17 ± 6.16	0.02:1
F3	272.13 ± 6.21	1059.70 ± 9.65	0.29 ± 0.11	0.38 ± 0.06	−25.60 ± 5.13	−28.15 ± 4.58	94.62 ± 6.58	93.08 ± 7.33	0.03:1
F4	224.67 ± 7.45	452.72 ± 8.12	0.25 ± 0.12	0.37 ± 0.05	−29.25 ± 6.95	−32.95 ± 5.08	94.62 ± 9.16	93.18 ± 6.74	0.03:1
F5	324.45 ± 7.44	817.75 ± 8.32	0.53 ± 0.09	0.43 ± 0.13	−26.45 ± 5.77	−27.35 ± 4.18	92.91 ± 5.49	91.07 ± 7.55	0.06:1
F6	310.15 ± 9.52	422.75 ± 7.54	0.46 ± 0.11	0.53 ± 0.04	−32.85 ± 5.34	−31.48 ± 6.58	91.16 ± 7.59	90.71 ± 6.49	0.06:1
F7	165.25 ± 8.25	202.25 ± 7.07	0.28 ± 0.03	0.20 ± 0.05	−32.18 ± 6.23	−31.03 ± 7.15	97.65 ± 8.25	98.22 ± 7.26	0.03:1
F8	136.48 ± 9.15	149.01 ± 9.73	0.19 ± 0.03	0.21 ± 0.05	−29.50 ± 4.42	−31.24 ± 6.72	97.73 ± 8.19	96.76 ± 6.59	0.03:1
F9	190.80 ± 8.55	231.25 ± 9.71	0.34 ± 0.08	0.25 ± 0.08	−36.15 ± 6.78	−34.67 ± 6.69	97.06 ± 6.23	96.16 ± 6.38	0.04:1
F10	163.80 ± 8.27	211.55 ± 7.92	0.29 ± 0.04	0.26 ± 0.05	−33.16 ± 6.62	−31.33 ± 5.92	95.19 ± 7.54	93.48 ± 7.09	0.04:1
F11	288.05 ± 6.79	516.25 ± 3.59	0.58 ± 0.27	0.41 ± 0.03	−25.52 ± 3.53	−25.80 ± 6.44	93.47 ± 6.85	91.28 ± 6.18	0.07:1
F12	206.05 ± 5.65	258.49 ± 7.29	0.44 ± 0.11	0.65 ± 0.33	−36.85 ± 6.69	−36.48 ± 7.06	93.82 ± 5.28	91.75 ± 6.68	0.07:1
F13	186.70 ± 4.78	254.23 ± 6.75	0.20 ± 0.05	0.25 ± 0.06	−30.15 ± 6.57	−32.39 ± 6.91	98.52 ± 5.97	97.55 ± 7.16	0.04:1
F14	142.41 ± 8.28	158.90 ± 7.99	0.15 ± 0.03	0.19 ± 0.11	−36.75 ± 6.86	−35.09 ± 7.98	98.17 ± 7.32	96.78 ± 5.91	0.04:1
F15	206.75 ± 7.25	298.76 ± 6.59	0.26 ± 0.06	0.34 ± 0.08	−30.60 ± 6.67	−29.07 ± 6.19	98.06 ± 4.16	95.72 ± 6.28	0.05:1
F16	182.80 ± 9.16	203.75 ± 7.47	0.21 ± 0.07	0.30 ± 0.09	−38.22 ± 7.36	−35.72 ± 6.69	96.24 ± 4.55	94.65 ± 5.53	0.05:1
F17	206.81 ± 7.26	492.25 ± 9.26	0.43 ± 0.02	0.24 ± 0.06	−34.81 ± 6.54	−31.65 ± 6.41	94.68 ± 5.62	92.26 ± 5.06	0.08:1
F18	187.19 ± 8.17	205.58 ± 9.48	0.28 ± 0.12	0.59 ± 0.25	−29.30 ± 7.97	−30.25 ± 6.98	94.55 ± 4.68	93.71 ± 6.26	0.07:1
F19	288.65 ± 7.63	346.77 ± 9.41	0.29 ± 0.06	0.32 ± 0.08	−25.85 ± 6.06	−29.45 ± 6.15	98.02 ± 5.05	98.82 ± 5.29	0.03:1
F20	265.70 ± 9.53	292.93 ± 8.09	0.25 ± 0.05	0.28 ± 0.04	−34.30 ± 4.68	−36.15 ± 6.46	98.48 ± 5.52	97.03 ± 5.18	0.03:1
F21	172.46 ± 6.55	379.95 ± 9.27	0.44 ± 0.09	0.32 ± 0.14	−30.25 ± 7.06	−32.65 ± 6.72	96.13 ± 4.87	98.27 ± 1.56	0.05:1
F22	144.54 ± 7.48	156.82 ± 8.39	0.17 ± 0.06	0.20 ± 0.03	−30.95 ± 6.88	−32.45 ± 7.70	97.34 ± 5.22	96.38 ± 4.51	0.05:1
F23	341.85 ± 7.84	393.65 ± 10.56	0.47 ± 0.05	0.44 ± 0.06	−30.42 ± 6.16	−27.15 ± 7.31	95.92 ± 5.72	94.27 ± 6.26	0.07:1
F24	202.59 ± 7.73	259.56 ± 8.62	0.39 ± 0.08	0.36 ± 0.11	−35.42 ± 6.67	−37.41 ± 5.86	95.44 ± 6.48	94.39 ± 4.71	0.07:1

Differences in particle size could be attributed to the solid lipid concentration, as this may affect the melting/solidification process during NLC production (Table 2), forming agglomerates when higher concentrations are used. Despite probe sonication, the agglomerates resisted breakdown, resulting in a wide PDI [13]. The effect of solid lipid concentration is evidenced in research conducted by Das, et al. [33] and Gokce, et al. [34], where increases in particle size have been observed. This increase in solid lipid concentration in the NLC formulations was posed to increase the dispersion viscosity, resulting in size increases [35,36]. A concentration-dependent relationship between surfactant and particle size has also been observed, with higher concentrations being associated with smaller particles [37]. This trend is also supported by previous findings [36,38].

Based on the particle size and PDI, TRES-NLC formulations F8, F14, and F22 (containing liquid lipid Lauroglycol 90, Miglyol 810, and Tributyrin) were selected, where the particle size of the freshly prepared samples was less than 150 nm, and the PDI value was less than 0.20. Particle sizes of 150 nm were used as a guide to compare formulation stability during storage conditions. Moreover, the formulations with a smaller particle size and lower PDI were preferred due to their large surface area as well as dose uniformity. Moreover, particle size is the major determinant in the deposition and distribution of inhaled drugs within the pulmonary system to achieve localized effects. Smaller particles possess the ability to reach the small airways and alveolar epithelium compared with larger particles with a wider PDI. This is attributed to the ability of nanoparticles to be incorporated into the "respirable" nebulized droplets. No significant difference ($p > 0.05$) was observed among the three selected formulations in terms of particle size or PDI when a comparison was conducted between freshly prepared formulations and formulations stored for four weeks at 25 °C (Table 2). Unlike the particle size findings, the zeta potentials were similar ($p > 0.05$) between the fresh TRES-NLC formulations and samples stored at 25 °C for four weeks (Table 2). The zeta potential values were more than −20 mV, due to the presence of the free hydroxyl group of the liquid lipids in the formulations [37].

Furthermore, no significant difference ($p > 0.05$) was observed in the entrapment efficiency (Table 2). The high entrapment efficiency was associated with using higher amounts of liquid and solid lipid (2000 mg in total), offering a large area for the drug to be encapsulated. There are other studies that have employed a higher amount of TRES and still achieved higher entrapment efficiencies. A study conducted by Mathew et al. [1] also used TRES (50 mg) with much lower amounts of solid and liquid lipids (i.e., 252 mg in total) in NLC formulations but still achieved a 95% entrapment efficiency, which is thus unlikely attributable to saturation. In the same study, liposomes and transfersomes were prepared with the same amounts of lipid phase and TRES, which still achieved high entrapment efficiency, demonstrating the ability of TRES to lodge within the vesicles. Similar results were also found by Houacine et al. [37] with regard to the entrapment efficiency of TRES in NLC formulations. The higher entrapment efficiency of TRES may be related to its high miscibility with lipids (i.e., solid and liquid) and surfactant. In general, the incorporation of higher concentrations of lipids may also reduce particle crystallinity and cause disorder in the crystal lattice, which allow greater accommodation of the drug (offering high solubility in the lipid matrix), leading to higher drug loading capacity and hence higher entrapment efficiency (>95%) (Table 2). Additionally, higher concentrations of liquid lipid and solid lipid may account for imperfections within the crystal matrix, providing more space in which the drug molecules can lodge [12,39,40]. The effect of liquid lipid on drug entrapment (i.e., increased with increasing concentration) has been previously reported [12,41–43].

Overall, it was found that higher concentrations of liquid lipid and surfactant in TRES-NLC formulations may be responsible for the higher drug entrapment, smaller particle size, and lower PDI. Therefore, based on the characterization studies, formulations F8, F14, and F22 were selected for further studies.

3.2. Surface Morphology Study of TRES-NLC Formulations

When the selected TRES-NLC formulations (F8, F14, and F22) were investigated for particle morphology, they were found to be spherical, within the nanosize range (Figure 1).

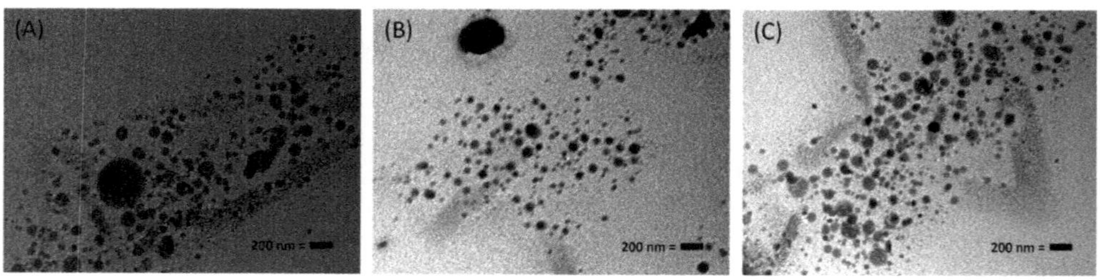

Figure 1. Transmission electron microscopy (TEM) images of TRES-NLC formulations (with 200 nm scale bar): (**A**) F8, (**B**) F14, and (**C**) F22. These images are typical of the three different batches.

3.3. Particle Size Analysis of TRES-NLC Formulations in NGI Stages

Aerosolization studies were conducted on the selected TRES-NLC formulations (i.e., F8, F14, and F22). Using the air-jet and ultrasonic nebulizers, the aerosol deposition of TRES-NLC formulations in the NGI was analyzed in terms of particle size. After aerosolization, a decreasing trend in particle size was observed when moving from stage 1 to stage 8 in the NGI (Figure 2); thus, larger droplets/particles were deposited in the initial stages, and smaller particles were deposited in the advanced stages of the NGI [12,44]. It is important to consider the inertial action of aero-dispersed particles, i.e., particles accelerate at a comparatively high speed under the influence of compressed air (in air-jet nebulizers) when compared to the piezoelectric crystal vibration (employed in ultrasonic nebulizers). Therefore, it is suggested that air stream/aerosols containing the droplets/particles are accelerated through the nozzle of the nebulizers, causing comparatively stronger abrupt movement of the particles in air-jet nebulizers than in ultrasonic nebulizers. Consequently, particle separation occurs based on the differences in the inertia of the particles (which depends on their size and speed) [45]. Thus, stage 1 demonstrated deposition of larger particles, which was observed more prominently when the air-jet nebulizer was used (Figure 2A).

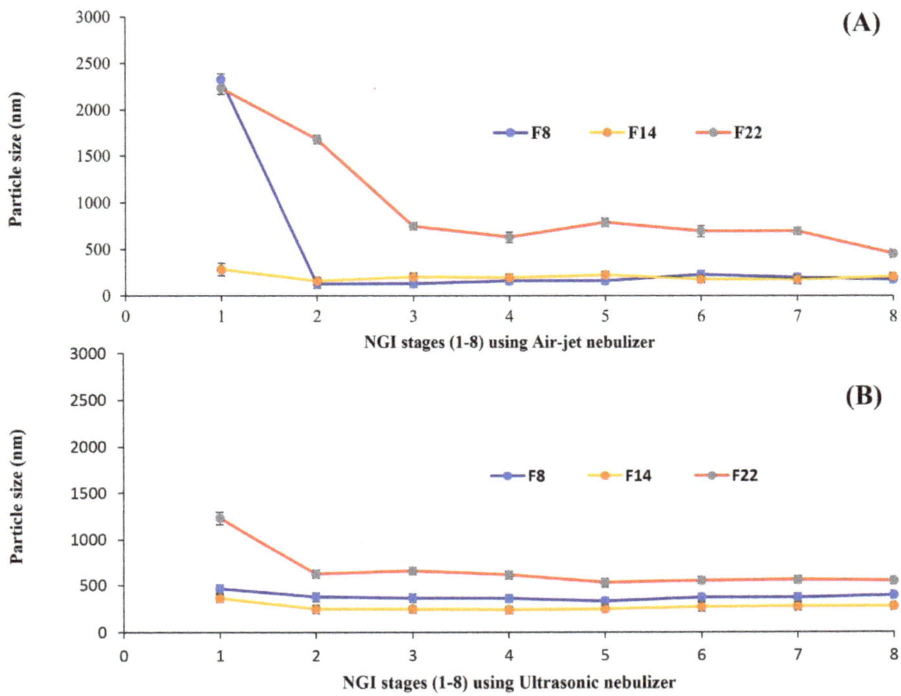

Figure 2. Deposition and analysis of aerosol droplets containing TRES-NLC particles of various formulations (F8, F14, and F22) in the various stages of a next-generation impactor (NGI) using (**A**) air-jet and (**B**) ultrasonic nebulizers at an airflow rate of 15 L/min. Data are presented as mean ± SD, n = 3.

According to the analysis of the TRES-NLC formulation deposition in the NGI stages, the performance of formulation F14 demonstrated greater stability and consistency compared to formulations F8 and F22 (Figure 2). Moreover, the particle size of formulation F14 was significantly smaller ($p < 0.05$) than that of the F8 and F22 formulations (in all eight stages of the NGI when the ultrasonic nebulizer was used) (Figure 2B).

3.4. TRES-NLC Formulation (F8, F14, and F22) Stability Study

TRES-NLC formulations F8, F14, and F22 were studied for stability via storage for six months at 4 or 25 °C. Particle size, PDI, Zeta potential, drug entrapment efficiency and drug recovery were determined to evaluate formulation stability at months 2, 4 and 6. It was noted that F8, F14, and F22 had significantly larger ($p < 0.05$) particle sizes at each time point when compared to their freshly prepared formulations. This instability related to particle size was significantly more pronounced ($p < 0.05$) at 25 °C than at 4 °C, which was also confirmed by the higher PDI values (Table 3). Higher temperatures caused migration of the surfactant molecules (Tween 80, SPC S-75) from the oil/water interface, causing particle coalescence [46]. Lower temperatures (e.g., 4 °C) are more favorable for the storage of nanoemuslions containing polysorbate surfactants (e.g., Tween 80). Additionally, it has been reported that the oxidative degradation of TRES is inhibited at 4 °C [47]. Similar nanoparticle stability at 4 °C has been reported by previous researchers [42].

Table 3. Particle size, polydispersity index (PDI), zeta potential, drug entrapment efficiency, and drug recovery of F8, F14, and F22 upon storage for 2, 4, or 6 months at 4 or 25 °C. Data are mean ± SD, n = 3.

Formulation	Storage Temperatures									
	4 °C					25 °C				
	Particle Size (nm)	PDI	Zeta Potential (mV)	Entrapment Efficiency (%)	Drug Recovery (%)	Particle Size (nm)	PDI	Zeta Potential (mV)	Entrapment Efficiency (%)	Drug Recovery (%)
2nd month										
F8	193.56 ± 7.74	0.32 ± 0.03	−27.83 ± 4.57	96.38 ± 5.75	94.52 ± 4.45	209.13 ± 6.65	0.38 ± 0.02	−23.72 ± 5.36	95.47 ± 4.12	93.40 ± 4.98
F14	175.26 ± 6.02	0.19 ± 0.03	−28.31 ± 6.44	97.22 ± 4.56	93.22 ± 4.97	206.46 ± 5.72	0.26 ± 0.03	−30.18 ± 6.16	96.12 ± 4.67	94.29 ± 3.10
F22	197.81 ± 7.28	0.24 ± 0.02	−30.05 ± 5.19	97.24 ± 4.01	94.41 ± 4.38	224.67 ± 7.69	0.32 ± 0.03	−26.84 ± 5.37	95.49 ± 4.09	96.27 ± 4.28
4th month										
F8	598.65 ± 9.16	0.36 ± 0.04	−25.92 ± 6.48	85.98 ± 5.36	78.37 ± 4.68	869.52 ± 9.26	0.38 ± 0.03	−29.82 ± 6.42	89.32 ± 3.59	67.97 ± 5.06
F14	196.35 ± 5.85	0.18 ± 0.03	−30.83 ± 5.71	94.51 ± 4.67	85.53 ± 5.46	224.68 ± 7.49	0.20 ± 0.04	−35.06 ± 6.55	95.79 ± 4.72	79.18 ± 4.88
F22	281.47 ± 8.09	0.42 ± 0.08	−35.28 ± 5.93	92.41 ± 4.18	68.97 ± 4.68	375.47 ± 7.67	0.46 ± 0.11	−34.87 ± 5.09	92.98 ± 4.21	55.19 ± 5.64
6th month										
F8	886.14 ± 7.55	0.41 ± 0.12	−25.38 ± 6.49	88.68 ± 4.15	60.04 ± 4.22	985.76 ± 7.16	0.42 ± 0.07	−28.52 ± 6.47	89.24 ± 4.55	55.78 ± 3.65
F14	199.64 ± 8.16	0.20 ± 0.06	−28.98 ± 5.71	95.38 ± 5.35	75.97 ± 4.31	245.45 ± 6.73	0.23 ± 0.06	−31.84 ± 5.46	94.89 ± 4.26	70.84 ± 4.52
F22	313.59 ± 7.34	0.51 ± 0.10	−31.46 ± 6.25	94.52 ± 4.43	52.16 ± 5.72	476.58 ± 6.92	0.46 ± 0.08	−30.44 ± 7.34	92.35 ± 5.17	45.43 ± 4.68

Zeta potential analysis and drug entrapment studies showed no significant difference ($p > 0.05$) between the freshly prepared and stored formulations (regardless of temperature) (Table 3). However, it is important to consider that slight changes in zeta potential values and entrapment efficiency may be related to storage temperature, where the temperature may marginally affect the crystallinity of lipid nanoparticles, which may cause minor disturbances in the electrical double diffuse layer of the formulation [48]. Notably, drug recovery was significantly affected at 4 and 6 months, especially at 25 °C, when compared to the freshly prepared TRES-NLC formulations (Table 3). TRES is not stable at alkaline pH, high temperatures, and during light exposure since the drug is prone to rapid degradation. Thus, drug recovery was significantly lower than for the freshly prepared TRES-NLC formulations. Additionally, TRES degradation was also found by Trela and Waterhouse [49], who reported the stability of TRES in buffers having pH 1, 3.5 or 7 upon storage for 28 days. Moreover, Liazid, et al. [50] reported that TRES can be degraded when exposed to high temperatures. The results from the current study were also confirmed and found to be in agreement with those of a previous study [47], where formulations were more stable at 4 °C than at 25 °C.

Overall, F14 demonstrated higher stability in terms of particle size, PDI, zeta potential, drug entrapment efficiency, and drug recovery (Table 3), as well as formulation deposition in various stages of the NGI (Section 3.3). TRES-NLC formulation F14 is comparatively more stable as it is composed of Miglyol 810 (liquid lipid), which is a medium-chain triglyceride, facilitating emulsification and reduced formulation aggregation; even when used at higher concentrations, the formulation was stable. These findings were also confirmed by Marzec, et al. [51], where lipid nanoparticles containing Miglyol 810 as a liquid lipid demonstrated greater stability. These findings indicate that the combination of Dynasan 116 and Miglyol 810 is compatible, producing stable NLC formulations for the delivery of TRES. Therefore, F14 was selected for subsequent studies.

3.5. Nebulization Performance of TRES-NLC Formulations

3.5.1. TRES-NLC Formulation F14 Deposition in Various Stages of NGI

According to the post-aerosolization analysis of the TRES-NLC formulation F14, the air-jet nebulizer demonstrated a lower deposition of TRES in the initial stages of the NGI and higher deposition in the middle to lower stages, which was significantly higher ($p < 0.05$) than that of the ultrasonic nebulizer (Figure 3). This could be attributed to the high velocity of the air compressed by the air-jet nebulizer, depositing larger droplets (containing a small mass of the formulation) in the initial stage and propelling smaller droplets (higher mass) in the later stages of the NGI [12]. Additionally, the presence of the baffle within the air-jet nebulizer plays an important role in TRES-NLC deposition. The smaller droplets generated by the air-jet nebulizer may escape the baffle, whereas larger droplets hit the baffle with high velocity, converting them into smaller droplets for inhalation, accounting for their deposition in the middle to later stages of the NGI, suggesting higher suitability for deep lung deposition. Similar results were observed when using the air-jet nebulizer, where two airflow rates (i.e., 15 and 60 L/min) were employed for beclometasone deposition [12]. The ultrasonic nebulizer produced significantly higher ($p < 0.05$) deposition of TRES in the early stages and lower deposition in the later stages of the NGI (Figure 3). This trend (opposite to the deposition trend of the air-jet nebulizer) may be related to the inconsistent and larger droplets formed by the ultrasonic nebulizer, resulting in deposition in the early stages.

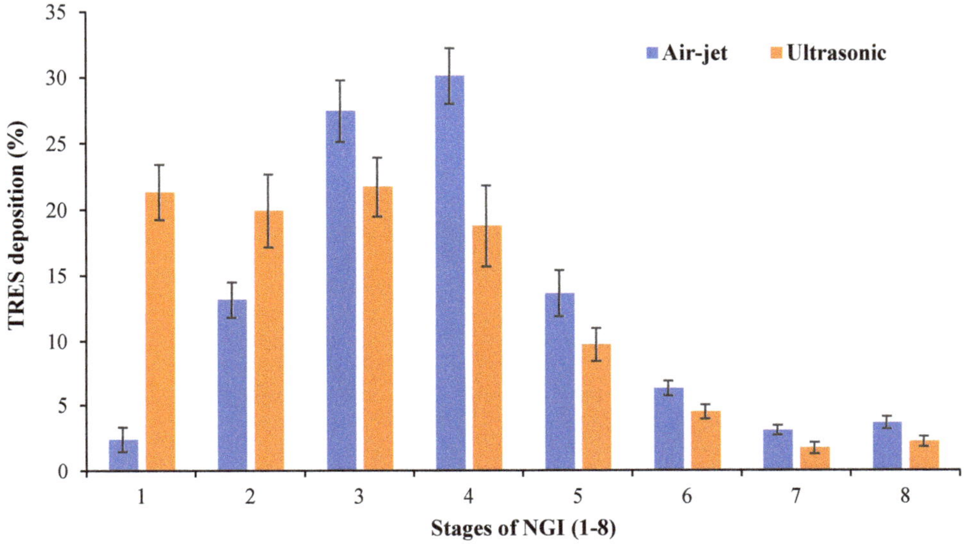

Figure 3. Deposition of TRES using TRES-NLC formulation F14 in various stages (1–8) of NGI via air-jet and ultrasonic nebulizers. Data are mean ± SD, n = 3.

3.5.2. Nebulization Time of F14

The nebulization time to "dryness" using the TRES-NLC formulation F14 was significantly higher ($p < 0.05$) for the air-jet nebulizer compared to the ultrasonic device (Figure 4A), agreeing with earlier findings reported by Harvey, et al. [52].

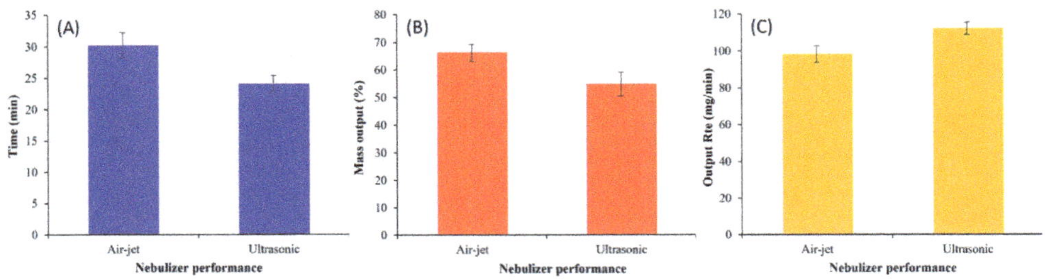

Figure 4. Nebulization performance, including the (**A**) nebulization time to "dryness" (min), (**B**) mass output (%), and (**C**) output rate (mg/min) of TRES-NLC formulation F14. Data are mean ± SD, n = 3.

The longer nebulization time for the air-jet nebulizer may be attributed to the latent heat of vaporization; this decreases the temperature of the nebulizer fluid, which in turn increases the fluid viscosity and decreases the nebulizer output. By contrast, the piezoelectric crystals of the ultrasonic nebulizer generate energy that increases the temperature of the nebulizer fluid, decreasing the content viscosity and shortening the nebulization time [7,53]. It is important to consider the design of the nebulizers, as air-jet nebulizers contain a baffle at the top of the venturi nozzle; as it produces fine droplets under the influence of highly compressed air flow, the smaller droplets escape for inhalation. By contrast, larger droplets impact the baffle and side walls, deflecting back into the nebulizer reservoir for further atomization into fine droplets; this increases the time needed to complete nebulization [54]. Overall, it can be concluded that the longer nebulization time of the air-jet nebulizer is associated with the deposition of higher drug amounts in the later stages of the NGI.

3.5.3. Nebulization Mass Output and Mass Output Rate of TRES-NLC Formulation

It is important to note that 100% mass output is not achievable after the total nebulization time; thus, some residual content remains in the nebulizer reservoir at the end of nebulization. Mass output represents the quantity of aerosolized formulation estimated via the gravimetric technique (by weighing nebulizers before and after nebulization) [55]. The air-jet nebulizer demonstrated significantly higher ($p < 0.05$) mass output (66.28 ± 3.03%) of the TRES-NLC formulation F14 when compared to the ultrasonic nebulizer (54.85 ± 4.23%) (Figure 4B). This difference in mass output was attributed to the dead/residual volume. The ultrasonic nebulizer retained higher residual volume, as well as generated heat during nebulization [5,56], causing particle fusion/aggregation. Similar findings were presented by Elhissi, et al. [57], where air-jet nebulizers were observed to exhibit higher mass output (i.e., less residual mass).

The mass output rate is a function of nebulization time. A significantly higher ($p < 0.05$) output rate was exhibited by the ultrasonic nebulizer when compared to the air-jet nebulizer (Figure 4C). Similar findings of higher mass output and lower mass output rate by the air-jet nebulizer have been demonstrated in previous studies [12,58].

3.5.4. Evaluation of ED, FPD, FPF, and RF of TRES-NLC Formulation F14

The total amount of TRES emitted and deposited in the various stages of NGI is referred to as the ED. A significantly higher ($p < 0.05$) ED was found when employing the air-jet nebulizer compared to the ultrasonic device (Table 4).

Table 4. Nebulization performance of air-jet and ultrasonic nebulizers employing TRES-NLC formulation F14 using NGI for emitted dose (ED), fine particle dose (FPD), fine particle fraction (FPF), and respirable fraction (RF). Data are mean ± SD, n = 3.

Characterization	Air-Jet Nebulizer	Ultrasonic Nebulizer
FPD (mg)	1.15 ± 0.05	0.78 ± 0.01
FPF (%)	24.74 ± 2.26	16.78 ± 1.38
RF (%)	94.05 ± 5.68	76.44 ± 3.75
ED (%)	80.95 ± 2.75	71.49 ± 2.06

Upon analysis of the FPD and FPF, the air-jet nebulizer was found to be more efficient in delivering and depositing the TRES-NLC formulation F14 in the "deep" NGI stages compared to the ultrasonic nebulizer (Table 4). Moreover, similar results were noted for the RF upon comparing the nebulizers (Table 4). It is important to note that droplets with an aerodynamic size of less than 5 μm possess the ability to travel further into the later stages of the NGI; therefore, these droplets are considered to be within the "respirable" fraction of the nebulized formulation [54]. However, droplets in excess of this size have a higher chance of deposition in the initial stages of the NGI (i.e., induction port and stage 1), which is related to inertial impaction (larger droplet possess lower maneuverability compared to smaller droplets) when employing an airflow rate of 15 L/min [12]. The smaller droplet size generated from air-jet nebulizers is also attributed to the built-in baffles positioned above its "venture" nozzle. During nebulization, as droplets are generated, smaller droplets are able to evade the baffle system for inhalation, whereas larger droplets impact the baffles, deflecting the primary aerosol back into the reservoir for further fragmentation into secondary aerosol droplets of "respirable" size.

Thus, although the air-jet nebulizer was associated with a prolonged nebulization time, it managed to generate smaller droplets that traveled deeper to the later stages of the impactor. The impact of droplets on the baffle in an ultrasonic nebulizer is milder (due to the distance between the generated droplets and the baffle position) than in an air-jet nebulizer. Thus, the generated droplets are propelled without restriction to the NGI despite their broad size distribution. Thus, the ultrasonic nebulizer is associated with a shorter nebulization time, with aerosol deposition across all NGI stages. Overall, it was found that the air-jet nebulizer exhibited superior aerosolization performance and hence is more appropriate for aerosolizing TRES-NLC formulations.

3.6. In Vitro Release Study of TRES-NLC Formulation F14

The sustained release profile of formulation F14 was analyzed in two different dissolution media, which were water (pH 7) (i.e., the suggested medium for the formulation) and acetate buffer (pH 5.4) (the pH physiologically reflective of the lungs in the presence of cancerous growth). Over a period of 24 h, the maximum release of TRES from NLC formulation F14 was found to be 58.02% and 95.79% in water and acetate buffer, respectively (Figure 5). It is noteworthy that TRES possesses phenate ions in its structure, which are susceptible to electrophilic attack and forms phenoxy radicals [59]. It was also identified that TRES is stable in acidic media up to pH 6, as, in acidic media, the hydroxyl group of TRES is protected from radical oxidation by the positively charged H_3O^+ [47]. Thus, TRES dissociates in neutral and basic media because of basic hydrolysis [60], and, in alkaline media, the dissociation of TRES follows first-order kinetics [47]. Overall, the ionization of TRES begins with the increasing pH in basic media, which marks the instability of the TRES [60].

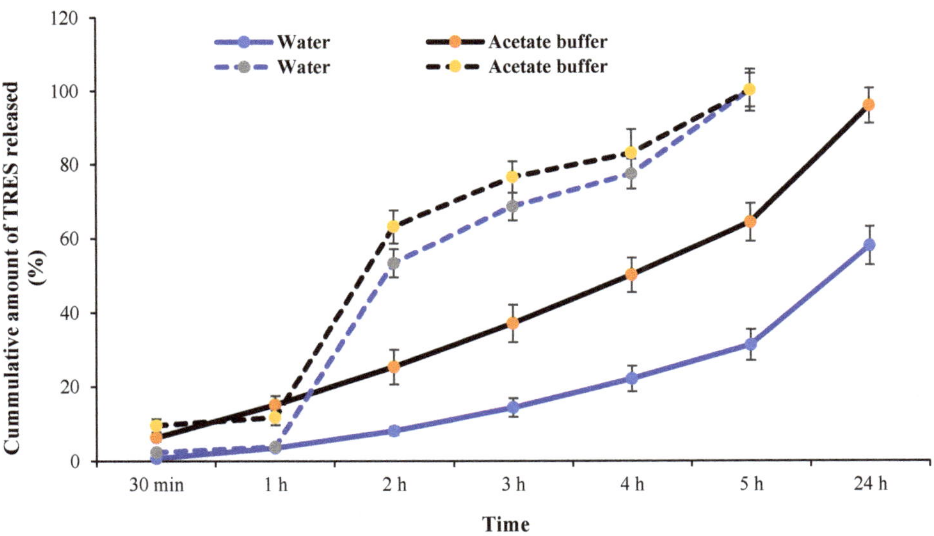

Figure 5. In vitro release of TRES from TRES-NLC formulation F14 (solid lines) and TRES as a free drug alone (doted lines) in two dissolution media, including water (pH 7) and acetate buffer (pH 5.4). Data are mean ± SD, n = 3.

Similar to formulation F14, the release profile of the free TRES drug was also assessed in water (pH 7) and acetate buffer (pH 5.4). The delayed release of the drug was observed in NLC formulations; this was markedly visible at the 3 h time point, where free TRES peaked to ~76% of the total drug concentration, whereas the NLC formulation had released ~37% (pH 5.4). This reduction is beneficial when considering the rapid metabolism of TRES (half-life of 1–2 h), potentially reducing the dosing frequency significantly. The present study demonstrates that the release of TRES is pH-dependent. Similar findings were also reported in the literature [47], where the TRES drug dissociation rate was observed in alkaline conditions; however, other researchers indicated the stability of TRES in acidic media [61–63]. Hence, it was found that TRES, as an anti-cancer drug, has better stability and sustained release in acidic media (i.e., pH 5) compared to pH 7 (causing drug degradation) [47]. Furthermore, the stability of TRES in pH 5 is preferable to target pulmonary system, since tumor growth causes the pH of the lungs to become acidic due to the excessive production of lactic acid, making it a suitable environment for TRES stability and sustained release [64].

4. Conclusions

In this study, 24 TRES-NLC formulations for pulmonary drug delivery were successfully prepared and optimized using a novel combination of solid lipid (Dynasan 116), liquid lipids (Capryol 90, Lauroglycol 90, Miglyol 810, and Tributyrin), surfactant (Tween 80), and co-surfactant (SPC S-75) in various ratios using probe sonication. Upon initial analysis of the freshly prepared formulations and formulations stored at 25 °C for four weeks, TRES-NLC formulations F8, F14, and F22 were selected based on their smaller particle size, lower polydispersity, and higher drug entrapment. The solid lipid type was deemed to not affect the physiochemical properties of the formulation. Contrastingly, the liquid lipid type, surfactant, and their ratios were noted to significantly influence the aforementioned formulation properties. After nebulization using the air-jet and ultrasonic nebulizers in the NGI stages, the F14 particles were consistent and smaller compared to the F8 and F22 formulations. Additionally, the F14 formulation demonstrated higher stability at 4 and 25 °C for six months, indicating a more appropriate combination of excipients for potential drug delivery when compared to the F8 and F22 formulations. This suggests that Dynasan 116 as the solid lipid, Miglyol 810 as the liquid lipid, and Tween 80 as the surfactant in formulation F14 are a promising combination that prevents particle aggregation/fusion and provides long-term storage stability. Upon comparison of the air-jet nebulizer with the ultrasonic nebulizer by employing formulation F14, the air-jet nebulizer exhibited lower amounts of TRES drug deposition in the initial stages and higher in the middle to later stages of the NGI. The air-jet nebulizer, although exhibiting prolonged nebulization, delivered higher mass output (retained less formulation F14 in the nebulizer reservoir, attributed to the mechanism of aerosol generation and the design of the nebulizer). During nebulization, the air-jet nebulizer exhibited superior performance in terms of higher ED, FPD, FPF, and RF when compared to the ultrasonic nebulizer using formulation F14. Moreover, the F14 formulation and TRES as a free drug showed higher sustained release and stability in acetate buffer. Thus, the air-jet nebulizer is suggested to be a significantly superior nebulizer when using TRES-NLC formulation F14 for pulmonary drug delivery.

Author Contributions: Conceptualization: I.K. and H.A.R.; methodology: S.S., H.K.O. and C.H.; investigation: S.S., N.R.H. and S.Y.; software: W.K. and H.K.O.; data curation: S.S. and C.H.; visualization: N.R.H. and W.K.; supervision: I.K. and A.E.; resources: H.A.R. and A.E.; funding acquisition: H.A.R.; project administration: I.K. and H.A.R.; writing—original draft preparation: I.K.; writing—review and editing: I.K., A.E. and H.A.R. All authors have read and agreed to the published version of the manuscript.

Funding: This publication was supported by Qatar University QUCG-CPH-24/25-547. The findings reported herein are solely the responsibility of the authors.

Institutional Review Board Statement: Not applicable.

Informed Consent Statement: Not applicable.

Data Availability Statement: The original contributions presented in this study are included in the article. Further inquiries can be directed to the corresponding author.

Conflicts of Interest: The authors declare no conflicts of interest.

References

1. Mathew Thevarkattil, A.; Yousaf, S.; Houacine, C.; Khan, W.; Bnyan, R.; Elhissi, A.; Khan, I. Anticancer drug delivery: Investigating the impacts of viscosity on lipid-based formulations for pulmonary targeting. *Int. J. Pharm.* **2024**, *664*, 124591. [CrossRef] [PubMed]
2. Cipolla, D. Will pulmonary drug delivery for systemic application ever fulfill its rich promise? *Expert. Opin. Drug Deliv.* **2016**, *13*, 1337–1340. [CrossRef] [PubMed]
3. Patton, J.S.; Fishburn, C.S.; Weers, J.G. The lungs as a portal of entry for systemic drug delivery. *Proc. Am. Thorac. Soc.* **2004**, *1*, 338–344. [CrossRef] [PubMed]
4. Scheuch, G.; Kohlhaeufl, M.J.; Brand, P.; Siekmeier, R. Clinical perspectives on pulmonary systemic and macromolecular delivery. *Adv. Drug Deliv. Rev.* **2006**, *58*, 996–1008. [CrossRef] [PubMed]
5. Khan, I.; Yousaf, S.; Alhnan, M.A.; Ahmed, W.; Elhissi, A.; Jackson, M.J. Design Characteristics of Inhaler Devices Used for Pulmonary Delivery of Medical Aerosols. In *Surgical Tools and Medical Devices*; Ahmed, W., Jackson, M.J., Eds.; Springer International Publishing: Cham, Switzerland, 2016; pp. 573–591. [CrossRef]
6. Yousaf, S.S.; Isreb, A.; Khan, I.; Mewsiga, E.; Elhissi, A.; Ahmed, W.; Alhnan, M.A. Impact of nanosizing on the formation and characteristics of polymethacrylate films: Micro- versus nano-suspensions. *Pharm. Dev. Technol.* **2021**, *26*, 729–739. [CrossRef]
7. Khan, I.; Yousaf, S.; Najlah, M.; Ahmed, W.; Elhissi, A. Proliposome powder or tablets for generating inhalable liposomes using a medical nebulizer. *J. Pharm. Investig.* **2020**, *51*, 61–73. [CrossRef]
8. Din, F.U.; Aman, W.; Ullah, I.; Qureshi, O.S.; Mustapha, O.; Shafique, S.; Zeb, A. Effective use of nanocarriers as drug delivery systems for the treatment of selected tumors. *Int. J. Nanomed.* **2017**, *12*, 7291–7309. [CrossRef]
9. Yousaf, S.S.; Houacine, C.; Khan, I.; Ahmed, W.; Jackson, M.J. Chapter 11—Importance of biomaterials in biomedical engineering. In *Advances in Medical and Surgical Engineering*; Ahmed, W., Phoenix, D.A., Jackson, M.J., Charalambous, C.P., Eds.; Academic Press: Cambridge, MA, USA, 2020; pp. 149–176. [CrossRef]
10. Umerska, A.; Mouzouvi, C.R.; Bigot, A.; Saulnier, P. Formulation and nebulization of fluticasone propionate-loaded lipid nanocarriers. *Int. J. Pharm.* **2015**, *493*, 224–232. [CrossRef]
11. Ansam, M.; Yousaf, S.; Bnyan, R.; Khan, I. Anti-aging Liposomal Formulation. Mini Review. *Nov. Approaches Drug Des. Dev.* **2018**, *3*, 66–68.
12. Khan, I.; Hussein, S.; Houacine, C.; Khan Sadozai, S.; Islam, Y.; Bnyan, R.; Elhissi, A.; Yousaf, S. Fabrication, characterization and optimization of nanostructured lipid carrier formulations using Beclomethasone dipropionate for pulmonary drug delivery via medical nebulizers. *Int. J. Pharm.* **2021**, *598*, 120376. [CrossRef]
13. Apostolou, M.; Assi, S.; Fatokun, A.A.; Khan, I. The Effects of Solid and Liquid Lipids on the Physicochemical Properties of Nanostructured Lipid Carriers. *J. Pharm. Sci.* **2021**, *10*, 2859–2872. [CrossRef] [PubMed]
14. Xu, L.; Wang, X.; Liu, Y.; Yang, G.; Falconer, R.J.; Zhao, C.-X. Lipid Nanoparticles for Drug Delivery. *Adv. NanoBiomed Res.* **2022**, *2*, 2100109. [CrossRef]
15. Lewis, P.O.; Khan, I.; Patel, P. Successful stepdown treatment of pulmonary histoplasmosis with thrice-weekly liposomal amphotericin B in a hospital-associated, outpatient infusion centre: A case report. *J. Clin. Pharm. Ther.* **2018**, *43*, 269–272. [CrossRef] [PubMed]
16. Barenholz, Y. Doxil®—The first FDA-approved nano-drug: Lessons learned. *J. Control. Release Off. J. Control. Release Soc.* **2012**, *160*, 117–134. [CrossRef] [PubMed]
17. Shukla, S.K.; Nguyen, V.; Goyal, M.; Gupta, V. Cationically modified inhalable nintedanib niosomes: Enhancing therapeutic activity against non-small-cell lung cancer. *Nanomedicine* **2022**, *17*, 935–958. [CrossRef]
18. Aparajay, P.; Dev, A. Functionalized niosomes as a smart delivery device in cancer and fungal infection. *Eur. J. Pharm. Sci.* **2022**, *168*, 106052. [CrossRef]
19. Ammar, H.O.; Tadros, M.I.; Salama, N.M.; Ghoneim, A.M. Ethosome-Derived Invasomes as a Potential Transdermal Delivery System for Vardenafil Hydrochloride: Development, Optimization and Application of Physiologically Based Pharmacokinetic Modeling in Adults and Geriatrics. *Int. J. Nanomed.* **2020**, *15*, 5671–5685. [CrossRef]
20. Świętek, M.; Panchuk, R.; Skorokhyd, N.; Černoch, P.; Finiuk, N.; Klyuchivska, O.; Hrubý, M.; Molčan, M.; Berger, W.; Trousil, J.; et al. Magnetic Temperature-Sensitive Solid-Lipid Particles for Targeting and Killing Tumor Cells. *Front. Chem.* **2020**, *8*, 205. [CrossRef]
21. Xu, Y.; Zheng, Y.; Wu, L.; Zhu, X.; Zhang, Z.; Huang, Y. Novel Solid Lipid Nanoparticle with Endosomal Escape Function for Oral Delivery of Insulin. *ACS Appl. Mater. Interfaces* **2018**, *10*, 9315–9324. [CrossRef]
22. Mishra, V.; Bansal, K.K.; Verma, A.; Yadav, N.; Thakur, S.; Sudhakar, K.; Rosenholm, J.M. Solid Lipid Nanoparticles: Emerging Colloidal Nano Drug Delivery Systems. *Pharmaceutics* **2018**, *10*, 191. [CrossRef]
23. Salvi, V.R.; Pawar, P. Nanostructured lipid carriers (NLC) system: A novel drug targeting carrier. *J. Drug Deliv. Sci. Technol.* **2019**, *51*, 255–267. [CrossRef]
24. Hollmerus, S.; Yousaf, S.; Islam, Y.; Khan, I. Isoflavones-based Liposome Formulations as Anti-aging for Skincare. *Nov. Approaches Drug Des. Dev.* **2018**, *3*, 28–37.
25. Axioti, E.; Apostolou, M.; Yousaf, S.; Khan, I. Skin Aging and Vesicular Delivery Systems. In *Science and Applications of Nanoparticles*; Jenny Stanford Publishing: New York, USA, 2022; pp. 309–368.
26. Chahinez, H.; Iftikhar, K.; Sakib Saleem, Y. Potential cardio-protective agents: A Resveratrol review (2000–2019). *Curr. Pharm. Des.* **2020**, *26*, 2943–2955. [CrossRef]

27. Ha, E.-S.; Kuk, D.-H.; Kim, J.-S.; Kim, M.-S. Solubility of trans-resveratrol in Transcutol HP + water mixtures at different temperatures and its application to fabrication of nanosuspensions. *J. Mol. Liq.* **2019**, *281*, 344–351. [CrossRef]
28. Vankayala, J.S.; Battula, S.N.; Kandasamy, R.; Mariya, G.A.; Franklin, M.E.E.; Pushpadass, H.A.; Naik, L.N. Surfactants and fatty alcohol based novel nanovesicles for resveratrol: Process optimization, characterization and evaluation of functional properties in RAW 264.7 macrophage cells. *J. Mol. Liq.* **2018**, *261*, 387–396. [CrossRef]
29. Darquenne, C. Deposition Mechanisms. *J. Aerosol Med. Pulm. Drug Deliv.* **2020**, *33*, 181–185. [CrossRef]
30. Marple, V.A.; Olson, B.A.; Santhanakrishnan, K.; Mitchell, J.P.; Murray, S.C.; Hudson-Curtis, B.L. Next generation pharmaceutical impactor (a new impactor for pharmaceutical inhaler testing). Part II: Archival calibration. *J. Aerosol Med. Off. J. Int. Soc. Aerosols Med.* **2003**, *16*, 301–324. [CrossRef]
31. Basso, J.; Mendes, M.; Cova, T.; Sousa, J.; Pais, A.; Fortuna, A.; Vitorino, R.; Vitorino, C. A Stepwise Framework for the Systematic Development of Lipid Nanoparticles. *Biomolecules* **2022**, *12*, 223. [CrossRef]
32. Zhang, N.; Liu, C.; Jin, L.; Zhang, R.; Siebert, H.C.; Wang, Z.; Prakash, S.; Yin, X.; Li, J.; Hou, D.; et al. Influence of Long-Chain/Medium-Chain Triglycerides and Whey Protein/Tween 80 Ratio on the Stability of Phosphatidylserine Emulsions (O/W). *ACS Omega* **2020**, *5*, 7792–7801. [CrossRef]
33. Das, S.; Ng, W.K.; Tan, R.B.H. Are nanostructured lipid carriers (NLCs) better than solid lipid nanoparticles (SLNs): Development, characterizations and comparative evaluations of clotrimazole-loaded SLNs and NLCs? *Eur. J. Pharm. Sci.* **2012**, *47*, 139–151. [CrossRef]
34. Gokce, E.H.; Sandri, G.; Bonferoni, M.C.; Rossi, S.; Ferrari, F.; Güneri, T.; Caramella, C. Cyclosporine A loaded SLNs: Evaluation of cellular uptake and corneal cytotoxicity. *Int. J. Pharm.* **2008**, *364*, 76–86. [CrossRef] [PubMed]
35. Jain, K.; Sood, S.; Gowthamarajan, K. Optimization of artemether-loaded NLC for intranasal delivery using central composite design. *Drug Deliv.* **2015**, *22*, 940–954. [CrossRef] [PubMed]
36. Varshosaz, J.; Tabbakhian, M.; Mohammadi, M.Y. Formulation and optimization of solid lipid nanoparticles of buspirone HCl for enhancement of its oral bioavailability. *J. Liposome Res.* **2010**, *20*, 286–296. [CrossRef]
37. Houacine, C.; Adams, D.; Singh, K.K. Impact of liquid lipid on development and stability of trimyristin nanostructured lipid carriers for oral delivery of resveratrol. *J. Mol. Liq.* **2020**, *316*, 113734. [CrossRef]
38. Niculae, G.; Lacatusu, I.; Badea, N.; Oprea, O.; Meghea, A. Optimization of lipid nanoparticles composition for sunscreen encapsulation. *UPB Sci. Bull. Ser. B* **2013**, *75*, 79–92.
39. Thatipamula, R.; Palem, C.; Gannu, R.; Mudragada, S.; Yamsani, M. Formulation and in vitro characterization of domperidone loaded solid lipid nanoparticles and nanostructured lipid carriers. *Daru* **2011**, *19*, 23–32.
40. Shah, N.V.; Seth, A.K.; Balaraman, R.; Aundhia, C.J.; Maheshwari, R.A.; Parmar, G.R. Nanostructured lipid carriers for oral bioavailability enhancement of raloxifene: Design and in vivo study. *J. Adv. Res.* **2016**, *7*, 423–434. [CrossRef]
41. Hu, F.-Q.; Jiang, S.-P.; Du, Y.-Z.; Yuan, H.; Ye, Y.-Q.; Zeng, S. Preparation and characteristics of monostearin nanostructured lipid carriers. *Int. J. Pharm.* **2006**, *314*, 83–89. [CrossRef]
42. Kelidari, H.R.; Saeedi, M.; Akbari, J.; Morteza-Semnani, K.; Valizadeh, H.; Maniruzzaman, M.; Farmoudeh, A.; Nokhodchi, A. Development and Optimisation of Spironolactone Nanoparticles for Enhanced Dissolution Rates and Stability. *AAPS PharmSciTech* **2017**, *18*, 1469–1474. [CrossRef]
43. Uprit, S.; Sahu, R.K.; Roy, A.; Pare, A. Preparation and characterization of minoxidil loaded nanostructured lipid carrier gel for effective treatment of alopecia. *Saudi Pharm. J.* **2013**, *21*, 379–385. [CrossRef]
44. Ali, M. CHAPTER 9—Pulmonary Drug Delivery. In *Handbook of Non-Invasive Drug Delivery Systems*; Kulkarni, V.S., Ed.; William Andrew Publishing: Boston, MA, USA, 2010; pp. 209–246. [CrossRef]
45. Araújo, L.M.P.d.; Abatti, P.J.; Araújo, W.D.d.; Alves, R.F. Performance evaluation of nebulizers based on aerodynamic droplet diameter characterization using the Direct Laminar Incidence (DLI). *Res. Biomed. Eng.* **2017**, *33*, 105–112. [CrossRef]
46. Sessa, M.; Tsao, R.; Liu, R.; Ferrari, G.; Donsì, F. Evaluation of the stability and antioxidant activity of nanoencapsulated resveratrol during in vitro digestion. *J. Agric. Food Chem.* **2011**, *59*, 12352–12360. [CrossRef] [PubMed]
47. Zupančič, Š.; Lavrič, Z.; Kristl, J. Stability and solubility of trans-resveratrol are strongly influenced by pH and temperature. *Eur. J. Pharm. Biopharm.* **2015**, *93*, 196–204. [CrossRef] [PubMed]
48. Carbone, C.; Campisi, A.; Manno, D.; Serra, A.; Spatuzza, M.; Musumeci, T.; Bonfanti, R.; Puglisi, G. The critical role of didodecyldimethylammonium bromide on physico-chemical, technological and biological properties of NLC. *Colloids Surf. B Biointerfaces* **2014**, *121*, 1–10. [CrossRef] [PubMed]
49. Trela, B.C.; Waterhouse, A.L. Resveratrol: Isomeric molar absorptivities and stability. *J. Agric. Food Chem.* **1996**, *44*, 1253–1257. [CrossRef]
50. Liazid, A.; Palma, M.; Brigui, J.; Barroso, C.G. Investigation on phenolic compounds stability during microwave-assisted extraction. *J. Chromatogr. A* **2007**, *1140*, 29–34. [CrossRef]
51. Marzec, M.; Dąbek, P.; Witkowski, A.; Monedeiro, F.; Pomastowski, P.; Buszewski, B.; Nowak, I. Lipid Constituents of Diatoms (Halamphora) as Components for Production of Lipid Nanoparticles. *Pharmaceutics* **2022**, *14*, 1171. [CrossRef]
52. Harvey, C.; O'Doherty, M.; Page, C.; Thomas, S.; Nunan, T.; Treacher, D. Comparison of jet and ultrasonic nebulizer pulmonary aerosol deposition during mechanical ventilation. *Eur. Respir. J.* **1997**, *10*, 905–909. [CrossRef]
53. Steckel, H.; Eskandar, F. Factors affecting aerosol performance during nebulization with jet and ultrasonic nebulizers. *Eur. J. Pharm. Sci.* **2003**, *19*, 443–455. [CrossRef]

54. O'Callaghan, C.; Barry, P.W. The science of nebulised drug delivery. *Thorax* **1997**, *52* (Suppl. 2), S31–S44. [CrossRef]
55. Tandon, R.; Smaldone, G.C.; McPeck, M. Measuring nebulizer output: Aerosol production vs. gravimetric analysis. *Chest* **1997**, *111*, 1361–1365. [CrossRef] [PubMed]
56. Dhand, R. Aerosol Delivery During Mechanical Ventilation: From Basic Techniques to New Devices. *J. Aerosol Med. Pulm. Drug Deliv.* **2008**, *21*, 45–60. [CrossRef] [PubMed]
57. Elhissi, A.; Hidayat, K.; Phoenix, D.A.; Mwesigwa, E.; Crean, S.; Ahmed, W.; Faheem, A.; Taylor, K.M.G. Air-jet and vibrating-mesh nebulization of niosomes generated using a particulate-based proniosome technology. *Int. J. Pharm.* **2013**, *444*, 193–199. [CrossRef] [PubMed]
58. Nafee, N.; Makled, S.; Boraie, N. Nanostructured lipid carriers versus solid lipid nanoparticles for the potential treatment of pulmonary hypertension via nebulization. *Eur. J. Pharm. Sci. Off. J. Eur. Fed. Pharm. Sci.* **2018**, *125*, 151–162. [CrossRef]
59. Graham, N.; Jiang, C.C.; Li, X.Z.; Jiang, J.Q.; Ma, J. The influence of pH on the degradation of phenol and chlorophenols by potassium ferrate. *Chemosphere* **2004**, *56*, 949–956. [CrossRef]
60. Robinson, K.; Mock, C.; Liang, D. Pre-formulation studies of resveratrol. *Drug Dev. Ind. Pharm.* **2015**, *41*, 1464–1469. [CrossRef]
61. Pentek, T.; Newenhouse, E.; O'Brien, B.; Chauhan, A.S. Development of a Topical Resveratrol Formulation for Commercial Applications Using Dendrimer Nanotechnology. *Molecules* **2017**, *22*, 137. [CrossRef]
62. Konopko, A.; Litwinienko, G. Unexpected Role of pH and Microenvironment on the Antioxidant and Synergistic Activity of Resveratrol in Model Micellar and Liposomal Systems. *J. Org. Chem.* **2022**, *87*, 1698–1709. [CrossRef]
63. Mota-Lugo, E.; Dolores-Hernández, M.; Morales-Hipólito, E.A.; Blanco-Alcántara, I.A.; Cuatecontzi-Flores, H.; López-Arellano, R. Development and Validation of a Stability-Indicating HPLC Method for the Simultaneous Determination of trans-Resveratrol and cis-Resveratrol in an Injectable Solution. *J. Anal. Methods Chem.* **2021**, *2021*, 8402157. [CrossRef]
64. Kato, Y.; Ozawa, S.; Miyamoto, C.; Maehata, Y.; Suzuki, A.; Maeda, T.; Baba, Y. Acidic extracellular microenvironment and cancer. *Cancer Cell Int.* **2013**, *13*, 89. [CrossRef]

pharmaceutics

Article

A Polysorbate-Based Lipid Nanoparticle Vaccine Formulation Induces In Vivo Immune Response Against SARS-CoV-2

Aishwarya Saraswat [1,†], Alireza Nomani [1,*,†], Lin-Kin Yong [2], Jimmy Chun-Tien Kuo [3], Heather Brown [3], Muralikrishna Narayanareddygari [2], Avery Peace [4], Rizan Fazily [1], Timothy Blake [3], Christopher D. Petro [4], Bindhu Rayaprolu [1], Johanna Hansen [2], Amardeep Singh Bhalla [1] and Mohammed Shameem [1]

1 Formulation Development Group, Regeneron Pharmaceuticals, Tarrytown, NY 10591, USA; aishwarya.saraswat@regeneron.com (A.S.)
2 Vaccine Technology, Regeneron Pharmaceuticals, Tarrytown, NY 10591, USA
3 Regeneron Genetic Medicines, Regeneron Pharmaceuticals, Tarrytown, NY 10591, USA
4 Infectious Diseases, Regeneron Pharmaceuticals, Tarrytown, NY 10591, USA
* Correspondence: alireza.nomani@regeneron.com
† These authors contributed equally to this work.

Abstract: Background: Lipid nanoparticles (LNPs) have proven effective in delivering RNA-based modalities. Rapid approval of the COVID-19 vaccines highlights the promise of LNPs as a delivery platform for nucleic acid-based therapies and vaccines. Nevertheless, improved LNP designs are needed to advance next-generation vaccines and other gene therapies toward greater clinical success. Lipid components and LNP formulation excipients play a central role in biodistribution, immunogenicity, and stability. Therefore, it is important to understand, identify, and assess the appropriate lipid components for developing a safe and effective formulation. Herein, this study focused on developing a novel Polysorbate-80 (PS-80)-based LNP. We hypothesized that substituting conventional linear PEG-lipids with PS-80, a widely used, biocompatible injectable surfactant featuring a branched PEG-like structure, may change the LNPs biodistribution pattern and enhance long-term stability. By leveraging PS-80's unique structural properties, this study aimed to develop an mRNA-LNP platform with improved extrahepatic delivery and robust freeze/thaw tolerance. **Methods**: We employed a stepwise optimization to establish both the lipid composition and formulation buffer to yield a stable, high-performing PS-80-based SARS-CoV-2 mRNA-LNP (SC2-PS80 LNP). We compared phosphate- versus tris-based buffers for long-term stability, examined multiple lipid ratios, and evaluated the impact of incorporating PS-80 (a branched PEG-lipid) on in vivo biodistribution. Various analytical assays were performed to assess particle size, encapsulation efficiency, mRNA purity, and in vitro potency of the developed formulation and a humanized mouse model was used to measure its immunogenicity over six months of storage at −80 °C. **Results:** Replacing the standard 1,2-dimyristoyl-rac-glycero-3-methoxy polyethylene glycol-2000 (PEG-DMG) lipid with PS-80 increased spleen-specific expression of the mRNA-LNPs after intramuscular injection. Formulating in a tris-sucrose-salt (TSS) buffer preserved the LNP's physicochemical properties and in vitro potency over six months at −80 °C, whereas a conventional PBS-sucrose (PSS) buffer was less protective under frozen conditions. Notably, TSS-based SC2-PS80 LNPs elicited potent humoral immunity in mice, including high anti-spike IgG titers and robust pseudovirus neutralization, comparable to freshly prepared formulations. **Conclusions:** A PS-80-based mRNA-LNP platform formulated in TSS buffer confers improved extrahepatic delivery, long-term frozen stability, and strong immunogenicity against SARS-CoV-2 following six months. These findings offer a promising pathway for the design of next-generation mRNA vaccines and therapeutics with enhanced stability and clinical potential.

Pharmaceutics **2025**, *17*, 441 https://doi.org/10.3390/pharmaceutics17040441

Keywords: mRNA lipid nanoparticles; vaccines; Polysorbate-80; SARS-CoV-2; gene therapy; storage stability; immunogenicity

1. Introduction

Gene therapy has drawn increasing attention over the past decade for its potential to treat both inherited and acquired diseases, including cancer and infectious disorders. Among the many approaches to gene therapy, lipid nanoparticles (LNPs) have emerged as effective and comparatively safe non-viral delivery vehicles [1]. Their clinical utility is highlighted by the success of multiple mRNA-LNP vaccines against COVID-19—most notably, Pfizer-BioNTech's Comirnaty®/BNT162b, and Moderna's Spikevax®/mRNA 1273, both of which have received full FDA and EMA approval. Also, Moderna recently secured FDA approval for an mRNA-based RSV vaccine (mRESVIA®/mRNA 1345) [2]. Before this wave of mRNA-LNP success, the first RNA-encapsulating LNP therapy (Onpattro®/Patisiran) was approved by the FDA to treat polyneuropathy caused by hereditary ATTR amyloidosis, laying a strong clinical foundation for the LNP platform [3].

Despite these achievements, several challenges continue to impede the full translational impact of mRNA-LNPs. For instance, nucleic acids (including mRNA) are prone to enzymatic degradation, and their uptake in target tissues is hampered by their large molecular weight and negative charge [4,5]. Many LNPs preferentially accumulate in the liver, meaning only a fraction of each dose reaches extrahepatic targets such as the spleen or lymph nodes which are critical sites for vaccine delivery. Moreover, long-term storage stability remains an obstacle and the LNP drug product must be protected from physical and chemical degradation to preserve its activity. Hence, it is pivotal to develop a formulation with suitable excipients to enhance both the activity and stability of LNPs.

Lipid components and formulation excipients are the most essential aspects of the LNP formulation design. Ionizable lipids (e.g., DLin-MC3-DMA), which can comprise $\geq$50% of the total lipid, are crucial for mRNA encapsulation and endosomal escape. Helper lipids (e.g., phospholipids and cholesterol) form a stable bilayer that supports LNP structure. Meanwhile, PEG-containing lipids, though used at the lowest molar percentage, have a significant effect on the physicochemical properties, shelf stability, and in vivo kinetics of LNPs [6–8]. Common PEG-lipids, such as DSPE-PEG2K or DMG-PEG2K, feature linear PEG chains of ~2 kDa. Additionally, ~30% of an mRNA-LNP is the aqueous phase, so the excipient system (buffer, ionic strength, cryoprotectants, pH, etc.) can profoundly affect LNP formation, size, structure, and overall quality [9,10].

In this study, we investigated Polysorbate-80 (PS-80), a branched PEG surfactant, as an alternative PEG-lipid in LNPs formulated for SARS-CoV-2 vaccine development. PS-80 contains branched PEG-like chains linked to mainly an oleic acid-based tail [11]. It is widely recognized as a biocompatible injectable excipient and is routinely used in protein-based therapeutics at low concentrations (<0.5% w/v) to prevent aggregation [12–14].

One of the key objectives of our research was to employ PS-80 to replace widely used PEG-lipids and subsequently study the physicochemical properties, stability, and biodistribution of RNA-LNPs. We evaluated the in vivo biodistribution of PS-80-based LNP formulation containing Firefly Luciferase reporter mRNA (Fluc-PS80 LNP) in comparison to the standard DMG-PEG2K-based LNPs when formulated in PBS buffer. Our results showed preferential LNP accumulation in the spleen for Fluc-PS80 LNP when compared to DMG-PEG2k LNP following intramuscular injection. We then studied the effect of formulation excipients (including cryoprotectant, salt, lipid ratios, buffer composition as formulation factors) and developed a suitable Tris Sucrose Saline (TSS)-based formulation buffer to improve the physicochemical properties and potency of Fluc-PS80 LNP formulation.

Subsequently, we assessed the therapeutic potential of this PS-80-based formulation platform by encapsulating SARS-CoV-2 spike mRNA (SC2-PS80 LNPs) and demonstrated its improved long-term storage stability in comparison to the conventional PBS-sucrose (PSS buffer). Following six months of storage at −80 °C, the in vivo potency of SC2-PS80 LNPs was evaluated in a COVID-19 disease model. Our results demonstrated high immunogenicity of SC2-PS80 LNPs in genetically humanized VelocImmune® mice [15]. Overall, we show that incorporating PS-80 as a branched PEG-lipid in an mRNA-LNP formulation resulted in enhanced spleen-targeted delivery as compared to the DMG-PEG2k LNPs and demonstrated acceptable storage stability in the TSS buffer. We hypothesize that PS-80's branched PEG-like structure can influence particle biodistribution, potentially improving extrahepatic (e.g., spleen) uptake. Moreover, its surfactant properties are known to mitigate particle aggregation of biologics under stress conditions, suggesting that replacing standard PEG-lipids with PS-80 could enhance mRNA-LNP stability while retaining or even boosting vaccine potency. Our data show that this unique formulation elicited robust immune responses against SARS-CoV-2 in the humanized mouse model.

2. Materials and Methods

2.1. Materials

DLin-MC3-DMA (CAS# 1224606-06-7) was acquired from BioFine International Inc. (Vancouver, BC, CA). DSPC (CAS# 816-94-4), cholesterol (CAS# 57-88-5) and DMG-PEG2K (CAS# 880-15-1) were procured from Avanti Polar Lipids, Inc. (Alabaster, AL, USA). Polysorbate-80 (PS-80, CAS# 9005-65-6), ethyl alcohol (200 Proof) (CAS# E7023) was bought from Sigma-Aldrich, Inc. (St. Louis, MO, USA). CleanCap® Firefly Luciferase (FLuc) mRNA (CAS# L-7602) was bought from TriLink BioTechnologies (San Diego, CA, USA). Quant-it™ RiboGreen RNA Assay Kit (CAS# R11490), sodium acetate (CAS# J63669.AK), molecular biology grade water (CAS# J71786.XCR), PBS (CAS# 14190144), and other cell culture reagents were purchased from Thermo Fisher Scientific (Fair Lawn, NJ, USA). Other solvents, chemicals and reagents were obtained from VWR International (Radnor, PA, USA).

2.2. Cell Culture

HEK-293 cells (CRL-1573) were purchased from ATCC (Manassas, VA, USA) and cultured in Dulbecco's Modified Eagle's Medium (DMEM, CAS#11995073 supplemented with 10% heat-inactivated fetal bovine serum (FBS) and 1× penicillin/streptomycin. The cells were maintained in an atmosphere of 5% CO_2 at 37 °C.

2.3. In Vitro Transcription of SARS-CoV-2 mRNA

Gene expressing SARS-CoV-2 6P [16,17] was cloned into a plasmid backbone, the coding sequence is flanked by 5′UTR and 3′UTR sequences. A T7 promoter is encoded upstream of the 5′UTR to initiate transcription using a T7 RNA polymerase. This promoter is compatible with CleanCAp AG reagent (TriLink BioTechnologies, San Diego, CA, USA) for co-transcriptional addition of the 5′ CAP during the in vitro transcription (IVT) reaction. The plasmid has a 104 nt segmented polyA tail that ends with a restriction site to allow for linearization of the plasmid at the end of the polyA tail. Plasmid was transformed into NEB stable *E. coli* cells and a colony was picked up and grown in LB media with 100 ug/mL ampicillin. Plasmid maxi prep was generated at our core facility and the sequence was verified using Sanger sequencing.

Further to this, mRNA was synthesized in an in vitro transcription reaction using T7 RNA polymerase (New England Biolabs, Ipswich, MA, USA) and linearized plasmid as a

DNA template. The transcription reaction was set up at 37 °C for 2 h in the presence of 5 mM each of ATP, CTP, GTP (New England Biolabs, Ipswich, MA, USA) and N1-methyl Pseudouridine triphosphate (TriLink BioTechnologies, San Diego, CA, USA), transcription buffer (40 mM Tris-HCl, 10 mM DTT, 2 mM Spermidine, 0.002% Triton and 16.5 mM Magnesium Acetate) and the reaction was supplemented with 4 mM Clean Cap AG reagent. After transcription, the DNA template was digested with TURBO DNase (Invitrogen, Waltham, MA, USA) for 30 min at 37 °C and cleaned up using RNAClean XP magnetic beads (Beckman Coulter Life Sciences, Jersey City, NJ, USA), RNA was eluted in the RNA storage solution (AM7000, Invitrogen). The synthesized mRNA was quantified using the Qubit™ RNA Extended Range (XR) Assay Kits (Invitrogen), and the integrity of the mRNA was evaluated on the 2100 Bioanalyzer instrument using the Agilent RNA 6000 Nano kit.

2.4. Formulation Development of Fluc-PS80 LNPs

2.4.1. Cryoprotectant Concentration Screening in PSS Buffer

Fluc-PS80 LNPs were prepared via microfluidic mixing using the NanoAssemblr® Ignite™ system (Precision NanoSystems Inc., Vancouver, BC, Canada) (Figure 1). A freeze/thaw study was performed to screen varied concentrations of sucrose as the cryoprotectant to maintain the stability of LNPs. Fluc-PS80 LNPs were prepared with the lipid composition of DLin-MC3-DMA/DSPC/Cholesterol/PS-80 in the molar percent ratio of 52/8/37/3. The lipid components were dissolved in 200 Proof absolute ethanol at a total lipid concentration of 50 mM, while Fluc mRNA (200 µg/mL) was diluted in 10 mM sodium acetate buffer pH 4.5. Lipids and Fluc mRNA solutions were both mixed at the previously optimized flow rate ratio of 3:1 (aqueous/organic), total flow rate of 12 mL/min, and N/P ratio of 14. Formulated LNPs were diluted with 1× PBS, pH 7.4, containing various sucrose concentrations (0, 5, 10, 15, 20% *w/v*). Diluted Fluc-PS80 LNPs were subjected to ultrafiltration for buffer exchange using Amicon Ultra centrifugal filter units (100 kDa MWCO) (Millipore, Burlington, MA, USA). All the formulations were sterile-filtered, filled in 2R vials, and subjected to one freeze/thaw cycle (overnight at −80 °C). Detailed analytical characterization was performed for the obtained Fluc-PS80 LNPs as described in Section 2.5.

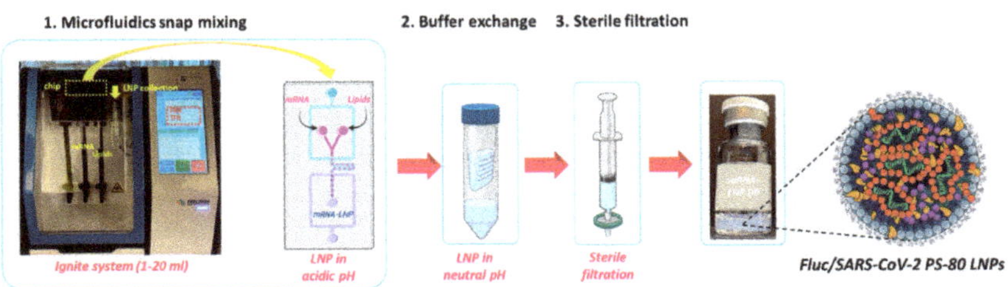

Figure 1. A schematic representation of the LNP manufacturing process using the NanoAssemblr® Ignite™ system. Constituent lipids and mRNA (acidic pH) are subjected to microfluidic mixing followed by buffer exchange using the formulation buffer for pH neutralization. The obtained neutral LNP solution is then sterile-filtered to produce the final mRNA-LNP DP. mRNA: Fluc or SARS-CoV-2; Lipids: DLin-MC3-DMA, DSPC, Cholesterol, PS-80; DP: drug product.

2.4.2. Lipid Combination Screening in TSS Buffer

We performed the lipid combination screening for Fluc-PS80 LNPs in TSS buffer. This TSS buffer was developed in a preliminary study (see Supplementary Information, Figures S1 and S2 for more details). Different lipid combinations were screened by modifying the molar ratios of the four lipid components in the Fluc-PS80 LNP formulation. Briefly, LNPs containing different lipid combinations (shown in Table 1) were prepared using the

NanoAssemblr® Ignite™ system (Precision NanoSystems Inc., Vancouver, BC, Canada). All six formulations (F1–F6) were prepared using similar mixing conditions described in Section 2.4.1. Following microfluidic mixing, LNPs were diluted with TSS buffer pH 7.4, and then subjected to buffer exchange using ultrafiltration followed by sterile filtration before filling into 2R vials. LNPs were tested in both frozen (one freeze/thaw cycle overnight at −80 °C) and liquid state (5 °C) to identify a stable formulation for further studies.

Table 1. Lipid composition of the screened Fluc-PS80 LNP formulations.

Formulations	Lipid Components (Molar Percent Ratio)			
	Dlin-MC3-DMA	DSPC	Cholesterol	PS-80
F1	52	8	37	3
F2	50	10	37	3
F3	48	12	37	3
F4	52	8	38.5	1.5
F5	50	10	38.5	1.5
F6	48	12	38.5	1.5

2.4.3. Formulation Buffer Screening for Long-Term Storage Stability of SC2-PS80 LNPs

SC2-PS80 LNPs containing the optimized lipid composition of DLin-MC3-DMA/DSPC/Cholesterol/PS-80 in the molar percent ratio of 52/8/37/3 and sucrose content (identified from the cryoprotectant screening study) were prepared using the same manufacturing method as explained in Section 2.4.1. LNPs prepared in the TSS buffer were tested for long-term storage in comparison to the PSS buffer at different temperatures (−80 °C, 5 °C, 25 °C) over six months of storage. Following microfluidic mixing, LNPs were diluted with either of the two buffers: PSS (1× PBS, 10% sucrose, pH 7.4) or TSS (50 mM Tris, 45 mM NaCl, 10% sucrose, pH 7.4). Diluted LNPs were subjected to buffer exchange using ultrafiltration, sterile-filtered, and filled into 2R vials. The SC2-PS80 LNP samples were taken at various timepoints over 6 months for detailed characterization according to the analytical panel explained in Section 2.5.

2.5. Analytical Characterization of mRNA-Loaded LNPs

A panel for testing various quality attributes was established to identify the drug product (DP) quality of all the manufactured mRNA-LNP formulations using various analytical techniques/assays as mentioned in Table 2 and the following sub-sections.

Table 2. Panel of quality attributes and respective analytical techniques/assays used to evaluate the mRNA-LNP drug product quality.

Quality Attribute	Analytical Techniques/Assays
Visual appearance	Manual
pH	pH meter
Particle size	Dynamic light scattering (DLS)
Surface charge	Electrophoretic mobility
Particle concentration	Nanoparticle tracking analysis (NTA)
Encapsulation efficiency	RiboGreen™ Assay
Particle morphology	Cryo-TEM
mRNA purity	Microchip capillary electrophoresis (MCE)
In vitro transfection efficiency	
Fluc-PS80 LNP	Cell-based luminescence assay
SC2-PS80 LNP	Immune staining and Flow cytometry
In vivo immunogenicity in mice	Luminex Spike Assay, Pseudovirus neutralization assay

2.5.1. Visual Inspection and pH

Fluc-PS80 LNP formulations prepared for lipid combinations screening in TSS buffer (−80 °C, 5 °C, and 25 °C) were assessed for their appearance in terms of color, clarity, and visible particulates by visual observation against a black background with white light illumination. Additionally, to measure the pH, 100 µL of LNPs were aliquoted in 0.5 mL Eppendorf tubes and the small pH meter probe (Mettler Toledo) was immersed in the LNP solution to read the final pH following buffer exchange and sterile filtration. Visual inspection and pH measurement for LNP formulations subjected to long-term storage stability were determined at D0, D30, D90, and D180 at different storage conditions (−80 °C, 5 °C, 25 °C).

2.5.2. Particle Size and Surface Charge

LNPs were analyzed for their particle size, polydispersity index by dynamic light scattering (DLS) and zeta potential using the electrophoretic mobility approach (Malvern Zetasizer Ultra). All the samples were measured in a disposable folded capillary cell (DTS1070) following 10 times dilution with sterile filtered 0.1× PBS, pH 7.4. Measurements were performed at 25 °C using a refractive index of 1.45 and an absorption of 0.001, with a viscosity of 0.8872 cP. Every sample was measured in triplicates, each with 5 runs and 5 s equilibration time, using a 173° backscatter detection angle.

2.5.3. Particle Concentration

Fluc-PS80 LNP formulations prepared for lipid combinations screening in TSS buffer (−80 °C, 5 °C) were assessed for their particle concentration using a nanoparticle tracking analysis (NTA) instrument, ZetaView® Z-NTA (Particle Metrix Inc., Mebane, NC, USA). Before running the LNPs, 100 nm polystyrene beads (AlphaNanoTech, Durham, NC, USA) were used for instrument QC, calibration, and auto-alignment. Then, LNPs were diluted between a range of 200,000×–500,000× in sterile-filtered 0.1× PBS pH 7.4 and injected into the cell for performing the measurements. Dilutions of each sample were identified to maintain 100–200 particles per frame to achieve accurate results. Particle count was performed for 11 positions/frames and three cycles, with a sensitivity of 85, shutter of 150, and laser wavelength of 488 nm for all the samples.

2.5.4. Encapsulation Efficiency

A Quant-IT™ RiboGreen RNA Assay Kit (Invitrogen™) was used to measure the encapsulation efficiency and mRNA concentration of Fluc-PS80 LNP and SC2-PS80 LNP formulations. Initially, two standard curves were generated for Fluc and SARS-CoV-2 mRNAs (50–200 ng/mL), each in 10 mM Tris/1 mM EDTA (TE) buffer and in 2% *w*/*v* Triton x-100/TE (TR) buffer. The total mRNA in the LNPs was diluted 5× in TE buffer and added in a 1:1 volume ratio to TE buffer in each well to determine the free mRNA concentration. Next, to analyze the total mRNA concentration, the LNPs were diluted 25 times in TE buffer and added in a 1:1 volume ratio to TR buffer in each well. Following the addition of samples and standards to the plate, it was incubated at 37 °C for 10 min to allow LNP dissociation and subsequent release of the total encapsulated mRNA for quantification. Ribogreen reagent diluted in TE buffer (1:200 *v*/*v*) was then added to each standard and sample well in a 1:1 volume ratio and the plates were immediately measured for fluorescence (Ex485/Em528) using the Synergy Neo2 Hybrid Multimode Reader (Biotek, Shoreline, WA, USA). Free and total mRNA concentrations were calculated using the two standard curves generated in TE and TR buffers, respectively. The encapsulation efficiency for each LNP formulation was calculated using the following equation:

$$Encapsulation\ efficiency\ (\%) = \frac{Total\ mRNA - Free\ mRNA}{Total\ mRNA} \times 100$$

2.5.5. mRNA Purity

Microchip capillary electrophoresis (MCE) was performed to determine the mRNA purity for all the tested LNP formulations. Fluc and SARS-CoV-2 mRNAs and their respective LNP samples were diluted with 2% Triton x-100 (w/v in nuclease-free water) to achieve a final concentration of 5 µg/mL. Next, 20 µL of the diluted samples were added to 80 µL of 1× Pico Sensitivity Sample Buffer into each well in a 96-well plate. Samples were denatured in a 70 °C heating block for 2 min, then snap-cooled on ice for 5 min. The RNA Pico ladder, Gel-Dye solution, and RNA Labchip were prepared by following the RNA Pico Sensitivity Assay Quick Guide (Perkin Elmer, Shelton, CT, USA) without any modifications. Briefly, 4 µL of RNA Pico ladder was added to 116 µL 1× Sample Buffer and transferred to the provided ladder tube. The Gel-Dye solution was prepared by transferring 90 µL of RNA Dye Concentrate to one RNA Pico Gel Matrix vial, followed by mixing and centrifugation in a microtube spin filter. The RNA Labchip was thoroughly washed with nuclease-free water, following which the Gel-Dye solution and RNA Pico marker were added to the designated wells. LabChip GXII Touch (Perkin Elmer, Shelton, CT, USA) was used to run the assay, which is based on the principle of mRNA electrophoresis that migrates across the sieving gel matrix to separate by size. The resultant mRNA signal was monitored by fluorescent detection. For each electropherogram obtained from running the Fluc or SARS-CoV-2 mRNA and their respective LNP samples, the main peak and the fragments were calculated as a percentage of the total peak area. The mRNA purity for both mRNA alone and mRNA encapsulated within LNPs is calculated as the percent peak area of the main peak.

2.5.6. Particle Morphology

Cryogenic transmission electron microscopy (cryo-TEM) was used to determine the effect of lipid combinations screening on the morphology of Fluc-PS80 LNPs prepared in TSS buffer (−80 °C, 5 °C). For that, the C-Flat 2/1 holey carbon, mesh copper grids (Electron Microscopy Sciences, Hatfield, PA, USA) were cleaned with a Solarus 950 Plasma Cleaner (Gatan, Pleasanton, CA, USA) or a PELCO easiGlow Glow Discharge Cleaning System (Ted Pella, Inc, Redding, CA, USA) before sample application. A Vitrobot Mark IV (Thermo Fisher Scientific, Waltham, MA, USA) with the environmental chamber set to 4 °C and 95% or 100% humidity was used to prepare the grids. A 3 µL sample in the original TSS buffer composition was applied to a grid for up to 30 s before blotting and plunge freezing in liquid ethane. Grids were stored under liquid nitrogen, clipped into cartridges, placed into a cassette, and transferred to the autoloader of the microscope while maintaining cryogenic temperatures (below −170 °C). Images were collected with a Glacios Cryo-Transmission Electron Microscope (Thermo Fisher Scientific, Waltham, MA, USA) equipped with a Falcon 3 or Falcon 4 camera (Thermo Fisher Scientific, Waltham, MA, USA) and operated at 200 kV. Leginon software (version 3.7) was used for semi-automated data collection. Areas of interest were targeted at lower magnifications (940×–8500×) before the acquisition of movies at nominal magnifications of 28,000× (~0.5 nm/pixel), 73,000× (~0.2 nm/pixel), and 150,000× (~0.1 nm/pixel). The 150,000× images were acquired with defocus between −2 µm to −4.5 µm and with an electron dose between 12–25 e−/Å2. Finally, the acquired movie frames were aligned with MotionCor2 (Version 1.6.4) and converted to a jpeg format.

2.6. In Vitro Transfection Efficiency of Fluc-PS80 LNP Formulations

The in vitro luciferase expression assay was performed in HEK-293 cells. Briefly, cells were seeded at a density of 10,000 cells per well in 96-well plates 24 h prior to the treatments. Following that, cells were treated with Fluc-PS80 LNPs containing different lipid combinations at 10 ng mRNA per well. Lipofectamine™ MessengerMAX™ Transfection Reagent (Invitrogen, Cat# LMRNA015) was used as a positive control, by following the manufacturer's instructions. After 24 h of treatment, ONE-Glo™ Luciferase Assay (Promega, Madison, WI, USA) was performed as per the manufacturer's protocol. For that, an equal volume of the assay reagent was added to each treatment and control wells and incubated for 3 min at room temperature. Following this step, 150 µL of the supernatant was transferred to a white opaque 96-well microplate and the luminescence was measured on a Tecan Infinite F500 Multimode Microplate Reader (Thermo Fisher Scientific, Waltham, MA, USA).

2.7. In Vivo Transfection of Fluc-PS80 LNP Versus DMG-PEG2K LNP Formulations

All animal studies were conducted according to Regeneron's and Institutional Animal Care and Use Committee (IACUC) for murine research (Protocol 303.4). The animal handling was performed in facilities accredited by the Association for Assessment and Accreditation of Laboratory Animal Care International in accordance with protocols approved by IACUC and the principles outlined in the Guide for the Care and Use of Laboratory Animals by the Institute for Laboratory Animal Resources. The 4–8-weeks-old, wild-type C57BL/6NTac female mice (Taconic Biosciences, Inc., Rensselaer, NY, USA) were IV (tail vein) or IM (hind limb) injected with 12 µg mRNA per mouse from Fluc mRNA formulated with PS-80 LNP or with conventional LNPs containing D-Lin-MC3-DMA and DMG-PEG lipids (Table 3). We used PBS solution to dilute the LNP samples and the maximum injection volume of samples was less than 100 µL per injection. Each treatment group contained four mice with an additional untreated mouse kept in the same cage as the control. The mice's whole-body images were collected 24 h post-LNP injection using IVIS. Before IVIS imaging, 100 µL of D-Luciferin substrate was injected per mouse. The mouse was maintained under 2% isoflurane anesthesia for 10 min. After whole-body imaging, the mice were sacrificed by exposing them to CO_2 gas for 10 min, and then their internal organs, including the liver, spleen, and lymph nodes, were dissected and subsequently imaged under the IVIS instrument.

Table 3. LNP formulations used for preliminary evaluation of the Fluc-PS80 LNPs versus DMG-PEG2K LNPs organ distribution.

LNP Formulation	Lipid Composition (MC3/DSPC/Chol/PEG-lipid mol%)	mRNA Buffer	Injection Route
1.5% DMG-PEG	52/8/38.5/1.5	10 mM Sodium Citrate, pH 5	IV
3% DMG-PEG	52/8/37/3	10 mM Sodium Acetate, pH 4.5	IV
1.5% DMG-PEG	52/8/38.5/1.5	10 mM Sodium Acetate, pH 4.5	IM
3%, DMG-PEG	52/8/37/3	10 mM Sodium Acetate, pH 4.5	IM
1.5% PS-80	52/8/38.5/1.5	10 mM Sodium Acetate, pH 4.5	IM
3% PS-80	52/8/37/3	10 mM Sodium Acetate, pH 4.5	IM

2.8. In Vitro Transfection Efficiency of SC2-PS80 LNP Formulations

2.8.1. Transfection of HEK-293 Cells with SC2-PS80 LNPs

The day before transfection, HEK-293 cells were seeded at 10,000 cells per well of a flat bottom 96-well plate and left to adhere overnight. Next, SC2-PS80 LNPs formulated in different buffers and stored at various temperatures were diluted with complete media to make 1 µg/mL mRNA, then added to HEK-293 cells in the 96-well plate. For the positive control, cells were transfected with mRNA formulated with Lipofectamine™

MessengerMAX™ (Invitrogen, Cat# LMRNA015), prepared according to the manufacturer's instructions. The resulting LNPs and Lipofectamine lipoplexes were added to the HEK-293 cells at 1/10th the media volume of the cells, at 1 μg/mL final mRNA concentration. After that, cells were incubated for 18–24 h at 37 °C, 5% CO_2 before being harvested to measure the expression of SARS-CoV-2 6P spike protein using flow cytometry.

2.8.2. Immunostaining of Transfected Cells and Analysis of SARS-CoV-2 6P Spike Protein Expression via Flow Cytometry

The transfected HEK-293 cells were washed by Mg/Ca-free DPBS (Gibco Cat# 14190144) then trypsinized, re-washed and transferred to a round bottom 96-well plate. Next, to measure the viability, 50 μL DPBS containing Live/Dead Fixable Violet (Invitrogen, Cat# L34964) viability dye was added to each well and incubated for 15 min at 37 °C in the dark. After that, the cells were washed with DPBS twice, and the primary antibody specific for SARS-CoV-2 6P spike protein was added to the cells at 4 μg/mL in 50 μL cell staining buffer (DPBS containing 1% FBS and 0.5 mM EDTA) and incubated for 20–30 min at room temperature in the dark. Cells were washed twice with DPBS, and an anti-human FcR secondary antibody conjugated to Alexa Fluor 647 (AF647) (Jackson Immunoresearch, Cat# 109-605-190) was added to the cells at 2 μg/mL in 50 μL cell staining buffer and incubated for 20–30 min at room temperature in the dark. Finally, the cells were washed twice with DPBS before resuspending in 80 μL of cell staining buffer for flow cytometry analysis on the Agilent Novocyte Penteon flow cytometer (Agilent Technologies, Santa Clara, CA). For flow cytometry, a minimum of 20,000 events were recorded and exported to FCS 3.0 files to be analyzed by the FlowJo software (version 9.9.6, BD, Ashland, OR) to quantify the expression of SARS-CoV-2 6P spike protein via AF647 gating. The Live/Dead Violet-negative and AF647-positive gating were used to quantify using FlowJo software. The level of spike protein expression was quantified by either the median fluorescence intensity (MFI) of AF647 in live cells, or the percentage of live cells that expressed AF647 relative to non-transfected cells.

2.9. *Mouse Immunization and In Vivo Immunogenicity of the Optimized SC2-PS80 LNP Formulation*

VelocImmune® mice (8–20 weeks of age) were immunized IM into the hind limb with 5 μg/mouse at 50 μL total volume diluted in PBS of SARS-CoV-2 mRNA encoding Wuhan-Hu-1 SARS-CoV-2 spike sequence (MN908947.3 with K986P + V987P stabilizing mutations) and SC2-PS80 LNP formulation. The mRNA/LNPs were either made fresh (n = 5/group) or stored at −80 °C or 5 °C (n = 3/group) for 6 months prior to vaccination. Sera was collected 26 days post single immunization and stored at 4 °C. Luminex spike assay was performed following previously published methods for polyclonal SARS-CoV-2 specific IgG binding on an INTELLIFLEX® Luminex™ instrument [18]. Sera samples were diluted to 1:6250 and reported as median fluorescence index (MFI) via an anti-mouse IgG-PE secondary antibody. Sera binding was to full-length Wuhan-Hu-1 SARS-CoV-2 spike protein.

Pseudovirus neutralization assays were performed on samples following previously published methods using non-replicative vesicular stomatitis virus (VSV) with firefly luciferase (Fluc) encoded and SARS-CoV-2 spike (aa 14-1255, D614G substitution, Wuhan-Hu-1; MN908947.3) replacing the native VSV glycoprotein (G) sequence [18]. Luciferase output was measured on a SpectraMax i3 plate reader with a MiniMax imaging cytometer. Sera samples are reported as pseudotyped virus neutralization titer 50 (pVNT50).

2.10. *Statistical Analysis*

Statistical analyses were performed for all the experiments using GraphPad Prism software (version: 10.1.0). All data were presented as mean ± SD for the in vitro assays, while that as mean ± SEM for any in vivo experiments. A p value of less than 0.05 was considered statistically significant.

3. Results

3.1. Fluc-PS80 LNPs Preferentially Accumulate in the Spleen Rather than the Liver

To gauge the effect of PS-80 on extrahepatic delivery, we formulated Fluc-PS80 LNPs at two PS-80 molar percentages (1.5% or 3%) in PBS buffer and compared their biodistribution with a conventional DMG-PEG2K LNP in mice (Table 3). All LNPs maintained a particle size below 100 nm and encapsulation efficiencies above 90%. We included IV administration of DMG-PEG LNPs as a baseline control to highlight the well-known liver accumulation typically seen with conventional PEG-lipid LNPs via IV injection. We showed that with the change of the administration route from IV to IM, the DMG-PEG2K LNPs' liver accumulation pattern did not change. Following IM injection of ~12 μg mRNA per mouse, ex vivo IVIS imaging (Figure 2) revealed that independent of the PS-80 percentage, Fluc-PS80 LNPs yielded, on average, a 3-to-5-fold higher luciferase signal in the spleen relative to DMG-PEG2K formulations (Figure 2c). Moreover, the spleen-to-liver expression ratio exceeded 50-fold in the PS-80 groups (Figure 2d), suggesting substantially enhanced extrahepatic uptake. Based on these promising results, we next refined the formulation buffer, cryoprotectant concentration, and lipid composition, to then evaluate the long-term stability of the optimized PS-80 LNP platform for the SARS-CoV-2 spike mRNA vaccine.

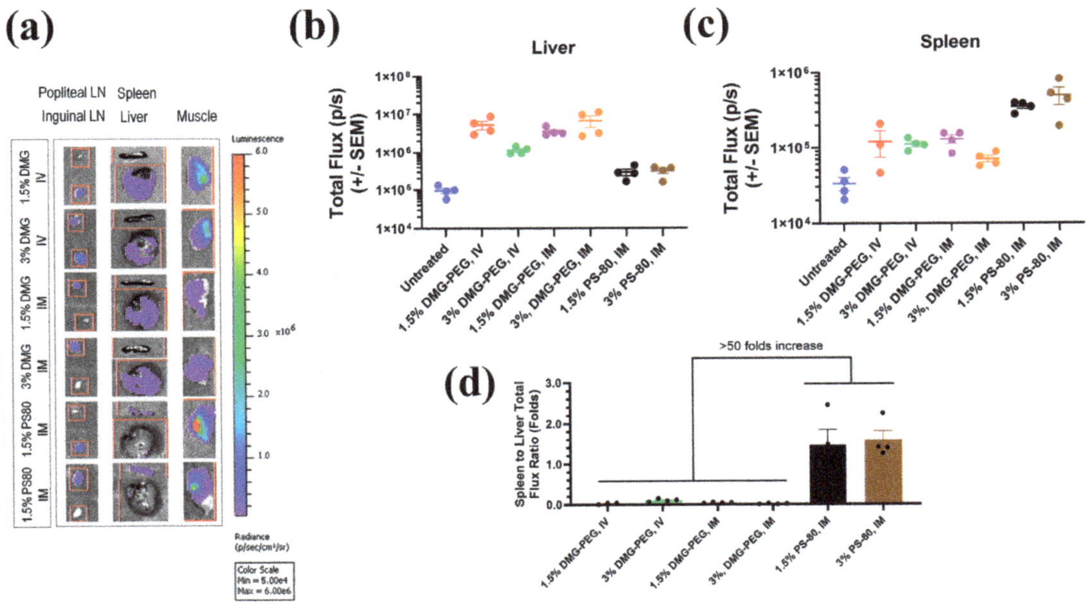

Figure 2. Organ transfection distribution of Fluc-PS80 LNPs compared to the DMG-PEG2K LNPs post-IV or IM administration in mice. (**a**) Luciferase expression of the dissected organs under IVIS; (**b**,**c**) quantified total flux for liver and spleen; and (**d**) Luciferase expression (total flux) fold ratios in the spleen compared to the liver. Four mice were injected per group and the data (**d**) were statistically compared using ANOVA with Bonferroni post hoc.

3.2. Optimization of Formulation Composition for Fluc-PS80 LNPs

Before optimizing other formulation variables (e.g., cryoprotectant levels, buffer types, and lipid compositions), we first tested how salt concentration affects the freeze/thaw stability of Fluc-PS80 LNPs. We found that 45 mM NaCl was necessary to maintain consistent particle attributes and potency, particularly in tris-based buffer (Figure S3). Consequently, all subsequent development of cryoprotectant and lipid composition was performed in the presence of ≥45 mM NaCl.

3.2.1. Buffer and Cryoprotectant Screening

Next, we screened sucrose levels ranging from 0% to 20% (*w*/*v*) in PBS (PSS) to identify the optimal cryoprotectant content for Fluc-PS80 LNPs under freeze/thaw stress. As shown in Figure 3, formulations containing ≥10% sucrose maintained a particle size ≤100 nm, encapsulation efficiency ≥90%, and mRNA purity higher than 70% following one freeze/thaw cycle (stored at −80 °C overnight and thawed at room temperature). By contrast, samples with <10% sucrose tended to aggregate or lose encapsulation upon the freeze/thaw cycle.

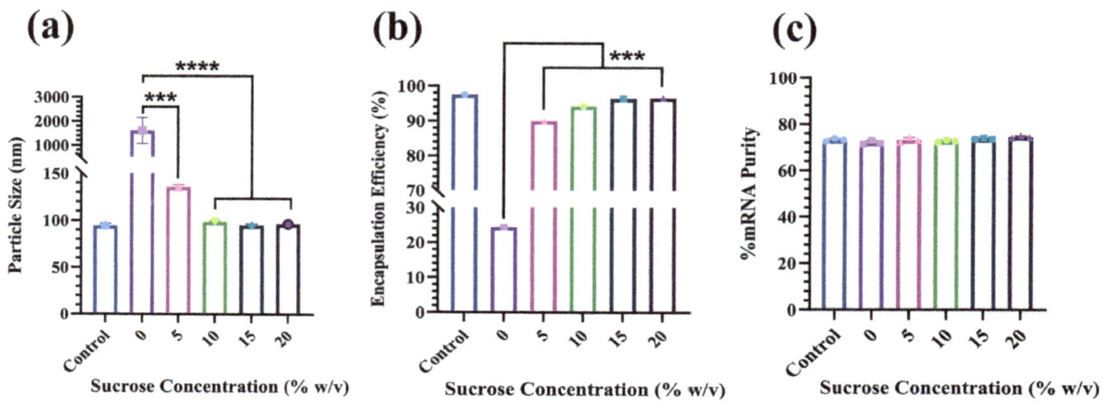

Figure 3. Screening of sucrose concentration to prepare stable Fluc-PS80 LNP formulation following one freeze/thaw cycle. LNP formulations containing ≥10% sucrose exhibited consistently smaller particle sizes of <100 nm, ≥90% encapsulation efficiency, and >70% mRNA purity. The control samples were the same LNPs stored at 5 °C overnight without the exposure to freeze/thaw cycle. The bars show the mean ± standard deviation of three independent measurements. Statistical comparison between samples was analyzed by performing one-way ANOVA with Bonferroni post hoc: *** *p* value < 0.001, **** *p* value < 0.0001.

In a separate set of experiments, we observed that a tris-sucrose-salt (TSS) buffer system (50 mM tris, 45 mM NaCl, 10% *w*/*v* sucrose) provided even better long-term stability for Fluc-PS80 LNPs than PSS (see Supplementary Information, Figures S1 and S2). As a result, TSS was selected for further in vitro and in vivo evaluations.

3.2.2. Lipid Combinations Screening

After establishing 10% sucrose in a tris-salt buffer (TSS) as optimal for freeze/thaw stability, we screened various PS-80 and helper-lipid ratios (Table 1) to determine their impact on Fluc-PS80 LNP quality and performance. Each formulation (F1–F6) was tested for physicochemical attributes (particle size, zeta potential, encapsulation efficiency, and particle concentration), then further examined via cryo-TEM and in vitro transfection.

Particle Size, Particle Concentration, and Encapsulation Efficiency

The particle size of all formulations was maintained below 100 nm pre- and post-freeze/thaw, albeit with different size distributions. Specifically, the polydispersity index (PDI) was lower (≤0.1) in F4–F6 (1.5% PS-80) compared to F1–F3 (3% PS-80), whose PDI was ≤0.2 (Figure 4a,b). Zeta potential remained near neutral (−3 to −10 mV), and encapsulation efficiencies exceeded 85% across all formulations, with no major changes from freeze/thaw (Figure 4c,d).

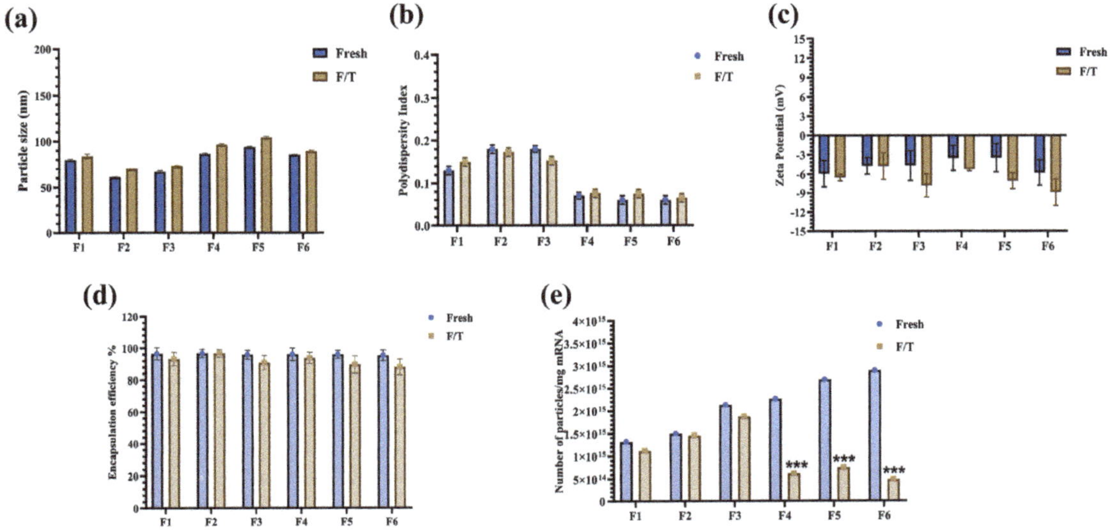

Figure 4. Physicochemical characterization of Fluc PS-80 LNP formulations containing various lipid combinations prepared in TSS buffer, including (**a**) Particle size, (**b**) Polydispersity index, (**c**) Zeta Potential, and (**d**) Encapsulation efficiency. F4–F6 formulations containing 1.5 mol% PS-80 demonstrated lower polydispersity index while the other analyses yielded similar results for all the formulations. (**e**) Particle concentration normalized to the mRNA content sharply reduced for F4-F6 formulations following freeze/thaw. The represented data are mean ± standard deviation of three independent measurements. Statistical comparison between samples was performed using one-way ANOVA with Bonferroni post hoc: *** p value < 0.001.

Despite these similarities, particle concentration differed markedly. Formulations F4–F6 lost 3- to 6-fold more particles upon one freeze/thaw than F1–F3 formulations did (Figure 4e). This suggests that lower PS-80 concentrations may yield narrower size distributions but could also compromise freeze/thaw robustness.

Particle Morphology by cryo-TEM

To visualize how lipid composition and freeze/thaw affected particle morphology, we examined F1 and F4–F6 by cryo-TEM (Figure 5). Both fresh F1 (3% PS-80) and F4 (1.5% PS-80) were generally spherical with minor internal blebs, suggesting PS-80 concentration alone did not drastically alter particle shape. However, increasing DSPC and reducing DLin-MC3-DMA (F5–F6) led to more elongated, polyhedral morphologies. After a single freeze/thaw cycle, the number of particles decreased for all samples, and F4–F6 displayed larger blebs with uneven surfaces—consistent with the observed decrease in particle concentration (Figure 4e). Considering the apparent particle sizes, it should be noted that Figure 4a shows the average hydrodynamic diameter in suspension (DLS), whereas cryo-TEM (Figure 5) images individual frozen particles, which can appear larger or more irregular than the DLS-measured mean size because the two techniques operate under different principles and conditions.

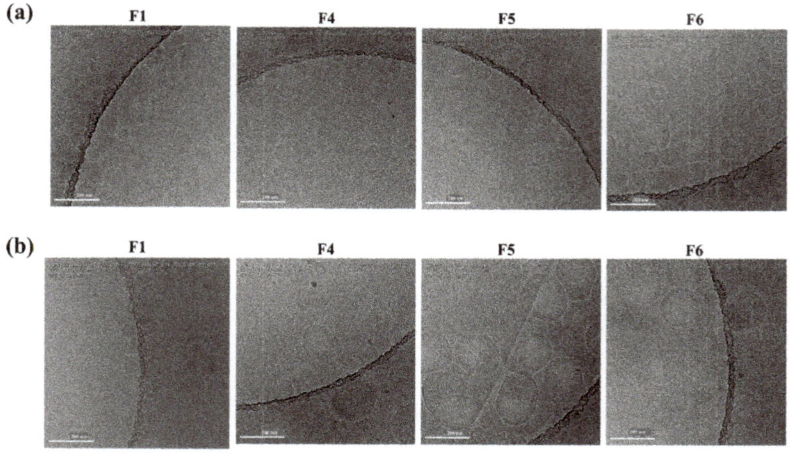

Figure 5. Representative cryo-TEM images of four Fluc-PS80 LNP formulations prepared in TSS buffer. (**a**) Fresh formulations, and (**b**) following one freeze/thaw cycle at −80 °C. For fresh formulations, F4–F6 formulations containing 1.5 mol% PS-80 showed a higher number of particles as compared to the F1 formulation containing 3 mol% PS-80. Increasing DSPC and simultaneously decreasing Dlin-MC3-DMA content resulted in changed particle morphology from circular to elongated LNPs with polyhedral shapes. For formulations subjected to freeze/thaw, F5 and F6 formulations showed a significant increase in the size of the particles as compared to the F1 formulation. The scale bar shows 200 nm for all presented images.

mRNA Purity and In Vitro Transfection

All LNPs preserved ≥80% mRNA purity, independent of formulation or freeze/thaw (Figure 6a). In contrast, in vitro transfection efficiency declined with rising DSPC and reduced DLin-MC3-DMA. Mean luminescence intensity dropped, for instance, from 4.48×10^6 a.u. (F1) to 1.51×10^6 a.u. (F3) in the 3% PS-80 series (Figure 6b). Additionally, LNPs with 1.5% PS-80 (F4-F6) suffered a further 1.5-fold reduction post-freeze/thaw, whereas 3% PS-80 formulations (F1–F3) remained unaffected. Overall, F1 offered the best balance of freeze/thaw stability and high transfection and was thus chosen to encapsulate SARS-CoV-2 mRNA for subsequent vaccine-related studies.

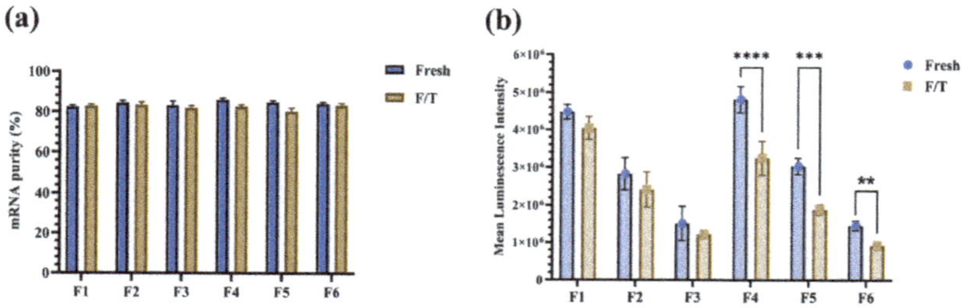

Figure 6. mRNA purity and in vitro transfection efficiency analyses of Fluc-PS80 LNP formulations containing various lipid combinations prepared in TSS buffer. (**a**) No substantial difference was observed between formulations in terms of mRNA purity, and (**b**) in vitro transfection efficiency was reduced with increased DSPC and decreased Dlin-MC3-DMA content. While F4–F6 formulations containing 1.5 mol% PS-80 showed higher transfection efficiency as compared to F1–F3 formulations, it significantly reduced following freeze/thaw. The formulations following freeze/thaw were significantly different in the mean luminescence intensity. The represented data are mean ± standard deviation of three independent measurements. Statistical comparison between samples was analyzed using Two-Way ANOVA with Bonferroni post hoc. ** *p* value <0.05, *** *p* value < 0.001, **** *p* value < 0.0001.

3.3. Storage Stability of SC2-PS80 LNPs In Tris vs. Phosphate-Based Buffers

Having identified F1 as the lead composition, we next encapsulated SARS-CoV-2 mRNA and compared the long-term stability of SC2-PS80 LNPs in PBS-sucrose (PSS) versus tris-sucrose-salt (TSS) buffers at −80 °C, 5 °C, or 25 °C for up to six months (Figure 7).

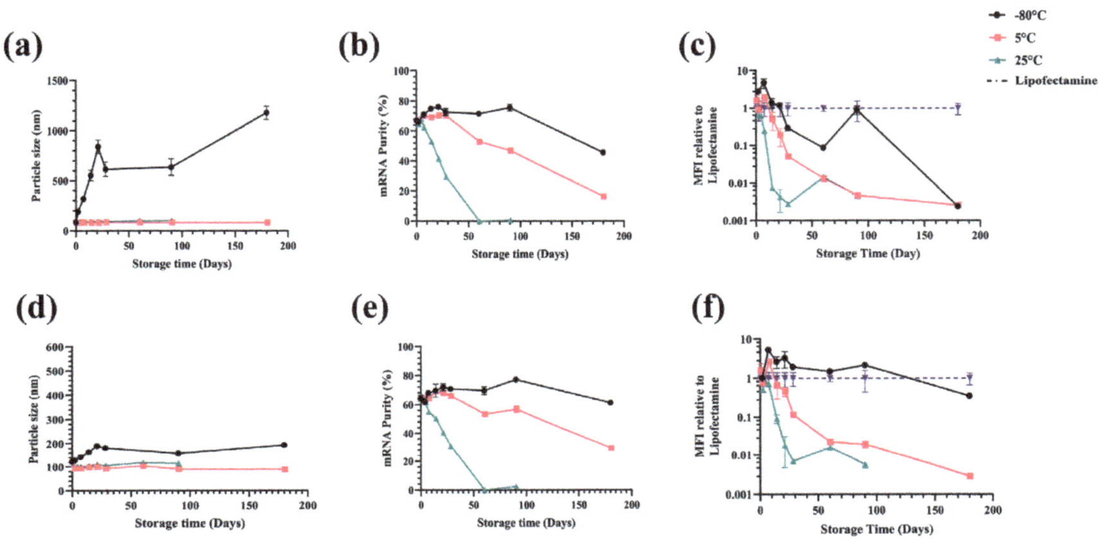

Figure 7. Storage stability of SC2-PS80 LNPs formulated in PSS (**a**–**c**) and TSS (**d**–**f**) buffers following six months when stored at different temperatures. SC2-PS80 LNPs formulated in PSS buffer and stored at −80 °C showed increased particle size and reduced mRNA purity as well as in vitro transfection efficiency. Most formulations depicted lower stability in terms of mRNA purity and in vitro transfection efficiency over time. SC2-PS80 LNPs formulated in TSS buffer and stored at −80 °C showed higher stability as compared to those prepared in PSS buffer with improved particle size, mRNA purity, and in vitro transfection efficiency over six months. The represented data are mean ± standard deviation of at least three independent measurements. MFI: Mean Fluorescence Intensity.

3.3.1. PSS-Formulated LNPs

SC2-PS80 LNPs in PSS showed significant instability when stored in a frozen state. Their particle size increased from ~85 nm to ~1180 nm at −80 °C, accompanied by an increase in polydispersity index (PDI) from 0.10 to 0.55 (Figures 7a and S6). While samples stored at 5 °C or 25 °C retained smaller sizes (85–100 nm), they demonstrated a notable reduction in mRNA purity (16.2% and 79% by six and three months, respectively; Figure 7b) and showed a significant loss in their in vitro transfection efficacy over time (Figure 7c). Overall, PSS-buffered LNPs did not maintain adequate particle properties at the tested temperatures.

3.3.2. TSS-Formulated LNPs

In contrast, TSS-based LNPs demonstrated substantially greater stability under frozen conditions. After six months at −80 °C, their size increased only to ~192 nm, with a PDI of ~0.13 (Figures 7d and S6c). Zeta potential also remained stable across all temperatures (Figure S6). Although mRNA purity at 5 °C or 25 °C gradually dropped (to 29.2% and 2.6%, respectively), the −80 °C samples retained ~61.2% (Figure 7e). Importantly, TSS-based LNPs stored at −80 °C preserved high in vitro transfection, comparable to that of Lipofectamine (used as positive control) (Figure 7f).

To contextualize our PS-80 based formulation, we performed a parallel stability assessment of conventional DMG-PEG2K LNPs in PSS versus TSS buffers (see Supplementary Figures S1 and S2). Although DMG-PEG2K LNPs also benefited from TSS in maintaining smaller particle sizes and higher in vitro potency over six months, their particle size was less affected by the buffer type under frozen storage compared to the PS-80-LNPs. Hence, while both formulations gain stability from TSS, PS-80-LNPs offer an added advantage of enhanced extrahepatic (spleen) localization (Figure 2), making them an attractive platform for mRNA vaccine applications.

Taken together, these data confirm that tris-sucrose-salt (TSS)-buffered PS-80 LNPs provide robust particle size control, mRNA integrity, and in vitro activity over extended storage at −80 °C, whereas freezing in phosphate-salt-sucrose (PSS) buffer leads to aggregation and reduced potency.

3.4. In Vivo Immunogenicity of the Optimized SC2-PS80 LNP Formulation

Following verification of the SC2-PS80 LNP's in vitro potency and stability, we assessed its immunogenicity in either a frozen state (−80 °C) or a liquid state (5 °C) after six months of storage in TSS buffer. At 26 days post-single immunization, serum samples were collected and evaluated for SARS-CoV-2-specific IgG binding and neutralization (Figure 8a). Results were compared to freshly prepared LNPs to detect any changes in vivo efficacy over storage time.

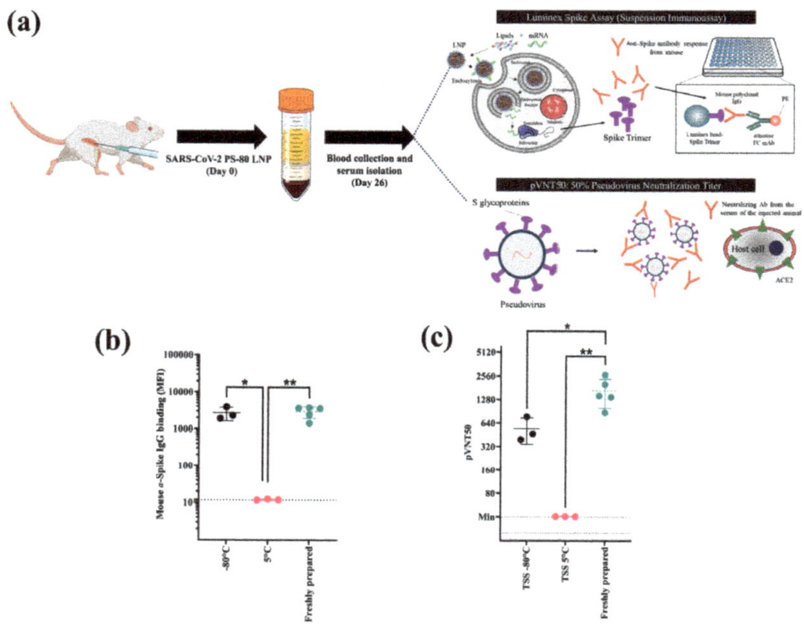

Figure 8. In vivo immunogenicity of the optimized SC2-PS80 LNPs in mice following six months of storage. (**a**) Schematics representing mice inoculation, sera collection and immunogenicity analyses following intramuscular administration of SC2-PS80 LNPs. (**b**) Anti-spike IgG antibodies were measured via a bead-based Luminex assay for spike in serum from mice immunized with the LNPs stored at −80 °C compared to the freshly prepared formulation at 1:6250 dilution of sera. (**c**) pVNT50 (50% pseudovirus neutralization titer) assay denoting the pVNT50 values of the formulation stored at −80 °C and 5 °C for 6 months in comparison to freshly prepared SC2-PS80 LNPs. The data on graphs (**b**) and (**c**) are mean ± standard deviations of at least three independent measurements. Statistical comparison between samples was analyzed using One-Way ANOVA with Bonferroni post hoc. * p value <0.1, ** p value < 0.05. The schematic was partially created with BioRender.com.

Mice that received LNPs stored at −80 °C for six months produced anti-spike IgG titers on par with those given freshly prepared formulations (Figure 8b). By contrast, the group stored at 5 °C showed minimal IgG binding, consistent with the drop in transfection efficiency seen in vitro for 5 °C samples. Similarly, pseudovirus neutralization titers (pVNT50) were robust in both freshly prepared and −80 °C–stored LNPs (average 540 and 1664 a.u., respectively), while 5 °C-stored LNPs induced negligible neutralization (Figure 8c). These findings confirm that formulating in TSS buffer and storing at −80 °C preserves the vaccine's ability to stimulate a strong SARS-CoV-2-specific humoral response.

4. Discussion

mRNA-LNPs have been extensively utilized as non-viral mRNA delivery systems both in preclinical and clinical studies given their safe and biodegradable nature, ease of manufacturing and scalability, low immunogenicity, as well as acceptable potency in delivering RNA therapeutics. LNPs have the capability to induce humoral and cellular immunity, which makes them an ideal carrier to fight against viruses that are easy to mutate. The recent approvals of Comirnaty®, Spikevax®, and mRESVIA® are prime examples of how LNPs can be harnessed for vaccine development. Nonetheless, improving extrahepatic targeting and long-term stability remains a key challenge, particularly for formulations intended as vaccines rather than therapies targeted to the liver.

In this study, we explored Polysorbate-80 (PS-80) as a branched PEG-lipid, and fine-tuned the formulation excipients to address both biodistribution and storage limitations. PS-80 has been used as a stabilizer in some FDA approved vaccine formulations such as those for H5N1 influenza (Adjuvant System 03/AS03), HPV (GARDASIL 9), DTaP (Infanrix), DTaP-IPV (Kinrix and Quadracel), DTaP-HepB-IPV (Pediarix), DTaP-IPV/Hib (Pentacel), Hep B (Heplisav-B), Meningococcal B (Trumenba), PCV13 (Prevnar 13), Rotavirus (RotaTeq), and Tdap (Boostrix) [19–25]. The role of the PEG-lipid in stabilizing lipid nanocarriers like liposomes and LNPs is also demonstrated in the literature [8,26]. The role of the PEG-lipid in stabilizing lipid nanocarriers like liposomes and LNPs is clearly demonstrated in the literature [8,26]. However, the structural conformation and the shedding nature of the PEG and their effect on the LNP biodistribution are among the less evaluated characteristics of the LNPs. Our initial comparisons of Fluc-PS80 LNPs against conventional DMG-PEG2K LNPs revealed a pronounced shift in organ distribution, with PS-80-containing formulations displaying a three- to five-fold higher accumulation in the spleen and reduced liver uptake (Figure 2). DMG-PEG2K was chosen as a standard of comparison, given that it is one of the commonly used PEG-lipids for LNP formulations. Also, DMG-PEG2K is part of the marketed drug products like Spikevax®, Onpattro®, and mRESVIA®. Nevertheless, these findings suggest that modifying the PEG-lipid structure can meaningfully alter LNP tropism, thereby improving vaccine relevant delivery to immune organs such as the spleen and lymph nodes. Notably, imaged capillary electrophoresis (iCE) measurements (see the Supplementary File, Section 2.6 and Figure S7) revealed that DMG-PEG LNPs have a slightly higher isoelectric point (pI) than PS80-based LNPs (7.96 vs. 7.63), indicating that the net charge of LNPs might have contributed to the observed LNP's biodistribution change. However, we speculate that alongside the lower net charge, PS-80's branched PEG-like headgroup can additionally alter how serum proteins adsorb to the LNP surface. This modified protein corona may favor spleen localization over hepatic clearance. In addition, PS-80 LNPs might have a reduced rate or extent of opsonization due mainly to their closer to the neutral charge relative to PEG-DMG LNPs, thereby promoting extrahepatic uptake. This hypothesis aligns with other reports indicating that subtle differences in PEG-lipid structure can significantly impact biodistribution [27]. Future mechanistic studies, including in-depth protein corona analysis, may clarify how PS-80 promotes extrahepatic uptake and improves immune-targeted delivery.

Beyond biodistribution, formulation stability is also pivotal for the long-term storage of LNPs. While cryoprotectants like sucrose are already known to preserve LNP quality during freezing [28], our systematic screening identified 10% (w/v) sucrose and 45 mM salt as a required combination to maintain particle size (<100 nm), encapsulation efficiency (>90%), and mRNA integrity (>70%) of PS-80-based formulations after a single freeze/thaw. Tailoring lipid composition—i.e., both lipid type and concentration—is another critical aspect when optimizing mRNA-LNP formulations for stability and potency [29]. Previously, PS-80 was shown to stabilize lipoplex formulations at 3 mol% and enhance the solubilization of other lipid components [30]. Building on that, we screened various molar ratios of DLin-MC3-DMA (48–52%), DSPC (8–12%), cholesterol (37–38.5%), and PS-80 (1.5–3%) in Fluc-PS80 LNPs to explore how each lipid affects particle quality and in vitro activity. The concentration of each of these lipid components was maintained within the acceptable range so that their function in encapsulating or delivering the mRNA was not impacted. Our data indicated that 3 mol% PS-80 (F1–F3) yielded smaller mean diameters (60–80 nm) with PDI $\leq$ 0.2, whereas dropping to 1.5 mol% (F4–F6) increased particle size slightly (80–100 nm) yet narrowed the distribution (PDI $\leq$ 0.1). All formulations maintained neutral zeta potential, high encapsulation efficiency, and mRNA purity before and after freeze/thaw. However, transfection efficiency declined when DLin-MC3-DMA content was lowered, indicating its essential role in mRNA encapsulation and endosomal escape.

Using cryo-TEM, we next examined how the freeze/thaw cycle and lipid composition influenced LNP morphology in F1-F6. In mRNA-LNPs, ionizable lipids like DLin-MC3-DMA typically form an electron-dense core by complexing with mRNA, cholesterol, and water, whereas peripheral blebs can harbor water and, in some cases, unencapsulated mRNA [31]. Consistent with other reports [32,33], both F1 and F4 showed a core-shell architecture with spherical shapes and smaller bleb-like regions. Notably, formulations with lower MC3 (i.e., higher DSPC) exhibited more pronounced blebs and diminished in vitro transfection. Although all LNPs underwent reduced particle concentration post-freeze/thaw, F1 (3% PS-80) still maintained a smaller particle size, robust freeze/thaw stability, and high luciferase expression and thus, was considered as the lead composition.

A key part of our optimization involved switching from a phosphate-sucrose (PSS) buffer to a tris-sucrose-salt (TSS) buffer. Phosphate-based systems frequently experience pH fluctuations (up to 3.5 pH units) upon freezing, which can degrade mRNA and alter LNP structure [10,34]. By contrast, TSS formulations were more "pH-resistant" and retained both structural and functional stability after long-term storage at −80 °C. Indeed, SC2-PS80 LNPs in TSS remained small in particle size (~192 nm), with high mRNA purity (61%) and robust in vitro transfection efficiency even after six months under frozen conditions, unlike their PSS counterparts, which aggregated and lost activity. However, SC2-PS80 LNPs stored in the liquid state (both 5 °C and 25 °C) showed a significant drop in their in vitro transfection following six months and might need further optimization to enhance their stability for long-term storage.

The in vivo immunogenicity experiments verified that SC2-PS80 LNPs stored at −80 °C in TSS elicited comparable anti-spike IgG binding antibodies and anti-SARS-CoV-2 neutralizing antibodies activity to freshly prepared formulations. By contrast, LNPs stored at 5 °C yielded negligible serologic responses, reflecting their poor in vitro transfection. These results demonstrate that formulating in TSS buffer with PS-80 as the PEG-lipid can not only redirect LNPs away from the liver but also preserve vaccine potency under frozen conditions. Finally, although we did not detect any visible injection-site reactions (e.g., swelling or limping) in our mouse studies, the detailed histopathological assessments or cytokine profiling remained to be comprehensively evaluated. Given PS-80's extensive clinical use in approved biologics, we anticipate a favorable safety profile for the PS-80-LNP platform. Overall, to the best of our knowledge, this is the very first study highlighting the potential of this novel lipid composition containing PS-80 as the PEG-lipid for vaccine applications of mRNA-LNPs, with acceptable stability over six months when stored in a frozen state.

5. Conclusions

Using a stepwise optimization strategy, we developed and characterized a new PS-80-based mRNA-LNP vaccine formulation aimed at immune-induction against SARS-CoV-2. Our findings demonstrate that incorporating PS-80 as a branched PEG-lipid and formulating in a tris-sucrose-salt (TSS) buffer mitigates two major limitations often faced by mRNA-LNP vaccines: preferential liver uptake and suboptimal freeze/thaw and storage stability. Specifically, PS-80-based LNPs exhibited enhanced spleen tropism over liver accumulation, maintained high mRNA encapsulation and activity after over six months of storage at −80 °C, and elicited potent in vivo humoral immune responses.

Notably, we confirmed that 10% sucrose and ≥45 mM NaCl in a tris buffer was crucial to preserving particle size and mRNA integrity of PS-80-based LNPs during the freeze/thaw cycle, and that 3 mol% PS-80 balanced robust transfection efficiency with smaller, well-defined LNPs. Extending these findings to SARS-CoV-2 spike mRNA-LNPs (SC2-PS80 LNPs), we observed stable physicochemical properties and strong immunogenicity which were comparable to freshly prepared formulations after six months of frozen storage. Taken together, these results indicate that a PS-80-based mRNA-LNP platform can improve extrahepatic delivery, offer durable frozen stability in tris-sucrose-salt based platform, and drive robust immune induction. Such improvements have the potential to streamline both the manufacturing and storage of next-generation mRNA vaccines, ultimately contributing to more effective and accessible prophylactic strategies against viral pathogens, including SARS-CoV-2.

Supplementary Materials: The following supporting information can be downloaded at https://www.mdpi.com/article/10.3390/pharmaceutics17040441/s1, Figure S1. Long-term storage stability results of Fluc-DMG-PEG LNPs formulated in PSS buffer following six months when stored at different temperatures. Figure S2. Long-term storage stability results of Fluc-DMG-PEG LNPs formulated in TSS buffer following six months when stored at different temperatures. Figure S3. Physicochemical characterization of Fluc-PS80 LNP formulations prepared in tris-sucrose (TS) and tris-sucrose containing 45 mM NaCl (TSS) buffers. Figure S4. Visual inspection of various Fluc-PS80 LNP formulations prepared in TSS buffer. Figure S5. Dynamic light scattering graphs depicting particle size and size distribution of Fluc-PS80 LNP formulations containing various lipid combinations prepared in TSS buffer. Figure S6. Long-term storage stability results of SC2-PS80 LNPs formulated in (a-b) PSS and (c-d) TSS buffers following six months when stored at different temperatures. Figure S7. Imaged capillary electrophoresis (iCE) of Fluc-PS80 LNPs and DMG-PEG LNPs.

Author Contributions: Conceptualization, A.N. and B.R.; formal analysis, A.S., A.N., L.-K.Y., J.C.-T.K., A.P., R.F. and T.B.; funding acquisition, B.R., J.H., A.S.B. and M.S.; investigation, A.S., A.N., L.-K.Y., J.C.-T.K., H.B., M.N. and A.P.; methodology, A.S., A.N., L.-K.Y., J.C.-T.K., H.B., M.N., A.P., R.F. and C.D.P.; project administration, B.R., J.H., A.S.B. and M.S.; resources, B.R., A.S.B. and M.S.; supervision, A.N., T.B., C.D.P., B.R., J.H., A.S.B. and M.S.; writing—original draft, A.S., A.N., L.-K.Y., J.C.-T.K., M.N. and A.P.; writing—review & editing, A.S., A.N., H.B., T.B., C.D.P., B.R., J.H., A.S.B. and M.S. All authors have read and agreed to the published version of the manuscript.

Funding: This research received no external funding.

Institutional Review Board Statement: The animal study protocol was approved by the Institutional Review Board (or Ethics Committee) of REGENERON PHARMACEUTICALS (Protocol 303.4, approved on 28 March 2021).

Data Availability Statement: The original contributions presented in this study are included in the article/Supplementary Material. Further inquiries can be directed to the corresponding author(s).

Acknowledgments: The authors would like to thank Katherine Cygnar, Andrew Baik, Jikang Wu, Suzanne Hartford (previous Regeneron employee), and Ying Wang (previous Regeneron employee) for their contributions to sample handling and for providing insights and comments on the manuscript.

Conflicts of Interest: All listed authors were employed by Regeneron Pharmaceuticals but have no potential conflicts of interest in data and scientific interpretation for this manuscript.

Abbreviations

The following abbreviations are used in this manuscript:

Cryo-TEM	Cryogenic transmission electron microscopy
DLin-MC3-DMA	[(6Z,9Z,28Z,31Z)-heptatriaconta-6,9,28,31-tetraen-19-yl]4-(dimethylamino)butanoate
DMEM	Dulbecco's Modified Eagle's Medium
DMG-PEG2K LNP	Fluc mRNA-LNP containing DMG-PEG2K as the PEG-lipid
DMG-PEG2K	1,2-dimyristoyl-rac-glycero-3-methoxypolyethylene glycol-2000
DSPC	Distearoylphosphatidylcholine
FBS	Fetal bovine serum
FLuc mRNA	Firefly luciferase mRNA
Fluc-PS80 LNP	Firefly luciferase reporter mRNA-LNP
HEK-293 cells	Human embryonic kidney 293 cells
LNPs	Lipid nanoparticles
MCE	Microchip capillary electrophoresis
PS-80	Polysorbate-80
PSS	Phosphate-saline-sucrose buffer
pVNT50	50% pseudovirus neutralization titer
SARS-CoV-2	Severe acute respiratory syndrome coronavirus 2
SC2-PS80 LNP	Polysorbate 80-based SARS-CoV-2 mRNA-LNP
TSS	Tris-saline-sucrose buffer

References

1. Liu, Y.; Huang, Y.; He, G.; Guo, C.; Dong, J.; Wu, L. Development of mRNA Lipid Nanoparticles: Targeting and Therapeutic Aspects. *Int. J. Mol. Sci.* **2024**, *25*, 10166. [CrossRef] [PubMed]
2. Wilson, E.; Goswami, J.; Baqui, A.H.; Doreski, P.A.; Perez-Marc, G.; Zaman, K.; Monroy, J.; Duncan, C.J.A.; Ujiie, M.; Ramet, M.; et al. Efficacy and Safety of an mRNA-Based RSV PreF Vaccine in Older Adults. *N. Engl. J. Med.* **2023**, *389*, 2233–2244. [CrossRef]
3. Li, S.; Hu, Y.; Li, A.; Lin, J.; Hsieh, K.; Schneiderman, Z.; Zhang, P.; Zhu, Y.; Qiu, C.; Kokkoli, E.; et al. Payload distribution and capacity of mRNA lipid nanoparticles. *Nat. Commun.* **2022**, *13*, 5561. [PubMed]
4. Ramachandran, S.; Satapathy, S.R.; Dutta, T. Delivery Strategies for mRNA Vaccines. *Pharm. Med.* **2022**, *36*, 11–20.
5. Mastrobattista, E.; Hennink, W.E.; Schiffelers, R.M. Delivery of nucleic acids. *Pharm. Res.* **2007**, *24*, 1561–1563.
6. Waggoner, L.E.; Miyasaki, K.F.; Kwon, E.J. Analysis of PEG-lipid anchor length on lipid nanoparticle pharmacokinetics and activity in a mouse model of traumatic brain injury. *Biomater. Sci.* **2023**, *11*, 4238–4253.
7. Kong, W.; Wei, Y.; Dong, Z.; Liu, W.; Zhao, J.; Huang, Y.; Yang, J.; Wu, W.; He, H.; Qi, J. Role of size, surface charge, and PEGylated lipids of lipid nanoparticles (LNPs) on intramuscular delivery of mRNA. *J. Nanobiotechnology* **2024**, *22*, 553.
8. Albertsen, C.H.; Kulkarni, J.A.; Witzigmann, D.; Lind, M.; Petersson, K.; Simonsen, J.B. The role of lipid components in lipid nanoparticles for vaccines and gene therapy. *Adv. Drug Deliv. Rev.* **2022**, *188*, 114416.
9. Carrasco, M.J.; Alishetty, S.; Alameh, M.G.; Said, H.; Wright, L.; Paige, M.; Soliman, O.; Weissman, D.; Cleveland, T.E.T.; Grishaev, A.; et al. Ionization and structural properties of mRNA lipid nanoparticles influence expression in intramuscular and intravascular administration. *Commun. Biol.* **2021**, *4*, 956.

10. Henderson, M.I.; Eygeris, Y.; Jozic, A.; Herrera, M.; Sahay, G. Leveraging Biological Buffers for Efficient Messenger RNA Delivery via Lipid Nanoparticles. *Mol. Pharm.* **2022**, *19*, 4275–4285.
11. Lind, T.K.; Nilsson, E.J.; Wyler, B.; Scherer, D.; Skansberger, T.; Morin, M.; Kocherbitov, V.; Engblom, J. Effects of ethylene oxide chain length on crystallization of polysorbate 80 and its related compounds. *J. Colloid Interface Sci.* **2021**, *592*, 468–484. [CrossRef] [PubMed]
12. Webster, G.K.; Chang, J.C.; Heflin, J.L. Stability Indicating Method for Polysorbate 80 in Protein Formulations. *J. Chromatogr. Sci.* **2021**, *59*, 706–713. [CrossRef]
13. Kozuch, B.; Weber, J.; Buske, J.; Mader, K.; Garidel, P.; Diederichs, T. Comparative Stability Study of Polysorbate 20 and Polysorbate 80 Related to Oxidative Degradation. *Pharmaceutics* **2023**, *15*, 2332. [CrossRef]
14. Le Basle, Y.; Chennell, P.; Tokhadze, N.; Astier, A.; Sautou, V. Physicochemical Stability of Monoclonal Antibodies: A Review. *J. Pharm. Sci.* **2020**, *109*, 169–190. [CrossRef]
15. Macdonald, L.E.; Karow, M.; Stevens, S.; Auerbach, W.; Poueymirou, W.T.; Yasenchak, J.; Frendewey, D.; Valenzuela, D.M.; Giallourakis, C.C.; Alt, F.W.; et al. Precise and in situ genetic humanization of 6 Mb of mouse immunoglobulin genes. *Proc. Natl. Acad. Sci. USA* **2014**, *111*, 5147–5152. [CrossRef] [PubMed]
16. Lai, C.J.; Kim, D.; Kang, S.; Li, K.; Cha, I.; Sasaki, A.; Porras, J.; Xia, T.; Jung, J.U. Viral codon optimization on SARS-CoV-2 Spike boosts immunity in the development of COVID-19 mRNA vaccines. *J. Med. Virol.* **2023**, *95*, e29183. [CrossRef]
17. Lu, M.; Chamblee, M.; Zhang, Y.; Ye, C.; Dravid, P.; Park, J.G.; Mahesh, K.C.; Trivedi, S.; Murthy, S.; Sharma, H.; et al. SARS-CoV-2 prefusion spike protein stabilized by six rather than two prolines is more potent for inducing antibodies that neutralize viral variants of concern. *Proc. Natl. Acad. Sci. USA* **2022**, *119*, e2110105119. [CrossRef] [PubMed]
18. Petro, C.D.; Hooper, A.T.; Peace, A.; Mohammadi, K.; Eagan, W.; Elbashir, S.M.; DiPiazza, A.; Makrinos, D.; Pascal, K.; Bandawane, P.; et al. Monoclonal antibodies against the spike protein alter the endogenous humoral response to SARS-CoV-2 vaccination and infection. *Sci. Transl. Med.* **2024**, *16*, eadn0396. [CrossRef]
19. GARDASIL 9. 2025. Available online: https://www.fda.gov/vaccines-blood-biologics/vaccines/gardasil-9 (accessed on 24 March 2025).
20. INFANRIX. 2025. Available online: https://www.fda.gov/vaccines-blood-biologics/vaccines/infanrix (accessed on 24 March 2025).
21. KINRIX. 2025. Available online: https://www.fda.gov/vaccines-blood-biologics/vaccines/kinrix (accessed on 24 March 2025).
22. HEPLISAV-B. 2025. Available online: https://www.fda.gov/vaccines-blood-biologics/vaccines/heplisav-b (accessed on 24 March 2025).
23. TRUMENBA. 2025. Available online: https://www.fda.gov/vaccines-blood-biologics/vaccines/trumenba (accessed on 24 March 2025).
24. RotaTeq. 2025. Available online: https://www.fda.gov/vaccines-blood-biologics/vaccines/rotateq (accessed on 24 March 2025).
25. BOOSTRIX. 2025. Available online: https://www.fda.gov/vaccines-blood-biologics/vaccines/boostrix (accessed on 24 March 2025).
26. Izumi, K.; Ji, J.; Koiwai, K.; Kawano, R. Long-Term Stable Liposome Modified by PEG-Lipid in Natural Seawater. *ACS Omega* **2024**, *9*, 10958–10966. [CrossRef]
27. Gautam, M.; Jozic, A.; Su, G.L.; Herrera-Barrera, M.; Curtis, A.; Arrizabalaga, S.; Tschetter, W.; Ryals, R.C.; Sahay, G. Lipid nanoparticles with PEG-variant surface modifications mediate genome editing in the mouse retina. *Nat. Commun.* **2023**, *14*, 6468. [CrossRef]
28. Kafetzis, K.N.; Papalamprou, N.; McNulty, E.; Thong, K.X.; Sato, Y.; Mironov, A.; Purohit, A.; Welsby, P.J.; Harashima, H.; Yu-Wai-Man, C.; et al. The Effect of Cryoprotectants and Storage Conditions on the Transfection Efficiency, Stability, and Safety of Lipid-Based Nanoparticles for mRNA and DNA Delivery. *Adv. Healthc. Mater.* **2023**, *12*, e2203022.
29. Schober, G.B.; Story, S.; Arya, D.P. A careful look at lipid nanoparticle characterization: Analysis of benchmark formulations for encapsulation of RNA cargo size gradient. *Sci. Rep.* **2024**, *14*, 2403.
30. Gretskaya, N.; Akimov, M.; Andreev, D.; Zalygin, A.; Belitskaya, E.; Zinchenko, G.; Fomina-Ageeva, E.; Mikhalyov, I.; Vodovozova, E.; Bezuglov, V. Multicomponent Lipid Nanoparticles for RNA Transfection. *Pharmaceutics* **2023**, *15*, 1289. [CrossRef] [PubMed]
31. Simonsen, J.B. A perspective on bleb and empty LNP structures. *J. Control. Release* **2024**, *373*, 952–961. [PubMed]
32. AboulFotouh, K.; Southard, B.; Dao, H.M.; Xu, H.; Moon, C.; Williams, R.O., III; Cui, Z. Effect of lipid composition on RNA-Lipid nanoparticle properties and their sensitivity to thin-film freezing and drying. *Int. J. Pharm.* **2024**, *650*, 123688. [CrossRef]

33. Sebastiani, F.; Arteta, M.Y.; Lerche, M.; Porcar, L.; Lang, C.; Bragg, R.A.; Elmore, C.S.; Krishnamurthy, V.R.; Russell, R.A.; Darwish, T.; et al. Apolipoprotein E Binding Drives Structural and Compositional Rearrangement of mRNA-Containing Lipid Nanoparticles. *ACS Nano* **2021**, *15*, 6709–6722.
34. Schoenmaker, L.; Witzigmann, D.; Kulkarni, J.A.; Verbeke, R.; Kersten, G.; Jiskoot, W.; Crommelin, D.J.A. mRNA-lipid nanoparticle COVID-19 vaccines: Structure and stability. *Int. J. Pharm.* **2021**, *601*, 120586.

pharmaceutics

Article

Characterization of VitE-TPGS Micelles Linked to Poorly Soluble Pharmaceutical Compounds Exploiting Pair Distribution Function's Moments

Liberato De Caro [1,*], Thibaud Stoll [2], Arnaud Grandeury [3], Fabia Gozzo [2] and Cinzia Giannini [1]

[1] Istituto di Cristallografia, Consiglio Nazionale delle Ricerche, Via Amendola 122/O, 70125 Bari, Italy; cinzia.giannini@cnr.it
[2] Excelsus Structural Solutions (Swiss) AG, Park Innovaare, Parkstrasse 1, 5234 Villigen, Switzerland; thibaud.stoll@excelsus2s.com (T.S.); fabia.gozzo@excelsus2s.com (F.G.)
[3] Novartis Pharma AG, Technical Research and Development, Material Science, Novartis Campus, Virchow 6.3.231, 4056 Basel, Switzerland; arnaud.grandeury@novartis.com
* Correspondence: liberato.decaro@cnr.it

Abstract: Background: Micelles have attracted significant interest in nanomedicine as drug delivery systems. This study investigates the morphology of micelles formed by the D-α-tocopherol polyethylene glycol 1000 succinate (VitE-TPGS) surfactant in the presence and absence of, respectively, a poorly soluble pharmaceutical compound (PSC), i.e., Eltrombopag (0.08 wt%) and $CaCl_2$ (0.03 wt%). The aim was to assess the micelles' ability to solubilize the PSC and potentially shield it from Ca^{2+} ions, simulating in vivo conditions. **Methods:** For this purpose, we have developed a novel theoretical approach for analyzing Pair Distribution Function (PDF) data derived from Small-Angle X-ray Scattering (SAXS) measurements, based on the use of PDF's moments. **Results:** Our spheroid-based model was able to characterize successfully the micellar morphology and their interactions with PSC and $CaCl_2$, providing detailed insights into their size, shape, and electron density contrasts. The presence of PSC significantly affected the shape and integral of the PDF curves, indicating incorporation into the micelles. This also resulted in a decrease in the micelle size, regardless of the presence of $CaCl_2$. When this salt was added, it reduced the amount of PSC within the micelles. This is likely due to a decrease in the overall PSC availability in solution, induced by Ca^{2+} ions. **Conclusions:** This advanced yet straightforward analytical model represents a powerful tool for characterizing and optimizing micelle-based drug delivery systems.

Keywords: drug delivery systems; surfactant; Small-Angle X-ray Scattering; micelles

1. Introduction

Micelles have attracted significant attention in nanomedicine, particularly for their potential as drug delivery systems [1–4]. These nanoscale structures, typically formed by the self-assembly of amphiphilic molecules in an aqueous environment, usually surfactants, exhibit a core–shell architecture that is highly conducive to encapsulating hydrophobic drugs. The core of the micelle provides a hydrophobic environment suitable for the entrapment of water-insoluble drugs, while the hydrophilic shell stabilizes its structure in biological fluids, thereby enhancing the solubility, bioavailability, and targeted delivery of therapeutic agents. Among the various factors that influence the efficacy of micelles as drug carriers, their morphology—encompassing both size and shape—plays a pivotal role [5].

 https://doi.org/10.3390/pharmaceutics17040431

The morphology of micelles directly impacts their drug-loading capacity and stability, in particular upon dilution, circulation time, and biodistribution, which are crucial parameters for effective drug delivery [6–11]. The size of the micelles is particularly important because it determines the ability of the micelles to pass through biological barriers, including cellular membranes, and to evade the reticuloendothelial system (RES), which is responsible for clearing foreign particles from the bloodstream. Micelles ranging in size from approximately 10 to 100 nm are often ideal for prolonged circulation, as well as for enhancing permeability and retention (EPR) effect, a phenomenon that enables nanoparticles to accumulate preferentially in tumor tissues due to their leaky vasculature and inefficient lymphatic drainage [7].

Although micelles have been traditionally approximated as spherical systems, recent research has revealed the existence of other shapes, such as ellipsoidal, rod-like, worm-like or even disk-like structures. These different shapes are mainly due to the structure of the micelle-forming surfactants used and to the characteristics of the surrounding environment (temperature, pH, and chemical composition). Non-spherical micelles have been shown to exhibit different cellular uptake mechanisms, circulation times, and biodistribution patterns compared to their spherical counterparts. For instance, they may exhibit prolonged circulation times due to reduced recognition and clearance by the RES, or they may demonstrate enhanced tissue penetration and cellular uptake via mechanisms that are less dependent on size, influencing the drug release profile, which is a critical factor affecting therapeutic efficacy. The internal structure of micelles, which is influenced by its size and shape, dictates the distribution of the drug within the micellar core and the interactions between the drug and the micelle-forming molecules. This, in turn, affects the rate at which the drug is released from the micelles. For example, smaller micelles may release their encapsulated drug more rapidly due to a higher surface-area-to-volume ratio, while larger or elongated micelles may provide a more sustained release profile. The ability to fine-tune the release kinetics through careful control of micelle morphology is particularly important for applications requiring a controlled and sustained release of the drug over time, such as in chronic disease management and chemotherapy. In these cases, minimizing side effects while maximizing therapeutic efficacy is paramount. Additionally, sustained-release drug delivery systems can improve the patients' quality of life by reducing dosing frequency, easing the burden of multiple daily administrations, and enhancing treatment adherence. This benefit is particularly important for patients with chronic conditions, as it ensures consistent medication delivery without the stress of managing multiple daily doses.

The size and shape of micelles influence their interaction with cell membranes, their uptake by cells, and their intracellular trafficking pathways [12]. These factors are crucial for ensuring that the drug reaches its target within the body, whether that target is a specific tissue, organ, or subcellular compartment. For example, smaller micelles are more readily taken up by cells via endocytosis, while larger or non-spherical micelles may interact differently with cell membranes, potentially leading to alternative uptake pathways or enhanced retention within specific tissues.

For the above reasons, an accurate and precise measurement of the micelle size and shape is essential. Various analytical techniques, such as dynamic light scattering (DLS), transmission electron microscopy (TEM), and cryogenic electron microscopy (cryo-EM), are commonly used for this purpose. They each have distinct advantages and provide complementary information about the size, shape, and internal structure of micelles. For instance, DLS is widely used for determining the hydrodynamic diameter of micelles in solution, while TEM and cryo-EM enable direct visualization of micelle morphology, providing detailed insights about their shape and internal organization.

In addition to these conventional techniques, emerging methods such as Small-/Wide-Angle X-ray Scattering (SAXS/WAXS) and atomic force microscopy (AFM) are being increasingly utilized to obtain more comprehensive and high-resolution data on micelle morphology [12]. These advanced techniques are particularly valuable for gaining a deeper understanding of the structural features that influence drug loading and release. SAXS is particularly suitable for the characterization of micelles in solution, under real conditions, requiring limited sample preparation.

In 2023, we developed a novel theoretical approach for analyzing Pair Distribution Function (PDF) data derived from SAXS measurements, based on a spherical core–shell model for micelles [13]. This method enables the determination of the core–shell and the shell–buffer electron density contrasts, as well as the core and shell sizes of micelles, by modeling the PDF data. The approach has been validated by applying it to VitE-TPGS micelles [13]. As a further development, we have extended our approach to model spheroidal core–shell micelles [14]. This new approach represents a significant improvement, as it uses the first derivative of the PDF and analytical equations to resolve the structure of spheroidal core–shell micelles. By applying these equations, we can determine key structural parameters, including the micelle's aggregation number, ellipticity, and electron density contrast between core and shell regions. The method was applied successfully to micelles formed by different surfactants, such as Polysorbate 20, Dodecyl phosphocholine, Sodium Dodecyl Sulfate, and VitE-TPGS.

In this work, assuming spheroidal-shaped micelles, we exploit nth-order moments of the PDF, with n ranging from 1 to 6, to perform the structural characterization of VitE-TPGS micelles both in the presence and absence of a poorly soluble pharmaceutical compound (PSC). In our study, the PSC was the active pharmaceutical ingredient Eltrombopag, a thrombopoietin receptor agonist, which is used to treat low blood platelet counts in adults with chronic immune (idiopathic) thrombocytopenia. It was approved by the FDA in 2008 [15]. Additionally, samples with and without $CaCl_2$ in the buffer solution have been measured, to assess the potential role of micelles to prevent the interaction reported when the formulated drug was administered with high-calcium-content food [16]. Unlike the previous method [14], which solved the micelle structure with a hybrid approach, i.e., partially graphical (first derivative of the PDF) and partially analytical, we present here a fully analytical method. It is described in Section 2 and Appendix A, while the experimental data are summarized in Section 3 and discussed in Section 4.

2. Analytical Method

For a two-component spheroidal micelle, we can derive the analytical expression of the following integrals, for any $n = 1, \ldots,$ N; they are reported explicitly in Appendix A:

$$R^n = \left(\int r^n(\rho(r) - \rho_s)d^3r\right) / \left(\int (\rho(r) - \rho_s)d^3r\right). \tag{1}$$

Here, ρ_s = solvent electron density, $\rho(r) = \rho_E$, the electron density inside the core, and $\rho(r) = \rho_P$, the electron density inside the shell. These integrals are a measure of the atomic electron density within the micelle as a function of the nth power distance r^n, like raw moments for a probability distribution calculated from zero and not with respect to the mean (central moments).

We can compare the analytical expression obtained by Equation (1) with the corresponding nth r-power integral of the PDF, derived from the experimental SAXS data:

$$R^n_{\text{PDF}} = \frac{\int_0^{D_{max}} PDF(r)r^n dr}{2^{n-1}\int_0^{D_{max}} PDF(r)dr}. \tag{2}$$

Here D_{max} is the maximum distance in the PDF. In this way, allowing n to range from 1 to N, we can derive a set of N independent equations with the following unknowns: the ellipticity ε; the core-solvent electron contrast $\Delta\rho_{ES} = \rho_E - \rho_s$; the shell-solvent electron contrast $\Delta\rho_{PS} = \rho_P - \rho_s$; the micelle size D_{max}; and the shell radius R_{SH}. Since we need at least 5 independent equations to determine the 5 unknown parameters defining the micelles' structure, we can also overdetermine the solution by solving a set of N equations with $N \geq 5$, by means of a least-square-minimum approach, as described in Appendix A. If $N > 5$, we would have an overdetermined system of equations.

3. Results

The micelles studied in this work are formed by VitE-TPGS surfactant monomers, with and without the presence in solution of a PSC, in order to study the level of incorporation of this compound into the micelles. SAXS data were collected at the SAXS Lab Sapienza with a Xeuss 2.0 Q-Xoom system (Xenocs SA, Grenoble, France). See details in [13]. We have considered four cases, summarized in Table 1. The nominal pH is 6.8. Samples 1 and 2 have been prepared with PSC, with and without $CaCl_2$ added to the buffer solution. Samples 3 and 4 have been prepared with PSC, with and without $CaCl_2$ added to the buffer. The nominal concentrations of VitE-TPGS and of the potassium phosphate buffer were kept constant across all experiments at 0.415% w/w and 50 mM, respectively. In subsequent solutions, concentration in PSC was maintained at 0.08% (w/w) and calcium chloride at about 0.03% (w/w). It corresponds to quite a large excess of calcium cations vs. PSC. The aim was to simulate digestive tract conditions, where high concentrations of Ca^{2+} from calcium-rich foods may be present and negatively affect the bioavailability and solubility of active pharmaceutical ingredients, and to evaluate the potential protective role of micelles. Samples 1–4 have been prepared according to the following protocol to maximize the sameness of the solution, minimizing experimental variability.

Table 1. Composition of samples 1–4, containing the VitE-TPGS surfactant in the buffer solution, without and with a poorly soluble compound (PSC), as well as without and with $CaCl_2$.

Sample		VitE-TPGS	PSC	$CaCl_2$	pH Measured
1	19.9 g of buffer 50 mM	82.6 mg (0.415 wt%)	No	No	6.87
2	2.4 g of sample 1	Yes (0.415 wt%)	No	0.55 mg (0.024 wt%)	6.82
3	10 g of sample 1	Yes (0.415 wt%)	8 mg (0.08 wt%)	No	6.91
4	2.8 g of sample 3	Yes (0.415 wt%)	Yes (0.08 wt%)	0.8 mg (0.029 wt%)	6.84

A buffer solution was prepared by mixing 682.7 mg of potassium hydrogen phosphate (K_2HPO_4) and 2.26 mmol of NaOH (added as 22.6 g of a 0.4 wt% solution) in Milli-Q water, to reach a final volume of 100 mL. The solution was stirred until a stable pH value was reached. The targeted value was 6.80 while the actual measured value was 6.81. The buffer solution was used to prepare all 4 samples, to ensure the same pH value. To prepare sample 1, 82.6 mg of VitE-TPGS was dissolved in 19.9 g of the pH 6.8 (50 mM) buffer solution to reach a concentration of 0.415 wt%. The sample was stirred at 500 rpm for 43 min to achieve complete dissolution. No significant variation was observed for the pH, in comparison to the buffer solution (as expected, since VitE-TPGS has no acidity/basicity). The final pH value was 6.87, before filtration. An aliquot of this sample was then filtered four times through Axiva sterile cellulose acetate syringe filters with pore diameters of 200 nm to remove any undissolved particulate matter and ensure a homogeneous solution. SAXS data collected on the unfiltered and filtered samples were superimposable, indicating that no undissolved surfactant in the form of particulate greater than 200 nm was present in the unfiltered sample. To prepare sample 2, 0.55 mg of $CaCl_2$ was dissolved in 2.4 g of the sample 1 solution, corresponding to 0.024 wt% of $CaCl_2$, and the solution was stirred at 500 rpm for 20 min. No significant variation was observed for the pH, as expected, since $CaCl_2$ has no particular acidity or basicity. To prepare sample 3, 8.0 mg of PSC was added to 10 g of the sample 1 solution to reach a concentration of 0.08 wt%. The solution was stirred at 500 rpm for 60 min to ensure complete dilution. After stirring, no significant deviation towards higher pH values was observed thanks to the buffer capacity. The final pH value was 6.91. To prepare sample 4, 0.8 mg of $CaCl_2$ was added to 2.8 g of the sample 3 solution, corresponding to a concentration of 0.415 wt% of VitE-TPGS, 0.08 wt% of PSC, and 0.029 wt% of $CaCl_2$. The solution was stirred at 500 rpm for 20 min. No significant variation was observed for the pH. The final pH value after filtration was 6.84. All preparations were performed at 25 °C. Table 1 summarizes the composition of the 4 samples.

The PDF curves, obtained for these samples, are shown in Figure 1; they describe the SAXS macroscopic cross-section as a function of the atom–atom distances r.

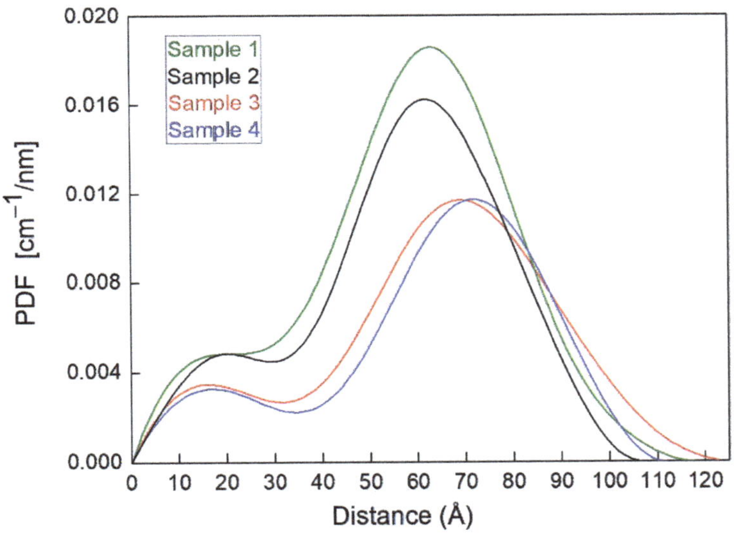

Figure 1. PDF curves, expressed on a quantitative scale, obtained for samples 1, 2, 3, and 4.

The PDFs, calculated by the software GNOM 47.5 [17], have been rescaled so that the integral of the PDFs plotted in Figure 1 is equal to the corresponding $I(0)$ [cm^{-1}] value, i.e., the SAXS macroscopic cross-section for the whole sample extrapolated to the scattering vector value q = 0. Figure 1 shows that the presence of the PSC significantly affects the shape and the integral of the PDF curve, which indicates that some PSC molecules have been incorporated into the micelles. The presence of $CaCl_2$ in solution reduces the integral of the macroscopic cross-section (cf green curve versus black curve in Figure 1), indicating that a smaller quantity of PSC could be incorporated into the VitE-TPGS micelles. A possible explanation for the observed reduction of the amount of PSC in the micelles (and possibly also outside, in the same buffer solution) in the presence of $CaCl_2$ is the occurrence of some specific interactions, eventually exemplified by the drug. Cation interactions are indeed known to reduce the bioavailability of the drug [18].

After having determined ε, $\Delta\rho_{ES}$, $\Delta\rho_{PS}$, D_M, R_{SH}, from Equations (1) and (2), via a least-square-minimum approach discussed in Appendix A, we can evaluate the aggregation number of monomers inside the micelles (N_{agg}), the number of water molecules inside the shell (N_{H2O}), and the number of PSC molecules per monomer inside the micelles ($x_{PSC} = N_{PSC}/N_{agg}$). All formulas are provided in Appendix A. Table 2 summarizes the micelles' parameters obtained for the 4 samples.

Table 2. Shell size (R_{SH}), maximum micelle size (D_{max}), ellipticity (ε), $\Delta\rho_{ES} = \Delta\rho_{EP} + \Delta\rho_{PS}$, $\Delta\rho_{PS}$, N_{agg}, N_{H2O}/N_{agg} obtained from the analysis of the PDF's moments of VitE-TPGS micelles. c_{mon} = 4.1 mg/mL. *cmc* = 0.02 mg/mL. R_g is the gyration radius. $I(0)$ is the PDF integral on an absolute scale. For prolate micelles, the minimum core size is in the equatorial plane (equatorial core radius).

Sample	R_{SH} (Å)	D_{max} (Å)	Equatorial Core Radius ($D_{max} - 2R_{SH}$)/2ε (Å)	$\Delta\rho_{ES}$ (n_e/Å^3)	$\Delta\rho_{PS}$ (n_e/Å^3)	ε	N_{agg}	N_{H2O}/N_{agg}	R_g(Å)	$I(0)$ (cm^{-1})
1 (without PSC and $CaCl_2$)	16.7 ± 0.1	122.0 ± 0.1	29.3 ± 0.2	−0.026 ± 0.001	0.032 ± 0.001	1.51 ± 0.01	127 ± 2	53 ± 4	47.3 ± 0.5	0.056 ± 0.001
2 (without PSC, with $CaCl_2$)	14.2 ± 0.1	113.8 ± 0.1	30.5 ± 0.2	−0.031 ± 0.001	0.039 ± 0.001	1.40 ± 0.01	122 ± 3	36 ± 4	47.3 ± 0.4	0.055 ± 0.001
3 (with PSC, without $CaCl_2$)	16.4 ± 0.1	116.7 ± 0.1	27.1 ± 0.2	−0.026 ± 0.001	0.036 ± 0.001	1.55 ± 0.01	118 ± 4	44 ± 4	43.5 ± 0.5	0.085 ± 0.001
4 (with PSC and $CaCl_2$)	12.3 ± 0.1	107.7 ± 0.1	27.7 ± 0.2	−0.030 ± 0.001	0.055 ± 0.001	1.51 ± 0.01	125 ± 4	12 ± 5	42.8 ± 0.3	0.079 ± 0.001

Figure 2 shows, for the four samples, the probability density function calculated by the SmoothDensityHistogram function implemented in Mathematica (Wolfram), associated with the histograms of least-square-root values (LSR) (cf Equation (A15)) obtained by the least-square approach discussed in Appendix A. We have set ten contour levels in the probability density function (P) at 10%, 20%, ..., 80%, 90% of the histogram maximum. The red color is associated with 90% of the maximum. The left column on Figure 2 shows P as a function of the variables D_M and R_{sh}. The enter column shows P as a function of the variables $\Delta\rho_{PS}$ and $-\Delta\rho_{EP} = -\Delta\rho_{ES} + \Delta\rho_{PS}$. The right column shows P as a function of the variables ε and N_{agg}.

It is interesting to note that in Figure 2, secondary maxima are occasionally observed in the two-dimensional P histograms. This is particularly evident for sample 4, suggesting that the presence of both PSC and $CaCl_2$ could cause a certain level of variability in the micelles' structure, which, in turn, could imply the occurrence of a certain level of interaction between the PSC and Ca^{2+} cations in solution during the formation of micelles. Further investigations would be needed to validate this hypothesis.

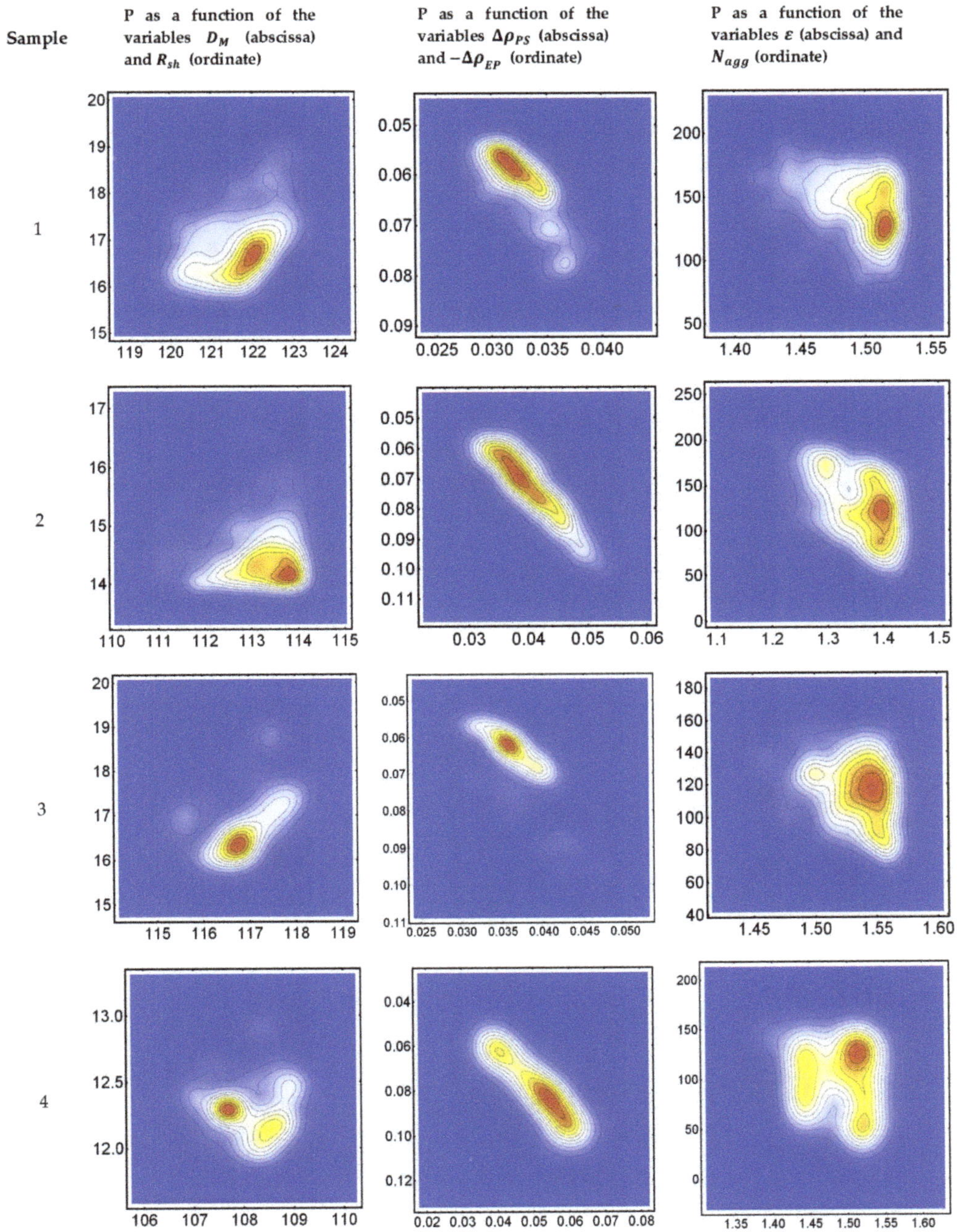

Figure 2. (**Left**): Probability density function (P), associated with the histograms of LRS values obtained from Equation (A15), for samples 1, 2, 3, and 4, as a function of the variables D_M and R_{sh}, expressed in Å. (**Center**): Probability density function, associated with the histograms of LSR values obtained from Equation (A15) as a function of the variables $\Delta\rho_{Ps}$ and $-\Delta\rho_{EP} = -\Delta\rho_E + \Delta\rho_P$, expressed in $n_e/\text{Å}^3$. (**Right**): Probability density function, associated with the histograms of LSR values obtained from Equation (A15) as a function of the variables ε and N_{agg}, expressed in dimensionless units. Ten contours have been determined, represented as 10%, 20%, ..., 80%, 90% levels of the histogram maximum. The red color is associated with 90% of the maximum.

4. Discussion

The comparison of the D_{max} and R_g values from Table 2 shows that the addition of PSC leads to the formation of smaller micelles, whether $CaCl_2$ is present or not. A similar effect can be seen on the shell size (R_{SH}) and the equatorial core radius. These observations are consistent with those made in our previous work [13], while our new spheroidal model provides here a more detailed characterization of the micelle morphological changes.

In our previous work [13], we assumed spherical-shaped micelles, following the suggestions in [19]. Under this hypothesis, we estimated, for sample 3, $x_{PSC,3} = 0.30 \pm 0.01$. By introducing, with y, the fraction of the PSC molecules per monomer inside the core (see Appendix A) and by relaxing the spherical-shape constraint by solving Equation (A22), we obtain the results shown in Figure 3, where x_{PSC} is represented as a function of y for samples 3 and 4. For sample 3 we obtain $x_{PSC,3}$ ranging between 0.47 and 0.53, as a function y. This difference with respect to the result obtained in [13] is mainly due to both the different number of monomers aggregated into the micelles and the different micelle shape given by the 2 models (spherical vs. spheroidal). Indeed in [13], from the difference of the PDF curves obtained with and without PSC in solution, we had estimated, under the hypothesis of spherical-shaped micelles, the localization of these molecules inside the micelles, close to the linker region, and a concentration $x_{PSC,3} = 0.30 \pm 0.01$. For spheroidal-shaped micelles, this approach is not possible, because differences in intensity of the PDF at the same distance from the center could also be due to both different number of aggregated monomers and to different ellipticity values, which, in turn, influence the distribution of distances in the PDF profile and the estimated value for x_{PSC}.

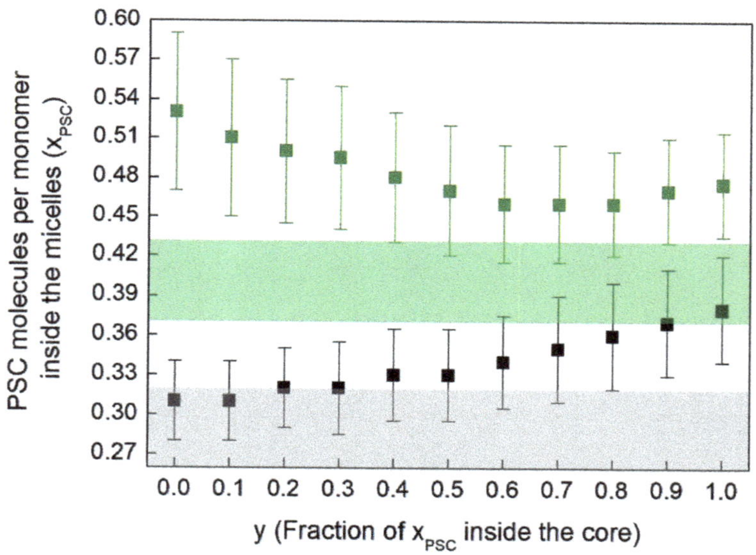

Figure 3. Number of PSC molecules x_{PSC} per monomer inside the micelles of sample 3 (green) and 4 (black) as a function of the fraction of x_{PSC} inside the core (denoted as y in Equation (A18)).

The colored bands in Figure 3 are the constraints for samples 3 (in green) and 4 (in grey), derived from Equation (A16) and developed in Equations (3) and (4) below. Indeed, from Equation (A16), it follows that the square difference of electrons per monomer, between the samples with and without PSC, must be equal to the difference of $I(0)/K$:

$$\left[827 + 232x_{PSC,3} - 10\frac{2327 + 554x_{PSC,3}}{29.9}\right]^2 N_{agg,3} - \left[827 - 10\frac{2327}{29.9}\right]^2 N_{agg,1} = [I(0)/K]_3 - [I(0)/K]_1; \tag{3}$$

$$\left[827 + 232x_{PSC,4} - 10\frac{2327 + 554x_{PSC,4}}{29.9}\right]^2 N_{agg,4} - \left[827 - 10\frac{2327}{29.9}\right]^2 N_{agg,2} = [I(0)/K]_4 - [I(0)/K]_2. \tag{4}$$

The numerical values 827, 232, and 10 correspond to the number of electrons of a VitE-TPGS, PSC, and water molecule, respectively; 2326 , 554, and 29.9 are the molecular volumes of these 3 species in Å^3 [13]. From Equation (3), we have, for samples 3 and 4, $x_{PSC,3} = 0.40 \pm 0.03$ and $x_{PSC,4} = 0.29 \pm 0.03$, respectively, which are represented as colored bands in Figure 3.

For sample 3, the middle value of the green band is 0.40; the upper value is 0.43 and the lower value is 0.37. We have obtained the grey band, for sample 4, similarly. The grey and green bands have to be compared with the black and green squares of Figure 3, respectively. The squares that are within the colored bands are possible solutions of all equations. By comparing these values with those obtained from Equation (A22), reported as squares in Figure 3, we obtain that for sample 3, the fraction of x_{PSC} inside the core should be $y_3 = 0.65 \pm 0.15$. For sample 4, we have $y_4 = 0.35 \pm 0.35$, a range that includes also 0. Therefore, in the presence of $CaCl_2$ in buffer solution, the PSC molecules are much less segregated into the core and not isolated from the external environment with respect to the hydrophobic core. They are almost all in the shell, still in interaction with the buffer, due to its hydration. This result is also supported by the very low shell hydration of the micelles of sample 4 (see Table 2), because the available space in the shell is effectively already occupied by the PEG-1000 tails and the PSC molecules. Conversely, in the absence of $CaCl_2$ in solution, the PSC molecules are almost all localized in the core and, partially, in the region of the linker, being hence much better isolated from the buffer.

As calculated in Appendix A, the ratio of N_{PSC} and N_{mon} in sample 3 is about 2/3. The addition of PSC in the solution leads to micelles of a smaller diameter, as can be seen from the results of Table 2 for samples 3 and 4. The addition of $CaCl_2$ in the solution reduces the hydration of the PEG-1000 shell too. Moreover, in the presence of PSC, the $CaCl_2$ in solution leads to the formation of micelles with a smaller fraction of PSC linked to them, as can be clearly seen in Figure 3. This observation could be explained by the fact that the presence of Ca^{2+} in solution reduces the incorporation of PSC molecules into the hydrophobic core of the micelles. Additionally, from the x_{PSC} and the N_{agg} values (Table 2), we can estimate the total number of PSC molecules per micelle to 47 in sample 3 and 36 in sample 4. These combined results suggest that the presence of $CaCl_2$ in the buffer solution reduces the incorporation of PSC molecules both specifically into the hydrophobic core and in total into the micelles. One possible mechanism could be the overall reduction of available PSC in solution, induced by the presence of Ca^{2+} ions.

5. Conclusions

Under the assumption of a spheroidal model for micelles, we have developed a new fully analytical method, which exploits nth-order moments of the PDF derived from SAXS measurements to determine the micelles' structural parameters. This model has been successfully applied to characterize the morphology of micelles with and without the presence of a poorly soluble API (PSC) and $CaCl_2$, respectively. We were able to confirm previous observations on the impact of PSC based on a simple spherical model, although now with many more details, thanks to our new spheroidal model. With this model, we were also able to estimate the relative fractions of the PSC incorporated in the core and in the shell of the micelles. The model also reveals that the presence of $CaCl_2$ reduces PSC incorporation, both within the hydrophobic core and the micelle as a whole. This advanced yet straightforward analytical model offers a powerful tool for characterizing micellar systems and guiding the development of optimized drug delivery strategies.

Future experiments, where the micelles' morphology is characterized with our model as a function of the $CaCl_2$ concentration, could help us further understand the role of Ca^{2+} in influencing the micelles' shape and size, and to which extent micelles can play a protective role for the PSC molecules. These studies could obviously be extended to other types of surfactants and PSC. The results of such in vitro studies could provide useful insights to understand in-vivo mechanisms. They could then help design drug delivery systems that can enhance the bioavailability of poorly soluble APIs and protect them against the detrimental effect of Ca^{2+} cations in vivo, which are known to impact significantly the absorption and effectiveness of some pharmaceuticals administered orally.

Author Contributions: Conceptualization, L.D.C., C.G., T.S., F.G. and A.G.; methodology, L.D.C., C.G. and T.S.; validation, L.D.C., C.G., T.S., F.G. and A.G.; writing—original draft preparation, L.D.C., C.G. and T.S.; funding acquisition, C.G. and F.G. All authors have read and agreed to the published version of the manuscript.

Funding: This research was funded by "Potentiating the Italian Capacity for Structural Biology Services in Instruct-ERIC", acronym "ITACA.SB" (Project No. IR0000009, CUP B53C22001790006), funded by the European Union's NextGenerationEU under the MUR call 3264/2021 PNRR M4/C2/L3.1.1. F.G. and T.S. contribution was funded by Excelsus R&D funds.

Institutional Review Board Statement: Not applicable.

Informed Consent Statement: Not applicable.

Data Availability Statement: No new data were created or analyzed in this study. Data sharing is not applicable to this article.

Conflicts of Interest: Thibaud Stoll and Fabia Gozzo were employed by Excelsus Structural Solutions (Swiss) AG, Arnaud Grandeury was employed by Novartis Pharma AG. The remaining authors declare that the research was conducted in the absence of any commercial or financial relationships that could be construed as a potential conflict of interest.

Abbreviations

The following abbreviations are used in this manuscript:

VitE-TPGS	D-α-tocopherol polyethylene glycol 1000 succinate
PSC	Poorly soluble pharmaceutical compound
PDF	Pair Distribution Function
SAXS	Small-Angle X-ray Scattering
WAXS	Wide-Angle X-ray Scattering
RES	Reticuloendothelial system
EPR	Enhanced permeability and retention
DLS	Dynamic light scattering
TEM	Transmission electron microscopy
Cryo-EM	Cryogenic electron microscopy
AFM	Atomic force microscopy
LSM	Least square minimum
PEG	Polyethylene glycol

Appendix A

Determination of the Micelles' Structure by Evaluating the PDF's Moments Through a Least-Square Approach

For two-component micelles with a prolate or oblate spheroid shape (ellipsoids of revolution around the polar axis), the electron density's contrasts can be defined through the following equations, where subscripts "*E*" and "*P*" refer to the core and shell regions, and ρ_E, ρ_P, and ρ_s are the core, the shell, and the buffer electron density, respectively:

$$\begin{aligned}\Delta\rho_{ES} &= \rho_E - \rho_s,\\ \Delta\rho_{PS} &= \rho_P - \rho_s.\end{aligned} \tag{A1}$$

The volumes of the whole micelle and of the core can be expressed as follows:

$$\begin{aligned}V_M &= \tfrac{4\pi}{3}\tfrac{D_M}{2}\left(\tfrac{D_E}{2\varepsilon} + R_{SH}\right)^2,\\ V_E &= \tfrac{4\pi}{3\varepsilon^2}\left(\tfrac{D_E}{2}\right)^3,\end{aligned} \tag{A2}$$

where D_M and $D_E = D_M - 2R_{SH}$ are the maximum sizes of the whole spheroid micelle and of its core along the polar axis, respectively. Here, $\varepsilon = R_{pol}/R_{eq}$ is the ratio between the polar R_{pol} and equatorial R_{eq} radius of the micelle's core, and $D_M = 2R_{pol} + 2R_{SH}$, $D_E = 2R_{pol}$, where R_{SH} is the shell size. For prolate spheroids ($\varepsilon > 1$), D_M coincides with the maximum size of the micelle, namely D_{max}. For oblate spheroids ($\varepsilon < 1$), $D_M = \varepsilon D_{max}$.

For positive integers n and for a two-component spheroid-shaped micelle, the integrals given by Equation (1) have an analytical expression. We have already derived the solutions of Equation (1) for n = 1, 2, 4, 6 [14]. For n = 2, from Equation (1), we have the analytical expression for the gyration radius. For the n = 3 and n = 5 cases, we obtain the new formulae. Putting

$$a = \frac{D_M - 2R_{SH}}{2}, \tag{A3}$$

$$b = \frac{D_M - 2R_{SH}}{2\varepsilon}, \tag{A4}$$

$$a_1 = \frac{D_M}{2}, \tag{A5}$$

$$b_1 = \frac{D_M + 2(\varepsilon - 1)R_{Sh}}{2\varepsilon}, \tag{A6}$$

for n = 1, 2, 3, 4, 5, and 6 we obtain the following equations:

$$R^1 = \frac{3\left\{ab^2\left(a + \frac{b^2 ArcCos[a/b]}{\sqrt{b^2-a^2}}\right)(\Delta\rho_{ES} - \Delta\rho_{PS}) + a_1 b_1^2 \Delta\rho_{PS}\left(a_1 + \frac{b_1^2 ArcCos[a_1/b_1]}{\sqrt{b_1^2-a_1^2}}\right)\right\}}{8\left[a_1 b_1^2 \Delta\rho_{PS} + ab^2(\Delta\rho_{ES} - \Delta\rho_{PS})\right]}, \tag{A7}$$

$$R^2 = \frac{ab^2(a^2 + 2b^2)(\Delta\rho_{ES} - \Delta\rho_{PS}) + a_1 b_1^2 \Delta\rho_{PS}(a_1^2 + 2b_1^2)}{5\left[a_1 b_1^2 \Delta\rho_{PS} + ab^2(\Delta\rho_{ES} - \Delta\rho_{PS})\right]}, \tag{A8}$$

$$R^3 = \frac{ab^2\left(2a^3 + 3ab^2 + \frac{3b^4 ArcCos[a/b]}{\sqrt{b^2-a^2}}\right)(\Delta\rho_{ES} - \Delta\rho_{PS}) + a_1 b_1^2 \Delta\rho_{PS}\left(2a_1^3 + 10a_1^3 b_1^2 + 15a_1 b_1^4 + \frac{15b_1^6 ArcCos[a_1/b_1]}{\sqrt{b_1^2-a_1^2}}\right)}{16\left[a_1 b_1^2 \Delta\rho_{PS} + ab^2(\Delta\rho_{ES} - \Delta\rho_{PS})\right]}, \tag{A9}$$

$$R^4 = \frac{ab^2(3a^4 + 4a^2b^2 + 8b^4)(\Delta\rho_{ES} - \Delta\rho_{PS}) + a_1 b_1^2 \Delta\rho_{PS}(3a_1^4 + 4a_1^2 b_1^2 + 8b_1^4)}{35\left[a_1 b_1^2 \Delta\rho_{PS} + ab^2(\Delta\rho_{ES} - \Delta\rho_{PS})\right]}, \tag{A10}$$

$$R^5 = \frac{ab^2\left(8a^5 + 10a^3b^2 + 15ab^4 + \frac{15b^6 ArcCos[a/b]}{\sqrt{b^2-a^2}}\right)(\Delta\rho_{ES} - \Delta\rho_{PS}) + a_1 b_1^2 \Delta\rho_P\left(8a_1^5 + 3a_1 b_1^2 + \frac{3b_1^4 ArcCos[a_1/b_1]}{\sqrt{b_1^2-a_1^2}}\right)}{128\left[a_1 b_1^2 \Delta\rho_{PS} + ab^2(\Delta\rho_{ES} - \Delta\rho_{PS})\right]}, \quad \text{(A11)}$$

$$R^6 = \frac{ab^2(5a^6 + 6a^4b^2 + 8a^2b^4 + 16b^6)(\Delta\rho_{ES} - \Delta\rho_{PS}) + a_1 b_1^2 \Delta\rho_{PS}(5a_1^6 + 6a_1^4 b_1^2 + 8a_1^2 b_1^4 + 16b_1^6)}{105\left[a_1 b_1^2 \Delta\rho_{PS} + ab^2(\Delta\rho_{ES} - \Delta\rho_{PS})\right]}. \quad \text{(A12)}$$

Equations (A7), (A8), (A10), and (A12) have been already derived and discussed in [14]. This approach, indeed, can be considered as a fully analytical generalization of the graphical–analytical approach of [14]. The graphical estimates of $D_{\max}$ and R_{SH}, derived from the derivative of the PDF, can be used as initial starting values for solving the following system of 6 equations (n = 1, . . ., 6) with the 5 unknowns ε, $\Delta\rho_{ES}$, $\Delta\rho_{PS}$, D_M, R_{SH},

$$\eta^{\frac{n}{2}} R^n_{\mathrm{PDF}} = R^n, \quad n = 1, \ldots, 6 \quad \text{(A13)}$$

where [14]

$$\eta = \frac{6R_{SH}D_M^2}{D_M^3 - D_E^3}. \quad \text{(A14)}$$

The overdetermined system of equations (more equations than unknowns) can be solved by searching the least squares associated with the solution of Equation (A13):

$$\mathrm{LSR} = \sqrt{\sum_{n=1}^{6}\left(\sqrt[n]{\eta^{n/2}R^n_{\mathrm{PDF}}} - \sqrt[n]{R^n}\right)^2}. \quad \text{(A15)}$$

Odd exponents could lead to imaginary solutions in Equations (A7), (A9), and (A11). We need to select only the solutions for which the imaginary components are zero. Obviously, by calculating additional analytical expressions for high-order moments of the PDF, a number of equations larger than 6 could be used to constrain the above 5 unknown quantities. However, moments of much higher order could not add further independent constraints, with respect to moments of lower order, because they would be dominated only by contributions of higher distances.

The solution is a function of 5 independent quantities. This 5-dimensional space can be visualized by means of suitable bidimensional sections, choosing several pairs of these 5 variables. To do this, the SmoothDensityHistogram function of the software Mathematica 14.1 (Wolfram) can be used. It allows the user to plot a smooth kernel histogram of data. The option "Probability Density Function" can be also activated. In this way, we can calculate several bidimensional histograms of the 5-dimensional *LRS* function given by Equation (A15), calculated close to the minimum, as shown in the main text.

Moreover, we can calculate the PDF on a quantitative scale. Its integral for a two-component spheroidal micelle can be expressed as follows:

$$I(0) = 4\pi\int_0^{D_{Max}} \mathrm{PDF}(r)dr = \frac{K}{N_{agg}} V_M^2 \left(\Delta\rho_{PS} + (\Delta\rho_{ES} - \Delta\rho_{PS})\frac{V_E}{V_M}\right)^2, \quad \text{(A16)}$$

where V_E, V_M are the volumes of the core and the whole micelles, respectively. Here

$$K = \frac{(c_{mon} - cmc)N_A {r_e}^2}{MW_{mon}}, \quad \text{(A17)}$$

where the surfactant concentration c_{mon} has been corrected by the critical micelle concentration *cmc*, both expressed in $\mathrm{g/cm^3}$, $N_A = 6.02214 \cdot 10^{23}/\mathrm{mol}$ is the Avogadro number, r_e is the classic radius of an electron ($2.81794 \cdot 10^{-13}$ cm), MW_{mon} is the molar mass of one monomer, and N_{agg} is the average number of monomers aggregating into micelles [13]. For the micelle under study, $K = 1.23 \times 10^{-7}$ cm^{-1} electrons^{-2}. Given the values of ε, $\Delta\rho_{ES}$, $\Delta\rho_{PS}$, D_M, R_{SH} obtained by minimizing Equation (A15), we can use Equations (A16) and (A17) to calculate N_{agg}.

In the presence of the PSC, the question is how to estimate N_{agg}. For sample 3, in the presence of PSC in the buffer, $I(0) = 0.085$ cm^{-1}. Thus, $\frac{I(0)}{K} \cong 831^2$. This is the average squared electron contrast per monomer of the micelles in solution, measured by SAXS. A PSC molecule has 232 electrons and a volume of 554 Å^3. A water molecule has 20 electrons and a volume of 29.9 Å^3, at room temperature [13]. Thus, a PSC molecule has a volume equivalent to 554/29.9 water molecules. Therefore, the squared electron contrast, due to a single PSC molecule, with respect to water, is $(232 - 10 \times 554/29.9)^2 \cong 47^2$. Since $47^2/831^2 \sim 0.003$, we can always use Equations (A16) and (A17) to calculate N_{agg}, even in the presence of PSC molecules in solution.

Generalizing the equation in ref. [20], the solvent fraction x_S in the shell, ranging from 0 to 1, can be put as a function of x_{PSC}, and it can be estimated as follows:

$$x_S(x_{PSC}, y) = \frac{\Delta\rho_{PS} + \rho_{H2O} - \rho_{sh} + x_{PSC} \times (1-y) \times (\Delta\rho_{PS} + \rho_{H2O} - \rho_{PSC})}{\rho_{H2O} - \rho_{sh} + x_{PSC} \times (1-y) \times (\rho_{H2O} - \rho_{PSC})}. \quad \text{(A18)}$$

Here, ρ_{sh} is the theoretical electron density due to the hydrophilic part of the monomer; x_{PSC} is the ratio of the number of PSC molecules divided by the number of monomers inside the micelle (x_{PSC} could be also greater than 1, because it is a ratio between the number of different molecules); y is the fraction of the PSC molecules per monomer inside the core and ρ_{PSC} is its electron density; $1 - y$ is the fraction inside the shell. Even if $x_{PSC} = 0$, for $\Delta\rho_{PS} = -\rho_{H2O} + \rho_{sh}$ in Equation (A18), we would have no solvent molecules inside the shell (no hydration of the shell). For $\Delta\rho_{PS} = 0$, we would have only solvent molecules inside the shell (no shell). Therefore, actual $\Delta\rho_{PS}$ values would fall between these two limits, due to the partial hydration of the hydrophilic part of the monomers and the eventual presence of PSC inside the shell.

An amount of 82.6 mg of TPGS in 19.9 g of solution (see Table 1) leads to 3.28×10^{19} monomers (55 μmol) in sample 1; 10 g of this solution was taken to realize sample 3. Thus, the number of monomers in 10 g of solution is $N_{mon} = 1.65 \times 10^{19}$ monomers. Instead, the number of PSC molecules in the 10 g solution is $N_{PSC} = 1.09 \times 10^{19}$ (18 μmol). Therefore, the ratio of N_{PSC} and N_{mon} in solution for samples 3 and 4 is $N_{PSC}/N_{mon} \cong 2/3$ [13]. Thus, we should expect $x_{PSC} \leq 2/3$.

Moreover, between the hydrophobic and the hydrophilic parts of the monomers constituting the investigated micelles, we have a succinate linker, with z = 60 total electrons, which, added to the 536 electron of PEG 1000 and divided by the molecular volumes for succinate (123.6 Å^3) plus PEG 1000 (1360.7 Å^3), gives [13]

$$\rho_{sh} \cong \frac{536 + 60}{123.6 + 1360.7} = 0.402\ n_e/\text{Å}^3. \quad \text{(A19)}$$

The above value is an estimate of the maximum electron density in the shell, for $x_{PSC} = 0$, whereas for PSC we have $\rho_{PSC} = 0.419\ n_e/\text{Å}^3$ [13].

Given $x_S(x_{PSC}, y)$ by Equation (A18), the number of solvent (H_2O) molecules inside the shell volume (V_M-V_E) can be estimated as follows:

$$N_{H2O}(x_{PSC}, y) = x_S(x_{PSC}, y) \times \frac{V_M - V_E - N_{agg} x_{PSC} V_{PSC}(1-y)}{V_{H20}}. \quad \text{(A20)}$$

Given the total N_{H2O} inside the shell, the number of PSC molecules x_{PSC} per monomer into the micelle can be evaluated by the constraint that the sum of the volumes of all molecules inside the micelle—i.e., the solvent, monomer and PSC molecules—has to be equal to the micelle's volume V_M:

$$N_{agg} x_{PSC} V_{PSC} + N_{agg} V_{mon} + N_{H2O}(x_{PSC}, y) V_{H20} = V_M. \quad \text{(A21)}$$

By inserting Equation (A20) into Equation (A21), we obtain the following equation:

$$N_{agg} x_{PSC} V_{PSC} + N_{agg} V_{mon} + x_S(x_{PSC}, y) \times (V_M - V_E - N_{agg} x_{PSC} V_{PSC}(1 - y)) - V_M = 0, \quad \text{(A22)}$$

with $x_S(x_{PSC}, y)$ given by Equation (A18). Equation (A22) can be solved numerically, after having determined ε, $\Delta\rho_{ES}$, $\Delta\rho_{PS}$, D_M, R_{SH}, and N_{agg}, as previously described, to obtain a value for x_{PSC} that depends on the fraction y of PSC molecules inside the core, as discussed in the main text.

References

1. Kabanov, A.V.; Alakhov, V.Y. Micelles of amphiphilic block copolymers as vehicles for drug delivery. *J. Control. Release* **2007**, *2000*, 347–376. [CrossRef]
2. Torchili, V.P. Micellar Nanocarriers: Pharmaceutical Perspectives. *Pharm. Res.* **2007**, *24*, 1–16. [CrossRef] [PubMed]
3. Lammers, T. Nanomedicine and tumor targeting. *Adv. Mater.* **2024**, *36*, 2312169. [CrossRef] [PubMed]
4. Blanco, E.; Shen, H.; Ferrari, M. Principles of nanoparticle design for overcoming biological barriers to drug delivery. *Nat. Biotechnol.* **2015**, *33*, 941–951. [CrossRef] [PubMed]
5. Discher, D.E.; Eisenberg, A. Polymer vesicles. *Science* **2002**, *297*, 967–973. [CrossRef] [PubMed]
6. Kinnear, C.; Moore, T.L.; Rodriguez-Lorenzo, L.; Rothen-Rutishauser, B.; Petri-Fink, A. Form Follows Function: Nanoparticle Shape and Its Implications for Nanomedicine. *Chem. Rev.* **2017**, *117*, 11476–11521. [CrossRef] [PubMed]
7. Fang, J.; Nakamura, H.; Maeda, H. The EPR effect: Unique features of tumor blood vessels for drug delivery, factors involved, and limitations and augmentation of the effect. *Adv. Drug Deliv. Rev.* **2011**, *63*, 136–151. [CrossRef] [PubMed]
8. Liu, Y.; Tan, J.; Thomas, A.; Ou-Yang, D.; Muzykantov, V.R. The Shape of Things to Come: Importance of Design in Nanotechnology for Drug Delivery. *Ther. Deliv.* **2012**, *3*, 181–194. [CrossRef] [PubMed]
9. Meng, F.; Zhong, Z.; Feijen, J. Stimuli-responsive polymersomes for programmed drug delivery. *Biomacromolecules* **2009**, *10*, 197–209. [CrossRef] [PubMed]
10. Petros, R.A.; De Simone, J.M. Strategies in the design of nanoparticles for therapeutic applications. *Nat. Rev. Drug Discov.* **2010**, *9*, 615–627. [CrossRef] [PubMed]
11. Verma, A.; Stellacci, F. Effect of surface properties on nanoparticle-cell interactions. *Small* **2010**, *6*, 12–21. [CrossRef] [PubMed]
12. Ghezzi, M.; Pescina, S.; Padula, C.; Santi, P.; Del Favero, E.; Cantù, L.; Nicoli, S. Polymeric micelles in drug delivery: An insight of the techniques for their characterization and assessment in biorelevant conditions. *J. Control. Release* **2021**, *332*, 312–336. [CrossRef] [PubMed]
13. De Caro, L.; Del Giudice, A.; Morin, M.; Reinle-Schmitt, M.; Grandeury, A.; Gozzo, F.; Giannini, C. Small Angle X-Ray Scattering Data Analysis and Theoretical Modelling for the Size and Shape Characterization of Drug Delivery Systems Based on Vitamin E TPGS Micelles. *J. Pharm. Sci.* **2023**, *112*, 243–249. [CrossRef] [PubMed]
14. De Caro, L.; Stoll, T.; Grandeury, A.; Gozzo, F.; Giannini, C. Characterization of Surfactant Spheroidal Micelle Structure for Pharmaceutical Applications: A Novel Analytical Framework. *Pharmaceutics* **2024**, *16*, 604. [CrossRef] [PubMed]
15. U.S. Food and Drug Administration. *Drug Approval Package: Promacta (Eltrombopag) NDA#022291*; U.S. Food and Drug Administration: Silver Spring, MD, USA, 2008. Available online: https://www.accessdata.fda.gov/drugsatfda_docs/nda/2008/022291s000_TOC.cfm (accessed on 18 February 2025).
16. Beth Wire, M.; Bruce, J.; Gauvin, J.; Pendry, C.J.; McGuire, A.; Qian, Y.; Brainsky, A. A Randomized, Open-Label, 5-Period, Balanced Crossover Study to Evaluate the Relative Bioavailability of Eltrombopag Powder for Oral Suspension (PfOS) and Tablet Formulations and the Effect of a High-Calcium Meal on Eltrombopag Pharmacokinetics When Administered with or 2 Hours Before or After PfOS. *Clin. Ther.* **2012**, *34*, 699–709. [CrossRef]
17. Svergun, D.I. Determination of the regularization parameter in indirect-transform methods using perceptual criteria. *J. Appl. Crystallogr.* **1992**, *25*, 495–503. [CrossRef]
18. Williams, D.D.; Peng, B.; Bailey, C.K.; Wire, M.B.; Deng, Y.; Park, J.W.; Collins, D.A.; Kapsi, S.G.; Jenkins, J.M. Effects of food and antacids on the pharmacokinetics of eltrombopag in healthy adult subjects: Two single-dose, open-label, randomized-sequence, crossover studies. *Clin. Ther.* **2009**, *31*, 764–776. [CrossRef] [PubMed]

19. Rathod, S.; Bahadur, P.; Tiwari, S. Nanocarriers based on vitamin E-TPGS: Design principle and molecular insights into improving the efficacy of anticancer drugs. *Int. J. Pharm.* **2021**, *592*, 120045. [CrossRef] [PubMed]
20. Puig-Rigall, J.; Grillo, I.; Dreiss, C.A.; González-Gaitano, G. Structural and Spectroscopic Characterization of TPGS Micelles: Disruptive Role of Cyclodextrins and Kinetic Pathways. *Langmuir* **2017**, *33*, 4737–4747. [CrossRef] [PubMed]

pharmaceutics MDPI

Article

Intravenous Nanoemulsions Loaded with Phospholipid Complex of a Novel Pyrazoloquinolinone Ligand for Enhanced Brain Delivery

Tijana Stanković [1], Tanja Ilić [1,*], Branka Divović Matović [2], Milos Petkovic [3], Vladimir Dobričić [4], Ivan Jančić [5], Biljana Bufan [5], Kristina Jezdić [2], Jelena Đoković [1], Ivana Pantelić [1], Danijela Randjelović [6], Dishary Sharmin [7], James M. Cook [7], Miroslav M. Savić [2] and Snežana Savić [1]

[1] Department of Pharmaceutical Technology and Cosmetology, Faculty of Pharmacy, University of Belgrade, 11211 Belgrade, Serbia; tijana.stankovic@pharmacy.bg.ac.rs (T.S.); jelena.djokovic@pharmacy.bg.ac.rs (J.Đ.); ivana.pantelic@pharmacy.bg.ac.rs (I.P.); snezana.savic@pharmacy.bg.ac.rs (S.S.)
[2] Department of Pharmacology, Faculty of Pharmacy, University of Belgrade, 11211 Belgrade, Serbia; branka.divovic@pharmacy.bg.ac.rs (B.D.M.); kristina.mirkovic@pharmacy.bg.ac.rs (K.J.); miroslav.savic@pharmacy.bg.ac.rs (M.M.S.)
[3] Department of Organic Chemistry, Faculty of Pharmacy, University of Belgrade, 11211 Belgrade, Serbia; milos.petkovic@pharmacy.bg.ac.rs
[4] Department of Pharmaceutical Chemistry, Faculty of Pharmacy, University of Belgrade, 11211 Belgrade, Serbia; vladimir.dobricic@pharmacy.bg.ac.rs
[5] Department of Microbiology and Immunology, Faculty of Pharmacy, University of Belgrade, 11211 Belgrade, Serbia; ivan.jancic@pharmacy.bg.ac.rs (I.J.); biljana.bufan@pharmacy.bg.ac.rs (B.B.)
[6] Institute of Chemistry, Technology and Metallurgy, National Institute of the Republic of Serbia, University of Belgrade, 11000 Belgrade, Serbia; danijela@nanosys.ihtm.bg.ac.rs
[7] Department of Chemistry and Biochemistry, Milwaukee Institute for Drug Discovery, University of Wisconsin-Milwaukee, Milwaukee, WI 53211, USA; dsharmin@uwm.edu (D.S.); capncook@uwm.edu (J.M.C.)
* Correspondence: tanja.ilic@pharmacy.bg.ac.rs; Tel.: +381-11-3951-365

Abstract: Background/Objectives: The novel pyrazoloquinolinone ligand CW-02-79 shows a unique profile of selective binding to σ2 receptors, but its poor solubility in both water and lipids makes its research and development a burdensome task. We aimed to develop a phospholipid-complex-based nanoemulsion formulation containing CW-02-79 suitable for intravenous administration in preclinical research. **Methods**: The decorated and undecorated nanoemulsions were formulated and subjected to detailed physiochemical characterization. The delivery and exposure to CW-02-79 from selected nanoemulsions were examined in the in vitro blood–brain barrier model based on human-induced pluripotent stem-cell-derived microvascular endothelial cells, astrocytes, and pericytes, and in vivo neuropharmacokinetic study in rats, respectively. **Results**: The developed biocompatible nanoemulsions loaded with a CW-02-79—phospholipid complex at a mass ratio of 1:10 exhibited a small droplet size and narrow size distribution, with satisfactory physicochemical stability during steam sterilization and short-term storage at 25 °C. The analysis of protein binding interactions revealed that the PEGylated nanoemulsions had fewer observable interactions compared to the undecorated nanoemulsions, especially when 0.2% DSPE-PEG2000 and 0.1% DSPE-PEG2000-mannose were combined. An in vitro BBB study demonstrated that a substantial part of CW-02-79 present in the applied nanoemulsion is able to permeate the barrier. The quantification of CW-02-79 in plasma/brain homogenate and calculated pharmacokinetic parameters confirmed good systemic and brain availability after intravenous administration. There were subtle differences in the pharmacokinetic parameters in favor of a dual surface-functionalized nanoemulson containing the glucose transporter-1-targeting ligand (mannose). **Conclusions**: The developed and characterized nanoemulsions enable substantial brain exposure to CW-02-79 as a prerequisite for a pharmacologically and clinically relevant selective modulation of σ2 receptors.

https://doi.org/10.3390/pharmaceutics17020232

Keywords: blood–brain barrier; droplet size; surface chemistry; neuropharmacokinetics; brain targeting

1. Introduction

Due to the substantial global burden and unmet needs of a variety of psychiatric and neurological disorders, tremendous efforts have been made to develop new chemical entities with novel or improved mechanisms of action. The pyrazoloquinolinone structure was recognized as the first non-benzodiazepine ligand to interact with the benzodiazepine site of $GABA_A$ receptors [1] and has more recently yielded new ligands with functional selectivity for $GABA_A$ receptors that contain the α6 subunit [2].

The primary screening of a novel pyrazoloquinolinone ligand CW-02-79 (7-methoxy-6-methyl-2-(4-(trifluoromethoxy)phenyl)-2,5-dihydro-3H-pyrazolo [4,3-c]quinolin-3-one) on 47 receptors and other targets within the Psychoactive Drug Screening Program (PDSP) discovered a total of five potential binding sites. Binding studies showed that CW-02-79 exerts at least a 20-fold selectivity for σ2 receptors. It has a substantial affinity for σ2 receptors (Ki value of 112 nM), with only low to negligible affinities at the other four hits discovered within the primary screen: 5-HT_7 receptor (Ki = 2.4 μM), the benzodiazepine binding site at $GABA_A$ receptors (Ki = 4.7 μM), histamine H_2 receptor (Ki = 5.2 μM), and dopamine transporter (Ki > 10 μM) (available at: https://pdspdb.unc.edu/databases/kidb.php (accessed on 28 December 2024)). In vitro electrophysiological data demonstrated that CW-02-79 at a high concentration (10 μM) does not at all modulate $GABA_A$ receptors that contain any of the α1 to α6 subunits (personal communication with Dr. Janet Fisher). Accordingly, the behavioral screening of this ligand in the wide range of doses (1 to 30 mg/kg) revealed no signs of sedation or motor incapacitation typical of commonly used benzodiazepines (unpublished data, MM Savić and B Divović Matović).

While σ2 receptors are mainly known for their high expression in rapidly proliferating cancer cells [3], they have increasingly been shown to play an important role in neuroprotection and neurological/cognitive disorders and are therefore potential targets for drug development for the treatment of brain diseases [4,5]. All these data point to CW-02-79 as a lead structure for the development of innovative psychopharmacological therapies that act via σ2 receptors. However, the undesirable physicochemical properties of CW-02-79, in particular its poor solubility in water and oils as well as in biocompatible organic solvents, jeopardize the development of a suitable parenteral formulation, which is required for extensive preclinical studies.

Phospholipid complex technology has been intensively investigated to address the poor solubility and permeability through the biological barriers of synthetic and naturally occurring active compounds, due to the high biocompatibility and biodegradability of the phospholipids. The numerous studies indicate that the formation of a phospholipid complex through the non-covalent interactions between drugs containing hydroxyl, carbonyl, and amine groups and the polar head of phospholipids can improve the lipophilicity of drugs and subsequently, their bioavailability [6–8]. However, due to stability issues (e.g., the risk of aggregation and chemical degradation) and formulation stickiness, drug-phospholipid complexes are commonly utilized as lipophilic intermediates for encapsulation into nanocarriers [9–11]. For example, the combinational approach based on drug–phospholipid complexes and intravenous nanoemulsions was shown to ensure an improved loading capacity for hydrophobic drugs without premature leakage, higher control over the drug release kinetics, and protection from undesirable hydrolytic and enzymatic degradation (e.g., [12–14]).

To achieve the efficient concentration of a drug in the brain after intravenous administration of nanoemulsions, multiple biological hurdles need to be overcome, including (i) opsonization and rapid clearance via the mononuclear phagocytic system (MPS) and (ii) the blood–brain barrier (BBB) [15,16]. The surface coating with PEGylated phospholipids is a commonly reported strategy to prolong the residence time of nanodroplets in the systemic circulation, thus increasing the likelihood for the brain's uptake of nanodroplets [17,18]. Due to the limited specificity of this approach for brain delivery, an additional modification of the nanodroplet surface with a suitable ligand that targets the specific receptors on the brain endothelial cells is commonly required. In this study, mannose was used as a brain-targeting ligand due to its high affinity for glucose transporter-1 (GLUT-1) receptors, overexpressed on the BBB luminal side [19,20]. Mannose-coated nanoparticles have been reported to be able to enhance the drug delivery to the brain (e.g., by Lei et al. [21]). Therefore, to facilitate the interaction between the anchored mannose and GLUT-1 receptors, we used a relatively novel, commercially available excipient, DSPE-PEG2000-mannose, containing mannose attached at the terminus of the PEG chain as a spacer. Although this excipient was successfully employed on polymer nanoparticles [22] and liposomes [23], to the best of our knowledge, there are no reports on its use in the lipid nanoemulsions for brain targeting.

In this research, we aimed to investigate the potential of a two-fold formulation strategy based on a phospholipid complex and nanoemulsion to overcome the poor aqueous and oil solubility of CW-02-79, and thus to obtain a stable formulation suitable for intravenous administration. In addition, some of nanoemulsions were surface-functionalized/decorated with the PEGylated phospholipid (DSPE-PEG2000), alone or in combination with the GLUT-1 targeting ligand (DSPE-PEG2000-mannose), to enhance the brain targeting. After the high-pressure homogenization, nanoemulsions were characterized in terms of critical quality attributes and stability after the storage and steam sterilization. The permeation of CW-02-79 across the BBB from dual-modified/decorated and plain, undecorated nanoemulsions was assessed using a novel in vitro BBB model based on human induced pluripotent stem cell (iPSC)-derived cells. Finally, we evaluated the complete neuropharmacokinetic profiles of CW-02-79 after the single intravenous administration of the two most promising nanoemulsions to male rats, to elucidate the feasibility of this formulation type for preclinical studies.

2. Materials and Methods

2.1. Materials

CW-02-79 was synthesized at the Department of Chemistry and Biochemistry, University of Wisconsin-Milwaukee, USA. The following excipients were used for the nanoemulsion preparation: medium-chain triglycerides and castor oil were obtained from Fagron GmbH & KG, Glinde, Germany; soybean oil (Lipoid Purified Soybean Oil 700), soybean lecithin (Lipoid S75), and DSPE-PEG2000 (N-(Carbonyl-methoxypolyethylenglycol-2000)-1,2-distearoyl-sn-glycero-3 phosphoethanolamine, sodium salt) were purchased from Lipoid GmbH (Ludwigshafen, Germany); DSPE-PEG2000-Mannose (1,2-distearoyl-sn-glycero-3-phosphoethanolamine-N-(polyethyleneglycol)-Mannose, sodium salt) was provided by Biopharma PEG Scientific Inc., Watertown, MA, USA; glycerol, polysorbate 80, and butylhydroxy toluene (BHT) were supplied by Sigma-Aldrich Co. (St. Louis, MO, USA). Organic solvents (absolute ethanol, methanol, ethanol, dimethyl sulfoxide) were obtained from Fisher scientific (Waltham, MA, USA). Ultrapure water obtained by employing a GenPure apparatus (TKA Wasseranfbereitungssysteme GmbH, Neiderelbert, Germany) was used.

2.2. Preformulation Study

2.2.1. Solubility Evaluation

The solubility of CW-02-79 in selected oils, organic solvents, and water solutions of various pH values was examined by using the shake-flask method, by adding an excess amount of CW-02-79. The blends were mixed on a vortex mixer for 24 h at 25 ± 2 °C to reach equilibrium. The samples were centrifuged (1000× *g*, 10 min, 25 °C) on a MiniSpin® plus centrifuge (Eppendorf, Hamburg, Germany). The concentration of CW-02-79 was determined after proper dilution of the supernatant with isopropanol using the LC-MS/MS method.

2.2.2. Polarization Microscopy

An initial insight into the physical state of CW-02-79 was obtained using polarized light microscopy. It was performed using an Olympus BX53-P microscope (Olympus, Tokyo, Japan) with cross polarizers. Photomicrographs were taken using the digital camera UPLFLN4XP and UPLFLN10XP, and processed with appropriate software, i.e., cellSens Entry Version 1.14 (Olympus, Tokyo, Japan).

2.2.3. X-Ray Powder Diffraction Analysis (XRPD)

CW-02-79 was further analyzed on a Rigaku Smartlab X-ray Diffractometer in θ-θ geometry (the sample in the horizontal position) by applying parafocusing Bragg–Brentano geometry using a D/teX Ultra 250 strip detector in the 1D standard mode with a CuKα1,2 radiation source (U = 40 kV and I = 30 mA). The XRPD patterns were collected in the 3–40° 2θ range, with steps of 0.01° and a data collection speed of 3°/min. To minimize the background, the low-background single-crystal silicon sample holder was used.

2.2.4. Melt-Quenching Approach

For this analysis, around 2 mg of the unprocessed CW-02-79 was heated to 330 °C, with a heating rate of 20 °C/min, then cooled to 25 °C with a cooling rate of 40 °C/min and finally heated again to 330 °C with a heating rate of 10 °C/min. The measurements were conducted under a nitrogen flow (50 mL/min) by using a DSC 1 (Mettler-Toledo AG, Analytical, Greifensee, Switzerland). The onset and peak temperature and enthalpy were evaluated by using STAR® SW 12.10 software.

2.3. Preparation and Characterization of Phospholipid Complexes

2.3.1. Preparation of Phospholipid Complexes

Phospholipid complexes of CW-02-79 were prepared by employing the solvent evaporation method, using soybean lecithin as the phospholipid in different mass ratios of 1:10, 1:15, and 1:20 (*w*/*w*). The required amount of CW-02-79 and lecithin was dissolved in absolute ethanol, and the obtained mixtures were refluxed for 2 h at 65 °C. After the evaporation of the solvent, using a rotary evaporator, the dried residues were gathered using a spatula and kept in Eppendorf tubes in a desiccator until characterization.

2.3.2. Differential Scanning Calorimetry (DSC)

Thermal analysis was performed on pure CW-02-79, soybean lecithin, prepared phospholipid complexes, and physical mixtures containing CW-02-79 and soybean lecithin in the mass ratios of 1:10, 1:15, and 1:20. About 10 mg of the samples was measured in aluminum pans and heated from 25 to 400 °C at a rate of 10 °C/min. The measurements were conducted under a nitrogen flow (50 mL/min) by using the DSC 1 and the appropriate parameters were determined.

2.3.3. Fourier Transform Infrared (FT-IR) Spectroscopy

FT-IR spectroscopy was used to investigate possible chemical interactions between CW-02-79 and soybean lecithin in the physical mixtures and obtained phospholipid complexes. For each spectrum, 10 scans were used and recorded between 4000 and 400 cm^{-1}. The spectra were recorded using a Nicolet iS10 FT-IR spectrometer (Thermo Fisher Scientific, Inc., Madison, WI, USA).

2.3.4. Nuclear Magnetic Resonance (NMR) Spectroscopy

This analysis was carried out on pure CW-02-79, soybean lecithin, physical mixtures, and prepared phospholipid complexes. All the compounds or mixtures were dissolved in 0.5 mL of CDCl3 and placed in an NMR tube. The proton nuclear magnetic resonance (^{1}H NMR) and phosphorus nuclear magnetic resonance (^{31}P NMR) spectra of the samples were acquired using a Bruker Ascend 400 spectrometer (Bruker, Berlin, Germany) at 400 MHz and 23 °C.

2.4. *Preparation and Characterization of Intravenous Lipid Nanoemulsions*

Blank and nanoemulsions loaded with CW-02-79-phospholipid complexes were prepared by using the hot high-pressure homogenization method (HPH). Briefly, an oil phase was prepared by mixing MCT and castor oil in a 1:1 (*w*/*w*) ratio, soybean lecithin, and BHT on the magnetic stirrer at 50 °C. For the CW-02-79 loaded samples, the components of the oil phase were added to the round-bottom flask containing the prepared CW-02-79-phospholipid complex and mixed until the complex was completely dissolved. An aqueous phase was prepared by dissolving polysorbate 80 as a hydrophilic stabilizer and glycerol as an isotonization agent in ultrapure water at 50 °C. Decorated nanoemulsions were prepared by adding DSPE-PEG2000 with/without DSPE-PEG2000-mannose to the oil phase. The oil phase was then added to the aqueous phase and mixed at 8000 rpm for 5 min using rotor-stator homogenizer (IKA Ultra-Turrax® T25 digital, IKA®-Werke GmbH and Co., KG, Staufen, Germany). The coarse pre-emulsions were further processed by using a high-pressure homogenizer (EmulsiFlex-C3, Avestin Inc., Ottawa, ON, Canada) for 10 discontinuous cycles at 800 bar. The complete composition of the tested formulations is given in Table 1.

Table 1. Composition of optimal placebo and nanoemulsions loaded with CW-02-79—phospholipid complex.

Composition (%, *w*/*w*)	NE1	CW_{PC}NE1	NE2	CW_{PC}NE2	NE3	CW_{PC}NE3	CW_{PC}NE4
Oil phase							
CW_{PC}	-	1.65	-	1.65	-	1.65	1.65
MCT	10	10	10	10	10	10	10
Castor oil	10	10	10	10	10	10	10
Soybean lecithin	0.5	0.5	0.5	0.5	0.5	0.5	0.5
DSPE-PEG2000	-	-	0.2	0.2	0.3	0.3	0.2
DSPE-PEG2000-mannose	-	-	-	-	-	-	0.1
BHT	0.05	0.05	0.05	0.05	0.05	0.05	0.05
Aqueous phase							
Polysorbate 80	2	2	2	2	2	2	2
Glycerol	1.7	1.7	1.7	1.7	1.7	1.7	1.7
Ultrapure water ad	100	100	100	100	100	100	100

CW_{PC}: CW-02-79-phospholipid complex in a mass ratio of 1:10 (*w*/*w*); MCT: medium-chain triglycerides; BHT: butylhydroxytoluene.

2.4.1. Size Measurements and the Polydispersity Index

The droplet size (intensity-weighted mean diameter, Z-Ave) and polydispersity index (PDI) of nanoemulsions were determined using the ZetasizerNano ZS90 (Malvern Instruments Ltd., Worcestershire, UK). All measurements were carried out after adequate dilution with ultrapure water (1:500 (*v*/*v*)) at 25 °C at a fixed scattering angle of 90° using a He–Ne laser at 633 nm.

2.4.2. Atomic Force Microscopy (AFM)

The morphology, shape, and size of the nanodroplets were investigated using an NTEGRA Prima Atomic Force Microscope (NT-MDT, Moscow, Russia). For the sample preparation, 10 μL of nanoemulsions diluted with ultrapure water (1:500, *v*/*v*) was placed on the circular mica substrate (Highest Grade V1 AFM Mica Discs, Ted Pella Inc., Redding, CA, USA) and dried in a vacuum dryer (2 h, 25 °C) to remove leftover water. The measurements were carried out in the intermittent contact AFM mode with NT-MDT NSGO1 silicon cantilevers (N-type, Antimony doped, Au reflective coating) using a nominal force constant of 5.1 N/m. The cantilever driving frequency was around 150 kHz throughout the testing. The topography of AFM images was analyzed using Gwyddion 2.61 (Free and Open Source software, Czech Metrology Institute, Brno, Czechia) software.

2.4.3. Zeta Potential

Zeta potential (ZP) was determined using a Zetasizer Nano ZS90 by measuring droplets' electrophoretic mobility at 25 °C and converting it into ZP by using software v7. 01. Before the measurements, the samples were diluted with ultrapure water at 1:500 (*v*/*v*) ratio.

2.4.4. pH and Electrical Conductivity Measurements

Measurements of pH values were conducted at 25 °C using an HI9321 pH meter (Hanna Instruments Inc., Woonsocket, RI, USA) via direct immersion of the pH electrode into the nanoemulsions. The electrical conductivity (EC) was easily determined using the Sensio + EC 71 conductivity meter (Hach Lange GmbH, Berlin, Germany) by simple plunging of the electrode into the investigated samples.

2.4.5. Osmolality

The osmolality of the samples was measured using the Advanced® Model 3320 Micro-Osmometer (Advanced Instruments, Inc., Norwood, MA, USA) with a single freezing point. The nanoemulsion samples (20 μL) were collected in an Ease-Eject™ Sampler, placed at the instrument cradle, and injected into the osmometer freezing chamber.

2.4.6. Encapsulation Efficacy

The encapsulation efficacy (EE) was evaluated using the Amicon Ultra-4; NMWL 10 kDa filter units (Merck Millipore, Burlington, MA, USA). Concisely, the tested nanoemulsions (2 mL) were placed in the tube and centrifuged at 2000 rcf for 45 min. The filtrate was mixed with an equal volume of isopropanol and analyzed for CW-02-79 content using the LC-MS/MS method.

2.4.7. Stability Studies

To evaluate the physicochemical stability of the prepared nanoemulsions, all the formulations were stored at room temperature for three months. The visual appearance and relevant physicochemical parameters (Z-ave, PDI, ZP, pH, EC, and osmolality) were monitored using the methods described above.

2.5. Evaluation of the Nanoemulsion Interactions with Proteins

The interactions of the developed nanoemulsions with proteins were investigated by analyzing the changes in droplet size using the Zetasizer Nano ZS90. The nanoemulsions were incubated with bovine serum albumin (BSA, 30 mg/mL) and fetal bovine serum (FBS, 10% *v*/*v*) in phosphate buffer saline (PBS, pH 7.4) at 37 °C for 24 h. The Z-ave and PDI were measured at the beginning and after 0.5 h, 1 h, 2 h, 4 h, 8 h, and 24 h of incubation at 37 °C and compared with those of nanoemulsions incubated under the same conditions in the PBS without proteins.

2.6. In Vitro Release Testing of CW-02-79 from Nanoemulsions

The direct dialysis method was used for the in vitro drug release assessment. A mixture of PBS pH 7.4 and ethanol 96% *v*/*v* in the ratio of 1:1 *v*/*v* was used as a receptor medium. The addition of ethanol was necessary to address the very poor solubility of CW-02-79 in aqueous medium and to ensure sink conditions throughout the experiment. Selected optimal nanoemulsions (2 mL) were placed in a dialysis bag (cellulose membrane MW cut-off 12,000, Sigma-Aldrich Co., St. Louis, MO, USA) and immersed in 200 mL of termostated medium (37 °C). Samples were taken at 0.5 h, 1 h, 2 h, 4 h, 8 h, and 24 h, and the concentration was determined using the LC-MS/MS technique. The release kinetics of CW-02-79 from developed nanoemulsions was evaluated by fitting the experimental data to various mathematical models (zero-order, first-order, Higuchi, Baker-Lonsdale, Korsmeyer-Peppas) using the DDSolver v. 1.0 add-in program for Microsoft Excel.

2.7. In Vitro Permeation Study Through the Blood–Brain Barrier

The in vitro BBB model based on the co-culture of iPSC-derived brain microvascular endothelial cells, astrocytes, and pericytes was used to estimate the transport of CW-02-79 into the brain from the developed nanoemulsions (the protocol used is available on the manufacturer's website: iCell Blood Brain Barrier Isogenic Kit protocol, FujiFilm Cellular Dynamic Inc., Madison, WI, USA) [24]. Cell culture inserts for BBB co-cultures (pore size 0.4 µm, effective cell growth area 0.33 cm^2, Falcon®, Corning Inc., Salt Lake City, UT, USA) were coated on the apical side with a fibronectin-collagen IV matrix and on the basolateral side with a 0.1% gelatin solution. Then, astrocyte and pericyte suspensions were seeded on the basolateral side, with brain microvascular endothelial cells in the apical region of inserts, followed by overnight incubation at 37 °C and 5% CO_2. Subsequently, the iCell BMEC Plating Medium was replaced with iCell BMEC Maintenance Medium on both the apical and basolateral sides, and the medium was refreshed daily during the subsequent cultivation of the BBB. The integrity of the formed BBB was confirmed by measuring the transendothelial electrical resistance (TEER) using the EVOM2 epithelial volt/ohm meter with a chopsticks electrode (World Precision Instruments, Inc., Sarasota, FL, USA).

Selected nanoemulsions were diluted with the maintenance medium to achieve a final concentration of CW-02-79 of 3 µM in the apical compartment of the Transwell inserts and incubated at 37 °C and 5% CO_2 for 24 h. At specific time points, after 2, 6, and 24 h, samples (100 µL) were taken from the basolateral side, and the concentration of CW-02-79 was determined by using the LC-MS/MS method. The total volume on the basolateral side was compensated with 100 µL of the fresh termostated medium. The endothelial permeability coefficient (Pe) was calculated as previously described by Heymans et al. [25]. The mass balance (%) was also determined based on the amount of CW-02-79 determined in both the apical and basolateral compartments at the end of the assay divided by the total amount of CW-02-79 placed in the apical compartment to assess the potential adsorption to plastic or non-specific binding to cells.

2.8. In Vivo Neuropharmacokinetic Study

A neuropharmacokinetic study was conducted in Sprague Dawley rats following intravenous administration of the selected undecorated ($CW_{PC}NE1$) and decorated nanoemulsion ($CW_{PC}NE4$). At the same time, the respective profiles of concentration changes in plasma were established. The study was conducted according to the National Institutes of Health Animal Care and Use Committee guidelines and approved by the Ethics Committee on Animal Experimentation of the University of Belgrade—Faculty of Pharmacy (Serbia) and Ministry of agriculture, forestry, and water management—Veterinary Directorate (323-07-10046/2020-05). Eight-week old male Sprague Dawley rats weighing 160–200 g were housed three animals per cage in the animal room, and the light/dark period was set on 12 h cycles, with the illumination 120 lx. The temperature was set at 22 ± 1 °C, with the relative humidity 40–70%. The test formulations were given intravenously in the tail vein in a volume of 5 mL/kg, obtaining a 7.5 mg/kg dose of CW-02-79. At 7 pre-determined time points (5 min, 20 min, 1 h, 3 h, 6 h, 12 h, and 24 h), 3 animals per time point were sacrificed and blood and brain samples were collected. The animals were anesthetized with ketamine hydrochloride (90 mg/kg, 10% Ketamidor, Richter Pharma AG, Wels, Austria). Blood samples were taken via cardiac puncture in heparinized syringes and spun at 1000× *g* for 10 min to separate the plasma. Simultaneously, brain was taken, weighed, and homogenized in 1 mL of methanol by using an ultrasonic probe. Homogenized samples were then centrifuged for 20 min at 3400× *g*, and the supernatants were separated. The CW-02-79 was extracted from the plasma, and the supernatants were obtained from brain via solid-phase extraction using Oasis HLB cartridges (Waters Corporation, Milford, MA, USA). Cartridges were preconditioned with methanol and water before loading the samples and internal standard. Endogenous impurities were eliminated via washing with water and methanol. The elution was performed with 1 mL of methanol for 1 min. The concentration of CW-02-79 in the eluates was determined using the LC-MS/MS technique. The concentration data were used to determine the pharmacokinetic parameters using Certara Phoenix WinNonlin™ software. v8.3.

2.9. LC-M/MS Method

The concentration of CW-02-79 was determined using a LC-MS/MS method. The analysis was performed on a UHPLC chromatograph ACELLA (Thermo Fisher Scientific Inc., Madison, WI, USA), coupled to a triple quadrupole mass spectrometer TSQ Quantum Access MAX (Thermo Fisher Scientific Inc., Madison, WI, USA) with a heated electrospray ionization (HESI) interface. The column was XTerra MS C18 (150 mm × 2.1 mm, 3.5 mm particle size). The mobile phase was acetonitrile/0.1% formic acid = 70:30 (v/v), the flow rate was 0.2 mL min^{-1}, the column temperature was set to 35 °C, and the injection volume was 10 µL. CW-02-79 and the internal standard were detected and quantified in the positive HESI mode (m/z = 389.90–345.90 and m/z = 349.00–304.11, respectively).

2.10. Statistical Analysis

Where applicable, measurements were performed in triplicate, and the outcomes are presented as mean ± standard deviation (SD). After verifying the normality of the data distribution, the statistical analysis was performed using a Student's *t*-test for two sets of results or analysis of variance (ANOVA) followed by Tukey post hoc test for more than two data sets. Statistical analysis was conducted using the IBM SPSS Statistics software (v. 25). p-values < 0.05 were considered statistically significant.

3. Results and Discussion

3.1. Preformulation Study

CW-02-79, the novel pyrazoloquinolinone ligand with a molecular mass of 389.33 and logP value of 2.60 (Figure 1a) appeared as a yellow powder, with a broad particle size distribution (Figure 1b). Due to the limited data available in the literature, special attention was initially paid to the detailed analysis of the key physicochemical descriptors (e.g., solubility in various solvents, i.e., lipid pharmaceutical excipients and common organic solvents, melting temperature, crystallinity, and amorphization ability) in order to select an optimal strategy for the formulation development. As shown in Table S1 (Supplementary Materials), CW-02-79 is practically insoluble in water, oils, and biocompatible organic solvents, except dimethyl sulfoxide (DMSO) which can be associated with various safety concerns. In addition, since no ionizable functional groups are present, the solubility of CW-02-79 does not change with alterations of pH value. These findings exclude salt formation as an approach to improve its solubility as well as the development of conventional water- and lipid-based formulations.

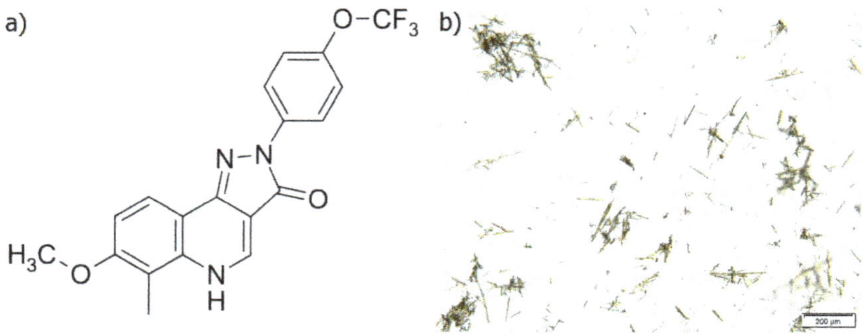

Figure 1. (**a**) Chemical structure of CW-02-79; (**b**) micrograph of coarse CW-02-79 powder.

To test the potential of CW-02-79 for amorphization, quenching of the melt was investigated providing an insight into the substance's ability to become amorphous upon cooling after melting. In the first heating cycle, the thermogram of CW-02-79 exhibited two endothermic peaks at 87.95 °C and 300.84 °C (Figure S1, Supplementary Materials). The first peak represents the glass transition temperature (Tg) and indicates the possible transition from the amorphous or semi-crystalline phase to a more disordered structure. The second peak at 301.98 °C corresponds to the melting point of the crystalline structure of CW-02-79. During the subsequent rapid cooling phase, crystallization occurred with decreasing temperature, which was evident from a sharp exothermic peak at 228.46 °C. In the second heating phase, a relatively broad endothermic peak at 269.92 °C could be attributed to the melting of the crystallized form formed during the rapid cooling. These results indicate that quenching of the melt allowed crystallization to a certain extent and prevented the substance from becoming completely amorphous, excluding amorphization as the strategy for overcoming the poor water solubility.

In addition, to obtain a more detailed insight into the physical state of unprocessed CW-02-79, XRPD analysis was performed. The diffractogram of CW-02-79 displays a significant number of sharp diffraction peaks, suggesting the existence of a significant proportion of crystalline material with a well-defined lattice structure (Figure S2, Supplementary Materials). Furthermore, a broad diffraction peak extending from 3 to 30° 2θ accompanied by a raised baseline is indicative of the absence of a long-range order in the structure, suggesting the presence of amorphous material [26]. In other words, this finding could mean that the ligand under investigation is not a purely crystalline or amorphous substance, and as such, is not suitable for the development of nanocrystalline dispersions.

3.2. Characterization of Prepared CW-02-79—Phospholipid Complexes

Analyzing the physicochemical properties of CW-02-79, phospholipid complexation was selected as a promising approach to overcome the poor oil solubility of CW-02-79 and to develop a suitable nanoemulsion carrier. Due to its relative simplicity, the solvent evaporation technique is most commonly used for the preparation of phospholipid complexes [27]. However, there is a lack of systematic studies in the current literature that provide the optimal conditions for the preparation of phospholipid complexes. This is mainly because each substance has unique physicochemical properties, making it difficult to apply a uniform set of parameters for the formation of phospholipid complexes, such as the type of reaction solvent, phospholipids, drug to phospholipid ratio, and reaction time [28]. Due to the solubility constraints of CW-02-79, absolute ethanol was used as an organic solvent in combination with soybean lecithin as a promising phospholipid for the preparation of complexes via solvent evaporation in the different mass ratios of 1:10, 1:15, and 1:20. The obtained complexes were analyzed via DSC, FT-IR spectrometry, and NMR spectroscopy.

DSC is considered a fast and reliable method to obtain information on the solid state of active substances and phospholipids and the interactions between them during the phospholipid complex formation [6]. The obtained DSC thermograms of CW-02-79, soybean lecithin, their physical mixtures, and the prepared complexes are shown in Figure 2a. No pronounced endothermic peaks were observed in the DSC curve of soybean lecithin; an exothermic peak around 325 °C could be attributed to its decomposition. On the other hand, the DSC thermograms of the physical mixtures and the CW-02-79 phospholipid complexes were highly similar and were superimposed by the lecithin curve. In other words, the characteristic sharp endothermic peak at 300.84 °C caused by the melting of CW-02-79 in its crystalline form had disappeared in both the physical mixtures and the complexes formed, probably due to masking by the soy lecithin. Therefore, additional characterization methods were required to prove the formation of the phospholipid complexes.

To identify the possible intermolecular interactions between the CW-02-79 and soybean lecithin in the physical mixtures and phospholipid complexes formed, FT-IR spectroscopy was used. The FT-IR spectrum of CW-02-79 (Figure 2b) revealed characteristic peaks at 3231 cm^{-1} (the N-H stretching vibrations), 1613 cm^{-1} (aromatic C=C stretching), 1464 cm^{-1} (C-H bending vibrations), 1254 cm^{-1} and 1092 cm^{-1} (C-O stretching vibration), and 771 cm^{-1} (out-of-plane C-H bending vibrations). The FT-IR spectrum of soybean lecithin shows characteristic peaks at 2922 cm^{-1} and 2852 cm^{-1} (C–H stretching vibration), 1737 cm^{-1} (C=O stretching), 1459 cm^{-1} (C-H bending vibrations), 1242 cm^{-1} (P=O stretching vibrations), and 1170 cm^{-1} and 1058 cm^{-1} (C-O stretching vibrations) (Figure 2b). The specific feature of CW-02-79—the N-H stretching vibration at 3231 cm^{-1}—was shifted to 3376 cm^{-1} in the physical mixtures, while it almost disappeared in the phospholipid complexes due to the delocalization of the vibrations, indicating the formation of hydrogen bonds. In addition, the stretching vibration P=O bond of soybean lecithin at 1242 cm^{-1} was shifted towards 1247 cm^{-1}, 1244 cm^{-1}, and 1249 cm^{-1} in physical mixtures with mass ratios of 1:10, 1:15, and 1:20, respectively, while the shift was more pronounced in the corresponding phospholipid complexes (1253 cm^{-1}, 1249 cm^{-1}, and 1255 cm^{-1}, respectively). These findings indicate that the aromatic amino group of CW-02-79 interacts with the oxygen atom of the phosphoryl group in phosphatidylcholine, the main component of soybean lecithin through hydrogen bonding in all the prepared complexes (Figure 2c).

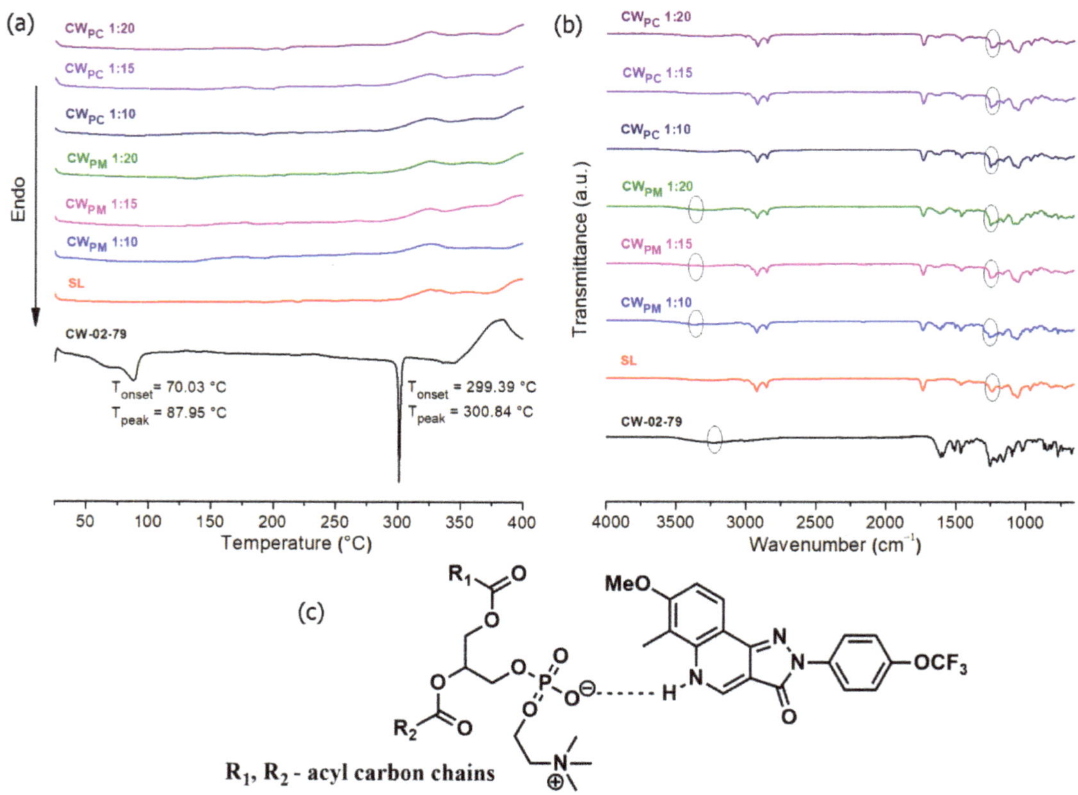

Figure 2. (**a**) DSC thermograms and (**b**) FT-IR spectra of pure CW-02-79, soybean lecithin (SL), physical mixtures (CW_{PM}) and phospholipid complexes (CW_{PC}) in investigated mass ratios of 1:10, 1:15, and 1:20; (**c**) graphical scheme of the proposed hydrogen bonding interactions between phosphatidylcholine from soybean lecithin and CW-02-79 during the CW-02-79 phospholipid complex formation.

NMR spectroscopy was used to confirm the formation of the phospholipid complex, providing an insight into the magnetic properties of hydrogen and phosphorus nuclei [6]. In the ^{1}H-NMR spectra, the changes in the chemical shifts of the significant protons involved in the interactions between CW-02-79 and soybean lecithin are shown in Table 2. All the protons revealed chemical shifts, whereby the highest shift of the protons of the secondary amino group attached to the aromatic ring was observed, from 9.03 (ppm) for unprocessed CW-02-79 to 12.40 (ppm), 12.40 (ppm), and 12.57 (ppm) upon the formation of complexes at different mass ratios with soybean lecithin of 1:10, 1:15, and 1:20, respectively. Also, H-2 attached to the aromatic ring of CW-02-79 revealed certain chemical shifts upon complex formation (Table 2). To further support the ^{1}H-NMR data, ^{31}P-NMR was also investigated to confirm the phosphorus group's chemical change. ^{31}P-NMR revealed a phosphorus chemical shift from 0.882 to 0.993, 0.874, and 0.999 upon complex formation with different ratios of soybean lecithin (1:10, 1:15, and 1:20, respectively). All the observed downfield shifts clearly support the existence of interactions between CW-02-79 and soybean lecithin. Overall, the results of DSC, FT-IR, and NMR spectroscopy clearly confirmed the formation of complexes between CW-02-79 and soybean lecithin at all the mass ratios tested.

Table 2. Overview of the chemical shifts (in ppm) of pure CW-02-79 or soybean lecithin compared to prepared phospholipid complexes (CW_{PC} 1:10, 1:15, and 1:20) using ^{1}H-NMR and ^{31}P-NMR.

	CW-02-79/SL *	CW_{PC} 1:10	CW_{PC} 1:15	CW_{PC} 1:20
		^{1}H-NMR		
NH	9.03, bs	12.40, bs	12.40, bs	12.57, bs
H-2	8.37 (d, J = 6.3 Hz),	8.63, s	8.69, s	8.66, s
H-5	8.28–8.23, m	8.07 (d, J = 8.8 Hz)	8.14 (d, J = 8.8 Hz)	8.11 (d, J = 8.8 Hz)
H-6	7.14 (d, J = 8.8 Hz),	6.98 (d, J = 9.0 Hz)	7.04 (d, J = 8.9 Hz)	7.01 (d, J = 9.1 Hz)
CH3	2.40, s	2.40, s	2.45, s	2.44, s
OCH3	3.97, s	3.85, s	3.90, s	3.88, s
H-2′ and H-6′	8.28–8.23, m	8.21 (d, J = 9.0 Hz)	8.25 (d, J = 9.0 Hz)	8.25 (d, J = 8.9 Hz)
H-3′ and H-5′	7.29 (d, J = 8.7 Hz)	7.23 (d, J = 8.6 Hz)	* covered by CDCl3 signal	7.24 (d, J = 8.6 Hz)
		^{31}P-NMR		
P=O	0.882	0.993	0.874	0.999

* ^{1}H-NMR refers to CW-02-79, while ^{31}P-NMR refers to soybean lecithin.

3.3. Preparation and Characterization of Nanoemulsions

The first step during the development of the nanoemulsions was to select the optimal oil core, allowing the adequate solubilization capacity for the developed phospholipid complexes as well as the stability of the nanoemulsion system per se. Among the tested oils, the highest solubility of CW-02-79 was obtained in the mixture of MCT and castor oil (1:1, *w/w*), and therefore, it was used as the oil phase for nanoemulsion development. The combination of MCT and castor oil, as a long-chain triglyceride, was also desirable because of the lower viscosity compared to pure castor oil as well as the free fatty acid in castor oil, which can act as co-surfactants and additional nanodroplet stabilizers [29].

Stabilizers were selected based on their suitability for parenteral administration and, more importantly, our goal to achieve the efficient delivery of CW-02-79 to the brain. Due to its biocompatibility, biodegradability, and safety reputation, soybean lecithin is the most commonly used stabilizer in commercial lipid nanoemulsions, ensuring the good stability of the system [30]. Therefore, soybean lecithin was not only used to form phospholipid complexes, but also played an important role in the stabilization of nanoemulsions. To improve the physicochemical stability during storage and thermal sterilization, polysorbate 80 was added as a co-stabilizer. In addition, numerous studies in the literature indicate that polysorbate 80 can improve the drug transport across the BBB by acting as a P-glycoprotein inhibitor, permeation enhancer, or promoter of receptor-mediated endocytosis [31]. To further facilitate the uptake of nanodroplets into the brain, a dual strategy based on passive targeting via PEGylated phospholipid (DSPE-PEG2000) and active targeting via GLUT-1 receptors using mannose at the end of the PEG chain (DSPE-PEG2000-mannose) was tested. However, due to the molecular weight and density of PEG chains, PEGylation can alter the droplet size, surface charge, and consequently the biological fate [17]. For this reason, special attention was paid to carefully selecting the optimal concentration of these PEGylated phospholipids when developing the formulation.

Immediately after preparation, all the nanoemulsions were highly fluid with a yellow appearance and characteristic bluish tint, without signs of phase separation. However, the precipitation of CW-02-79 was observed within 7 days of storage in the nanoemulsions loaded with phospholipid complexes prepared at mass ratios of 1:15 and 1:20, regardless of the stabilizer mixture used. In contrast, formulations prepared with the 1:10 CW-02-79-phospholipid complex were homogeneous with no evidence of the precipitation of CW-02-

79. Therefore, the formulations prepared with 1:15 and 1:20 phospholipid complexes were excluded from further investigations.

The Z-ave and PDI of the placebo and nanoemulsions loaded with the 1:10 CW-02-79-phospholipid complex, differing in the surface composition (undecorated, decorated by DSPE-PEG2000 with/without mannose), are summarized in Table 3. The Z-ave of all the formulations tested was in the nanometer range, between 145 and 165 nm, with a PDI < 0.25, typical of a narrow size distribution, indicating good stability and suitability for intravenous administration and brain delivery (to achieve efficient brain delivery, the Z-ave of nanoparticles should be in the range of 100 to 200 nm [32]). Incorporation of the phospholipid complex into the oil core did not change the Z-ave compared to the corresponding blanks. Interestingly, no significant difference in the Z-ave and PDI was also observed between the undecorated and PEGylated formulations. Moreover, the addition of DSPE-PEG2000-mannose ($CW_{PC}NE4$) had no effect on the Z-ave and PDI compared to the corresponding formulation prepared with DSPE-PEG2000 only ($CW_{PC}NE2$).

Table 3. Droplet size (Z-ave), polydispersity index (PDI), zeta potential (ZP), pH, and electrical conductivity (EC) of autoclaved and non-autoclaved blank and nanoemulsions loaded with CW-02-79–phospholipid complex after preparation and after three months of storage at 25 °C.

Sample		Z-ave (nm)	PDI	ZP (mV)	pH	EC (μS/cm)
One day after preparation						
NE1	n	152.8 ± 1.3	0.148 ± 0.016	−45.1 ± 0.2	6.70 ± 0.02	81.4 ± 0.2
	a	152.6 ± 0.5	0.148 ± 0.016	−37.8 ± 1.1 ^{e}	5.54 ± 0.01 ^{f}	82.5 ± 0.6 ^{e}
$CW_{PC}NE1$	n	151.3 ± 1.3	0.174 ± 0.035	−42.3 ± 1.2 ^{a}	6.19 ± 0.01 ^{c}	79.2 ± 1.0 ^{b}
	a	148.0 ± 1.0	0.143 ± 0.010	−32.6 ± 1.3	5.56 ± 0.01	72.3 ± 0.2
NE2	n	145.5 ± 1.8	0.112 ± 0.019	−46.0 ± 0.4	6.90 ± 0.01	82.4 ± 0.3
	a	144.1 ± 0.2	0.104 ± 0.018	−43.1 ± 1.4	5.53 ± 0.01	90.6 ± 0.4
$CW_{PC}NE2$	n	158.4 ± 3.4 ^{b}	0.217 ± 0.007 ^{b}	−48.0 ± 0.4 ^{c}	6.33 ± 0.02	90.9 ± 0.2 ^{c}
	a	155.0 ± 0.1	0.140 ± 0.005 ^{f}	−40.9 ± 1.2 ^{e}	5.54 ± 0.02 ^{e}	94.9 ± 0.1 ^{f}
NE3	n	161.2 ± 2.0	0.158 ± 0.025	−37.5 ± 0.4	6.65 ± 0.03	96.9 ± 0.3
	a	159.7 ± 1.4	0.133 ± 0.011	−39.2 ± 0.2	5.76 ± 0.01	102.1 ± 0.4
$CW_{PC}NE3$	n	144.7 ± 2.5 ^{b}	0.173 ± 0.025	−42.0 ± 0.5 ^{c}	6.14 ± 0.02 ^{c}	96.6 ± 0.3 ^{c}
	a	139.3 ± 2.1	0.119 ± 0.034	−42.7 ± 0.7	5.85 ± 0.02 ^{e}	100.4 ± 0.3 ^{e}
$CW_{PC}NE4$	n	153.4 ± 0.9	0.113 ± 0.090	−37.9 ± 0.3	6.31 ± 0.01	101.7 ± 0.2
	a	155.2 ± 1.7	0.129 ± 0.024	−40.1 ± 0.3	5.90 ± 0.03 ^{e}	113.3 ± 0.1 ^{f}
After three months of storage						
NE1	n	150.0 ± 2.3	0.139 ± 0.014	−31.5 ± 0.7	5.92 ± 0.04	126.6 ± 0.9
	a	146.5 ± 1.7	0.135 ± 0.008	−31.7 ± 0.5	5.17 ± 0.01	89.0 ± 0.9
$CW_{PC}NE1$	n	146.7 ± 1.4	0.108 ± 0.022	−40.6 ± 1.9	4.75 ± 0.04 ^{i}	135.4 ± 1.9 ^{i}
	a	142.4 ± 1.0	0.122 ± 0.021	−30.9 ± 0.6	4.97 ± 0.04	84.7 ± 1.5
NE2	n	142.7 ± 1.8	0.111 ± 0.008	−30.3 ± 0.3	4.68 ± 0.01	115.4 ± 0.3
	a	145.6 ± 0.6	0.092 ± 0.006	−43.1 ± 1.1	5.17 ± 0.00	112.1 ± 0.3
$CW_{PC}NE2$	n	154.8 ± 0.8	0.146 ± 0.01 ^{h}	−40.3 ± 0.3 ^{i}	5.73 ± 0.01 ^{i}	123.5 ± 0.6 ^{i}
	a	153.2 ± 1.0	0.135 ± 0.026	−31.2 ± 1.9	5.22 ± 0.01	114.0 ± 0.7
NE3	n	165.5 ± 1.2	0.129 ± 0.026	−40.0 ± 0.2	5.12 ± 0.02	179.9 ± 0.1
	a	164.6 ± 1.1	0.159 ± 0.008	−46.0 ± 0.3	5.14 ± 0.01	120.9 ± 0.5
$CW_{PC}NE3$	n	148.5 ± 1.8	0.166 ± 0.009	−49.7 ± 1.9 ^{h}	5.17 ± 0.03 ^{i}	147.8 ± 1.1 ^{i}
	a	139.6 ± 1.0	0.147 ± 0.023	−36.3 ± 1.2	5.25 ± 0.01	113.0 ± 0.7
$CW_{PC}NE4$	n	158.0 ± 1.8 ^{g}	0.152 ± 0.017 ^{g}	−40.6 ± 0.5 ^{i}	5.13 ± 0.01 ^{h}	171.1 ± 0.9 ^{h}
	a	155.0 ± 2.0	0.137 ± 0.035	−39.9 ± 0.3	4.94 ± 0.02	107.9 ± 1.1

n—non-autoclaved nanoemulsion sample, a—autoclaved nanoemulsion sample. ^{a} $p < 0.05$, ^{b} $p < 0.01$, ^{c} $p < 0.001$ compared to corresponding blank sample. ^{d} $p < 0.05$, ^{e} $p < 0.01$, ^{f} $p < 0.001$ compared with corresponding non-autoclaved sample. ^{g} $p < 0.05$, ^{h} $p < 0.01$, ^{i} $p < 0.001$ compared with the same sample one day after preparation.

Although dynamic light scattering (DLS) is the most commonly used method for particle sizing, it is considered a low-resolution technique that is unable to distinguish different particle populations [16,33]. Therefore, AFM analysis was performed as a complementary method to gain further insight into the droplet size, size distribution, shape, and possible aggregation in the nanoemulsions loaded with the CW-02-79 phospholipid complex. The AFM images illustrating the 2D and 3D topography of the $1.0 \times 1.0\ \mu m^2$ area from the selected samples are presented in Figures 3a and 3b, respectively. The height profiles of individual nanodroplets are shown in Figure 3c. The AFM micrographs showed droplet sizes of around 140–180 nm, with a spherical droplet morphology and a uniform shape for both PEGylated and non-PEGylated samples, which was consistent with the DLS measurements. In the formulations with 0.2% DSPE-PEG2000 as well as in the 0.1% DSPE-PEG2000-mannose combination, some sample preparation artifacts (hole-like structures) can be seen after drying, but droplets with a size of around 180 nm were still visible (Figure 3). In addition, AFM analysis proved the absence of larger droplets, aggregates, and undissolved CW-02-79 crystals in all the formulations tested.

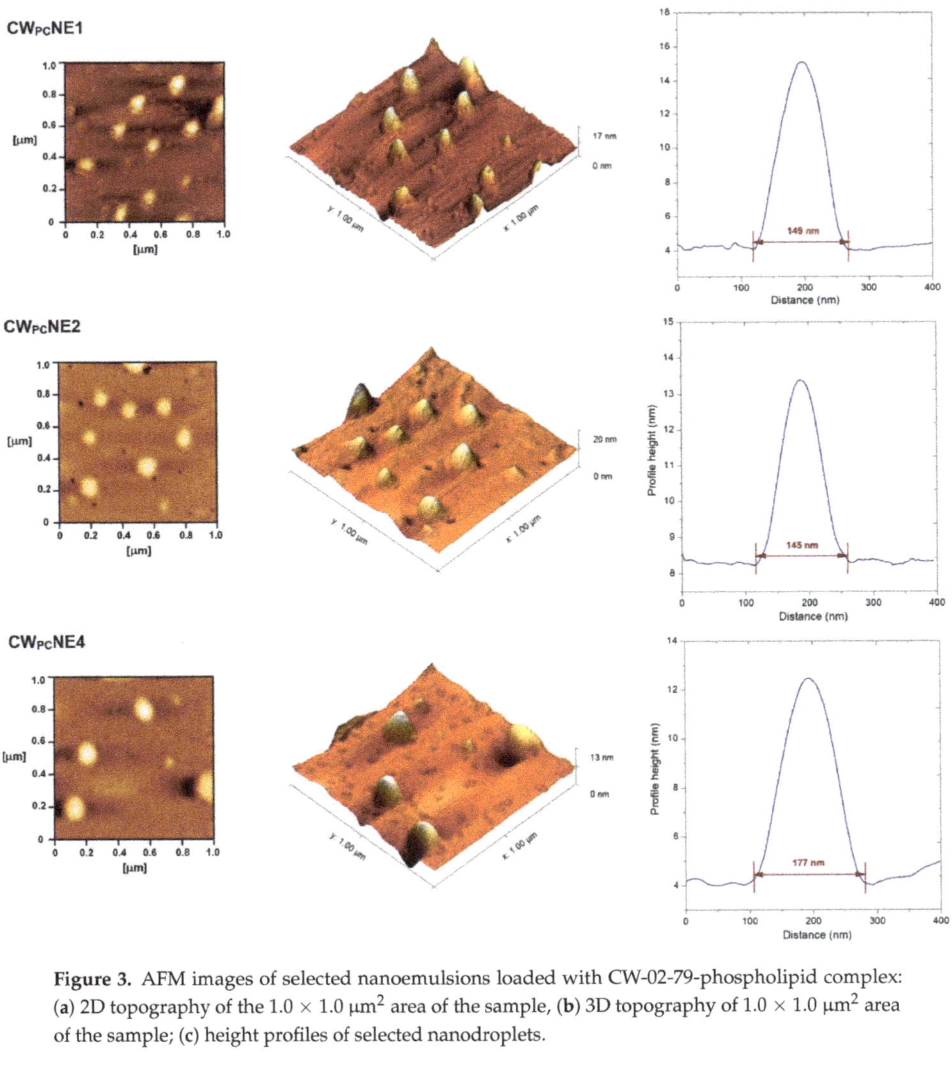

Figure 3. AFM images of selected nanoemulsions loaded with CW-02-79-phospholipid complex: (**a**) 2D topography of the $1.0 \times 1.0\ \mu m^2$ area of the sample, (**b**) 3D topography of $1.0 \times 1.0\ \mu m^2$ area of the sample; (**c**) height profiles of selected nanodroplets.

The ZP of all the formulations developed was also measured, as absolute values of more than 30 mV indicate the good stability of the nanoemulsion system [31]. One day after preparation, the ZP values for all the tested nanoemulsions were in the range of –37.5 to –48 mV (Table 3), indicating a high negative surface charge and consequently, a strong electrostatic repulsion between the nanodroplets. In view of the fact that all the formulations were stabilized by soybean lecithin, these high values were to be expected. Interestingly, the incorporation of the CW-02-79-phospholipid complex led to a slight, but statistically significant increase in negative ZP values in all the formulations tested compared to the corresponding blank samples. In addition, the significant reduction in ZP after the addition of PEGylated phospholipids has already been described in the literature and could be attributed to the shielding effect of the PEG chains on the droplet surface.

The pH value of nanoemulsions is crucial for the physiological compatibility during administration, and particularly, for the long-term stability of the nanoemulsion system. As shown in Table 3, the pH values of all the tested nanoemulsions were suitable for parenteral administration. However, it should be noted that the pH values of the blank formulations (6.65–6.90) were higher than those of the corresponding formulations (6.14–6.33) containing the CW-02-79-phospholipid complex. This difference cannot be attributed to CW-02-79, as there are no ionizable functional groups in its structure, but to the different spatial arrangement of the lecithin molecules within the nanoemulsion system. On the other hand, the EC of the nanoemulsions loaded with CW-02-79 was similar to that of the corresponding blank samples. Finally, to avoid local damage to the vascular endothelium and circulating blood cells, the isotonicity of the nanoemulsions was adjusted by adding glycerol (1.7%, *w*/*w*). The measured osmolality of all the developed formulations was in the range of 280–300 mOsm/kg, which proves their suitability for intravenous administration.

The determination of the EE is an integral part of the physicochemical properties of the nanosystems and was performed to acquire quantitative data on the amount of encapsulated CW-02-79. The obtained results indicate that the CW-02-79-phospholipid complex was completely encapsulated in the oil phase (98.33%, 96.33%, 96.37%, and 97.89% for $CW_{PC}NE1$, $CW_{PC}NE2$, $CW_{PC}NE3$, and $CW_{PC}NE4$, respectively), with minor differences between the tested formulations. This finding clearly confirmed that the formation of phospholipid at the ratio of 1:10 significantly improved the lipophilicity of CW-02-79, retaining it in the oil core of the nanoemulsions.

3.4. Stability Study—Impact of Steam Sterilization and Storage

The preliminary stability study of the optimal formulations was conducted during three months of storage at 25 °C analyzing the visual appearance and the following physicochemical parameters: Z-ave, PDI, ZP, pH value, EC, and osmolality. Considering the parenteral route of administration and strict requirements for the product's sterility, the impact of steam sterilization (autoclave, 15 min at 121 °C) was also monitored.

Interestingly, autoclaving did not significantly change the physicochemical properties of any of the developed nanoemulsions, neither immediately after preparation nor during the three-month storage period. In fact, all the nanoemulsions retained their original appearance after three months of storage, and no difference was observed between the non-autoclaved and autoclaved samples. Importantly, no CW-02-79 crystals were detected using polarization microscopy, confirming the absence of CW-02-79 precipitation. Moreover, the Z-ave and PDI remained almost unchanged during the storage period, indicating the homogeneous distribution of nanodroplets and a lack of coalescence within the system. On the other hand, immediately after autoclaving, the ZP of the undecorated formulations decreased significantly, but it changed only slightly in the PEGylated formulations. The same trend was observed over the course of three months, suggesting that PEGylated phospholipids at the droplet surface protect the negative surface charge provided by the phospholipids. However, it is important to note that the absolute ZP values of the autoclaved and non-autoclaved samples were still higher than $|-30 \text{ mV}|$ after three months of storage, demonstrating sufficient electrostatic forces for droplet repulsion.

Similarly, the pH decreased significantly after autoclaving in all the developed formulations, although the decrease was more pronounced in the undecorated formulation. This phenomenon is well described in the literature and can be attributed to the hydrolysis of phospholipids and castor oil and thus the release of fatty acids during exposure to heat [16]. The decrease in pH was accompanied by an increase in the EC, as a greater amount of free H^+ was present in the aqueous phase. During the three-month storage period, a significant drop in pH was observed in all the formulations tested, indicating the need for variation in the selection of antioxidants. Osmolality remained in the same range suitable for intravenous administration. Overall, the results obtained indicate a satisfactory preliminary physicochemical stability of the developed nanoemulsions containing the phospholipid complex of CW-02-79. Importantly, they can withstand heat stress during steam sterilization, which is of paramount importance to ensure an adequate level of sterility, which is required for intravenous administration products.

3.5. Protein Binding Studies

After an intravenous injection, depending on the size, charge, and surface chemistry of the nanodroplets, proteins can bind to the their surfaces immediately after entering the bloodstream, and form a shell, the so-called protein corona. This layer can change the droplet size and their recognition via MPS, thus impairing their functionality and biological distribution. Likewise, a protein corona may trigger droplet aggregation, influencing the nanoemulsion safety [34]. To predict the behavior of the developed nanoemulsions in biological systems, we analyzed the interactions with the proteins by measuring the change in droplet size as a function of time after incubation with (i) the PBS containing BSA as the most abundant protein in plasma as well as with (ii) the PBS containing FBS, a more complex medium used in cell cultures, and rich in growth factors, hormones, amino acids, proteins, and vitamins [35].

During the 24 h incubation of the tested nanoemulsions with the pure PBS, the Z-ave and PDI were almost constant. Therefore, the changes in these parameters after incubation with the BSA-containing medium are due to albumin binding on the surface of the nanodroplets (Figure 4). A statistically significant increase in the Z-ave and PDI was observed primarily in the undecorated $CW_{PC}NE1$ formulation, indicating that the undecorated droplet surface has a high affinity for albumin binding. It has been shown that PEG chains can sterically hinder the access of serum proteins to the nanodroplet surface if PEGylated phospholipids are present in the optimal concentrations in the nanoformulation [18]. However, when 0.2% and 0.3% DSPE-PEG2000 ($CW_{PC}NE2$ and $CW_{PC}NE3$ formulations) were used, the droplet size and PDI statistically increased after incubation with BSA, indicating albumin binding to the surface. On the other hand, the interactions were less pronounced in the formulations prepared with 0.2% DSPE-PEG2000 and 0.1% DSPE-PEG2000-mannose. These results suggest that the addition of DSPE-PEG2000-mannose improves the stability of the nanodroplets in protein-enriched medium by providing additional hydrophilicity and steric hindrance.

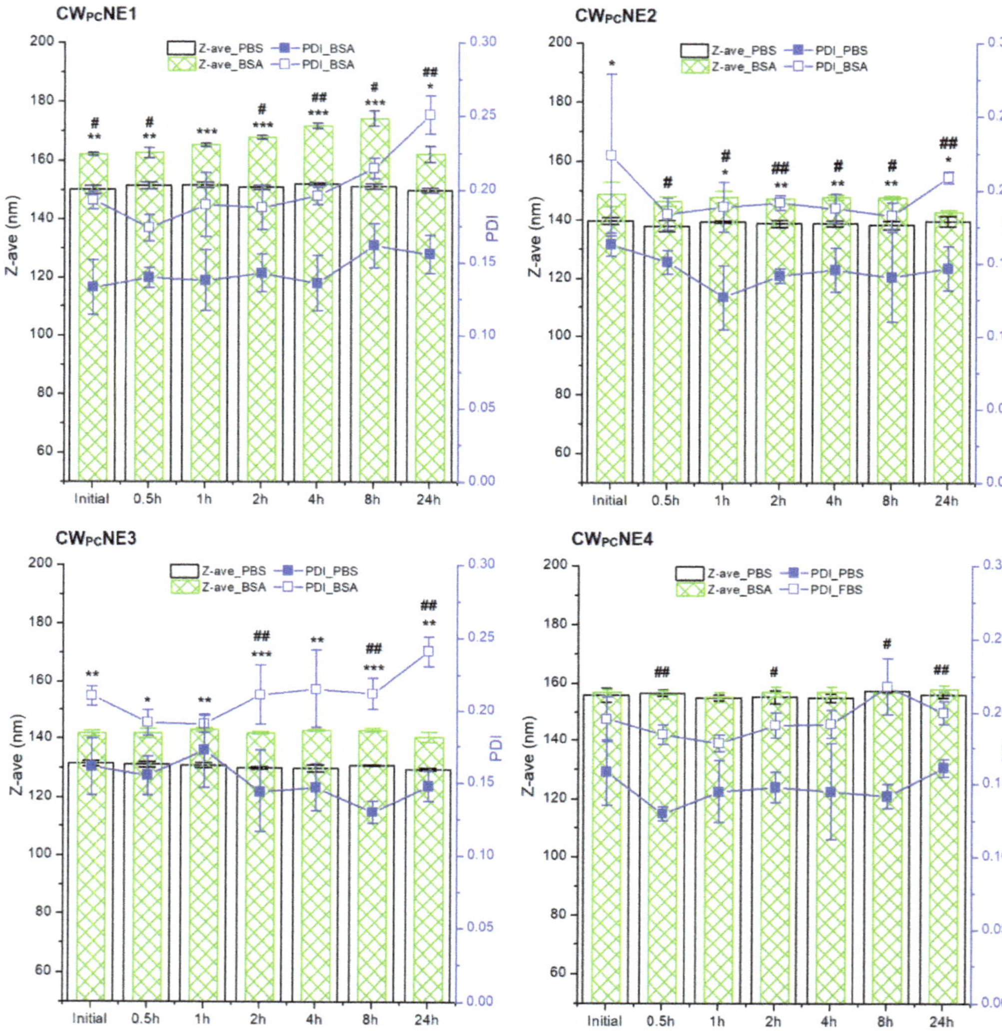

Figure 4. The changes in droplet size (Z-ave) and polydispersity index (PDI) of developed nanoemulsions during 24 h incubation in phosphate buffer saline (PBS)- and bovine serum albumin (BSA)-enriched PBS, reflecting the interactions of the nanodroplets with the protein-enriched media. * $p < 0.05$, ** $p < 0.01$, *** $p < 0.001$ compared to the Z-ave in PBS for each time point; # $p < 0.05$, ## $p < 0.01$, compared to the PDI values in PBS for each time point.

After the incubation of the tested formulations with a medium containing FBS (10%), no significant changes were observed in the Z-ave and PDI compared to the values of these parameters measured after incubation with pure PBS (Figure S3, Supplementary Materials). Furthermore, a very slight difference was detected between the undecorated and PEGylated formulations, suggesting that FBS does not bind strongly to the surface of nanodroplets. This could be ascribed to a lower protein concentration in the FBS medium and/or competing effects between different biomolecules on the droplet surface limiting protein binding.

In summary, the results of the comprehensive characterization revealed that the dual surface decoration with DSPE-PEG2000 and DSPE-PEG2000-mannose resulted in a nanoemulsion with satisfactory physicochemical properties, stability, and low protein binding affinity ($CW_{PC}NE4$). Therefore, it was selected as promising for evaluating the transport of CW-02-79 across the BBB in vitro and in vivo, compared to the undecorated formulation ($CW_{PC}NE1$).

3.6. In Vitro Release Study

Although not a direct indication of the drug bioavailability in vivo, the in vitro release data obtained by the direct dialysis bag method was used to evaluate how the internal structure and formulation composition of the tested nanoemulsions affect the release rate of CW-02-79, providing a deeper understanding of the complexity of the factors involved in the delivery of CW-02-79 to the brain. The obtained in vitro release profiles are shown in Figure 5. After 24 h, 67.26 ± 4.28 and 56.64 ± 2.84 (%) of CW-02-79 was released from the $CW_{PC}NE1$ and $CW_{PC}NE4$ formulations, respectively, indicating the sustained release of CW-02-79 from both formulations tested. It seems that CW-02-79 needs time to dissociate from the phospholipid complex, then diffuse from the oil core through the interfacial stabilizer layer and finally reach the aqueous medium [36]. However, it should be noted that the addition of PEGylated phospholipids remarkably restricted the release of CW-02-79 compared to the undecorated nanoemulsion. Since both nanoemulsions exhibited similar physicochemical properties (Z-ave, PDI, ZP, pH, and EE), the formation of a more densely packed layer at the oil–water interface could be responsible for the observed lower release rate of CW-02-79 from the $CW_{PC}NE4$ formulation. In addition, the modeling of the release data (Table S2, Supplementary Materials) revealed that the release of CW-02-79 from both tested nanoemulsions can be best described by a first-order kinetic model. According to the literature data, this means that the release of CW-02-79 from the tested nanoemulsions follows a concentration gradient—the amount released is directly proportional to the amount remaining in the nanoemulsion and decreases with time, leading to the sustained release profile [37].

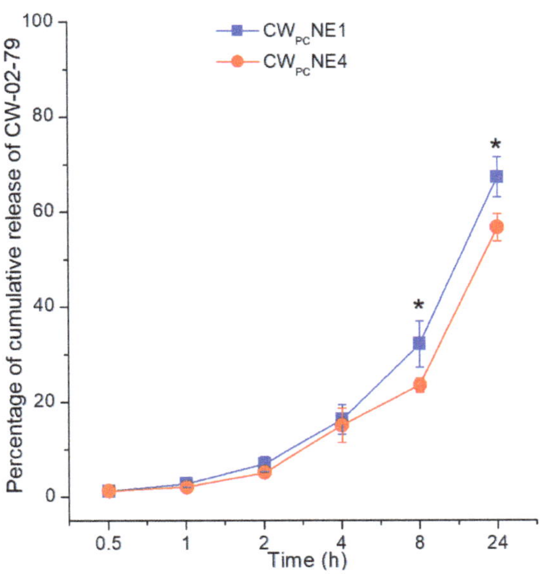

Figure 5. Cumulative release profile of CW-02-79 from selected nanoemulsions ($CW_{PC}NE1$ and $CW_{PC}NE4$). Values are shown as means ± SD ($n = 3$); * $p < 0.05$, $CW_{PC}NE1$ vs. $CW_{PC}NE4$.

3.7. In Vitro Permeation Through the Blood–Brain Barrier

The BBB is responsible for the high failure rate of most new drug candidates targeting CNS disorders, as it hinders their entry into the brain in a therapeutically effective amount. Therefore, a vigorous in vitro BBB model that closely resembles the structure and functions of the human BBB is needed in the early stages of new drug/delivery system development [38]. Most BBB models declared to assess the permeability of parenteral nanoparticles are based on a monolayer of endothelial cells in the Transwell inserts [16]. However, these models do not adequately reflect the complex structure of the BBB, as barriergenic modulatory stimuli from neighboring cells are missing. Namely, a close collaboration between endothelial cells and adjacent astrocytes and pericytes is required to control the function of the tight junctions [39]. To investigate the ability of the dual-modified nanoemulsion loaded with the phospholipid complex to efficiently transport CW-02-079 across the BBB, we used an advanced in vitro iPSC-derived BBB model consisting of the co-culture of brain microvascular endothelial cells, astrocytes, and pericytes. Compared to other similar models described in the literature, the main advantages of this model are its human origin (all three cell types were differentiated from human iPSCs of the same donor), and its functional performance as assessed by the transendothelial electrical resistance (TEER) assay (>1500 $\Omega \cdot cm^2$) (iCell Blood-Brain Barrier Isogenic Kit) [24]. Prior to the application of the nanoemulsions, TEER measurements were performed, and the values obtained (1616.34 $\pm$ 184.17 $\Omega \cdot cm^2$) indicated satisfactory barrier integrity, according to the manufacturer's specification. In addition, to gain insight into the status of the BBB model upon exposure to the nanoformulations, TEER values were also measured at the end of the experiment, 24 h after the application of the tested nanoemulsions. The TEER values obtained (1801.8 $\pm$ 171.23 $\Omega \cdot cm^2$) did not differ remarkably, demonstrating the preserved barrier integrity and the absence of a cytotoxic effect of the tested nanoemulsions in the concentration used.

The Pe of CW-02-79 from the dual functionalized nanoemulsion containing 0.2% PEG2000-DSPE and 0.1% DSPE-PEG2000-mannose (0.232 $\times$ 10^{-3} cm/min) was slightly lower compared to the plain, undecorated formulation (0.432 $\times$ 10^{-3} cm/min). No statistically significant difference was found between these two formulations in terms of the amount of CW-02-79 permeating through the BBB model used (Figure 6). These results, showing the limited permeability of CW-02-79 through the BBB, were in good agreement with the release profiles of the investigated nanoemulsions. It appears that the rate of release was the limiting factor for the efficient uptake of CW-02-79 across the BBB. Similarly, the mass balance calculations (73.58% and 78.18% for $CW_{PC}NE1$ and $CW_{PC}NE4$, respectively) revealed that a certain amount of CW-02-79 was retained in the endothelial cells, astrocytes, and pericytes of the BBB. Since the recovery of CW-02-79 without cells was nearly 100%, these results demonstrate the absence of non-specific binding to plastic inserts and the slower diffusion through the BBB model used. A similar result was reported for the permeation of diazepam through the BBB model consisting of bovine brain capillary endothelial cells (bBCECs) co-cultured with primary rat glial cells (astrocytes, oligodendrocytes, and microglia) [25]. However, it is evident that the expected permeation-enhancing effect of the mannose ligand, targeting the GLUT-1 receptors at the BBB, was completely absent. Therefore, the in vivo neuropharmacokinetic study provided further insights into the delivery of CW-02-79 to the brain.

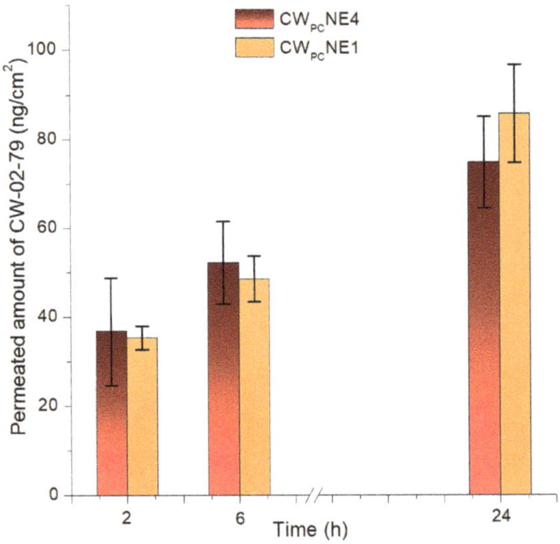

Figure 6. Transport of CW-02-79 through the in vitro iPSC-based blood–brain barrier model from the selected decorated (CW$_{PC}$NE4) and undecorated (CW$_{PC}$NE1) nanoemulsions. Values are shown as mean ± SD (n = 3).

3.8. Neuropharmacokinetic Study

To investigate the potential of the dual modification of the nanoemulsion surface with PEGylated phospholipid and the GLUT-1 targeting ligand DSPE-PEG2000-mannose to improve the delivery of CW-02-79 to the brain and its suitability for preclinical testing, a neuropharmacokinetic study was conducted in adult male rats. Based on previous studies, two favorable formulations of CW-02-79, mannose-decorated (CW$_{PC}$NE4) and undecorated (CW$_{PC}$NE1), were administered intravenously at a well-tolerated dose of 7.5 mg/kg. Due to the limited solubility of CW-02-79, it was not possible to prepare a solution of CW-02-79 without using a high concentration of both dimethyl sulfoxide and surfactants, so making it non-biocompatible/toxic for intravenous administration to animals.

The mean plasma concentration curves in male rats after intravenous administration are presented in Figure 7a, and the calculated pharmacokinetic parameters were estimated via non-compartmental analysis and are summarized in Table 4. No adverse events were observed in either group after intravenous administration of the selected nanoemulsions. Blood concentrations of CW-02-79 tended to be slightly higher after administration of the decorated compared to undecorated formulation, but a statistically significant difference was found only after 3 h (t-test, $p < 0.05$). The area under the curve ($AUC_{0\text{–}24}$) of CW-02-79 in plasma from CW$_{PC}$NE4-treated rats was 1.13-fold higher than that from CW$_{PC}$NE1 rats. On the other hand, Cmax was 1.43-fold lower in CW$_{PC}$NE4-treated rats. These apparently discordant findings are consistent with the data on in vitro release and permeation across the BBB. The decorated nanoemulsion exhibits a slow release, as CW-02-79 must first dissociate from the phospholipid complex into oil droplets, then diffuse through the interfacial layer and finally enter the bloodstream [12]. Nevertheless, the half-life ($t_{1/2}$) of CW-02-79 in plasma was shorter in rats treated with CW$_{PC}$NE4 than in those treated with CW$_{PC}$NE1. The shorter half-life of the decorated nanoemulsion could be explained by the brain delivery targeted by binding to GLUT-1 and endocytosis-mediated transport across the BBB [40], and also by the distribution of the nanodroplets in other organs and tissues.

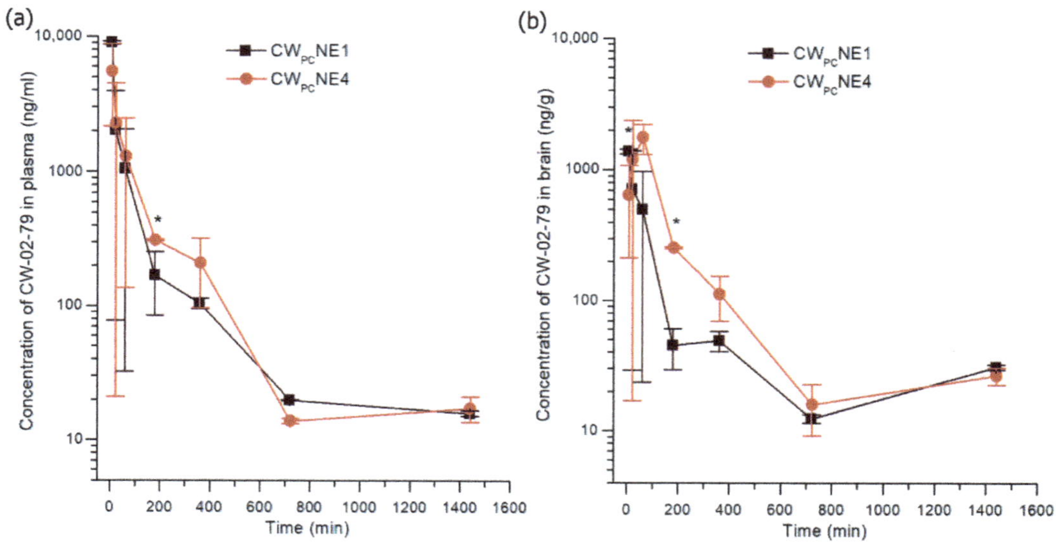

Figure 7. Plasma (**a**) and brain (**b**) concentration time curve after intravenous administration of selected nanoemulsions ($CW_{PC}NE1$ and $CW_{PC}NE4$) to male rats. Values are shown as means ± SD, $n = 3$. * $p < 0.05$ compared with $CW_{PC}NE1$.

Table 4. Calculated pharmacokinetic parameters of CW-02-79 after intravenous administration of selected nanoemulsions $CW_{PC}NE1$ and $CW_{PC}NE4$. Values are shown as means ± SD, $n = 3$.

Parameter	**Formulation**	
	CW_{PC} NE1	**CW_{PC} NE4**
Plasma		
C_{max} (ng/mL)	8964.35 ± 250.78	6280.30 ± 2265.22
T_{max} (h)	0.083 ± 0.00	0.16 ± 0.14
$AUC_{0–24}$ (h·ng/mL)	5934.46 ± 1082.25	6680.29 ± 1396.42
$t_{1/2}$ (h)	6.48 ± 1.35	3.53 ± 0.63 *
Brain		
C_{max} (ng/g)	1377.53 ± 58.32	1279.49 ± 1069.41
T_{max} (h)	0.083 ± 0.0	1.22 ± 1.53 *
$AUC_{0–24}$ (h·ng/g)	1961.74 ± 712.00	2913.77 ± 985.67
$t_{1/2}$ (h)	6.37 ± 3.13	4.78 ± 0.93

C_{max}: maximum concentration; T_{max}: maximum concentration; $t_{1/2}$: elimination half-life; $AUC_{0–t}$: area under the curve from time zero to 24 h. * $p < 0.05$ compared with $CW_{PC}NE1$.

The neuropharmacokinetic profile of CW-02-79 after the intravenous administration of a dose of 7.5 mg/kg is shown in Figure 7b. The brain concentrations were slightly higher after the administration of the decorated compared to the undecorated nanoemulsion, with the difference being significant only after 3 h (*t*-test, $p < 0.05$), which follows the pattern seen in plasma. The brain-to-plasma partition coefficients for the decorated and undecorated nanoemulsion were 43.6% and 33.1%, respectively, and reflect moderate levels of brain exposure [41]. Introducing dual surface decoration with PEGylated phospholipids and DSPE-PEG2000-mannose in the nanoemulsion preparation resulted in an increase in brain $AUC_{0–24}$ values of 48.5%; however, the difference was statistically insignificant.

When interpreting the presented partial proof of concept that the surface decoration of the nanoemulsion with the GLUT-1-targeting ligand DSPE-PEG2000-mannose can enhance the GLUT-1-mediated permeation through the BBB, two caveats should be noted. First, for a complete insight into the brain exposure, the ratio of unbound drug in the brain to unbound drug in the plasma would need to be determined [42]. Second, a recent study by Lei et al. [21] showed that the glycemic control strategy plays an important role in shifting GLUT-1 from the apical to the basolateral side of the BBB, allowing the mannose-decorated nanodroplets to penetrate the BBB and accumulate in the brain. In addition, the complex and sex-dependent role of σ2 receptors in metabolic regulation was recently discovered in mice [43]. In our study, the blood glucose level of rats was not controlled, which might be related to the suboptimal permeation of mannose-decorated nanoemulsions into the brain. Therefore, further studies should aim to evaluate the unbound brain-to-plasma partition coefficients of the discovered σ2 receptor ligand in the settings of controlled glycemia in rats of both sexes and possibly with different concentrations of DSPE-PEG2000-mannose.

4. Conclusions

Due to its limited water and oil solubility, it was not possible to prepare a conventional delivery vehicle for the novel pyrazoloquinolinone ligand CW-02-79 without using non-biocompatible solvents. Based on systemic exploration, a two-fold formulation strategy was applied, combining phospholipid complexes and lipid nanoemulsions to improve the liposolubility of CW-02-79 by introducing decoration to enhance the brain-targeting efficiency. The developed biocompatible nanoemulsion loaded with the CW-02-079—phospholipid complex at a mass ratio of 1:10 exhibited a small droplet size and narrow size distribution as well as satisfactory physicochemical stability during steam sterilization and short-term storage at 25 °C, making it suitable for intravenous administration. The analysis of protein-binding interactions revealed that the PEGylated nanoemulsions had fewer observable interactions compared to the undecorated nanoemulsions, especially when 0.2% DSPE-PEG2000 and 0.1% DSPE-PEG2000-mannose were combined. The neuropharmacokinetic study showed that there were minor differences in the pharmacokinetic parameters favoring the dual surface-functionalized nanoemulsion with PEGylated phospholipids and the GLUT-1-targeting ligand DSPE-PEG2000-mannose to facilitate BBB crossing and enhance transport into the brain. The study suggests, overall, that this formulation is suitable for the preclinical testing of ligands such as CW-02-79, but further research is required to optimize their targeted delivery to the brain.

Supplementary Materials: The following supporting information can be downloaded at: https://www.mdpi.com/article/10.3390/pharmaceutics17020232/s1. Table S1. Solubility of CW-02-79 in the selected solvents, Table S2. Interpretation the release kinetics of selected nanoemulsions by fitting in vitro drug release data to different models, Figure S1. XRPD pattern of unprocessed CW-02-79, Figure S2. DSC thermograms showing the crystallization tendency of CW-02-79 after melt quenching, Figure S3. The changes of droplet size (Z-ave) and polydispersity index (PDI) of developed nanoemulsions during 24-h incubation in phosphate buffer saline (PBS) and fetal bovine serum (FBS) enriched PBS, reflecting the interactions of the nanodroplets with the biological media.

Author Contributions: Conceptualization, T.S., T.I., M.M.S. and S.S.; methodology T.S., T.I., B.D.M., M.P., V.D., I.J., B.B., K.J., J.Đ., I.P., D.R., D.S. and M.M.S.; validation, V.D. and D.S., formal analysis, T.S. and T.I.; investigation, T.S., T.I., B.D.M., M.P., V.D., I.J., B.B., K.J., J.Đ., I.P., D.R. and M.M.S.; resources, D.S. and J.M.C.; data curation, T.S.; writing—original draft preparation, T.S. and T.I.; writing—review and editing, M.M.S. and S.S.; visualization, T.S. and T.I.; supervision, T.I., M.M.S. and S.S.; project administration, M.M.S.; funding acquisition, J.M.C. and M.M.S. All authors have read and agreed to the published version of the manuscript.

Funding: This research was funded by the Science Fund of the Republic of Serbia, Grant No. 7749108, Neuroimmune aspects of mood, anxiety and cognitive effects of leads/drug candidates acting at GABAA and/or sigma-2 receptors: In vitro/in vivo delineation by nano- and hiPSC-based platform-NanoCellEmoCog and supported by the Ministry of Education, Science and Technological

Development, Republic of Serbia, through two Grant Agreements with the University of Belgrade's Faculty of Pharmacy, No. 451-03-65/2024-03/200161 and No. 451-03-66/2024-03/200161 and with the Institute of Chemistry, Technology and Metallurgy, No. 451-03-66/2024-03/200026. We would also like to acknowledge the National Institutes of Health, USA (2R01 DA043204-06A1 (NIDA), R01 AA029023 (NIAAA) and R01 DA054177 (NIDA) subawarded to JMC).

Institutional Review Board Statement: The study was conducted according to the National Institutes of Health Animal Care and Use Committee guidelines and approved by the Ethics Committee on Animal Experimentation of the University of Belgrade-Faculty of Pharmacy (Serbia) and Ministry of agriculture, forestry and water management-Veterinary Directorate (323-07-10046/2020-05).

Informed Consent Statement: Not applicable.

Data Availability Statement: The original contributions presented in this study are included in the article/Supplementary Materials. Further inquiries can be directed to the corresponding author(s).

Acknowledgments: We thank PDSP services and Bryan Roth (UNC Chapel Hill) for profiling CW-02-79 against 47 CNS receptors and other targets. CW-02-79 (10 μM) binding to receptors in the NIMH PDSP was performed in technical quadruplicate per SOPs in the PDSP assay protocol book, which can be found at https://pdspdb.unc.edu/pdspweb/ (accessed on 29 December 2024).

Conflicts of Interest: JMC and MMS are listed inventors on patents covering the syntheses and use of the compound.

Abbreviations

The following abbreviations are used in this manuscript:

AFM	Atomic Force Microscopy
BBB	Blood Brain Barrier
bBCEC	Bovine Brain Capillary Endothelial Cell
BHT	Butylhydroxyltoluene
BMEC	Brain Microvascular Endothelial cells
BSA	Bovine Serum Albumin
CW_{PC}	CW-02-79—phospholipid complex
CW_{PM}	CW-02-79—physical mixture
DLS	Dynamic Light Scattering
DMSO	Dimethyl Sulfoxide
DSC	Differential Scanning Calorimetry
EC	Electrical Conductivity
EE	Encapsulation Efficiency
FBS	Fetal Bovine Serum
FT-IR	Fourier Transform Infrared Spectroscopy
$GABA_A$	γ-aminobutyric acid type A
GLUT-1	Glucose Transporter-1
HLB	Hydrophilic–Lipophilic Balance
HPH	High-Pressure Homogenization
iPSCs	Induced Pluripotent Stem Cells
LC-MS/MS	Liquid Chromatography with Tandem Mass Spectrometry
MCT	Medium-Chain Triglycerides
MPS	Mononuclear Phagocytic System
MW	Molecular Weight
NMR	Nuclear Magnetic Resonance
PBS	Phosphate Buffer Saline
PDI	Polydispersity Index
PDSP	Psychoactive Drug Screening Program
Pe	Permeability Coefficient
ppm	Parts Per Million

SD	Standard Deviation
TEER	Trans Endothelial Electrical Resistance
UHPLC	Ultra-High-Performance Liquid Chromatography
XRPD	X-Ray Powder Diffraction
Z-ave	Intensity-Weighted Mean Hydrodynamic diameter
ZP	Zeta Potential
σ2	Sigma-2 Receptors

References

1. Czernik, A.J.; Petrack, B.; Kalinsky, H.; Psychoyos, S.; Cash, W.D.; Tsai, C.; Rinehart, R.K.; Granat, F.R.; Lovell, R.A.; Brundish, D.E.; et al. CGS 8216: Receptor binding characteristics of a potent benzodiazepine antagonist. *Life Sci.* **1982**, *30*, 363–372. [CrossRef]
2. Knutson, D.E.; Kodali, R.; Divović, B.; Treven, M.; Stephen, M.R.; Zahn, N.M.; Dobričić, V.; Huber, A.T.; Meirelles, M.A.; Verma, R.S.; et al. Design and Synthesis of Novel Deuterated Ligands Functionally Selective for the γ-Aminobutyric Acid Type A Receptor (GABAAR) α6 Subtype with Improved Metabolic Stability and Enhanced Bioavailability. *J. Med. Chem.* **2018**, *61*, 2422–2446. [CrossRef]
3. Takchi, R.; Prudner, B.C.; Gong, Q.; Hagi, T.; Newcomer, K.F.; Jin, L.X.; Vangveravong, S.; Van Tine, B.A.; Hawkins, W.G.; Spitzer, D. Cytotoxic sigma-2 ligands trigger cancer cell death via cholesterol-induced-ER-stress. *Cell Death Dis.* **2024**, *15*, 309. [CrossRef]
4. Piechal, A.; Jakimiuk, A.; Mirowska-Guzel, D. Sigma receptors and neurological disorders. *Pharmacol. Rep.* **2021**, *73*, 1582–1594. [CrossRef]
5. Malar, D.S.; Thitilertdecha, P.; Ruckvongacheep, K.S.; Brimson, S.; Tencomnao, T.; Brimson, J.M. Targeting Sigma Receptors for the Treatment of Neurodegenerative and Neurodevelopmental Disorders. *CNS Drugs* **2023**, *37*, 399–440. [CrossRef]
6. Kuche, K.; Bhargavi, N.; Dora, C.P.; Jain, S. Drug-Phospholipid Complex-a Go Through Strategy for Enhanced Oral Bioavailability. *AAPS PharmSciTech* **2019**, *20*, 43. [CrossRef]
7. Waghule, T.; Saha, R.N.; Alexander, A.; Singhvi, G. Tailoring the multi-functional properties of phospholipids for simple to complex self-assemblies. *J. Control. Release* **2022**, *349*, 460–474. [CrossRef]
8. Patil, J.; Pawde, D.M.; Bhattacharya, S.; Srivastava, S. Phospholipid Complex Formulation Technology for Improved Drug Delivery in Oncological Settings: A Comprehensive Review. *AAPS PharmSciTech* **2024**, *25*, 91. [CrossRef]
9. Dora, C.P.; Kushwah, V.; Yadav, V.; Kuche, K.; Jain, S. Gemcitabine-Phospholipid Complex Loaded Lipid Nanoparticles for Improving Drug Loading, Stability, and Efficacy against Pancreatic Cancer. *Mol. Pharm.* **2024**, *21*, 2699–2712. [CrossRef]
10. Dong, W.; Ye, J.; Wang, W.; Yang, Y.; Wang, H.; Sun, T.; Gao, L.; Liu, Y. Self-Assembled Lecithin/Chitosan Nanoparticles Based on Phospholipid Complex: A Feasible Strategy to Improve Entrapment Efficiency and Transdermal Delivery of Poorly Lipophilic Drug. *Int. J. Nanomed.* **2020**, *15*, 5629–5643. [CrossRef]
11. Zhang, Z.; Chen, Y.; Deng, J.; Jia, X.; Zhou, J.; Lv, H. Solid dispersion of berberine-phospholipid complex/TPGS 1000/SiO_2: Preparation, characterization and in vivo studies. *Int. J. Pharm.* **2014**, *465*, 306–316. [CrossRef] [PubMed]
12. Lu, Y.; Zhang, Y.; Yang, Z.; Tang, X. Formulation of an intravenous emulsion loaded with a clarithromycin-phospholipid complex and its pharmacokinetics in rats. *Int. J. Pharm.* **2009**, *366*, 160–169. [CrossRef] [PubMed]
13. Li, Y.; Jin, W.; Yan, H.; Liu, H.; Wang, C. Development of intravenous lipid emulsion of vinorelbine based on drug-phospholipid complex technique. *Int. J. Pharm.* **2013**, *454*, 472–477. [CrossRef] [PubMed]
14. Li, Y.; Yin, H.; Wu, C.; He, J.; Wang, C.; Ren, B.; Wang, H.; Geng, D.; Zhang, Y.; Zhao, L. Preparation and in vivo evaluation of an intravenous emulsion loaded with an aprepitant-phospholipid complex. *Drug Deliv.* **2023**, *30*, 2183834. [CrossRef]
15. Bisso, S.; Leroux, J.C. Nanopharmaceuticals: A focus on their clinical translatability. *Int. J. Pharm.* **2020**, *578*, 119098. [CrossRef]
16. Ilić, T.; Đoković, J.B.; Nikolić, I.; Mitrović, J.R.; Pantelić, I.; Savić, S.D.; Savić, M.M. Parenteral Lipid-Based Nanoparticles for CNS Disorders: Integrating Various Facets of Preclinical Evaluation towards More Effective Clinical Translation. *Pharmaceutics* **2023**, *15*, 443. [CrossRef]
17. Gajbhiye, K.R.; Pawar, A.; Mahadik, K.R.; Gajbhiye, V. PEGylated nanocarriers: A promising tool for targeted delivery to the brain. *Colloids Surf. B Biointerfaces* **2020**, *187*, 110770. [CrossRef]
18. Đoković, J.B.; Demisli, S.; Savić, S.M.; Savić, S.R.; Randjelović, D.V.; Marković, B.M.; Pantelić, I.; Mitrović, J.R.; Stanković, T.; Papadimitrou, V.; et al. Evaluation of PEGylation efficacy of curcumin-loaded nanoemulsions using complementary methods to assess protein interactions and physicochemical properties. *J. Mol. Liq.* **2024**, *404*, 124888. [CrossRef]
19. Arora, S.; Sharma, D.; Singh, J. GLUT-1: An Effective Target to Deliver Brain-Derived Neurotrophic Factor Gene Across the Blood Brain Barrier. *ACS Chem. Neurosci.* **2020**, *11*, 1620–1633. [CrossRef]

20. Du, D.; Chang, N.; Sun, S.; Li, M.; Yu, H.; Liu, M.; Liu, X.; Wang, G.; Li, H.; Liu, X.; et al. The role of glucose transporters in the distribution of p-aminophenyl-α-d-mannopyranoside modified liposomes within mice brain. *J. Control. Release* **2014**, *182*, 99–110. [CrossRef]
21. Lei, T.; Yang, Z.; Jiang, C.; Wang, X.; Yang, W.; Yang, X.; Xie, R.; Tong, F.; Xia, X.; Huang, Q.; et al. Mannose-Integrated Nanoparticle Hitchhike Glucose Transporter 1 Recycling to Overcome Various Barriers of Oral Delivery for Alzheimer's Disease Therapy. *ACS Nano* **2024**, *18*, 3234–3250. [CrossRef] [PubMed]
22. Ruge, C.A.; Hillairea, H.; Grabowski, N.; Beck-Broichsitter, M.; Cañadas, O.; Tsapis, N.; Casals, C.; Nicolas, J.; Fattal, E. Pulmonary Surfactant Protein A-Mediated Enrichment of Surface-Decorated Polymeric Nanoparticles in Alveolar Macrophages. *Mol. Pharm.* **2016**, *13*, 4168–4178. [CrossRef] [PubMed]
23. Ye, J.; Yang, Y.; Jin, J.; Ji, M.; Gao, Y.; Feng, Y.; Wang, H.; Chen, X.; Liu, Y. Targeted delivery of chlorogenic acid by mannosylated liposomes to effectively promote the polarization of TAMs for the treatment of glioblastoma. *Bioact. Mater.* **2020**, *5*, 694–708. [CrossRef] [PubMed]
24. iCell Blood-Brain Barrier Isogenic Kit. Available online: https://www.fujifilmcdi.com/icell-blood-brain-barrier-isogenic-kit-01279-r1241 (accessed on 27 December 2024).
25. Heymans, M.; Sevin, E.; Gosselet, F.; Lundquist, S.; Culot, M. Mimicking brain tissue binding in an in vitro model of the blood-brain barrier illustrates differences between in vitro and in vivo methods for assessing the rate of brain penetration. *Eur. J. Pharm. Biopharm.* **2018**, *127*, 453–461; Erratum in *Eur. J. Pharm. Biopharm.* **2018**, *133*, 200–202. [CrossRef]
26. Rantanen, J.; Rades, T.; Strachan, C. Solid-state analysis for pharmaceuticals: Pathways to feasible and meaningful analysis. *J. Pharm. Biomed. Anal.* **2023**, *236*, 115649. [CrossRef]
27. Freag, M.S.; Saleh, W.M.; Abdallah, O.Y. Self-assembled phospholipid-based phytosomal nanocarriers as promising platforms for improving oral bioavailability of the anticancer celastrol. *Int. J. Pharm.* **2018**, *535*, 18–26. [CrossRef]
28. Ebada, H.M.K.; Nasra, M.M.A.; Elnaggar, Y.S.R.; Abdallah, O.Y. Novel rhein-phospholipid complex targeting skin diseases: Development, in vitro, ex vivo, and in vivo studies. *Drug Deliv. Transl. Res.* **2021**, *11*, 1107–1118. [CrossRef]
29. Rachmawati, H.; Arvin, Y.A.; Asyarie, S.; Anggadiredja, K.; Tjandrawinata, R.R.; Storm, G. Local sustained delivery of bupivacaine HCl from a new castor oil-based nanoemulsion system. *Drug Deliv. Transl. Res.* **2018**, *8*, 515–524. [CrossRef]
30. Pires, P.C.; Paiva-Santos, A.C.; Veiga, F. Antipsychotics-Loaded Nanometric Emulsions for Brain Delivery. *Pharmaceutics* **2022**, *14*, 2174. [CrossRef]
31. Đorđević, S.M.; Cekić, N.D.; Savić, M.M.; Isailović, T.M.; Ranđelović, D.V.; Marković, B.D.; Savić, S.R.; Timić Stamenić, T.; Daniels, R.; Savić, S.D. Parenteral nanoemulsions as promising carriers for brain delivery of risperidone: Design, characterization and in vivo pharmacokinetic evaluation. *Int. J. Pharm.* **2015**, *493*, 40–54. [CrossRef]
32. Yokoyama, R.; Taharabaru, T.; Nishida, T.; Ohno, Y.; Maeda, Y.; Sato, M.; Ishikura, K.; Yanagihara, K.; Takagi, H.; Nakamura, T.; et al. Lactose-appended β-cyclodextrin as an effective nanocarrier for brain delivery. *J. Control. Release* **2020**, *328*, 722–735. [CrossRef] [PubMed]
33. Varenne, F.; Makky, A.; Gaucher-Delmas, M.; Violleau, F.; Vauthier, C. Multimodal Dispersion of Nanoparticles: A Comprehensive Evaluation of Size Distribution with 9 Size Measurement Methods. *Pharm. Res.* **2016**, *33*, 1220–1234. [CrossRef] [PubMed]
34. Khan, S.; Sharifi, M.; Gleghorn, J.P.; Babadaei, M.M.N.; Bloukh, S.H.; Edis, Z.; Amin, M.; Bai, Q.; Ten Hagen, T.L.M.; Falahati, M.; et al. Artificial engineering of the protein corona at bio-nano interfaces for improved cancer-targeted nanotherapy. *J. Control. Release* **2022**, *348*, 127–147. [CrossRef]
35. Ferreira, L.F.; Picco, A.S.; Galdino, F.E.; Albuquerque, L.J.C.; Berret, J.F.; Cardoso, M.B. Nanoparticle-Protein Interaction: Demystifying the Correlation between Protein Corona and Aggregation Phenomena. *ACS Appl. Mater. Interfaces* **2022**, *14*, 28559–28569. [CrossRef]
36. Buyukozturk, F.; Benneyan, J.C.; Carrier, R.L. Impact of emulsion-based drug delivery systems on intestinal permeability and drug release kinetics. *J. Control. Release* **2010**, *142*, 22–30. [CrossRef]
37. Costa, P.; Sousa Lobo, J.M. Modeling and comparison of dissolution profiles. *Eur. J. Pharm. Sci.* **2001**, *13*, 123–133. [CrossRef]
38. Zhu, Q.; Huang, Y.; Zhu, X.; Peng, L.; Wang, H.; Gao, S.; Yang, Z.; Zhang, J.; Liu, X. Mannose-coated superparamagnetic iron oxide nanozyme for preventing postoperative cognitive dysfunction. *Mater. Today Bio* **2023**, *19*, 100568. [CrossRef]
39. Song, Y.; Du, D.; Li, L.; Xu, J.; Dutta, P.; Lin, Y. In Vitro Study of Receptor-Mediated Silica Nanoparticles Delivery across Blood-Brain Barrier. *ACS Appl. Mater. Interfaces* **2017**, *9*, 20410–20416. [CrossRef]
40. Handa, M.; Sanap, S.N.; Bhatta, R.S.; Patil, G.P.; Ghose, S.; Singh, D.P.; Shukla, R. Combining donepezil and memantine via mannosylated PLGA nanoparticles for intranasal delivery: Characterization and preclinical studies. *Biomater. Adv.* **2023**, *154*, 213663. [CrossRef]
41. Rankovic, Z. CNS drug design: Balancing physicochemical properties for optimal brain exposure. *J. Med. Chem.* **2015**, *58*, 2584–2608. [CrossRef]

42. Loryan, I.; Reichel, A.; Feng, B.; Bundgaard, C.; Shaffer, C.; Kalvass, C.; Bednarczyk, D.; Morrison, D.; Lesuisse, D.; Hoppe, E.; et al. Unbound Brain-to-Plasma Partition Coefficient, $K_{p,uu,brain}$—A Game Changing Parameter for CNS Drug Discovery and Development. *Pharm. Res.* **2022**, *39*, 1321–1341. [CrossRef] [PubMed]
43. Li, J.; Félix-Soriano, E.; Wright, K.R.; Shen, H.; Baer, L.A.; Stanford, K.I.; Guo, L.W. Differential Responses to Sigma-1 or Sigma-2 Receptor Ablation in Adiposity, Fat Oxidation, and Sexual Dimorphism. *Int. J. Mol. Sci.* **2022**, *23*, 10846. [CrossRef] [PubMed]

pharmaceutics

MDPI

Article

Bioactive Hydrogel Supplemented with Stromal Cell-Derived Extracellular Vesicles Enhance Wound Healing

Matteo Galbiati [1], Fabio Maiullari [1,2], Maria Grazia Ceraolo [3], Salma Bousselmi [3,4], Nicole Fratini [5], Klajdi Gega [1], Sandro Recchia [6], Anna Maria Ferretti [7], Giovanni Scala [8], Marco Costantini [2], Tommaso Sciarra [9], Roberto Rizzi [10,*] and Claudia Bearzi [1,*]

1 Institute for Biomedical Technologies, National Research Council, Via Fratelli Cervi, 93, Segrate, 20054 Milan, Italy; galbiati@ingm.org (M.G.); fabio.maiullari3d@gmail.com (F.M.); claudiogega@live.com (K.G.)
2 Institute of Physical Chemistry, Polish Academy of Sciences, Marcina Kasprzaka 44/52, 01-224 Warsaw, Poland; mcostantini@ichf.edu.pl
3 Neurology Unit, Fondazione IRCCS Ca' Granda Ospedale Maggiore Policlinico, 20122 Milan, Italy; ceraolo@ingm.org (M.G.C.); salma.bousselmi@students.uniroma2.eu (S.B.)
4 Ph.D. Program in Cellular and Molecular Biology, Department of Biology, University of Rome "Tor Vergata", Via della Ricerca Scientifica, 1, 00133 Rome, Italy
5 Department of Molecular Medicine, Sapienza University, Viale Regina Elena, 324, 00161 Rome, Italy; nicole.fratini@uniroma1.it
6 Department of Science and High Technology, University of Insubria, 22100 Como, Italy; sandro.recchia@uninsubria.it
7 CNR-SCITEC Istituto di Scienze e Tecnologie Chimiche "G. Natta", Via G. Fantoli 16/15, 20138 Milan, Italy; anna.ferretti@scitec.cnr.it
8 Department of Biology, University Federico II, 80128 Naples, Italy; giovanni.scala@unina.it
9 Joint Veteran Center, Scientific Department, Army Medical Center, 00184 Rome, Italy; tommaso.sciarra@esercito.difesa.it
10 Department of Medical-Surgical Sciences and Biotechnologies, Sapienza University, Corso della Repubblica 79, 04100 Latina, Italy
* Correspondence: roberto.rizzi@uniroma1.it (R.R.); claudia.bearzi@itb.cnr.it (C.B.); Tel.: +39-3395371377 (R.R.); +39-3335693093 (C.B.)

Abstract: Background/Objectives: Skin regeneration is a rapidly advancing field with significant implications for regenerative medicine, particularly in treating wounds and burns. This study explores the potential of hydrogels functionalized with fibroblast-derived extracellular vesicles (EVs) to enhance skin regeneration in vivo. Being immunoprivileged, EVs minimize immune rejection, offering an attractive alternative to whole-cell therapies by replicating fibroblasts' key roles in tissue repair. **Methods**: To promote EVs' versatility and effective application across different conditions, a lyophilization method with lyoprotectants was optimized. Then, EVs were used to functionalize a hydrogel to perform experiments on murine cutaneous wound models. **Results**: Gelatin methacrylate (GelMA) was selected as the polymeric hydrogel due to its biocompatibility, tunable mechanical properties, and ability to support wound healing. Mechanical tests confirmed GelMA's strength and elasticity for this application. Fibroblast-derived EVs were characterized using Western blot, Transmission Electron Microscopy, and NanoSight analysis, proving their integrity, size distribution, and stability. miRNome profiling identified enriched biological pathways related to cell migration, differentiation, and angiogenesis, emphasizing the critical role of EV cargo in promoting wound repair. In a murine model, hydrogels loaded with fibroblast-derived EVs significantly accelerated wound healing compared to controls (mean wound area 0.62 mm^2 and 4.4 mm^2, respectively), with faster closure, enhanced epithelialization, increased vascularization, and reduced fibrosis. Notably, the lyoprotectants successfully preserved the EVs' structure and bioactivity during freeze-drying, reducing EVs loss by 35% compared to the control group and underscoring the feasibility of this approach for long-term storage and clinical application. **Conclusions**: This study introduces a novel scalable and adaptable strategy for regenerative medicine by combining fibroblast-derived EVs with GelMA, optimizing EVs' stability and functionality for enhanced wound healing in clinical settings, even in challenging contexts such as combat zones or large-scale natural disasters.

Keywords: regenerative medicine; wound healing; extracellular vesicles; bioactive hydrogel; lyoprotectants

1. Introduction

Regenerative medicine and tissue engineering have transformed healthcare by introducing advanced solutions for tissue repair and organ regeneration [1–3]. Wound healing is a pivotal area of research, given its significant influence on patient recovery and healthcare expenses. Despite significant advancements, improving wound healing remains challenging, particularly in managing scar formation and reducing infection risks [4]. The wound healing process is complex, involving coordinated cellular activities such as migration, proliferation, extracellular matrix remodeling, angiogenesis, and re-epithelialization [5]. However, natural healing is often slow, and various factors, including chronic inflammation, infections, and pre-existing medical conditions, can hinder effective wound closure, leading to scarring that may progress to pathological fibrosis. Several traditional approaches, including laser therapies [6,7], growth factor-based treatments [8], and cell-based therapies [9–11], have been explored to enhance wound healing. While promising, these methods face notable limitations, such as invasiveness, low effectiveness, risks of tumorigenicity, and potential immune rejection, which limit their clinical utility.

In recent years, advances in bioengineering have driven the development of biomaterials specifically designed to support regeneration [12]. Among these, hydrogels have emerged as one of the most promising due to their biocompatibility, antibacterial properties, and ease of application [13,14]. These three-dimensional scaffolds absorb large amounts of water, creating an ideal environment for cellular proliferation and enabling the controlled delivery of therapeutic agents directly to the wound site [15,16]. Although hydrogels have typically been studied when combined with cells, recent advancements are shifting toward functionalizing these biomaterials with bioactive molecules to enhance their efficacy [17,18]. An in vivo study revealed that hydrogel scaffolds functionalized with Cannabidiol-Loaded Lipid Nanoparticles improved dermal architecture, collagen deposition, enhanced angiogenesis, and reduced inflammation, thus significantly accelerating wound healing [19].

Our study explores an innovative strategy to enhance wound healing by functionalizing hydrogels with extracellular vesicles (EVs), which we hypothesize could yield improved therapeutic outcomes. EVs are nanosized particles secreted by various cell types that mediate intercellular communication and have demonstrated remarkable potential in tissue regeneration [20–22]. These vesicles function as key mediators in numerous essential biological processes, carrying a rich and heterogeneous cargo that includes growth factors, proteins, cytokines, lipids, and nucleic acids. EVs have emerged as a promising cell-free alternative for therapeutic applications. Unlike whole-cell therapies, EVs have several advantages, including reduced immunogenicity, making them an immunoprivileged approach. Furthermore, EVs retain the bioactive properties of their originating cells without the risks associated with direct cell transplantation [23]. Exploiting the complexity of their cargo, which to date is almost impossible to replicate in vitro, can open important scenarios and overcome the limitations of using single factors as bioactive molecules. In a previous study, we demonstrated the therapeutic potential of EVs derived from HUVECs to enhance tissue regeneration following myocardial infarction [24], laying the groundwork for exploring this approach in other pathological contexts.

One of the primary challenges in translating EVs-based therapies to the clinic is the preservation and storage of these particles without compromising their biological activity. Lyophilization has shown promise as a technique for maintaining the structural integrity and bioactivity of EVs during long-term storage at ambient temperatures [25]. By stabilizing EVs through lyophilization, their potential use in diverse clinical settings, including resource-limited environments, becomes more feasible [26]. Despite the limited studies on EV lyophilization, this strategy holds great promise for preserving their stability and functionality, making them more suitable for storage and therapeutic use. However, lyophilization can pose challenges, such as EV degradation or a loss of functionality due to stresses like ice crystallization and protein denaturation. To overcome these hurdles, lyoprotectants, which are substances that shield biological materials during freeze-drying, have proven to be indispensable [27,28]. These protective agents stabilize EVs membranes and prevent protein aggregation, ensuring the preservation of their structural and functional integrity throughout the process [29]. Motivated by these advantages, we sought to evaluate the effectiveness of lyophilization for EVs preservation, aiming to establish a reliable method to maintain their bioactivity and potential for clinical applications.

In this study, Gelatin methacrylate (GelMA) was selected to deliver and support the EVs in skin wound healing. GelMA hydrogels mimic the natural extracellular matrix, offering structural support for cell growth and tissue regeneration [30]; they are particularly suitable due to their adjustable mechanical properties, biocompatibility, and biodegradability, making them ideal for wound healing. Additionally, they act as a protective matrix for EVs, allowing sustained release and reducing rapid degradation in biological fluids [18]. This controlled release helps to maintain the bioactivity of EVs components, enhancing their therapeutic potential in tissue repair. Beyond structural support, these biomaterials also provide cell-anchoring sites that facilitate cell migration and proliferation, essential for effective tissue regeneration [31,32].

Primary human dermal fibroblasts were used as the source of the EVs, as they play a central role in wound healing. These cells secrete essential extracellular matrix components, growth factors, and cytokines that are critical for tissue repair [33,34]. They are pivotal in synthesizing and remodeling the matrix by producing collagen, elastin, and glycoproteins alongside signaling molecules that drive regeneration [35,36]. Additionally, fibroblasts are readily isolable and highly adaptable to culture conditions, making them accessible for research and therapeutic use and enabling innovative wound healing strategies. Thus, fibroblast-derived EVs could potentially replicate many essential functions of fibroblasts by encapsulating bioactive molecules that mimic their paracrine signaling. This approach may enhance angiogenesis, cell proliferation, and matrix remodeling, positioning EVs as promising therapeutic agents that offer the advantages of fibroblasts without the limitations of whole-cell therapies, such as storage challenges and immune rejection [37].

Based on these premises, the present work aims to address EVs preservation and delivery challenges by exploring lyophilized fibroblast-derived EVs within GelMA hydrogels for improved wound healing. We expect this combination to synergistically boost tissue regeneration, accelerate wound closure, and improve tissue properties and functionality.

2. Materials and Methods

2.1. Human Fibroblasts Culture

Primary human dermal fibroblasts were grown in a complete growth medium, composed of Dulbecco's Modified Eagle Medium High Glucose (DMEM, L0101-500,

BioWest, Nuaillé, France) supplemented with 10% Fetal Bovine Serum (FBS, 10270106, Gibco, Waltham, MA, USA), 1% penicillin/streptomycin (P/S stock solution 10,000 U/mL, 15140122, Gibco), and 1% Sodium Pyruvate (100 mM, 11360070, Gibco) at 37 °C and 5% CO_2. When the cells achieved 70–80% confluence, they were collected through trypsinization and subsequently expanded.

2.2. Isolation of Human Fibroblast-Derived EVs

Human dermal fibroblasts (ATCC) were seeded in 150 mm dishes and cultured in the complete growth medium. Once the cells reached a confluence state of ~60%, they were washed twice with sterile phosphate buffer saline (PBS, L0615-500, BioWest) and then cultured in an EV-free complete medium for 48 h. FBS was ultracentrifuged to remove EVs and obtain EV-free FBS, which was then used to prepare the EV-free complete medium. The EVs were pelleted using a Beckman L-90 centrifuge (Beckman Instruments, Inc., Fullerton, CA, USA) equipped with a Ti-70 rotor (Beckman Instruments) at 125,000× g for 90 min at 4 °C using 25 mL polycarbonate tubes (Beckman Coulter, Brea, CA, USA). After 48 h of culture, the conditioned medium of fibroblasts was collected from each dish and centrifuged at 500× g for 15 min and subsequently at 2000× g for 25 min at 4 °C to remove cell debris and organelles. Afterwards, the supernatants were transferred into 25 mL polycarbonate tubes and ultracentrifugated at 125,000× g for 90 min at 4 °C. Next, the supernatants were discarded and the obtained EVs pellets were resuspended in 1.25 mL of sterile PBS and collected in 1.5 mL polycarbonate. To concentrate the EVs into a smaller volume, another ultracentrifuge was performed at 125,000× g for 90 min at 4 °C. The pellets were resuspended either in 80 µL of PBS for NanoSight and TEM analysis, 80 µL of RIPA buffer for protein extraction for Western blot analysis, or in 700 µL of Qiazol for miRNome analysis.

2.3. Western Blotting

Western blotting was performed using a sodium dodecyl sulfate–polyacrylamide gel electrophoresis (SDS–PAGE) system. EVs were lysed in RIPA buffer, containing 50 mM Tris HCl pH 7.6, 150 mM NaCl, 0.5% sodium deoxycholate (264103, Merck Millipore, Burlington, MA, USA), 0.1% sodium dodecyl sulfate (SDS, 10% #1610416, BIO RAD), 1% Triton X-100 (Sigma-Aldrich), 1 mM EDTA (0.5 M, 324506, Merck Millipore), protease inhibitor cocktail (04693116001, Roche, Basel, Switzerland), and 1 mM phenylmethylsulphonyl fluoride (36978, Thermo Scientific, Waltham, MA, USA). Proteins were quantified with Qubit Protein Assay Kits (Q33212, Invitrogen, Carlsbad, CA, USA), and 20 µg were loaded on Bolt 4–12% Bis-Tris gel (NW04125BOX, Thermo Fisher Scientific, Waltham, MA, USA), transferred to nitrocellulose membranes (GE10600079, Amersham Protran, Johns Creek, GA, USA), and blocked with 5% non-fat dry milk powder (1.15363, Merck Millipore) in 1X Tris-buffered saline. Membranes were incubated with the following primary antibodies: anti-CD9 (1:1000, Cell Signaling, Danvers, MA, USA), anti-CD81 (1:100, Cell Signaling), anti-TSG101 (1:1000, Abcam, Cambridge, UK), and then with the corresponding anti-rabbit peroxidase-linked secondary antibodies (1:2000, GE Healthcare Life Sciences, Havelock, NE, USA). Signal detection was performed via chemiluminescence reaction (ECL, GE Healthcare) using the iBright (Thermo Fischer Scientific) Western blot imaging system.

2.4. NanoSight Analysis

Nanoparticle Tracking Analysis was performed using a NanoSight NS300 instrument (Malvern Panalytical, Malvern, UK). Five 30 s videos were recorded for each sample with a camera level set at 14/15 and a detection threshold set at 2. The EVs concentration and size distribution were subsequently analyzed with NTA 3.2 software.

2.5. Transmission Electron Microscope Acquisition

Vesicles isolated from the three experimental conditions were analyzed with a Zeiss LIBRA 200FE-HR TEM, operating at 200 kV and equipped with a second-generation in-column W filter. Sample preparation followed the freeze-drying protocol previously described. A drop of vesicle suspension (3×10^6 particles/µL) was placed onto a Carbon/Formvar TEM grid, left to air-dry, and then stained with UranyLess (EMS-Electron Microscopy Science, St. Louis, MO, USA).

2.6. EVs Freeze-Drying

Trehalose (182550250, Thermo Fisher Scientific) and PVP40 (PVP40-50G, Sigma Aldrich, St. Louis, MO, USA) were used as lyoprotectants in the preparation of the freeze-drying solution. To maintain the overall osmolality of the lyophilization solutions at around 290 mOsm/kg, the strength of PBS was adjusted according to trehalose concentration, while PVP40 concentration was excluded due to its irrelevant contribution to the overall osmolality. The final concentrations of trehalose and PVP40 were 100 mM and 5%, respectively. The EV samples were divided into two groups and resuspended in either 600 µL of lyophilization solution with lyoprotectants or in 600 µL µl of PBS. The EV samples were placed in safe-lock polypropylene microcentrifuge tubes and were frozen overnight at −80 °C. The samples were closed with a perforated parafilm membrane immediately before being loaded into the Benchtop Freeze Dryer (LIO-5P, 5pascal, Trezzano sul Naviglio, Milan, Italy). The samples were lyophilized overnight and stored at −80 °C. Before use, the lyophilized EVs were rehydrated with bidistilled water to restore the original volume and then resuspended. Next, trehalose and PVP40 were removed by centrifugation with concentrator tubes (UFC905024, Merck, St. Louis, MO, USA) with a 50 kDa MWCO membrane, and NanoSight analysis was performed.

2.7. miRNome Analysis

Total RNA was extracted from fibroblast-derived EVs (n = 3) using the commercial miRNeasy Mini Kit (217004, Qiagen, Hilden, Germania). The concentration and purity of the total RNA were assessed using Nanodrop 2000 and Bioanalyzer 2100. Samples were then sequenced using NGS technology. Briefly, 3′ and 5′ adaptors were ligated to 3′ and 5′ end of small RNA, respectively. Then, the first strand cDNA was synthesized after hybridization with reverse transcription primer. The double-stranded cDNA library was generated through PCR enrichment. After purification and size selection, libraries with insertions between 18~40 bp were ready for sequencing with Illumina Sequencing SE50, generating approximately 20 million reads. The NGS data were generated by Novogene Co., Ltd. (Cambridge, UK) Small RNA sequencing data for the three replicates were processed using the nf-core/smrnaseq pipeline version 2.4.0 [38]. In particular, FastP [39] was used to perform adapter trimming and quality and length filtering on raw fastq files. Bowtie1 [40] was used to perform the alignment of filtered reads against miRBase mature miRNA catalog. Samtools [41] was used for the sorting and indexing of BAM files and to quantify miRBase miRNA abundances. Edger was used to compute normalized counts [42]. RNA categories for each sample were obtained using the miRTace tool [43]. Gene Ontology enrichment analysis was performed using the miEAA [44] online tool. In particular, the miEAA "miRNA enrichment analysis ((G)SEA)" was performed by passing an ordered miRNA id list based on their average TPM values among the three replicates and choosing the following parameters: annotations derived from the miRTarBase (Gene Ontology Consortium) as the category, the Bonferroni adjustment method used for multiple testing, a minimum of at least 2 hits per sub-category, and 0.05 as the significance threshold.

2.8. Bioactive Hydrogel Formulation

Gelatin methacrylate (GelMA) was prepared following a previously published protocol [18]. Briefly, gelatin (type A3 from porcine skin; Sigma-Aldrich, 9000-70-8) was reacted with methacrylic anhydride. Gelatin was dissolved in phosphate buffer (1 g/10 mL, pH 7.5) at 50 °C, and 0.8 mL methacrylic anhydride was added dropwise under vigorous stirring. After 2 h of reaction, the mixture was diluted, dialyzed (MWCO = 2 kDa) against distilled water for 3 days at 40 °C, and subsequently freeze-dried. The bioink stock solution was prepared by dissolving 7% of GelMA *w*/*v* in 25 mM HEPES buffer (Sigma-Aldrich, 7365-45-9). After biopolymer dissolution, the pH of the polymeric stock solution was brought to 7.2 and filtered (0.22 μm) to guarantee sterile conditions. To obtain a 5% GelMA working solution, the stock solution (GelMA 7%) was diluted with phosphate buffer or phosphate buffer + EVs at a final concentration of 9×10^9 particles/mL. Thus, we obtained a control hydrogel (GelMA) and a functionalized hydrogel (GelMA + EVs), respectively. The EVs' concentration was obtained by analyzing and quantifying through NanoSight technology, which allowed the precise measurement of the particle amount (Section 2.4 of materials and methods). Finally, photopolymerization was achieved by adding 1 mg/mL of Irgacure 2959 to the bioinks.

2.9. Scanning Electron Microscopy (SEM) Analysis

The SEM imaging of the polymer, both with and without EVs, was carried out using an FEI ESEM-FEG XL30 microscope. The parameters were set as described in a previous study [18]. The system was operated at an acceleration voltage of 10 kV in low vacuum mode, with the chamber pressure maintained at 1 torr and equipped with a gas secondary electron detector. Imaging conditions were optimized, including a working distance of 8 mm, a spot size of 3, and a sample temperature of 20 °C. Samples were individually mounted on stubs using carbon-based conductive double-sided adhesive tape. The samples remained stable under the electron beam without requiring cooling, even at magnifications reaching 40,000×.

2.10. Bioactive Hydrogel Mechanical Testing

Compressive stress–strain measurements were conducted as previously described [45]. In short, samples including 5% GelMA (*w*/*v*) and 5% GelMA (*w*/*v*) with EVs (9×10^9 particles/mL) were both cross-linked under UV light at 365 nm (intensity of 4–5 mW/cm^2) for 5 min. Compression testing was performed using a DMA Q800 Dynamic Mechanical Analyzer (TA Instruments, New Castle, DE, USA) operating in strain rate mode. The tests were conducted at a constant temperature of 25 °C under the following conditions: an initial preloading force of 0.003 N, a strain rate of 5% per minute, and a maximum deformation of 30%. Young's modulus was calculated from the linear portion of the stress–strain curve corresponding to 0–5% strain. All experiments were conducted in triplicate, and the data are reported as mean values accompanied by standard deviation.

2.11. PDMS O-Ring Preparation

O-rings for in vivo implants were prepared using polydimethylsiloxane (PDMS). The PDMS was prepared by mixing the Silicone Elastomer Base (Sylgard 184) and Silicone Elastomer Curing Agent in a 10:1 ratio. The obtained mixture was poured into a 1 mm thick polycarbonate mold designed to create a PDMS sheet. After degassing to remove the air bubbles, the molds were placed in a stove at 65 °C for 3 h. Finally, the O-rings were prepared using punches with a defined diameter. For the external circumference, a punch with a diameter of 1 cm was used, while for the internal circumference, a punch with a diameter of 5 mm.

2.12. Cutaneous Implantation in Mice

C57/BL6 mice (Jackson Laboratory, Bar Harbor, ME, USA) were used to evaluate the in vivo induced skin regeneration through EVs-functionalized hydrogel. Four-month-old male mice (n = 9) were anesthetized by 2% isoflurane inhalation. The backs of the animals were carefully shaved with an electric shaver and sterilized with ethanol solution. Afterward, the mice were placed on the operating table. Two limited skin incisions on the back medial sides were performed with biopsy punches with a diameter of 4 mm. An O-ring with a 5 mm diameter was placed on each wound, secured with surgical glue, and sutured with four stitches using 4-0 suture thread (Ethicon, Raritan, NJ, USA). The experimental conditions were the following: (i) saline solution (NT), (ii) GelMA, and (iii) GelMA + EVs. Three animals for a total of six wounds were considered for each treatment. The cross-linking of the hydrogel was performed using a UV gun (Electro-Lite Corporation mod. LED-200, Bethel, CT, USA) for 2 min. After the treatment, the implants were covered and protected by a transparent water-repellent wound plaster (Tegaderm, 3M, London, UK). The surgical procedure is reported in Figure 1. Mice were housed individually for 15 days. Finally, the mice were sacrificed via cervical dislocation, and the samples along with the surrounding tissue were excised and processed for histological and molecular analysis. All experiments involving animals were conducted according to the protocols of good animal experimentation under the Italian Health Minister approval n° 324/2024-PR-Risp. a prot. 8C65E.13-3 April 2024.

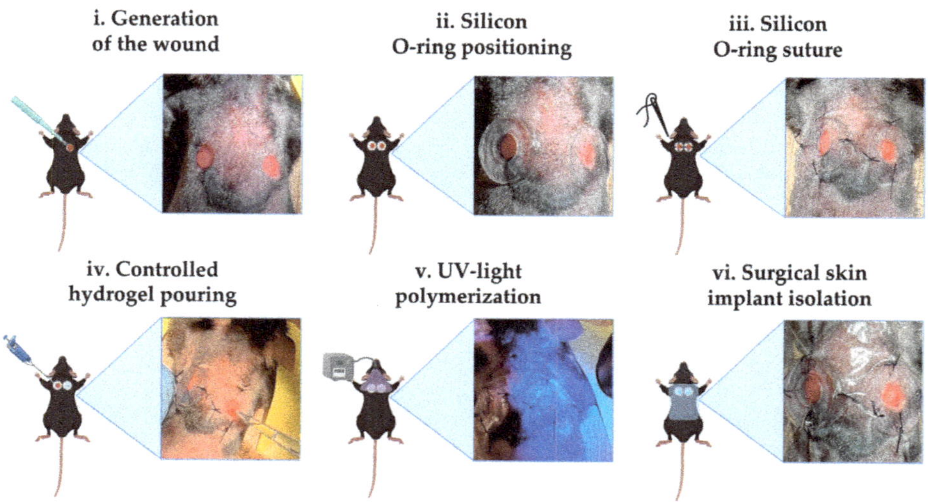

Figure 1. Surgical procedure. Schematic representation of the various steps of the protocol for cutaneous implantation in mice (created with Biorender.com) alongside the real image. Limited skin incisions on the back medial sides were performed with biopsy punches with a diameter of 4 mm (**i**); an O-ring with a 5 mm diameter was placed at each wound (**ii**) and then was fixed with surgical glue and four stitches (**iii**). In every wound, 20 μL of bioink was administered (**iv**). GelMA hydrogels were polymerized using a UV gun (**v**). The implants were covered and protected by a transparent water-repellent wound plaster (**vi**).

2.13. Confocal Microscopy Acquisition

The fibroblasts were expanded in μ-Slide (80 426, Ibidi, Gräfelfing, Germany) and when they reached 80% of confluence they were fixed in 4% Paraformaldehyde (PFA, 047347.9M1, Thermo Scientific) for 15 min at room temperature and washed three times with PBS and then stained with Vimentin (Ms, V5255, Sigma) for 2 h at room temperature;

this was followed by the secondary antibody (1:1000, A32766, Invitrogen) for 1 h at room temperature. DAPI (4′, 6-Diamidino-2-Phenylindole, D1306, Life Technology, Carlsbad, CA, USA) was used for labeling the nuclei. The EVs were stained with a deep-red cell mask (C10046, Invitrogen), then ultracentrifuged and used to produce the bioactive bioink. A 50 μL sample was polymerized using UV light (VILBER LOURMAT mod. VL-6.L) at 365 nm (intensity 4–5 mW/cm^2) for 2 min and imaged using confocal microscopy to assess the distribution of EVs within the hydrogel. The images of the samples were acquired using a Leica Confocal Microscope (Leica Microsystem Srl, Buccinasco, Milan, Italy).

2.14. H&E Staining and Masson's Trichrome

The skin tissues were collected on day 14 and fixed in 4% PFA. Subsequently, the tissues were embedded in Tissue Freezing Medium Optimal Cutting Temperature (OCT, 14020108926, Leica Biosystem, Buccinasco, Milan, Italy) and sectioned using a cryostat (Leica Microsystem, Wetzlar, Germania). The sections (10-μm) were stained with Masson's Trichrome KIT (04-010802, BioOptica, Milan, Italy) according to the manufacturer's protocol, or using a hematoxylin and eosin KIT (BioOptica). Healthy skin (WT) sections taken from the same animals were used as controls.

2.15. Immunofluorescence Assay

OCT-embedded skin sections were first washed with PBS and then permeabilized with 0.2% Triton X-100 to gain access to the intracellular antigens. Sections were then incubated in 5% Bovine Serum Albumin (BSA, A1470, Sigma-Aldrich) blocking solution for 3 h to saturate the nonspecific sites, and thereafter with anti-smooth muscle actin (α-SMA, 1:1000, A2547, Sigma-Aldrich) and anti-Ki-67 (Ki-67, 1:1000, AB15580, Abcam) primary antibody diluted in 0.5% BSA solution overnight at 4 °C. Subsequently, the primary antibody solution was removed, and slides were washed two times in PBS for 5 min and incubated with 488-conjugated Isolectin B4 antibody (S-L2895, Sigma-Aldrich) and fluorescent-conjugated secondary antibodies (1:1000, A10042, Invitrogen) for 2 h. Cell nuclei were counterstained with DAPI (4′, 6-Diamidino-2-Phenylindole, D1306, Life Technology), and the slides were mounted with ProLong Glass Antifade Mountant (P36984, Invitrogen). Healthy skin (WT) sections taken from the same animals were used as controls. A TCS SP5 confocal microscope was employed to acquire the labeled sample images.

2.16. Statistical Analysis

Statistical analysis was carried out using Prism 5 software (GraphPad, La Jolla, CA, USA). Data are presented as mean ± SD (Standard Deviation). Differences between the sample mean at each time point were evaluated with Two-Way ANOVA. A p-value < 0.05 was considered statistically significant.

3. Results and Discussion

3.1. Isolation and Characterization of Human Fibroblast-Derived EVs

EVs were successfully isolated from the conditioned medium of human dermal fibroblasts (Figure 2A). To assess the proper morphology and cell type-specific marker expression, we stained them with Vimentin, which allowed us to confirm the expected elongated and spindle-like morphology and the positivity for the fibroblast marker (Figure 2B). The pellet of EVs was re-suspended, and the vesicles were characterized using NanoSight NS300 and Western blot analysis. The purified EVs had a size range of 100 to 150 nm with a homogeneous distribution, similar to the EVs present in the supernatant prior to isolation. However, the concentration of vesicles in the supernatant was significantly lower, with a peak of 1.3×10^6 particles/mL, compared to the higher peak concentration of 2.7 × 10^8 particles/mL observed in the sample after purification (Figure 2C). Notably, the isolated population was significantly enriched in exosomes, identified by their size of 40–120 nm [46,47]. Western blot analysis confirmed the presence of tetraspanin proteins (CD9, CD81, and TSG-101), which are hallmark markers of EVs, further validating the successful isolation of these vesicles (Figure 2D). The confirmation of tetraspanin expression reflects the proper biogenesis of EVs and aligns with the previously reported data in the literature, supporting their role in cell-to-cell communication, their relevance in biological processes [48], and their suitability for downstream applications in tissue engineering and regenerative medicine fields.

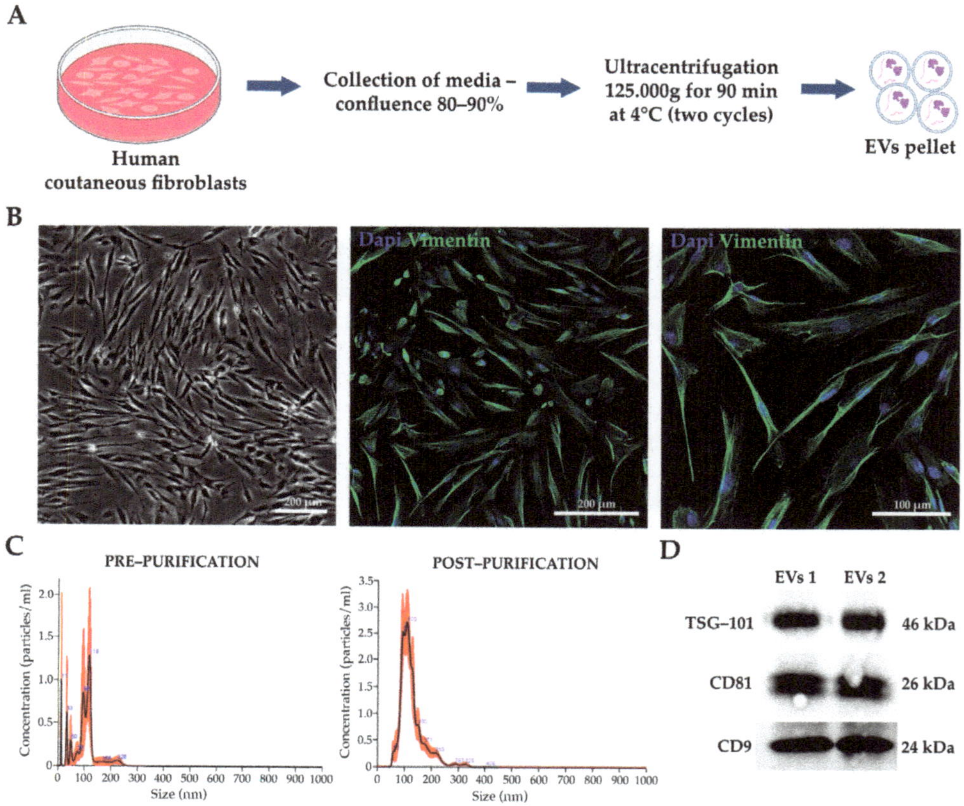

Figure 2. EVs characterization. (**A**) Schematic diagram of EVs isolation from fibroblasts (generated with Biorender.com). (**B**) Bright-field and immunofluorescence representative acquisition of human cutaneous fibroblasts. The scale bar represents 200 and 100 µm. (**C**) The size distribution and concentration profiles of fibroblast-derived EVs analyzed by NanoSight NS300 before and after purification. (**D**) Anti-CD9, anti-CD81, and anti-TSG-101 antibodies were used for the Western blot analysis of fibroblast-derived EVs.

3.2. *Effects of Freeze-Drying on Fibroblast-Derived EVs*

Freeze-drying is a critical method for the long-term preservation of EVs, yet it poses challenges to maintaining vesicle integrity. In this study, the lyoprotectants trehalose and PVP40 were used for their ability to stabilize the lipid bilayer and prevent ice crystal formation. The selection of these specific lyoprotectants and their optimal concentrations (100 mM trehalose and 5% PVP40) for the freezing-drying process were selected based on evidence from the literature [29]. Three groups of EVs were analyzed: (i) EVs resuspended in PBS and frozen, (ii) EVs resuspended in PBS and freeze-dried, and (iii) EVs resuspended with lyoprotectants (trehalose and PVP-40) and freeze-dried. Macroscopically, the lyophilized pellet in the lyoprotectant group appeared more cohesive and denser compared to the PBS group. Post-freeze-drying, the EVs were rehydrated and analyzed using NanoSight NS300 and TEM. NanoSight revealed a heterogeneous size distribution in the PBS group, with a statistically significant 35% loss of EVs after freeze-drying (Figure 3A,B), from a total particle number of approximately 2×10^{10} to 1×10^{10} (Figure 3B). In contrast, no significant changes in size or concentration were observed in the group with lyoprotectants. Indeed, the total number of pre- and post-freeze-drying EVs remained almost unchanged at roughly 2×10^{10} particles, indicating that adding lyoprotectants preserved the structure of the EVs. TEM analysis confirmed these results, revealing that freeze-dried EVs without lyoprotectants had a smaller diameter compared to the other groups (Figure 3C,D). A high percentage of the freeze-drying EVs without lyoprotectants were around 30 nm in size, with diameters ranging from a minimum of 13.60 nm to a maximum of 77.67 nm, probably due to vesicle fragmentation (Figure 3C,D). On the other hand, the group treated with lyoprotectants maintained a more uniform population of vesicles, with a similar diameter distribution to the control (Figure 3C,D). The peak frequency is around 55 nm, while the maximum and minimum are 105.81 nm and 13.80 nm, respectively. These results highlight the importance of lyoprotectants in maintaining vesicle integrity, as their absence leads to increased vesicle rupture and the formation of smaller particles [49]. Overall, these data demonstrate that lyoprotectants are essential for preserving EVs' structural and functional characteristics during freeze-drying, ensuring their long-term stability.

3.3. *miRNome Profiling of Fibroblast-Derived EVs*

We conducted an in-depth molecular characterization of fibroblast-derived EVs using miRNome profiling to evaluate their potential as bioadditives for enhancing hydrogel functionality. A comprehensive analysis of vesicle contents revealed the distribution of nucleic acids, including the proportions of miRNA (10.8%), tRNA (27.5%), and rRNA (20.5%) (Figure 4A). To identify the most abundant miRNAs, we quantified the expression levels of mature miRNAs using normalized TPM (Transcripts Per Million) values obtained from our sequencing data. The normalization process accounted for library size and sequencing depth, enabling a reliable comparison of miRNA abundance across samples. We compiled a table reporting the TPM values for all detected mature miRNAs and ranked them based on their expression levels. This allowed us to identify the top expressed miRNAs, which were considered for further pathway enrichment analyses. To explore the biological implications of these miRNAs, we performed miRNA enrichment analysis using the Gene Set Enrichment Analysis (GSEA) module of the MiEAA tool. The results revealed enriched biological pathways associated with the overall miRNA expression profile, including cell migration, differentiation, and angiogenesis (Figure 4B). Based on these findings, and through an analysis utilizing the miRBase database, we identified 30 miRNAs with critical roles in these processes (Figure 4C). Subsequent Over-Representation Analysis (ORA) further highlighted the principal pathways that involved these miRNAs (Figure 4D). We focused on four highly expressed miRNAs, including miR-10a-5p, miR-10b-5p, miR-29a-3p, and miR-21-5p, which play crucial roles in angiogenesis, extracellular matrix remodeling, and cell proliferation—processes essential for tissue development and repair. Specifically, miR-10a-5p and hsa-miR-10b-5p are involved in vascular remodeling and angiogenesis by regulating endothelial cell migration and function [50]. miR-29a-3p contributes to extracellular matrix rearrangement by facilitating tissue reorganization and cell growth. During the remodeling phase, these miRNAs regulate fibroblast differentiation, collagen deposition, and wound contraction, directly affecting collagen expression [51,52]. Lastly, miR-21 promotes the migration of keratinocytes and fibroblasts, enhances cell survival, proliferation, and angiogenesis, while its inhibition delays re-epithelialization and wound contraction [53,54]. The cargo of fibroblast-derived EVs, enriched with key miRNAs, highlights their potential as bioactive agents capable of enhancing tissue repair and promoting optimal healing outcomes by supporting vascular development, cell survival, and tissue homeostasis.

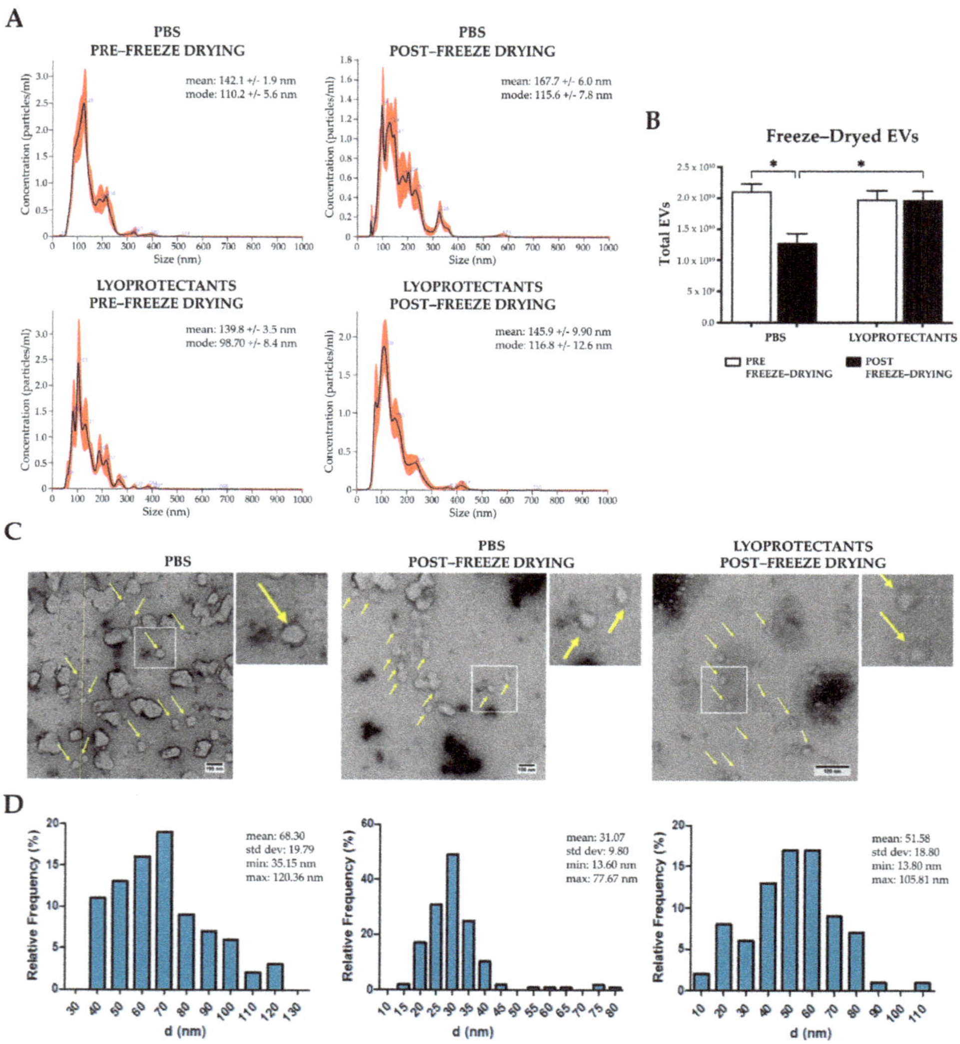

Figure 3. EVs freeze-drying analysis. (**A**) Size distribution profiles of fibroblast-derived EVs pre- and post-lyophilization with and without lyoprotectants analyzed by NanoSight NS300. (**B**) Histogram of EV total number in different experimental conditions, pre- and post-lyophilization. Error bars represent ± SD. Two-Way ANOVA, * $p < 0.05$. (**C**) Representative TEM images of the EVs in the three different experimental conditions. Yellow arrows show the vesicles. (**D**) Histograms displaying the diameter (nm) distribution of vesicles obtained from the diverse experimental contexts.

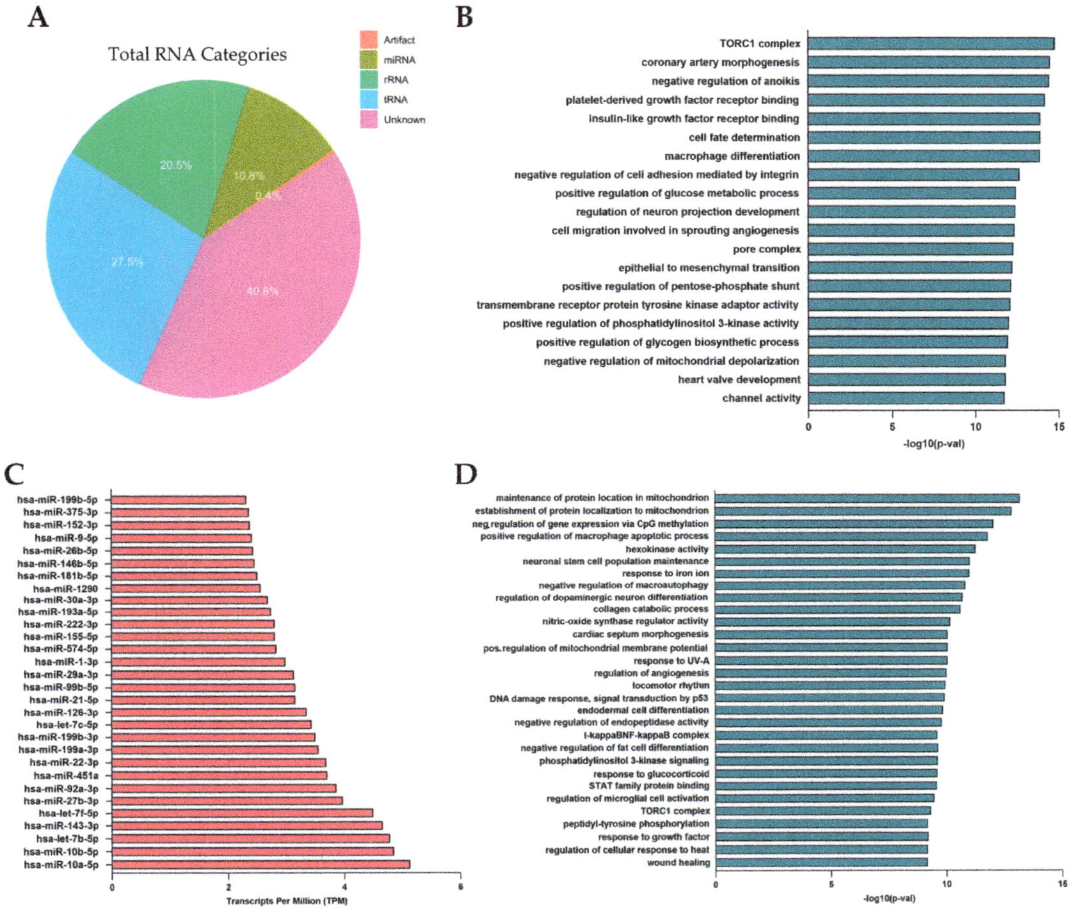

Figure 4. miRNome characterization of EVs derived from human dermal fibroblasts. (**A**) Pie chart describing the percentages of RNA within vesicles. (**B**) Enrichment analysis of total miRNAs using (Gene) Set Enrichment Analysis ((G)SEA). (**C**) Graphical representation of 30 selected miRNAs, identified for their key roles in the wound healing process. (**D**) Over-Representation Analysis (ORA) performed on the selected miRNAs.

3.4. Characterization of Bioactive Hydrogel

GelMA hydrogels were analyzed by confocal microscopy, SEM, and mechanical tests to assess vesicle incorporation and the structural characteristics of the biomaterial. All experiments were performed using hydrogels loaded with extracellular vesicles at a concentration of 9×10^9 EVs/mL. The confocal microscopy analysis of the EVs labeled with Cell Mask Deep Red revealed their clear visibility and uniform distribution within the hydrogel matrix (Figure 5A). SEM images also confirm the presence of EVs in the functionalized matrices in contrast to the pure matrices (Figure 5B). This analysis also visualized a porous network in both types of hydrogels, an essential feature for tissue integration. Mechanical compression tests (Figure 5C) showed that the incorporation of EVs did not significantly affect the Young's modulus value, with both pure GelMA hydrogels and those loaded with EVs presenting values between 2 and 2.5 kPa (Figure 5D). This stability highlights that the mechanical properties of GelMA remain unchanged despite EV incorporation, making these hydrogels very suitable for soft tissue engineering applications where mechanical integrity is critical. The stiffness of the skin, characterized by Young's modulus in the range optimal for maintaining cell viability and promoting tissue regeneration [55], aligns well with the mechanical properties of GelMA hydrogels, further supporting their application in regenerating the target tissue.

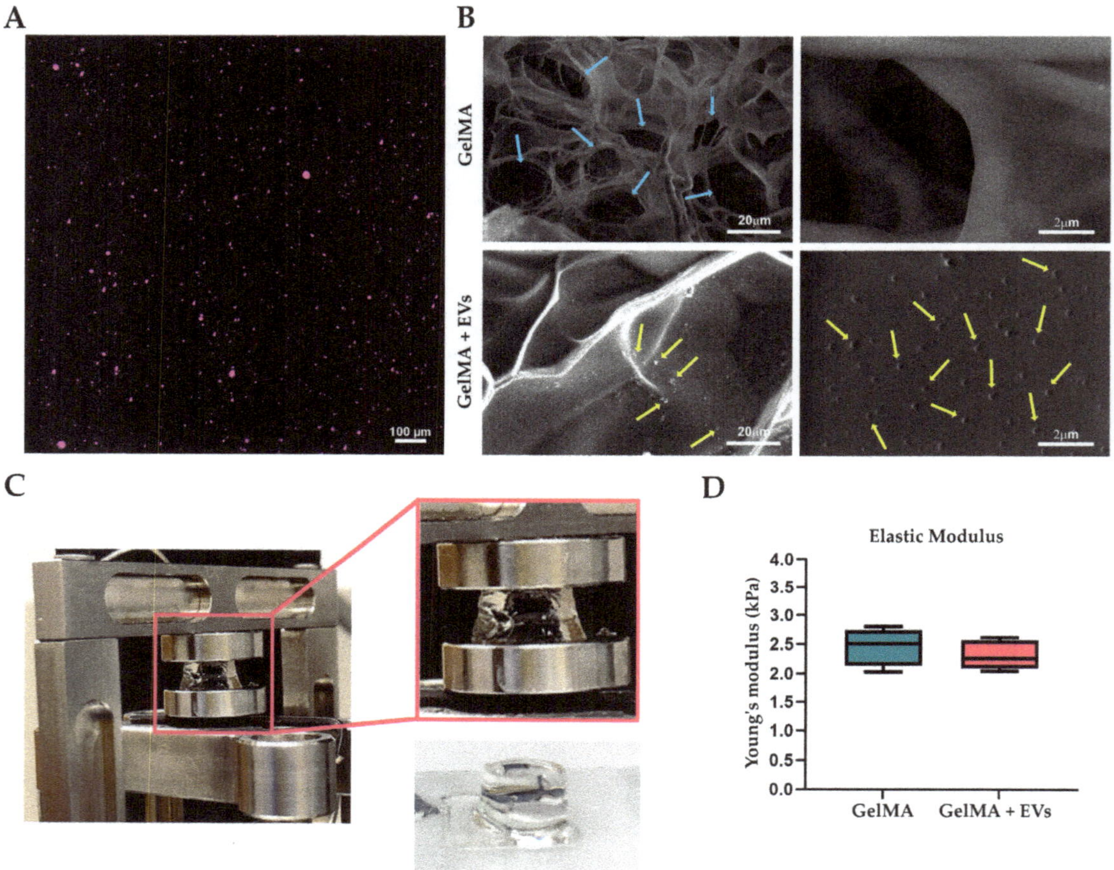

Figure 5. Bioactive hydrogel characterization. (**A**) Representative fluorescence images of bioactive bioink. EVs labeled with Cell Mask Deep Red (magenta) plasma membrane stain were effectively encapsulated into GelMA hydrogel. Scale bars represent 100 µm. (**B**) SEM images of 5% GelMA-based hydrogel with and without EVs. Blue and yellow arrows show the porosity of the hydrogel and the morphology of EVs, respectively. The scale bars represent 20 µm and 2 µm. (**C**) Actual image of the GelMA hydrogel during compression test in the DMA Q800 Dynamic Mechanical Analyzer and after UV polymerization. (**D**) Values of the compressive modulus of elasticity as calculated from stress–strain curves for 5% GelMA hydrogels both pure and loaded with EVs.

3.5. Evaluation of EVs-Loaded Hydrogels in Skin Wound Healing In Vivo

This study focused on evaluating the in vivo efficacy of fibroblast-derived EV-functionalized hydrogels. To this end, dorsal skin wounds were created on C57/BL6 mice and treated with (i) saline solution (NT), (ii) GelMA, or (iii) GelMA + EVs (9×10^9 particles/mL). Wound healing was assessed via macroscopic analysis on days 2 and 14 post-treatment, supported by histological data (Figure 6A,B). On day 2, wounds treated with GelMA + EVs showed a more marked reduction in wound area compared to the other groups, with a mean wound area of 11.5 mm^2 in the GelMA + EVs group versus 12.8 mm^2 and 12.2 mm^2 for the NT and GelMA groups, respectively. This trend persisted through day 14, where wounds in the GelMA + EVs group exhibited almost complete closure with a mean wound area of 0.62 mm^2, which was significantly smaller compared to 4.4 mm^2 in the NT group and 3.12 mm^2 in the GelMA group. The quantitative analysis of wound area and closure rate revealed a statistically significant improvement in closure for GelMA + EVs compared to NT on day 2. By day 14, GelMA + EVs showed a significantly higher closure rate than both GelMA and NT (Figure 6C), underscoring the enhanced healing efficacy of EV-functionalized hydrogels across the healing timeline. These findings suggest that EVs support critical stages of the regenerative process, comprising inflammation resolution, angiogenesis, granulation tissue formation, and ECM remodeling, highlighting EV-functionalized hydrogels as a promising therapeutic approach for enhanced wound healing.

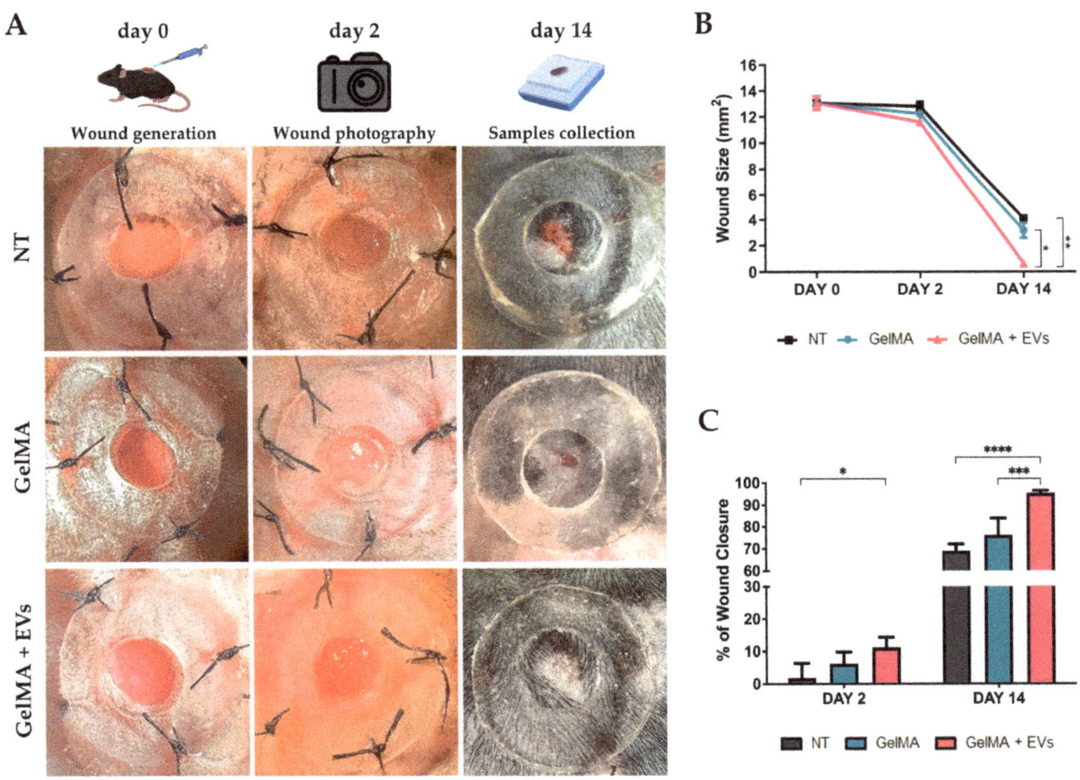

Figure 6. Wound healing in vivo. (**A**) Representative images displaying the wound healing process of mice under the three experimental conditions: NT, GelMA, and GelMA + EVs (day 0, 2, and 14). The rendering figures at the top, "wound generation", "wound photography" and "sample collection" were created with BioRender.com. (**B**) Graph of wound closure progress in mice under the diverse experimental contexts: NT, GelMA, and GelMA + EVs from day 0 to day 14. Error bars represent ± SD. Two-Way ANOVA, * $p < 0.05$, ** $p < 0.01$. (**C**)Percentage of wound closure in mice in the different treatments: NT, GelMA, and GelMA + EVs. Error bars represent ± SD. Two-Way ANOVA, * $p < 0.05$, *** $p < 0.001$, **** $p < 0.0001$.

3.6. Regenerative Effects of Bioactive Hydrogels in Skin Wound Healing

The hematoxylin–eosin (H&E) staining revealed distinct tissue organization among the NT, GelMA, and GelMA + EVs groups when compared to healthy tissue (WT). The

GelMA + EVs group exhibited a denser cellular arrangement and more mature tissue architecture than the GelMA and NT groups on day 14 post-treatment. Specifically, the NT group displayed delayed and non-functional wound closure, characterized by extensive fibrotic areas at the injury site (Figure 7A). In contrast, structures resembling normal skin appendages (e.g., hair follicles, sebaceous glands, and sweat glands) were clearly visible in the GelMA + EVs group, whereas they were sparse or absent in the GelMA and NT groups. The epidermis was notably thin or absent in the NT group, while GelMA-treated wounds displayed partial epidermal regeneration without full re-epithelialization. Notably, the GelMA + EVs group achieved both full epidermal and dermal regeneration, closely mirroring the architecture of WT tissue. These findings suggest that the presence of EVs enhances cellular communication, promotes cell proliferation, and regulates ECM deposition, supporting an organized healing process more akin to natural tissue architecture [56,57]. Further validation by Masson's trichrome evaluation demonstrated improved structural organization in the GelMA + EVs group, aligning with WT tissue composition. The analysis revealed minimal collagen disarray in GelMA + EVs-treated tissue, in contrast to the NT and GelMA groups, which exhibited prominent collagen deposits indicative of fibrotic scar formation (Figure 7B). Additionally, the GelMA + EVs-treated tissues retained the characteristic epidermal and dermal functions of WT tissue, underscoring its regenerative potential. These data suggest that our bioactive hydrogel offers a promising avenue for effective tissue regeneration by fostering re-epithelialization and controlled collagen deposition, essential for preserving skin integrity and function [58]. These observations were further supported by immunofluorescence staining for Ki-67, an established marker of proliferating cells. WT samples exhibited Ki-67 in the basal epidermis near hair follicles, a pattern replicated in the GelMA + EVs group (Figure 8A), indicating an enhanced cell proliferation relative to NT and GelMA groups (Figure 8B). This result reflects the ability of the bioactive hydrogel to support the cellular proliferation necessary for transitioning from granulation tissue to functional tissue remodeling [59]. Finally, immunofluorescence staining for α-SMA and isolectin B4, markers for myofibroblasts and endothelial cells, respectively, confirmed heightened vascularization in the GelMA + EVs group on day 14. The GelMA + EVs-treated tissue showed a marked increase in blood vessel density relative to NT and GelMA groups, which is critical for nutrient and oxygen supply during tissue repair (Figure 8C). The restored vascular network supports normal skin functions and underscores the bioactive hydrogel's role in facilitating comprehensive skin regeneration, thus offering an effective strategy for improved wound healing outcomes [60]. It should be noted that some non-specific signals observed in the immunofluorescence staining could be attributed to the composition of the epidermis, which includes desquamated and non-viable keratinocytes. Additionally, potential background autofluorescence or antibody cross-reactivity in these complex tissue sections may have contributed to the observed signals.

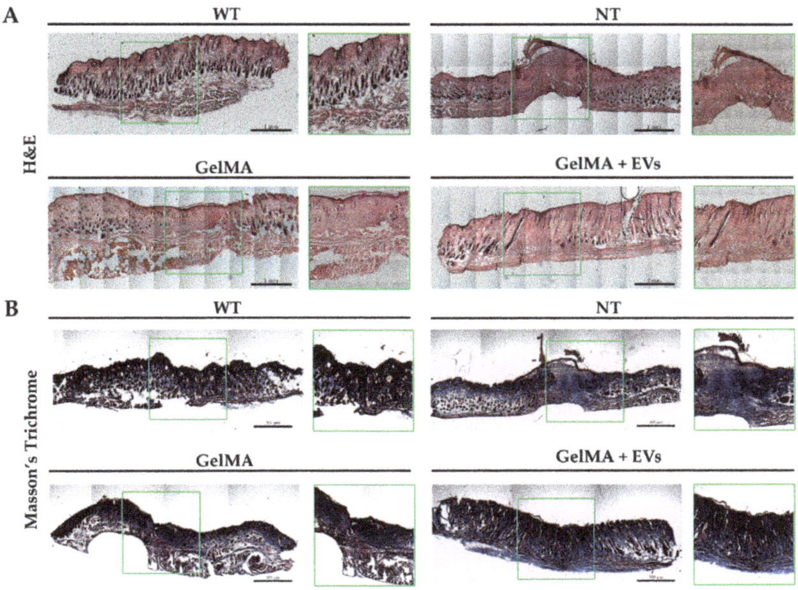

Figure 7. Histological analysis of skin. (**A**) H&E staining of wound sections WT, NT, GelMA, and GelMA + EVs groups at day 14. The scale bars represent 1 mm. (**B**) Masson's trichrome staining of wound sections WT, NT, GelMA, and GelMA + EVs groups at day 14. The scale bars represent 500 μm.

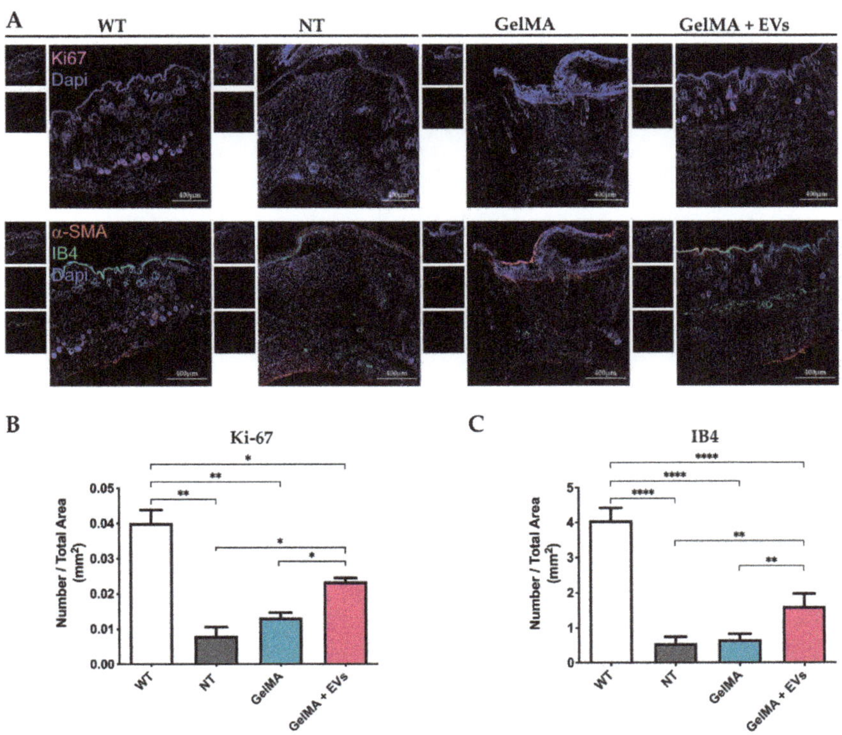

Figure 8. Immunofluorescence analysis on skin. (**A**) Representative immunofluorescence images of staining against Ki-67 (magenta) on skin sections of the four experimental conditions WT, NT, GelMA,

and GelMA + EVs at day 14. The scale bars represent 400 μm. Nuclei were counterstained with DAPI (blue) (**upper panels**). Representative immunofluorescence images of staining against α-SMA (red) and IB4 (green) on skin sections of the different experimental conditions WT, NT, GelMA, and GelMA + EVs at day 14. The scale bars represent 400 μm. Nuclei were counterstained with DAPI (blue) (**lower panels**). (**B**,**C**) Diagrams represent the ratio between the number of Ki-67 positive cells (**B**) or the number of ISO/B4 positive capillaries (**C**) and the total area (mm2) in the different experimental groups. Error bars represent ± SD. Two-Way ANOVA, * $p < 0.05$, ** $p < 0.01$, **** $p < 0.0001$.

4. Conclusions

Wound healing remains a complex and challenging process, particularly in chronic or severe wounds, where the natural healing mechanisms are often impaired. Functionalized hydrogels incorporating EVs represent a promising solution to enhance tissue regeneration, offering a cell-free, immune-tolerant approach. Our results indicate that the hydrogels functionalized with fibroblast-derived EVs significantly accelerated skin repair in an immunocompetent mouse model, promoting the formation of skin appendages, improving tissue architecture, and reducing fibrosis. Importantly, this delivery strategy supports the sustained release of bioactive EVs at the wound site, addressing the limitations of previous EV-based therapies that struggled with poor retention [61–63]. Furthermore, the application of freeze-drying with lyoprotectants successfully preserved the structural integrity and bioactivity of EVs, overcoming key challenges related to long-term storage and transport and allowing immediate wound management This approach holds significant promise for the scalability and clinical translation of EV-based therapies, making them more accessible and practical for use in diverse medical environments. Specifically, it provides solutions for peculiar acute wounds, such as combat injuries, which require rapid and straightforward interventions. Moreover, one key finding from the miRNome analysis of EVs is the significant involvement of miRNAs in the wound healing process. In particular, several highly expressed miRNAs, including miR-10a-5p, miR-10b-5p, miR-29a-3p, and miR-21-5p, were identified. These results highlight the functional relevance of EV-derived miRNAs in orchestrating complex biological processes associated with tissue repair. Further investigation into their specific molecular mechanisms could provide valuable insights into the development of miRNA-based therapeutic strategies for enhanced wound healing and regenerative medicine. The generation of biofunctional hydrogel enriched with EVs represents a significant advancement in the field of regenerative medicine, combining the strengths of bioengineering, materials science, and cellular biology. This bioengineered scaffold not only enhances the speed and quality of healing but also supports the development of more functional tissue. Future work should focus on optimizing this system for human applications and exploring its utility in treating complex wounds or large-scale tissue damage. The potential to develop portable, EV-loaded hydrogels for immediate, on-site application could have profound implications for military medicine, emergency care, and other areas where rapid intervention is critical. This approach also holds potential for chronic wound management. Chronic wounds often arise as complications from conditions such as vascularization insufficiency, diabetes, and neuropathies. They are typically characterized by a prolonged inflammatory phase that hinders the natural healing process. The miRNome profile results support the potential use of our functionalized hydrogel to regulate persistent inflammation, thereby preventing complications such as infections or limb amputations.

Additionally, investigating the production of EVs from cells under stress conditions [24] could open new avenues for enhancing the therapeutic potential of this system. Stress-induced EVs may carry unique bioactive molecules that can further modulate the healing process, improve cellular communication, and promote tissue regeneration.

Another promising direction could involve the development of multilayered hydrogels composed of layers with distinct biomechanical properties and functionalized with EVs derived from diverse cellular sources. This approach would allow the production of a tailored healing environment, enhancing the integration of the regenerating tissue while promoting functional recovery. By mimicking the complexity of native tissue architecture and combining the specialized bioactivity of EVs, such systems could redefine the landscape of advanced regenerative therapies. Our formulation is easy to produce and cost efficient since it does not require high-level biosafety laboratories. Moreover, it has the advantage of not being restricted to patient-specific EVs. This flexibility allows for the preparation of large quantities in advance, making it highly scalable for clinical applications. In conclusion, the study lays the foundation for a transformative approach to wound healing, seamlessly integrating advanced biological technologies with innovative biomaterials. By bridging, potentially, the gap between regenerative medicine and tissue engineering, our findings could open new horizons for developing innovative therapies that not only accelerate healing but also restore tissue functionality.

Author Contributions: Conceptualization: C.B. and R.R.; data curation: C.B., R.R., M.G., F.M., M.G.C., S.B., A.M.F., M.C. and G.S.; formal analysis: M.G., K.G., S.R., A.M.F., G.S. and T.S.; funding acquisition: C.B. and R.R.; methodology: M.G., F.M., M.G.C., N.F., S.B., K.G., M.C., A.M.F. and S.R.; supervision: C.B., R.R. and F.M.; writing—original draft: M.G., F.M. and M.G.C.; writing—review and editing: C.B., R.R., T.S. and S.B. All authors have read and agreed to the published version of the manuscript.

Funding: This research was supported by the Italian Ministry of Defense by the funding scheme PNRM 2019 for the project GRENADE No. 2019.038.

Institutional Review Board Statement: The animal study protocol was approved by the Italian Health Minister (protocol n° 324/2024-PR-Risp. a prot. 8C65E.13-3 April 2024).

Informed Consent Statement: Not applicable.

Data Availability Statement: The data supporting the findings of this article will be made available by the authors on request.

Acknowledgments: We are grateful to the Imaging Facility of Fondazione Istituto Nazionale di Genetica Molecolare for their assistance during image acquisition and to Mannella Valeria (Center for Omics Sciences, IRCCS, San Raffaele Scientific Institute, Milan, Italy) for her valuable help. During the preparation of this manuscript, the authors used ChatGPT (OpenAI, GPT-4o) to perform grammar checking and language improvement in English. The authors have reviewed and edited the output and take full responsibility for the content of this publication.

Conflicts of Interest: The authors declare no conflicts of interest.

References

1. Wardhana, A.; Valeria, M. Tissue Engineering and Regenerative Medicine: A Review. *J. Plast. Rekonstr.* **2020**, *7*, 10–17. [CrossRef]
2. McKinley, K.L.; Longaker, M.T.; Naik, S. Emerging Frontiers in Regenerative Medicine: Bridging Knowledge Gaps Could Enable Regenerative Therapy. *Science* **2023**, *380*, 796–798. [CrossRef] [PubMed]
3. Edgar, L.; Pu, T.; Porter, B.; Aziz, J.M.; Pointe, C.L.; Asthana, A.; Orlando, G. Regenerative Medicine, Organ Bioengineering and Transplantation. *Br. J. Surg.* **2020**, *107*, 793–800. [CrossRef]
4. Gurtner, G.C.; Werner, S.; Barrandon, Y.; Longaker, M.T. Wound Repair and Regeneration. *Nature* **2008**, *453*, 314–321. [CrossRef] [PubMed]
5. Sorg, H.; Sorg, C.G.G. Skin Wound Healing: Of Players, Patterns, and Processes. *Eur. Surg. Res. Eur. Chir. Forsch. Rech. Chir. Eur.* **2023**, *64*, 141–157. [CrossRef]
6. Andrade, F.d.S.d.S.D.; Clark, R.M.d.O.; Ferreira, M.L. Effects of Low-Level Laser Therapy on Wound Healing. *Rev. Colégio Bras. Cir.* **2014**, *41*, 129–133. [CrossRef]

7. Yoon, S.H.; Huh, B.K.; Abdi, S.; Javed, S. The Efficacy of High-Intensity Laser Therapy in Wound Healing: A Narrative Review. *Lasers Med. Sci.* **2024**, *39*, 208. [CrossRef] [PubMed]
8. Dolati, S.; Yousefi, M.; Pishgahi, A.; Nourbakhsh, S.; Pourabbas, B.; Shakouri, S.K. Prospects for the Application of Growth Factors in Wound Healing. *Growth Factors* **2020**, *38*, 25–34. [CrossRef]
9. Dehkordi, A.N.; Babaheydari, F.M.; Chehelgerdi, M.; Dehkordi, S.R. Skin Tissue Engineering: Wound Healing Based on Stem-Cell-Based Therapeutic Strategies. *Stem Cell Res. Ther.* **2019**, *10*, 111. [CrossRef]
10. Guillamat-Prats, R. The Role of MSC in Wound Healing, Scarring and Regeneration. *Cells* **2021**, *10*, 1729. [CrossRef]
11. Mazini, L.; Rochette, L.; Admou, B.; Amal, S.; Malka, G. Hopes and Limits of Adipose-Derived Stem Cells (ADSCs) and Mesenchymal Stem Cells (MSCs) in Wound Healing. *Int. J. Mol. Sci.* **2020**, *21*, 1306. [CrossRef]
12. Farahani, M.; Shafiee, A. Wound Healing: From Passive to Smart Dressings. *Adv. Healthc. Mater.* **2021**, *10*, 2100477. [CrossRef] [PubMed]
13. Vannozzi, L.; Ricotti, L.; Cianchetti, M.; Bearzi, C.; Gargioli, C.; Rizzi, R.; Dario, P.; Menciassi, A. Self-Assembly of Polydimethyl-siloxane Structures from 2D to 3D for Bio-Hybrid Actuation. *Bioinspir. Biomim.* **2015**, *10*, 5. [CrossRef] [PubMed]
14. Fuoco, C.; Sangalli, E.; Vono, R.; Testa, S.; Sacchetti, B.; Latronico, M.V.G.; Bernardini, S.; Madeddu, P.; Cesareni, G.; Seliktar, D.; et al. 3D Hydrogel Environment Rejuvenates Aged Pericytes for Skeletal Muscle Tissue Engineering. *Front. Physiol.* **2014**, *5*, 203. [CrossRef]
15. Liu, Y.; Su, G.; Zhang, R.; Dai, R.; Li, Z. Nanomaterials-Functionalized Hydrogels for the Treatment of Cutaneous Wounds. *Int. J. Mol. Sci.* **2023**, *24*, 336. [CrossRef]
16. Kolimi, P.; Narala, S.; Nyavanandi, D.; Youssef, A.A.A.; Dudhipala, N. Innovative Treatment Strategies to Accelerate Wound Healing: Trajectory and Recent Advancements. *Cells* **2022**, *11*, 2439. [CrossRef] [PubMed]
17. Liang, Y.; He, J.; Guo, B. Functional Hydrogels as Wound Dressing to Enhance Wound Healing. *ACS Nano* **2021**, *15*, 12687–12722. [CrossRef]
18. Maiullari, F.; Chirivì, M.; Costantini, M.; Ferretti, A.M.; Recchia, S.; Maiullari, S.; Milan, M.; Presutti, D.; Pace, V.; Raspa, M.; et al. In Vivo Organized Neovascularization Induced by 3D Bioprinted Endothelial-Derived Extracellular Vesicles. *Biofabrication* **2021**, *13*, 035014. [CrossRef]
19. Lapmanee, S.; Bhubhanil, S.; Charoenphon, N.; Inchan, A.; Bunwatcharaphansakun, P.; Khongkow, M.; Namdee, K. Cannabidiol-Loaded Lipid Nanoparticles Incorporated in Polyvinyl Alcohol and Sodium Alginate Hydrogel Scaffold for Enhancing Cell Migration and Accelerating Wound Healing. *Gels* **2024**, *10*, 843. [CrossRef]
20. Théry, C.; Witwer, K.W.; Aikawa, E.; Alcaraz, M.J.; Anderson, J.D.; Andriantsitohaina, R.; Antoniou, A.; Arab, T.; Archer, F.; Atkin-Smith, G.K.; et al. Minimal Information for Studies of Extracellular Vesicles 2018 (MISEV2018): A Position Statement of the International Society for Extracellular Vesicles and Update of the MISEV2014 Guidelines. *J. Extracell. Vesicles* **2018**, *7*, 1535750. [CrossRef]
21. Yáñez-Mó, M.; Siljander, P.R.M.; Andreu, Z.; Zavec, A.B.; Borràs, F.E.; Buzas, E.I.; Buzas, K.; Casal, E.; Cappello, F.; Carvalho, J.; et al. Biological Properties of Extracellular Vesicles and Their Physiological Functions. *J. Extracell. Vesicles* **2015**, *4*, 27066. [CrossRef] [PubMed]
22. Baci, D.; Chirivì, M.; Pace, V.; Maiullari, F.; Milan, M.; Rampin, A.; Somma, P.; Presutti, D.; Garavelli, S.; Bruno, A.; et al. Extracellular Vesicles from Skeletal Muscle Cells Efficiently Promote Myogenesis in Induced Pluripotent Stem Cells. *Cells* **2020**, *9*, 1527. [CrossRef]
23. Rani, S.; Ritter, T. The Exosome—A Naturally Secreted Nanoparticle and Its Application to Wound Healing. *Adv. Mater.* **2016**, *28*, 5542–5552. [CrossRef] [PubMed]
24. Maiullari, F.; Milan, M.; Chirivì, M.; Ceraolo, M.G.; Bousselmi, S.; Fratini, N.; Galbiati, M.; Fortunato, O.; Costantini, M.; Brambilla, F.; et al. Enhancing Neovascularization Post-Myocardial Infarction through Injectable Hydrogel Functionalized with Endothelial-Derived EVs. *Biofabrication* **2024**, *16*, 045009. [CrossRef]
25. Charoenviriyakul, C.; Takahashi, Y.; Nishikawa, M.; Takakura, Y. Preservation of Exosomes at Room Temperature Using Lyophilization. *Int. J. Pharm.* **2018**, *553*, 1–7. [CrossRef]
26. Wisdom, E.C.; Lamont, A.; Martinez, H.; Rockovich, M.; Lee, W.; Gilchrist, K.H.; Ho, V.B.; Klarmann, G.J. An Exosome-Laden Hydrogel Wound Dressing That Can Be Point-of-Need Manufactured in Austere and Operational Environments. *Bioengineering* **2024**, *11*, 804. [CrossRef]
27. Yuan, F.; Li, Y.-M.; Wang, Z. Preserving Extracellular Vesicles for Biomedical Applications: Consideration of Storage Stability before and after Isolation. *Drug Deliv.* **2021**, *28*, 1501–1509. [CrossRef]
28. Elliott, G.D.; Wang, S.; Fuller, B.J. Cryoprotectants: A Review of the Actions and Applications of Cryoprotective Solutes That Modulate Cell Recovery from Ultra-Low Temperatures. *Cryobiology* **2017**, *76*, 74–91. [CrossRef] [PubMed]
29. El Baradie, K.B.Y.; Nouh, M.; O'Brien Iii, F.; Liu, Y.; Fulzele, S.; Eroglu, A.; Hamrick, M.W. Freeze-Dried Extracellular Vesicles From Adipose-Derived Stem Cells Prevent Hypoxia-Induced Muscle Cell Injury. *Front. Cell Dev. Biol.* **2020**, *8*, 181. [CrossRef] [PubMed]

30. Yue, K.; Trujillo-de Santiago, G.; Alvarez, M.M.; Tamayol, A.; Annabi, N.; Khademhosseini, A. Synthesis, Properties, and Biomedical Applications of Gelatin Methacryloyl (GelMA) Hydrogels. *Biomaterials* **2015**, *73*, 254–271. [CrossRef]
31. Marin, E.; Boschetto, F.; Pezzotti, G. Biomaterials and Biocompatibility: An Historical Overview. *J. Biomed. Mater. Res. A* **2020**, *108*, 1617–1633. [CrossRef] [PubMed]
32. Revete, A.; Aparicio, A.; Cisterna, B.A.; Revete, J.; Luis, L.; Ibarra, E.; González, E.A.S.; Molino, J.; Reginensi, D. Advancements in the Use of Hydrogels for Regenerative Medicine: Properties and Biomedical Applications. *Int. J. Biomater.* **2022**, *2022*, 3606765. [CrossRef]
33. Bainbridge, P. Wound Healing and the Role of Fibroblasts. *J. Wound Care* **2013**, *22*, 407–408, 410–412. [CrossRef]
34. Talbott, H.E.; Mascharak, S.; Griffin, M.; Wan, D.C.; Longaker, M.T. Wound Healing, Fibroblast Heterogeneity, and Fibrosis. *Cell Stem. Cell* **2022**, *29*, 1161–1180. [CrossRef]
35. Jiang, D.; Guo, R.; Machens, H.-G.; Rinkevich, Y. Diversity of Fibroblasts and Their Roles in Wound Healing. *Cold Spring Harb. Perspect Biol.* **2023**, *15*, a041222. [CrossRef] [PubMed]
36. Cañedo-Dorantes, L.; Cañedo-Ayala, M. Skin Acute Wound Healing: A Comprehensive Review. *Int. J. Inflamm.* **2019**, 2019. [CrossRef]
37. Welsh, J.A.; Goberdhan, D.C.; O'Driscoll, L.; Théry, C.; Witwer, K.W. MISEV2023: An Updated Guide to EV Research and Applications. *J. Extracell. Vesicles* **2024**, *13*, e12416. [CrossRef] [PubMed]
38. Peltzer, A.; Trigila, A.; Pantano, L.; Ewels, P.; Wang, C.; Espinosa-Carrasco, J.; Schcolnicov, N.; Mohr, C.; bot, nf-core; Menden, K.; et al. Nf-Core/Smrnaseq: V2.4.0–2024-10-14–Gray Zinc Dalmation Patch 2024. Available online: https://zenodo.org/records/13928318 (accessed on 14 October 2024).
39. Chen, S. Ultrafast One-Pass FASTQ Data Preprocessing, Quality Control, and Deduplication Using Fastp. *iMeta* **2023**, *2*, e107. [CrossRef] [PubMed]
40. Langmead, B.; Trapnell, C.; Pop, M.; Salzberg, S.L. Ultrafast and Memory-Efficient Alignment of Short DNA Sequences to the Human Genome. *Genome Biol.* **2009**, *10*, R25. [CrossRef]
41. Li, H.; Handsaker, B.; Wysoker, A.; Fennell, T.; Ruan, J.; Homer, N.; Marth, G.; Abecasis, G.; Durbin, R. The Sequence Alignment/Map Format and SAMtools. *Bioinformatics* **2009**, *25*, 2078–2079. [CrossRef] [PubMed]
42. Chen, Y.; Chen, L.; Lun, A.T.L.; Baldoni, P.L.; Smyth, G.K. edgeR v4: Powerful Differential Analysis of Sequencing Data with Expanded Functionality and Improved Support for Small Counts and Larger Datasets 2024. Available online: https://www.biorxiv.org/content/10.1101/2024.01.21.576131v2 (accessed on 24 November 2024).
43. Kang, W.; Eldfjell, Y.; Fromm, B.; Estivill, X.; Biryukova, I.; Friedländer, M.R. miRTrace Reveals the Organismal Origins of microRNA Sequencing Data. *Genome Biol.* **2018**, *19*, 213. [CrossRef]
44. Aparicio-Puerta, E.; Hirsch, P.; Schmartz, G.P.; Kern, F.; Fehlmann, T.; Keller, A. *miEAA* 2023: Updates, New Functional microRNA Sets and Improved Enrichment Visualizations. *Nucleic Acids Res.* **2023**, *51*, W319–W325. [CrossRef]
45. Chirivì, M.; Maiullari, F.; Milan, M.; Presutti, D.; Cordiglieri, C.; Crosti, M.; Sarnicola, M.L.; Soluri, A.; Volpi, M.; Święszkowski, W.; et al. Tumor Extracellular Matrix Stiffness Promptly Modulates the Phenotype and Gene Expression of Infiltrating T Lymphocytes. *Int. J. Mol. Sci.* **2021**, *22*, 5862. [CrossRef] [PubMed]
46. Zhang, Y.; Liu, Y.; Liu, H.; Tang, W.H. Exosomes: Biogenesis, Biologic Function and Clinical Potential. *Cell Biosci.* **2019**, *9*, 19. [CrossRef]
47. Dilsiz, N. A Comprehensive Review on Recent Advances in Exosome Isolation and Characterization: Toward Clinical Applications. *Transl. Oncol.* **2024**, *50*, 102121. [CrossRef]
48. Han, Q.-F.; Li, W.-J.; Hu, K.-S.; Gao, J.; Zhai, W.-L.; Yang, J.-H.; Zhang, S.-J. Exosome Biogenesis: Machinery, Regulation, and Therapeutic Implications in Cancer. *Mol. Cancer* **2022**, *21*, 207. [CrossRef]
49. Susa, F.; Limongi, T.; Borgione, F.; Peiretti, S.; Vallino, M.; Cauda, V.; Pisano, R. Comparative Studies of Different Preservation Methods and Relative Freeze-Drying Formulations for Extracellular Vesicle Pharmaceutical Applications. *ACS Biomater. Sci. Eng.* **2023**, *9*, 5871–5885. [CrossRef] [PubMed]
50. Hassel, D.; Cheng, P.; White, M.P.; Ivey, K.N.; Kroll, J.; Augustin, H.G.; Katus, H.A.; Stainier, D.Y.R.; Srivastava, D. miR-10 Regulates the Angiogenic Behavior of Zebrafish and Human Endothelial Cells by Promoting VEGF Signaling. *Circ. Res.* **2012**, *111*, 1421–1433. [CrossRef] [PubMed]
51. Meng, Z.; Zhou, D.; Gao, Y.; Zeng, M.; Wang, W. miRNA Delivery for Skin Wound Healing. *Adv. Drug Deliv. Rev.* **2018**, *129*, 308–318. [CrossRef]
52. Van Rooij, E.; Sutherland, L.B.; Thatcher, J.E.; DiMaio, J.M.; Naseem, R.H.; Marshall, W.S.; Hill, J.A.; Olson, E.N. Dysregulation of microRNAs after Myocardial Infarction Reveals a Role of miR-29 in Cardiac Fibrosis. *Proc. Natl. Acad. Sci. USA* **2008**, *105*, 13027–13032. [CrossRef]
53. Yang, X.; Wang, J.; Guo, S.-L.; Fan, K.-J.; Li, J.; Wang, Y.-L.; Teng, Y.; Yang, X. miR-21 Promotes Keratinocyte Migration and Re-Epithelialization During Wound Healing. *Int. J. Biol. Sci.* **2011**, *7*, 685–690. [CrossRef] [PubMed]

54. Madhyastha, R.; Madhyastha, H.; Nakajima, Y.; Omura, S.; Maruyama, M. MicroRNA Signature in Diabetic Wound Healing: Promotive Role of miR-21 in Fibroblast Migration. *Int. Wound J.* **2012**, *9*, 355–361. [CrossRef] [PubMed]
55. Pawlaczyk, M.; Lelonkiewicz, M.; Wieczorowski, M. Age-Dependent Biomechanical Properties of the Skin. *Adv. Dermatol. Allergol. Dermatol. Alergol.* **2013**, *30*, 302–306. [CrossRef]
56. Rodrigues, M.; Kosaric, N.; Bonham, C.A.; Gurtner, G.C. Wound Healing: A Cellular Perspective. *Physiol. Rev.* **2018**, *99*, 665–706. [CrossRef] [PubMed]
57. Weng, T.; Wu, P.; Zhang, W.; Zheng, Y.; Li, Q.; Jin, R.; Chen, H.; You, C.; Guo, S.; Han, C.; et al. Regeneration of Skin Appendages and Nerves: Current Status and Further Challenges. *J. Transl. Med.* **2020**, *18*, 53. [CrossRef]
58. Xue, M.; Jackson, C.J. Extracellular Matrix Reorganization During Wound Healing and Its Impact on Abnormal Scarring. *Adv. Wound Care* **2015**, *4*, 119. [CrossRef]
59. Velnar, T.; Bailey, T.; Smrkolj, V. The Wound Healing Process: An Overview of the Cellular and Molecular Mechanisms. *J. Int. Med. Res.* **2009**, *37*, 1528–1542. [CrossRef]
60. Peña, O.A.; Martin, P. Cellular and Molecular Mechanisms of Skin Wound Healing. *Nat. Rev. Mol. Cell Biol.* **2024**, *25*, 599–616. [CrossRef]
61. Xing, H.; Zhang, Z.; Mao, Q.; Wang, C.; Zhou, Y.; Zhou, X.; Ying, L.; Xu, H.; Hu, S.; Zhang, N. Injectable Exosome-Functionalized Extracellular Matrix Hydrogel for Metabolism Balance and Pyroptosis Regulation in Intervertebral Disc Degeneration. *J. Nanobiotechnology* **2021**, *19*, 264. [CrossRef] [PubMed]
62. Lazar, S.; Mor, S.; Chen, J.; Hao, D.; Wan, A. Bioengineered Extracellular Vesicle-Loaded Bioscaffolds for Therapeutic Appli-cations in Regenerative Medicine. *EVCNA* **2021**, *2*, 175–178. [CrossRef]
63. Debnath, K.; Las Heras, K.; Rivera, A.; Lenzini, S.; Shin, J.-W. Extracellular Vesicle–Matrix Interactions. *Nat. Rev. Mater.* **2023**, *8*, 390–402. [CrossRef] [PubMed]

pharmaceutics

MDPI

Article

Future-Oriented Nanosystems Composed of Polyamidoamine Dendrimer and Biodegradable Polymers as an Anticancer Drug Carrier for Potential Targeted Treatment

Katarzyna Strzelecka [1], Adam Kasiński [1], Tadeusz Biela [2], Anita Bocho-Janiszewska [3], Anna Laskowska [4], Łukasz Szeleszczuk [5], Maciej Gawlak [6], Marcin Sobczak [1] and Ewa Oledzka [1,*]

1 Department of Pharmaceutical Chemistry and Biomaterials, Faculty of Pharmacy, Medical University of Warsaw, Banacha 1 Str., 02-097 Warsaw, Poland; katarzyna.strzelecka@wum.edu.pl (K.S.); adam.kasinski@wum.edu.pl (A.K.); marcin.sobczak@wum.edu.pl (M.S.)

2 Department of Polymer Chemistry, Centre of Molecular and Macromolecular Studies, Polish Academy of Sciences, Sienkiewicza 112 Str., 90-363 Lodz, Poland; tadeusz.biela@cbmm.lodz.pl

3 Faculty of Applied Chemistry, Casimir Pulaski Radom University, Chrobrego 27 Str., 26-600 Radom, Poland; a.janiszewska@uthrad.pl

4 Department of Pharmaceutical Microbiology, Centre for Preclinical Research, Medical University of Warsaw, Banacha 1b Str., 02-097 Warsaw, Poland; anna.laskowska@wum.edu.pl

5 Department of Organic and Physical Chemistry, Faculty of Pharmacy, Medical University of Warsaw, Banacha 1 Str., 02-093 Warsaw, Poland; lukasz.szeleszczuk@wum.edu.pl

6 Laboratory of Physiology and Pathophysiology, Centre for Preclinical Research, Medical University of Warsaw, Banacha 1b Str., 02-097 Warsaw, Poland; maciej.gawlak@wum.edu.pl

* Correspondence: eoledzka@wum.edu.pl or eoledzka@wp.pl; Tel.: +48-22-572-07-55; Fax: +48-22-572-07-84

Abstract: Background/Objectives: Camptothecin (CPT) is a well-known chemical compound recognized for its significant anticancer properties. However, its clinical application remains limited due to challenges related to CPT's high hydrophobicity and the instability of its active form. To address these difficulties, our research focused on the development of four novel nanoparticulate systems intended for either oral or intravenous administration. **Methods**: These nanosystems were based on a poly(amidoamine) (PAMAM) dendrimer/CPT complex, which had been coated with biodegradable homo- and copolymers, designed with appropriate physicochemical properties and chain microstructures. **Results**: The resulting nanomaterials, with diameters ranging from 110 to 406 nm and dispersity values between 0.10 and 0.67, exhibited a positive surface charge and were synthesized using biodegradable poly(L-lactide) (PLLA), poly(L-lactide-*co*-ε-caprolactone) (PLACL), and poly(glycolide-*co*-ε-caprolactone) (PGACL). Biological assessments, including cell viability and hemolysis tests, indicated that all polymers demonstrated less than 5% hemolysis, confirming their hemocompatibility for potential intravenous use. Furthermore, fibroblasts exposed to these matrices showed concentration-dependent viability. The entrapment efficiency (*EE*) of CPT reached up to 27%, with drug loading (*DL*) values as high as 17%. The in vitro drug release studies lasted over 400 h with the use of phosphate buffer solutions at two different pH levels, demonstrating that time-dependent processes allowed for a gradual and controlled release of CPT from the developed nanosystems. The release kinetics of the active compound at pH 7.4 ± 0.05 and 6.5 ± 0.05 followed near-first-order or first-order models, with diffusion and Fickian/non-Fickian transport mechanisms. Importantly, the nanoparticulate systems enabled the stabilization of the pharmacologically active form of CPT, while providing protection against hydrolysis, even in physiological environments. **Conclusions**: In our opinion, these results underscore the promising future of biodegradable nanosystems as effective drug delivery systems (DDSs) for targeted cancer treatment, offering stability and efficacy over short, medium, and long-term applications.

Keywords: nanopharmacy; camptothecin; PAMAM dendrimer; biodegradable polyesters; controlled drug delivery systems; targeted therapy

1. Introduction

The field of nanotechnology focuses on the molecular creation of a wide range of functional systems. These systems exhibit unique physical, electrical, and optical properties that make them appealing in a wide range of applications [1]. Nanopharmacy is one of the most well-known nanotechnology study areas. It employs nanotechnology to provide precisely tailored pharmaceutical treatments for illness diagnosis, prevention, and therapy. Over the last several decades, there has been an increase in nanopharmacy research, which is now being translated into commercialization efforts around the world, culminating in the selling of a variety of products [2,3]. Drug delivery systems (DDSs) currently dominate nanopharmacy, accounting for more than 75% of total sales [4].

The term DDSs refers to a wide variety of vehicles developed to increase the selectivity of action and improve the drug's pharmacological and pharmacokinetic characteristics. Most of the drugs in use today are classified as low-molecular-weight compounds. These substances are characterized by their quick metabolism and elimination from the human body, along with a lack of selectivity in their pharmacodynamic effects. This highlights the necessity for the development of formulations that can address these challenges [5]. The idea of DDSs originated as early as 1891, when German scientist Paul Erlich proposed a paradigm for selectively delivering drugs to their site of action, in the right concentration, and at the appropriate time [6].

Traditional ways of drug administration are frequently inefficient and pose a significant risk of side effects. DDSs allow for the alteration of drug characteristics, such as increasing solubility, preventing the drug from being transformed into an inactive form, and improving pharmacokinetic parameters and biodistribution [7]. DDSs are most commonly employed to develop systems that provide controlled or prolonged release of the active substance, known as therapeutic systems. Therapeutic systems are designed to maintain a constant drug concentration throughout time and to make the release rate independent of the amount of drug left in the system (achieving zero-order kinetics). The time required for the therapeutic system to release the drug is highly associated with the type of carrier used, which is the factor that controls the release [2]. The polymeric, inorganic, or composite material that acts as the drug's carrier must fulfill certain requirements, including biocompatibility, non-toxicity, non-immunogenicity, and no accumulation in the body. Furthermore, its size, surface character, method of binding the active substance, and presence of functional groups on the surface all play an important role in DDSs functioning [8].

Recent focus has been directed towards the chemistry of biocompatible and biodegradable polymers, often referred to as "biomedical polymers". These materials are advantageous due to their ability to be easily hydrolyzed into non-toxic, removable products that can be eliminated through metabolic processes [9,10]. Furthermore, it is essential that biomedical polymers are synthesized with the use of natural initiators, co-initiators, and/or catalysts that are both effective and safe for the environment and human health [11]. Most significantly, these materials have great potential for various medical applications, including tissue engineering, gene therapy, temporary implanted devices, regenerative medicine, nanopharmacy, and coatings on implants [12]. Biodegradable and/or bioresorbable polymers such as polyglycolide (PGA), polylactide (PLA), poly(ε-caprolactone) (PCL), poly(trimethylene carbonate) (PTMC) and copolymers of glycolide (GL), L-lactide (LA), *rac*-lactide (*rac*-LA), ε-caprolactone (CL), trimethylene carbonate (TMC), or others cyclic esters and carbonates are most commonly used in nanopharmacy to develop DDSs and other therapeutic systems [13].

Dendrimers, especially poly(amidoamine) (PAMAM) dendrimers, also known as tree-shaped, stellar, hyperbranched, or cascading polymers, are unique carriers that require particular attention. These are spherical structures with greatly branching arms that terminate in functional groups [14]. The presence of peripheral functional groups (e.g., amine, hydroxyl) as well as internal cavities in PAMAM dendrimers can be adopted to encapsulate drugs or other active compounds. The encapsulation of the active component within the PAMAM dendrimer cavity is a typical idea for drugs with a low molecular weight and poor water solubility. A host-guest interaction occurs inside dendrimer cavities due to the hydrogen bonds between dendrimer and the drug molecules, resulting in a highly soluble complex [15]. Furthermore, the empty spaces in the dendrimer structure are frequently hydrophobic, allowing for interactions with poorly soluble molecules via hydrophobic interactions [16]. The active substance might be additionally conjugated to the peripheral functional groups via covalent bonding. This strategy is preferred, since it provides more precise control over the drug release, enabling its delivery to the target site [17]. Last but not least, the main benefits of using PAMAM dendrimers as drug carriers include improved solubility of hydrophobic drugs, drug protection during transport in the body, a longer period of drug activity, improved pharmacodynamics, reduced side effects, and the possibility of prolonged and controlled drug release [18].

Cancer is a prevalent cause of mortality worldwide. The American Cancer Society predicts that in 2024, 2,001,140 new cancer cases and 611,720 cancer deaths will occur in the United States [19]. According to the National Cancer Registry data, the overall number of malignant tumor cases in Poland in 2020 was over 146,000, with about 100,000 deaths. Unfortunately, the disease structure in Poland is remarkably similar to that of other countries [20].

The main objective of oncological therapy is to bring the tumor under control to ensure better life expectancy and quality. In addition to surgical therapy and radiotherapy, chemotherapy includes a wide range of drugs from various groups, each with a different mechanism of action. All three treatment procedures carry a significant risk of major side effects, as well as limited specificity and selectivity [21].

Chemotherapeutic drug treatment is associated with high toxicity, which is a severe clinical issue that has a considerable impact on the patient's quality of life [22]. Furthermore, the anticancer drugs utilized exhibit rapid renal clearance, making it difficult to achieve the appropriate therapeutic concentration, thus necessitating the use of higher doses. Also, the majority of drugs taken systemically are lipophilic, tend to accumulate in the liver, and, as a result, may lead to hepatic steatosis [23]. In order to improve the efficacy and safety of therapy, scientists are searching for carriers that would allow targeted drug delivery to cancer cells as well as controlled drug release.

One of the most promising anticancer drugs is camptothecin (CPT), a pentacyclic alkaloid isolated from the *Camptotheca acuminata* tree [24]. The α-hydroxylactone ring in the CPT's structure plays a crucial role in sustaining the anticancer efficiency, since its opening leads to deactivation [25]. CPT provides a high cytotoxic effect, and its mechanism of action relies on the suppression of topoisomerase I activity, which results in DNA damage and, consequently, cell death [26]. Nonetheless, CPT's therapeutic usage, however, is challenging due to its low solubility in water, high cellular toxicity, and hydrolytic cleavage of the lactone ring to the inactive carboxyl form in vivo [27]. In recent years, extensive research has been conducted to generate novel formulations of CPT, which could address the aforementioned concerns [24]. It involves the development of polymer nanoparticles, micelles, liposomes, and lipid nanoparticles [28–32]. Another alternative strategy is to encapsulate CPT inside the cavity of a PAMAM (polyamidoamine) dendrimer, which has minimal cytotoxicity and is able to penetrate biological membranes [33].

In our previous investigation, we examined PAMAM dendrimer/CPT complex for non-small-cell lung cancer cell targeting [34]. Considering that the findings we obtained were highly promising and revealed an opportunity for further study, we decided to develop innovative PAMAM dendrimer/biodegradable polymer nanosystems as a CPT carrier in the present research. To date, there have been no reports in the literature of nanosystems that encapsulate both CPT and its derivatives inside a PAMAM dendrimer, with a biodegradable polymer serving as the carrier. We suspected that encapsulating CPT inside a PAMAM dendrimer would improve its solubility and the therapeutic bioavailability, while utilizing a biodegradable material with a predicted microstructure and topology would allow for controlled and sustained drug release. Furthermore, the acidic microenvironment formed by the hydrolytic degradation of the biodegradable matrix will inhibit the active lactone form of CPT from converting to its inactive carboxyl form. As a result, the developed novel nanosystems may allow for oral or intravenous administration, while maintaining the therapy's effectiveness and biosafety.

2. Materials and Methods

2.1. Materials

(*S*)-(+)-Camptothecin ((*S*)-4-Ethyl-4-hydroxy-1H-pyrano-[3′,4′:6,7]indolizino [1,2-b] quinoline-3,14(4H,12H)-dione) (CPT) (purity: >97.0% (HPLC)) was purchased from TCI Europe N.V. (Zwijndrecht, Belgium). PAMAM dendrimer, ethylenediamine core, generation 4.0, 10 wt.% solution in methanol was obtained from Merck, Poznan, Poland. L-lactide ((3S)-*cis*-3,6-dimethyl-1,4-dioxane-2,5-dione) (LA) (purity: 100%), ε-caprolactone (2-oxepanone) (CL) (purity: 100%), glycolide (1,4-dioxane-2,5-dione) (GL) (purity: 100%), diethylzinc solution 1.0 M in hexanes (Et_2Zn), poly(ethylene glycol) average M_n 400 (PEG-400), Tween® 80 (polyethylene glycol sorbitan monooleate, polysorbate 80) were also obtained from Merck, Poznan, Poland. *N,N*-dimethylformamide (DMF, anhydrous, 99%, Avantor Performance Materials S.A., Gliwice, Poland), dimethyl sulphoxide (DMSO, anhydrous, 99%, Avantor Performance Materials S.A., Gliwice, Poland), methanol (anhydrous, 99.9%, Avantor Performance Materials S.A., Gliwice, Poland), dichloromethane (DCM, anhydrous, 99.8%, Chempur, Piekary Śląskie, Poland), chloroform (pure, stabilized with amylen, 98.5%, Chempur, Piekary Śląskie, Poland), petroleum ether boiling range 60–90 °C (Chempur, Piekary Śląskie, Poland), liquid paraffin (Chempur, Piekary Śląskie, Poland), hydrochloric acid (≥37%, Merck, Poznan, Poland) and acetonitrile ((ACN), anhydrous, 99.8%, Avantor Performance Materials S.A., Gliwice, Poland) were used as received. Dimethyl-d_6-sulfoxide (DMSO-d_6) in ampoules, for NMR measurements (99.9 atom% D), was purchased from ARMAR Chemicals (Döttingen, Switzerland), whereas chloroform-d (deuterochloroform, $CDCl_3$ 99.8 atom% D) was purchased from Merck, Poznan, Poland. Phosphate buffer solutions (PBS, pH 7.40 ± 0.05 and pH 6.50 ± 0.05, 20 °C, Avantor Performance Materials S.A., Gliwice, Poland) were also used as received.

2.2. Synthesis of PAMAM Dendrimer/CPT Complex

The synthesis was carried out according to a previously established method by Oledzka et al. [34]. Briefly, 9.1 mg of CPT was placed in a 5.0 mL round-bottom flask and dissolved in 2 mL of DMF. Then, 1 mL of PAMAM dendrimer (G4, 10 wt.% in methanol) was added, and the prepared reaction mixture was incubated in the dark for 24 h at 37 °C, at a rotational speed of 130 rpm. Following that, the DMF was evaporated, and 2.0 mL of distilled water was added to the solid residue and stirred for 1 h in order to remove the unreacted CPT. The obtained suspension was filtered using a 0.45 μm syringe filter, and the supernatant was evaporated using a rotary evaporator. The resulting solid compound was dried in a vacuum oven at 40 °C for 72 h, until the constant weight was achieved. The PAMAM dendrimer/CPT complex synthesis yielded 84.85%. The synthesised complex was stored in the dark in an inert gas atmosphere until it was used. Subsequent analyses were conducted within 24 h of synthesis.

The ^1H NMR spectrum of the synthesized PAMAM dendrimer/CPT complex (DMSO-d_6, 400 MHz; δH): 8.69 ppm (G, B-ring of CPT), 7.93 ppm (H and K, A-ring of CPT), 7.70 ppm (I and J, A-ring of CPT), 7.34 ppm (A, D-ring of CPT), 5.42 ppm (E, E-ring of CPT), 5.29 ppm (F, C-ring of CPT), 4.87 ppm (6 (-CH_2-CH_2-C(O)-N($\underline{H}$)-) of PAMAM dendrimer), 4.67 ppm (7 (-C(O)-N(H)-CH_2-CH_2-N$\underline{H_2}$) of PAMAM dendrimer), 2.00–3.62 ppm (2 (-C$\underline{H_2}$-CH_2-C(O)-N(H)-), 3 (-CH_2-C$\underline{H_2}$-C(O)-N(H)-), 4 (-C(O)-N(H)-C$\underline{H_2}$-CH_2-) and 5 (-C(O)-N(H)-CH_2-C$\underline{H_2}$-NH_2) of PAMAM dendrimer), 1.86 ppm (B, E-ring of CPT, methylene group), 1.22 ppm (1 (-N-C$\underline{H_2}$-C$\underline{H_2}$-N-) and 1′ (-C(O)-N(H)-CH_2-C$\underline{H_2}$-) of PAMAM dendrimer), 0.87 ppm (C, E-ring of CPT, methylene group) (Figure S1, Supplementary Materials).

2.3. Synthesis of Biodegradable Polymers

The Ring-Opening Polymerisation (ROP) process was applied to produce four polymers, with $ZnEt_2$ acting as a catalyst and PEG-400 serving as a co-initiator. The reactions were carried out in bulk. Briefly, carefully weighted amounts of monomers—LA (M1), LA and CL (M2), and CL and GL (M3, M4) (1 g total)—were placed in glass ampoules and vacuum dried to remove trace amounts of moisture. After that, calculated amounts of $ZnEt_2$ and PEG-400 were added in an argon atmosphere via the Schlenk line, and the ampoules were safely sealed. Reactions were carried out in an oil bath at 130 °C for 24 h. The post-reaction mixtures of M1 and M2 were then dissolved in 6.0 mL of DCM, while M3 and M4 were dissolved in 6.0 mL of a 1:1 mixture consisting of DCM and chloroform. Following that, the dissolved polymers were transferred to beakers and precipitated using an ice-cold 5% HCl solution in methanol. The precipitates were subsequently washed twice more with pure, ice-cold methanol. The collected products were vacuum-dried for 24 h at 30 °C.

The ^1H NMR spectrum of the synthesized PLLA (M1, $CDCl_3$, 400 MHz; δH): 5.15 ppm (2, $(-O(O)C-(\underline{H})C(CH_3)-)$), 4.31 ppm (5, $(-O(O)C-(\underline{H})C(CH_3)-OH)$), 3.63 ppm (PEG, $(-C\underline{H_2}-C\underline{H_2}-)$), 2.17 ppm (1, $(-O(O)C-(H)C(CH_3)-O\underline{H})$), 1.42 ppm (3, $(-O(O)C-(H)C(C\underline{H_3})-)$), 1.25 ppm (4, $(-O(O)C-(H)C(C\underline{H_3})-OH)$) (Figure S2, Supplementary Materials).

The ^{13}C NMR spectrum of the synthesized PLLA (M1, $CDCl_3$, 400 MHz; δH): 169.7 ppm $(-O(O)\underline{C}-(H)C(CH_3)-)$, 69.0 ppm $(-O(O)C-(H)\underline{C}(CH_3)-)$, 16.7 ppm (2, $(-O(O)C-(H)C(\underline{C}H_3)-)$) (Figure S3, Supplementary Materials).

The ^1H NMR spectrum of the synthesized PLACL (M2, $CDCl_3$, 400 MHz; δH): 5.15 ppm (2, $(-O(O)C-(\underline{H})C(CH_3)-)$), 5.06 ppm (3, $(-O-(\underline{H})C(CH_3)-C(O)O-(CH_2)_5-)$), 4.12 ppm (5, $(-(H)C(CH_3)-C(O)O-C\underline{H_2}-CH_2-CH_2-CH_2-CH_2-C(O)O-)$), 4.05 ppm (10, $(-(CH_2)_5-C(O)O-C\underline{H_2}-CH_2-CH_2-CH_2-CH_2-)$), 3.64 ppm (PEG, $(-C\underline{H_2}-C\underline{H_2}-)$), 2.38 ppm (9, $(-(H)C(CH_3)-C(O)O-CH_2-CH_2-CH_2-CH_2-C\underline{H_2}-C(O)O-)$), 2.29 ppm (14, $(-(CH_2)_5-C(O)O-CH_2-CH_2-CH_2-CH_2-C\underline{H_2}-)$), 1.45–1.71 ppm (1, $(-O(O)C-(H)C(C\underline{H_3})-)$, 4, $(-O-(H)C(C\underline{H_3})-C(O)O-(CH_2)_5-)$, 6, $(-(H)C(CH_3)-C(O)O-CH_2-C\underline{H_2}-CH_2-CH_2-C\underline{H_2}-C(O)O-)$, 8, $(-(H)C(CH_3)-C(O)O-CH_2-CH_2-CH_2-C\underline{H_2}-CH_2-C(O)O-)$, 11, $(-(CH_2)_5-C(O)O-CH_2-C\underline{H_2}-CH_2-CH_2-CH_2-)$, 13 $(-(CH_2)_5-C(O)O-CH_2-CH_2-CH_2-C\underline{H_2}-CH_2-)$), 1.39 ppm (7, $(-(H)C(CH_3)-C(O)O-CH_2-CH_2-C\underline{H_2}-CH_2-CH_2-C(O)O-)$, 12, $(-(CH_2)_5-C(O)O-CH_2-CH_2-C\underline{H_2}-CH_2-CH_2-)$) (Figure S4, Supplementary Materials).

The ^{13}C NMR spectrum of the synthesized PLACL (M2, $CDCl_3$, 400 MHz; δH): 172.6–173.9 ppm (1, $(-(CH_2)_5-\underline{C}(O)O-(CH_2)_5-)$, carbonyl carbon atoms of oxycaproyl unit), 169.3–171.2 ppm (2, $(-O(O)\underline{C}-(H)C(CH_3)-)$, carbonyl carbon atoms of lactidyl unit), 67.8–69.9 ppm (4, $(-O(O)C-(H)\underline{C}(CH_3)-)$, methine carbon atoms of lactidyl unit), 63.4–65.9 ppm (9, $(-C(O)O-CH_2-CH_2-CH_2-CH_2-\underline{C}H_2-)$, ε-carbon atoms of oxycaproyl unit), 33.1–33.4 ppm (5, $(-C(O)O-\underline{C}H_2-CH_2-CH_2-CH_2-CH_2-)$, α-carbon atoms of oxycaproyl unit)), 28.2 ppm (8, $(-C(O)O-CH_2-CH_2-CH_2-\underline{C}H_2-CH_2-)$, δ-carbon atoms of oxycaproyl unit), 23.9–25.9 ppm (6, $(-C(O)O-CH_2-\underline{C}H_2-CH_2-CH_2-CH_2-)$, β-carbon atoms of oxycaproyl unit, 7, $(-C(O)O-CH_2-CH_2-\underline{C}H_2-CH_2-CH_2-)$, γ-carbon atoms of oxycaproyl unit), 16.6 ppm (3, $(-O(O)C-(H)C(\underline{C}H_3)-)$, methyl carbon atoms of lactidyl unit) (Figure S5, Supplementary Materials).

The ^1H NMR spectrum of the synthesized PGACL (M3 and M4, $CDCl_3$, 400 MHz; δH): 4.60 ppm (1, $(-O-C\underline{H_2}-C(O)-)$, glycolidyl unit), 4.05 ppm (2, $(-C(O)O-C\underline{H_2}-CH_2-CH_2-CH_2-CH_2-)$, caproyl unit), 3.65 ppm (PEG, $(-C\underline{H_2}-C\underline{H_2}-)$), 2.30 ppm (6, $(-C(O)O-CH_2-CH_2-CH_2-CH_2-C\underline{H_2}-)$, caproyl unit), 1.65 ppm (6, $(-C(O)O-CH_2-C\underline{H_2}-CH_2-CH_2-CH_2-)$, caproyl unit, 5, (6, $(-C(O)O-CH_2-CH_2-CH_2-C\underline{H_2}-CH_2-)$, caproyl unit), 1.38 ppm (4, $(-C(O)O-CH_2-CH_2-C\underline{H_2}-CH_2-CH_2-)$, caproyl unit) (Figure S6, Supplementary Materials).

The ^{13}C NMR spectrum of the synthesized PGACL (M3 and M4, $CDCl_3$, 400 MHz; δH): 172.8–173.5 ppm ($(-O-CH_2-\underline{C}(O)-)$, glycolidyl unit), 167.9 ppm ($(-\underline{C}(O)O-CH_2-CH_2-CH_2-CH_2-CH_2-)$, caproyl unit), 64.2–65.2 ppm ($(-C(O)O-CH_2-CH_2-CH_2-CH_2-\underline{C}H_2-)$, ε-carbon atoms of oxycaproyl unit), 60.2–60.5 ppm ($(-O-\underline{C}H_2-C(O)-)$, glycolidyl unit), 33.6–34.1 ppm ($(-C(O)O-\underline{C}H_2-CH_2-CH_2-CH_2-CH_2-)$, α-carbon atoms of oxycaproyl unit)), 28.2 ppm ($(-C(O)O-CH_2-CH_2-CH_2-\underline{C}H_2-CH_2-)$, δ-carbon atoms of oxycaproyl unit), 25.4 ppm ((-C(O)O-CH2-CH2-

$\underline{C}H_2$-CH_2-CH_2-), γ-carbon atoms of oxycaproyl unit), 24.4 ppm ((-C(O)O-CH_2-$\underline{C}H_2$-CH_2-CH_2-CH_2-), β-carbon atoms of oxycaproyl unit) (Figure S7, Supplementary Materials).

The conversion of monomers was determined from ^{1}H NMR spectra of post-reaction, by comparing the integrated signals of equivalent protons from the monomer and polymer, according to the following formula (Equation (1)):

$$Conv_i = \frac{I_i}{I_i + I_I} \quad (1)$$

where I_i and I_I represent the integral intensities of signals from equivalent protons in the monomer and polymer, respectively.

The microstructural analysis of the obtained polymers was carried out with ^{13}C NMR spectra in the methine and carbonyl regions for PLLA and the carbonyl region for PLACL. The microstructure of PGACL matrices was examined using ^{1}H NMR spectra in the region of methylene protons of glycolidyl units (*GG*) and ε-methylene proton region of caproyl units (*Cap*). By comparison with the available literature, relevant spectral lines were assigned to the respective sequences [35–37].

With the use of ^{1}H and ^{13}C spectra, the experimental lengths of glycolidyl units ($L^e{}_{GG}$) and lactydyl units ($L^e{}_{LL}$) were calculated according to Equation (2), whereas experimental lengths of caproyl units were calculated with the use of Equation (3) for ^{1}H NMR spectrum and Equation (4) for ^{13}C NMR spectrum, respectively:

$$L^e_{XX} = \frac{CapXCap + CapXX + XXCap + XXX}{CapXCap + \frac{1}{2}(CapXX + XXCap)} \times \frac{1}{2} \quad (2)$$

$$L^e_{Cap} = \frac{XCap + CapCap}{XCap} \quad (3)$$

$$L^e_{Cap} = \frac{CapCapCap + XCapCap + CapCapX + XCapX}{XCapX + \frac{1}{2}(XCapCap + CapCapX)} \quad (4)$$

where X represents lactydyl unit -OCH(CH_3)CO- (*L*) or glycolidyl unit -OCH_2CO- (*G*), *Cap* represents caproyl unit -O(CH_2)$_5$CO-, and *CapXX*, *CapXCap*, *XCap*, *CapCapX*, and so on represent particular sequences in the polymeric chain.

The transesterification of the second mode (T_{II}) may cause a break in the *L* or *G* units within the copolymeric chain, resulting in the formation of distinct *CapLCap* or *CapGCap* sequences. To quantitatively determine the yield of T_{II} in the copolymeric chains, the following Equation (5) was applied:

$$T_{II} = \frac{[CapXCap]}{[CapXCap]_R} \quad (5)$$

where [*CapXCap*] represents the experimental concentration of *CapXCap* sequences, and $[CapXCap]_R$ is the concentration of *CapXCap* sequences in a completely random copolymeric chain.

The $[CapXCap]_R$ can be described using the following formula (Equation (6)), where the ratio of [Cap]/[X] is denoted as k′:

$$[CapXCap]_R = \frac{k'^2}{\left(k' + 1\right)^3} \quad (6)$$

The degree of the randomness (*R*) of the copolymeric chain was calculated according to Equation (7):

$$R = \frac{L^R_{XX}}{L^e_{XX}} \quad (7)$$

where L^R_{XX} represents the average lengths of lactydyl or glycolidyl blocks (Equation (8)) and caproyl blocks (Equation (9)), respectively, in a completely randomized copolymeric chain.

$$L^R_{XX} = \frac{k' + 1}{2k'} \tag{8}$$

$$L^R_{Cap} = k' + 1 \tag{9}$$

2.4. In Vitro Hydrolytic Degradation of Polymerics

In brief, 10 mg of the produced polymers were weighed into prepared and labelled glass vials. The experiment was conducted simultaneously in two series: 10.0 mL of buffer pH 7.4 ± 0.05 was added to the first series, and 10.0 mL of buffer pH 6.5 ± 0.05 was used in the second series. The prepared samples were placed in an incubator set to 37 °C with a rotational speed of 100 rpm. The measurement points for each sample were set at 7, 14, 21, 28, 56, and 77 days. The pH of the sample was determined at each time point using the Volcraft pH-100ATC pH-meter.

2.5. Synthesis of the Nanosystems Composed of PAMAM Dendrimer/CPT Complex and Biodegradable Polymer

The beaker was filled with 49.5 mL of liquid paraffin and 0.5 mL of Tween 80 to produce a 0.5% solution, which was then placed on a magnetic stirrer. Two glass vials were weighed with 200 mg of the proper biodegradable polymer (M1, M2, M3, or M4) and 20 mg of the PAMAM/CPT complex. The appropriate amount of DCM was poured to the vials with the matrices, followed by methanol to the vial with complex. All vials spent 30 min in an ultrasonic cleaner. The contents of the vials were then mixed and withdrawn using a syringe. The contents of the syringe were added in a dropwise manner to the Tween 80 solution in liquid paraffin at a constant mixing speed of 1000 rpm. Subsequently, the beaker was placed in an ultrasonic homogeniser for 5 min, while cooling in an ice bath. The beaker was then put back on the magnetic stirrer at 400 rpm, covered with parafilm, and left for about 3 h. Following this, n-hexane was poured in the beaker and kept at room temperature for 24 h. The precipitate solution was then decanted, and the resulting products (denoted as NP1, NP2, NP3, NP4) were washed seven times with petroleum ether before drying.

To determine the drug loading (*DL*) and the entrapment efficiency (*EE*) of CPT in the obtained nanosystems, the accurately weighted amounts of the developed products (~10 mg) were dissolved in 5 mL of ACN and sonicated for 30 min in an ice bath. The resulting solutions were filtered through 0.45 μm syringe filters to the HPLC vials.

The *DL* was calculated using the following Equation (10):

$$DL = \frac{Measured\ CPT\ content}{Nanosystem\ weight} \times 100\% \tag{10}$$

whereas the *EE* was determined using Equation (11):

$$EE = \frac{Measured\ CPT\ content}{Theoretical\ CPT\ content} \times 100\% \tag{11}$$

2.6. In Vitro Release Study of CPT from the Developed Nanosystems

The obtained nanosystems (~50 mg) were suspended in PBS at pH 6.50 ± 0.05 and 7.40 ± 0.05. The resulting suspensions were transferred to dialysis membranes with pore diameters of 3.50 kDa and immersed in appropriate buffer solution. The release experiment lasted 23 days and involved constant rotating at 100 cycles per min at 37 °C. At each time point, 1.5 mL of samples were collected and supplemented with 1.5 mL of fresh pH-appropriate PBS. The collected samples were then subjected to HPLC analysis to assess the amount of CPT released as well as the percentage amount of lactone and carboxylic form of CPT. The analysis was performed using gradient elution and UV detector at a wavelength of 363 nm. The calibration curve was designed between 0.46 and 46.55 µg/mL (R^2 = 1.000, y = 2.3926x − 0.2040). Each of the collected samples was tested three times, and the outcome of the analysis was expressed as an amount of CPT released (in µg).

2.7. Mathematical Models

The release data points were subjected to zero-order, first-order kinetics, Higuchi, and Korsmeyer–Peppas models, respectively. The calculations were performed according to the formulas provided below:

Zero-order:

$$F = kt \tag{12}$$

First-order:

$$\log F = \log F_0 - \frac{kt}{2.303} \tag{13}$$

Higuchi model:

$$F = k\sqrt{t} \tag{14}$$

Korsmeyer–Peppas model:

$$F = kt^n \ (F < 0.6) \tag{15}$$

where:
F is the fraction of drug released from the matrix after time t;
F_0 is the initial amount of the drug;
k is a model constant; and n is drug release exponent in the Korsmeyer–Peppas model [34,38–41].

2.8. Hemolysis

Defibrinated sheep blood was purchased from Graso, Starogard Gdański, Poland. Blood was centrifuged at 2000 rpm for 10 min (RT). The supernatant was carefully removed without disturbing the RBC pellet. Samples were resuspended in 5 mL of PBS (pH 7.40 ± 0.05) and centrifuged at 2000 rpm for 10 min. The washing step was repeated three times until the supernatant was clear. The remaining RBC pellet was diluted in PBS (pH 7.4, RT) to obtain a 2% suspension. Next, 2% RBC suspension was incubated with serial dilution of the proper matrix (M1, M2, M3, or M4, 0.05–0.5 mg/mL) in a 1:1 ratio for 1 h at 37 °C. Positive control (100% hemolysis) was prepared with distilled water and negative control (0% hemolysis) with PBS (pH 7.40 ± 0.05). Next, samples were centrifuged at 2000 rpm for 5 min (RT), and 100 µL of supernatant from each sample was transferred to a 96-well F-bottom plate. Optical density (OD) was measured at 540 nm in a microplate reader (BioTek Synergy HTX Multimode Reader, Agilent, Santa Clara, CA, USA). The value of compound-induced hemolysis was calculated according to Equation (16) [42]:

$$\text{Hemolysis [\%]} = (A - A_{0\%})/(A_{100\%} - A_{0\%})\cdot 100\% \tag{16}$$

where A is the absorbance of the sample, $A_{100\%}$ is the absorbance of the positive control (100% hemolysis), and $A_{0\%}$ is the absorbance of the negative control (0% hemolysis).

2.9. Cell Culture and Viability Assay

Normal human dermal fibroblasts (Promocell) were maintained in Dulbecco's Modified Eagle Medium (DMEM) (Biowest, Nuaillé, France) containing 10% fetal bovine serum (FBS) (Biowest, Nuaillé, France) and 1% penicillin-streptomycin solution (Biowest, Nuaillé, France). Cells were incubated at 37 °C in humidifying conditions with 5% CO_2. At confluency of 80% cells were harvested and seeded in 96-well plates at a density of $3\cdot 10^3$ per well and incubated overnight. The growth media was then changed to DMEM at pH 7.40 ± 0.05 or DMEM at pH 6.50 ± 0.05 with serial dilutions of M1, M2, M3, or M4 (0.05–50 µg/mL). Plates were incubated at 37 °C for 72 h. After the incubation period, 20 µL of

CellTiter 96® AQueous One Solution Cell Proliferation Assay (MTS) (Promega, Walldorf, Germany) was added to each well, and the plates were incubated for an additional 2 h at 37 °C. The absorbance was measured at λ = 490 nm. The viability of untreated cells (negative control) was defined as 100%.

2.10. Statistical Analysis

The in vitro experiment findings were provided as a mean and standard deviation of mean (SEM). The normality of distribution was tested first, followed by one-way ANOVA or the non-parametric Kruskal–Walli's test to determine the statistical significance of mean differences. To compare the different circumstances, two-way ANOVA was employed, followed by Bonferroni's multiple comparisons. $p < 0.05$ was deemed statistically significant. The data was analysed with GraphPad Prism 5.0 (GraphPad Software, San Diego, CA, USA).

2.11. Molecular Modelling of the Nanosystems Composed of PAMAM Dendrimer/CPT Complex and Biodegradable Polymer

The structure of PAMAM dendrimer generation 4.0 was built using the Build Polymers module within the Biovia Materials Studio 2020 software suite (https://www.3ds.com/products-services/biovia/products/molecular-modeling-simulation/biovia-materials-studio/, accessed on 20 October 2024). The terminal, primary amino groups of dendrimers are demonstrated to be protonated and thereby positively charged at pH ranges between 6.5 ± 0.05 and 9.0 ± 0.05 [43]. Since the dissolution analyses conducted for this study were done at pH 6.5 ± 0.05 and 7.4 ± 0.05, all of the terminal amino groups of the modeled PAMAM structure have been protonated to improve comparability with those studies.

The Forcite Plus module has been used to optimize the structures, applying ultra-fine-quality settings of geometry optimization and smart algorithm. The convergence tolerance values were set to $2 \cdot 10^{-5}$ kcal/mol for energy, $1 \cdot 10^{-3}$ kcal/(Å · mol) for force, and $1 \cdot 10^{-5}$ Å for displacement, with $5 \cdot 10^{4}$ maximum iterations. All calculations have been performed using the COMPASS II forcefield [44], which has been shown to provide accurate results when modeling PAMAM dendrimers [45]. As charge assignments are one of the characteristics provided in this forcefield specification, the charges have been allocated using the COMPASS II forcefield. The electrostatic and van der Waals summation methods were both atoms-based with cubic spline truncation of non-bond energy terms, 18.5 Å cutoff distance, 1 Å spline width, and 0.5 Å buffer width.

Molecular docking calculations were conducted utilizing the Adsorption Locator module, a part of the Biovia Materials Studio 2020 software suite. The Adsorption Locator module identifies potential adsorption sites through Monte Carlo searches of the configurational space of the substrate (PAMAM) and adsorbate (CPT) system, as the temperature is gradually lowered during the simulated annealing process of a molecular dynamics simulation. This approach offers the advantage of allowing for the simultaneous docking of the designated quantities of CPT, specifically three molecules of API in this study. The Adsorption Locator makes use of a simulation of annealing with geometry adjustments in-between repeating heat-cool cycles. For repeatable results, 10 cycles with 100,000 steps each and annealing temperatures ranging from 100 to 5000 K were utilized. For "conformer", "rotate", and "translate", the Monte Carlo parameters were set to a probability of 0.32 (ratio = 1), whereas "regrow" was set to 0.1 (ratio = 0.03). The computations employed the identical geometry optimization parameters from the preceding paragraph's detailed description of geometry optimization and the COMPASS II force field.

To calculate the stoichiometry of the PAMAM dendrimer/CPT complex, the formula below was used (Equation (17)):

$$L = \frac{m_{CPT} \times M_{PAMAM} \times EE}{M_{CPT} \times V_{PAMAM} \times d_{PAMAM} \times C_{PAMAM}} = 3.1 \quad (17)$$

where L represents the loading (average number of CPT molecules per one PAMAM molecule), m_{CPT} denotes the mass of added CPT ($9.1 \cdot 10^{-3}$ g), M_{PAMAM} indicates the molar mass of PAMAM (14,214.17 g/mol), *EE* refers to the encapsulation efficiency (84.85%), M_{CPT} signifies the molar mass of CPT (348.35 g/mol), V_{PAMAM} is the volume of added PAMAM methanol solution ($1 \cdot 10^{-3}$ dm^3), d_{PAMAM} represents the density of the PAMAM methanol solution (0.813 g/cm^3), and C_{PAMAM} is the percentage concentration of PAMAM methanol solution (10%).

The optimised systems, which included three molecules of CPT, were then analysed using molecular dynamics (MD) simulations with periodic boundary conditions [34]. First, the MODELS 1–4 were created using the Amorphous Cell module of Materials Studio. This application provides a comprehensive set of tools to construct three-dimensional periodic structures of polymeric systems. The module builds molecules in a cell in a Monte Carlo fashion, by minimizing close contacts between atoms, whilst ensuring a realistic distribution of torsion angles for any given forcefield. The output of such simulations is a single periodic structure, which in the case of the present study served as the basic input to MD simulations. The composition of the cubic unit cells of MODELS 1–4 included PAMAM G4.0/3 molecules of CPT complex, surrounded by the polymer. After construction, the systems MODELS 1–4 were subjected to geometry optimization, including unit cell dimensions optimization, using the parameters from the preceding paragraph's detailed description of geometry optimization setup and the COMPASS II force field as well.

A simulated annealing process was conducted in five cycles of 10,000 steps, within a temperature range of 300–500 K, utilizing the NVT ensemble mode, five heating ramps per cycle, 100 dynamics steps per run, and the Berendsen thermostat with a 0.1 ps decay constant. A production run lasting 100 ns was conducted in NVT mode, utilizing the Nosé–Hoover thermostat for temperature regulation, with a Q-ratio set at 2 and a time step of 1 fs. The MD calculations employed the COMPASS II force field, utilizing parameters identical to those applied during geometry optimization.

2.12. Measurements

All ^{1}H and ^{13}C NMR measurements were performed using a Varian 300 MHz (Palo Alto, Santa Clara, CA, USA) and Agilent Technologies 400 MHz (Santa Clara, CA, USA) spectrometer.

The quantitative analysis of CPT content in the samples was determined using previously developed and described method by Oledzka et al. [34]. The study was performed using HPLC apparatus (Beckman Coulter, Miami, Florida, USA) equipped with a UV/Vis detector (Beckman Coulter System Gold® 166, Fullerton, CA, USA), an autosampler (Triathlon 900, Spark Holland B.V., Emmen, Netherlands) and a pump (Beckman Coulter System Gold® 125NM Solvent Module, Fullerton, CA, USA). The C18 column (Luna 25 cm, 5 μm, 100 A, Phenomenex, Basel, Switzerland) was placed at 30 °C, and the injection volume was 20 μL. The gradient mobile phase consisting of acetonitrile (ACN): phosphate buffer solution (pH 6.50 ± 0.05 or 7.40 ± 0.05) (*v*/*v*) was delivered at a flow rate of 1.0 mL/min (ACN concentration varied with time: 5% ACN after 0 min, 15% ACN after 5 min, 35% ACN after 15 min, 50% ACN after 20 min, and 5% ACN after 22 and 25 min). The retention time of CPT's carboxylic form was 13.90 ± 0.1 min and 20.69 ± 0.1 min for the lactone form of CPT.

The number-average molecular weight (M_n) and dispersity index (*Đ*) of the polymeric materials were measured by the SEC-MALLS instrument (Wyatt Technology Corporation, Santa Barbara, CA, USA), composed of an autosampler, degasser, 1100 Agilent isocratic pump, thermostatic box for columns, a photometer MALLS DAWN EOS (Wyatt Technology Corporation, Santa Barbara, CA, USA), and differential refractometer Optilab Rex (Wyatt Technology Corporation, Santa Barbara, CA, USA). For data collecting and processing, the ASTRA 4.90.07 software (Wyatt Technology Corporation, Santa Barbara, CA, USA) was used. For separation the two 2 × PLGel 5 microns MIXED-C columns were used. The samples were injected as a solution in methylene chloride, and the volume of the injection loop was 100 mL. The mobile phase consisting of methylene chloride was delivered at a flow rate of 0.8 mL/min.

The dynamic light scattering studies of hydrodynamic diameters and zeta potential were performed using the Zetasizer Nano ZS (Malvern, UK). The excitement wavelength of the DLS instrument was 633 nm (He-Ne laser, power = 5 W), and the measurement angle was 173. Polystyrene disposable cuvettes were used during hydrodynamic diameter determination, while the zeta potential measurements were performed using standard dip cells equipped with palladium electrodes. The assessments were conducted at 25 °C in aqueous solutions, using an excitation wavelength of 633 nm (He-Ne laser, power = 5 W) of DLS instrument. Prior to measurement, the samples were briefly sonicated. All experiments were replicated three times.

Transmission electron microscopy (TEM) was used to assess the shape morphology and size of the developed nanosystems. The developed products that had been synthesized were collected on TEM grids. TEM studies were carried out using equipment installed in the Laborarory of Electron Microscopy, Nencki Institute of Experimental Biology, Polish Academy of Sciences, Warsaw, Poland. Electron micrographs were taken using a CCD MORADA G2 (EMSIS GmbH, Münster, Germany) camera on a JEM 1400 (JEOL Co., Tokyo, Japan) transmission electron microscope sponsored by the EU Structural Funds: Centre of Advanced Technology BIM—Equipment purchase for the Laboratory of Biological and Medical Imaging.

Concerning confocal fluorescence microscopy, the samples were mounted (Chemland, Stargard, Poland) and sealed with #1.5 coverslips (Epredia, Braunschweig, Germany). The fluorescent signal was acquired with an Olympus Fluoview FV1000 confocal microscope (EVIDENT Europe GmbH, Hamburg, Germany) and with 10× and 60× objectives. Fluorescence was excited with 488 nm line of an Argon laser, and the emission was detected at 461 nm.

3. Results and Discussion

3.1. Synthesis and Characterization of Biodegradable Polymers

As a first approach, four biodegradable homo- and copolymers were synthesized via ROP of LA, CL, and GL in the presence of $ZnEt_2$ as a catalyst and PEG-400 as a biosafe co-initiator. The polymerization process was carried out at 130 °C for 24 h. The molar ratio of the monomers to the catalyst and co-initiator was constant and equal to 100:1:1. The reactions were carried out in bulk. The polymers were synthesized with a moderate high monomer conversion, satisfactory yield, reasonably narrow $Đ$, and M_n ranged from 8700 to 21,300 g/mol (Table 1). It is well established in the scientific literature that polymeric matrices characterized by a higher M_n tend to demonstrate slower drug release profiles compared to those with lower M_n values [46]. Therefore, our primary intention in this study was to develop PAMAM dendrimer/biodegradable polymer nanosystems that are proficient in releasing CPT in a controlled manner over varying durations, including short, medium, and long periods.

Table 1. Homo- and copolymerization of CL, GL, and LA. The characteristics of the obtained biodegradable polymers.

Code	Matrix	Monomer Molar Ratio	Yield [%]	$Conv_i$ [a] [%]	M_n [b] [g/mol]	$Đ$ [b]
M1	PLLA poly(L-lactide)	LA = 1.0	78	97	13,600	1.23
M2	PLACL poly(L-lactide-*co*-ε-caprolactone)	LA = 0.40 CL = 0.60	78	83 (LA) 82 (CL)	8700	1.77
M3	PGACL poly(glycolide-*co*-ε-caprolactone)	CL = 0.85 GL = 0.15	83	86 (CL) 74 (GL)	16,100	1.57
M4		CL = 0.90 GL = 0.10	90	85 (CL) 63 (GL)	21,300	1.52

[a]—calculated from ^{1}H NMR; [b]—determined by SEC-MALLS.

The ^{1}H and ^{13}C NMR spectra of the synthesized materials were utilized to determine the structural properties of the polymeric matrices (Figure S2, ^{1}H NMR spectra of PLLA; Figure S3, ^{13}C NMR spectra of PLLA; Figure S4, ^{1}H NMR spectra of PLACL; Figure S5, ^{13}C NMR spectra of PLACL; Figure S6, ^{1}H NMR spectra of PGACL; Figure S7, ^{13}C NMR spectra of PGACL, Supplementary Materials). The characteristic signals observed in the spectra were assigned according to the literature, which confirmed the structures of the produced PLLA, PLACL, and PGACL [35–37,47].

As seen in Figure S8 (Supplementary Materials), which displays the PLLA carbonyl and methine regions, the only spectral lines that could be assigned represent *iiiii* hexad and *iii* tetrad. Accordingly, our data indicates that transesterification has no effect on the stereoregularity of the produced PLLA. Consequently, the synthesized PLLA exhibited high isotacticity.

The examination of the copolymer spectra, particularly the ^{13}C NMR spectrum of PLACL (M2) (Figure 1) and the ^{1}H NMR spectra of PGACL (M3 and M4) (Figure 2), were supported in the identification of spectral lines corresponding to distinct comonomeric sequences within the PGACL and PLACL copolymeric chains. The ^{1}H NMR spectra of M3 and M4 revealed the presence of a signal generated from the *-GCapG-* triad, with *G* representing the glycolidyl unit -OCH_2CO- and *Cap* (*C*) representing the caproyl unit -$O(CH_2)_5CO$-. The presence of this signal indicated that type II intermolecular transesterification occurred during the synthesis. Furthermore, the presence of the *-CapLCap-* triad in the ^{13}C NMR spectrum of PLACL, where *L* represents the lactydyl unit -$OCH(CH_3)CO$-, suggests that in this case, type II intermolecular transesterification also took place. The distribution of comonomeric units in the polymer chains was calculated according to the literature and using the relevant equations (2–8, Experimental section) [36,37]. The average block lengths, transesterification of the second mode, and degree of randomness are provided in Table 2. The estimated findings indicate that the resultant copolymers have an atactic chain microstructure.

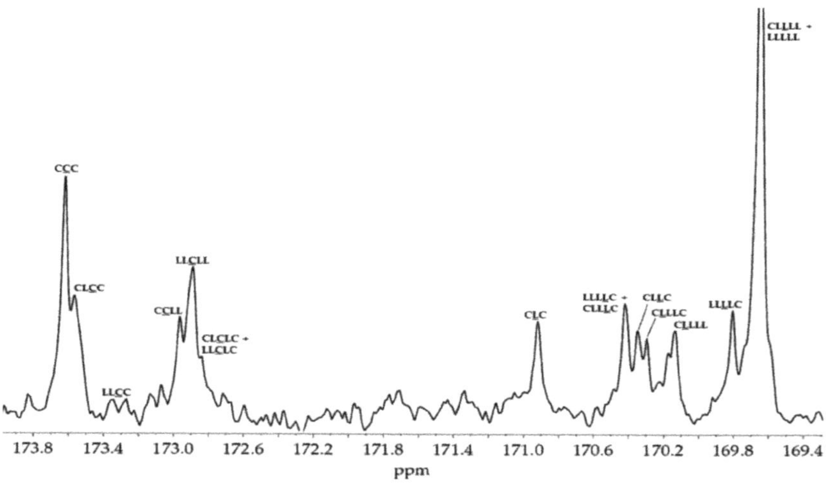

Figure 1. Expansion of the domain of interest in ^{13}C NMR spectrum of carbonyl region for PLACL copolymer (M2).

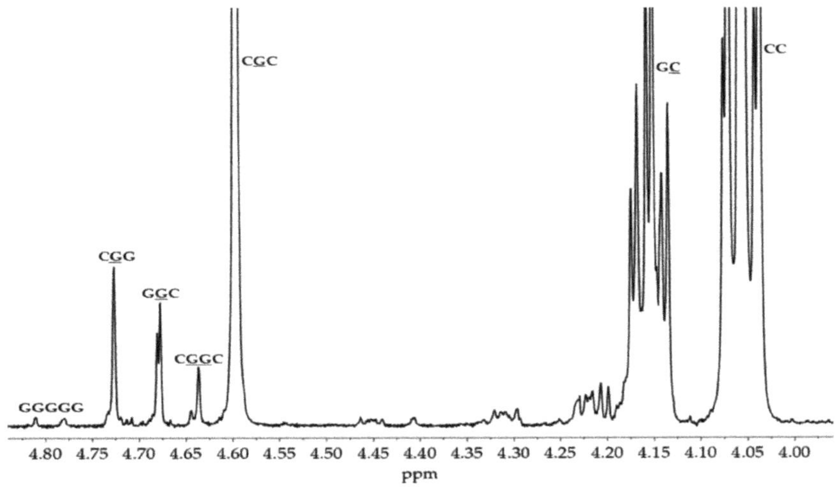

Figure 2. Expansion of the domain of interest in ^{1}H NMR spectrum of PGACL copolymer (M3 and M4).

Table 2. Analysis of the chain microstructure of the synthesized copolymers.

Code	Polymer	Average Block Length	T_{II}	R
M2	poly(L-lactide-*co*-ε-caprolactone) PLACL/40:60	$L^e_{LL} = 1.27$ $L^e_{Cap} = 0.99$	0.49	1.00
M3	poly(glycolide-*co*-ε-caprolactone) PGACL/15:85	$L^e_{GG} = 1.67$ $L^e_{Cap} = 4.43$	0.73	0.60
M4	poly(glycolide-*co*-ε-caprolactone) PGACL/10:90	$L^e_{GG} = 1.46$ $L^e_{Cap} = 8.81$	0.94	0.68

L^e_{LL}—experimental average length of lactydyl blocks; L^e_{Cap}—experimental average length of caproyl blocks; L^e_{GG}—experimental average length of glycolidyl blocks; T_{II}—yield of the second mode of transesterification; R—the degree of randomness.

Given that it is commonly known that materials used in the medical and pharmaceutical fields must fulfil certain criteria, the resulting polymer matrices were subjected to biological tests, namely cell viability and hemolysis.

The level of RBC hemolysis was matrix-dependent ($p = 0.0982$), but concentration-independent (Figure 3). Among tested polymeric matrices, the lowest hemolysis was induced by M3 (max. 0.3%) followed by M1 (max. 1%) and M4 (max. 1.2%). The highest hemolytic activity was observed for M2 (max. 2.85%). No statistically significant differences in the level of hemolysis were observed between all matrices except the highest concentration. At a concentration of 0.5 mg/mL, M2-induced hemolysis was significantly higher compared to M1, M3, and M4.

A hemolysis assay is an indispensable initial step in evaluating the blood compatibility of polymers to identify severe acute toxic reactions in RBCs in vivo [48]. Furthermore, many studies have reported that in vitro hemolysis assays have good correlations with in vivo toxicity considering the hemolytic effect [49,50]. Importantly, if the hemolysis rate is less than 5%, medicinal products are termed non-hemolysis under national biological safety guidelines. In our study, all tested matrices revealed results of less than 5%, meeting the national regulatory requirements for biological materials and establishing their hemocompatibility for possible intravenous application (Figures 3 and S9, Supplementary Materials).

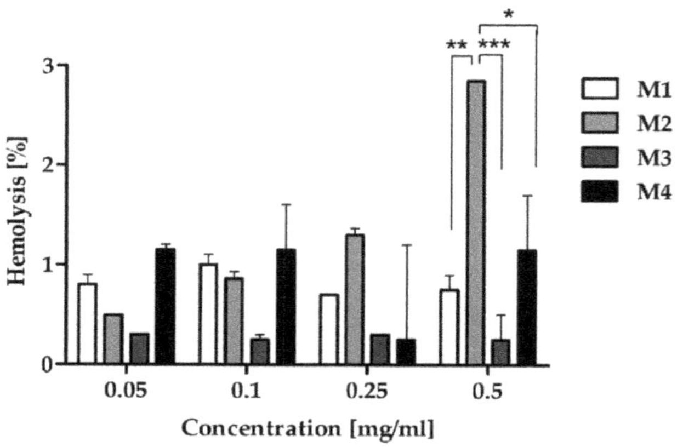

Figure 3. Hemolytic activity of the synthesized biodegradable polymers: M1, M2, M3, and M4 after 1 h of incubation. The graph depicts the level of hemolysis of RBC treated with increasing concentrations of the complex after 1 h of treatment. Two-way ANOVA followed by the Bonferroni post-test was used for statistical analysis. The results were considered statistically significant: * $p < 0.05$; ** $p < 0.01$; *** $p < 0.005$.

As seen in Figure 4, the fibroblasts treated with polymers exhibited comparable concentration-dependent viability. The pH of the cultures had no significant influence on the activity of the polymer samples, except for M4, which caused a greater decrease in viability at pH 6.5 ± 0.05 (see Figure S10, Supplementary Materials). The viability of polymers-treated cells reached approximately 90% viability level of control cells (the concentration ranged from 0.01 to 5 µg/mL). However, at higher concentrations (10–50 µg/mL), the fibroblast viability was reduced to around 80% after 72 h of treatment. A statistically significant difference in cell viability was noted for M1 and M2 matrices at a concentration of 0.5 µg/mL and between M3 and M4 at 10 µg/mL.

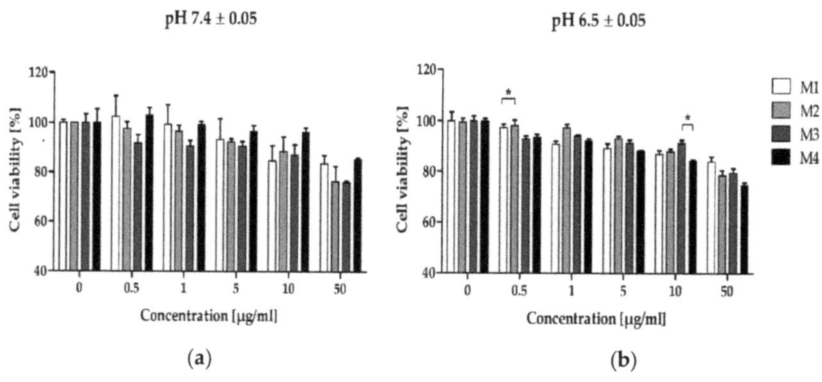

Figure 4. The viability of normal fibroblasts treated for 72 h with the synthesized biodegradable polymers at pH 7.4 ± 0.05 (**a**) and pH 6.5 ± 0.05 (**b**). The graphs depict differences in the susceptibility of cells to the complex. The MTS assay was used to determine the relative cell number. The results are given as mean ± SEM. Two-way ANOVA was used for statistical analysis, followed by Bonferroni post-tests. When the following conditions were met, the results were considered statistically significant: * $p < 0.05$.

3.2. Synthesis and Characterization of the Nanosystems Composed of PAMAM Dendrimer/CPT Complex and Biodegradable Polymers

In the second step of the investigation, the synthesized and characterized polymers, as well as the PAMAM dendrimer/CPT complex, were employed to develop nanoparticulate systems for targeted therapy. Based on the previous optimization findings, four nanosystems were produced, each employing a different biodegradable polymer (Table 3).

Table 3. Characterization of the developed nanosystems composed of PAMAM dendrimer/CPT complex and biodegradable polymer.

Code	Polymer Used	Entrapment Efficiency (*EE*) [a] [%]	Drug Loading (*DL*) [a] [%]	Size [b] [nm]	Zeta Potential [b] [mV]	PDI [b]
NP1	PLLA (M1)	25 ± 2.51	16 ± 1.35	190	5.24 ± 2.34	0.51
NP2	PLACL/40:60 (M2)	27 ± 1.94	17 ± 0.94	110	34.40 ± 2.14	0.52
NP3	PGACL/15:85 (M3)	22 ± 2.42	14 ± 1.78	284	23.43 ± 3.11	0.67
NP4	PGACL/10:90 (M4)	11 ± 2.91	7 ± 3.59	406	26.83 ± 1.79	0.10

[a]—determined by HPLC; [b]—determined by DLS.

As shown in Table 3, the *EE* value ranged from 11 ± 2.91 to 27 ± 1.94%. The highest value was observed for the NP2 sample (27 ± 1.94%), and the lowest for the NP4 (11 ± 2.91%). We suspect that these variations are most likely caused by the varied types of polymeric materials used to obtain nanosystems. Furthermore, the DLS analysis indicated that the developed nanosystems had an average size of 190 nm (NP1), 110 nm (NP2), 284 nm (NP3), and 406 nm (NP4). The dispersity values ranged from 0.10 to 0.67, showing a rather broad particle size distribution. Zeta potential experiments indicated that all produced nanoparticulate systems have a positive surface charge (ranging from 5.24 to 24.4 mV), which is most likely explained by the presence of protonated primary amino groups in PAMAM dendrimer macromolecules [51]. It is also important to note that the TEM images of the produced nanomaterials supported the DLS results. Figure 5 shows that the size range of the nanosystems was below 500 nm.

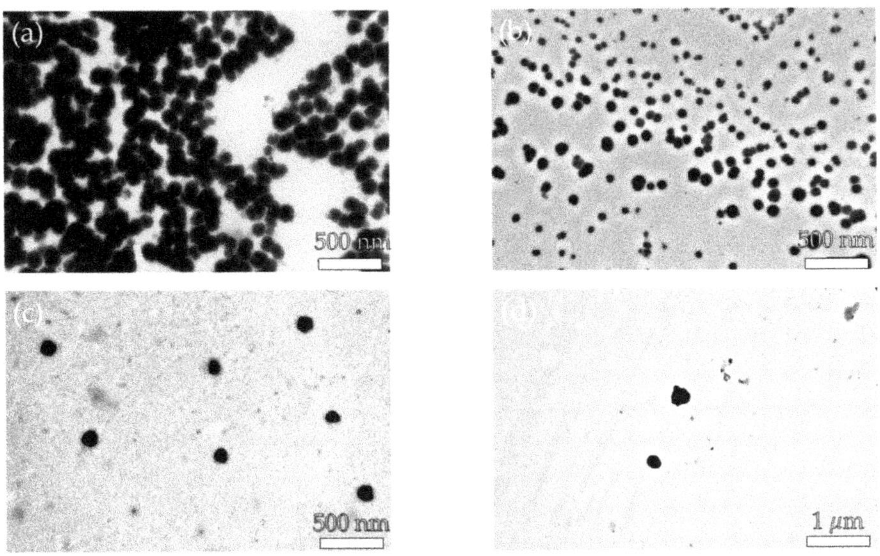

Figure 5. TEM image of: (**a**) NP1 sample, (**b**) NP2 sample, (**c**) NP3 sample, (**d**) NP4 sample.

To confirm the presence of CPT more clearly in the prepared nanosystems and roughly determine its location, the confocal microscopy was applied (Figure 6). Given that CPT is a naturally fluorescent substance (Figure 6a) [52], this technique appears to be suitable for this specific application. The confocal microscopic images showed an effective entrapment of this drug into the PAMAM dendrimer cavity as fluorescence was detected in all nanoparticulate materials.

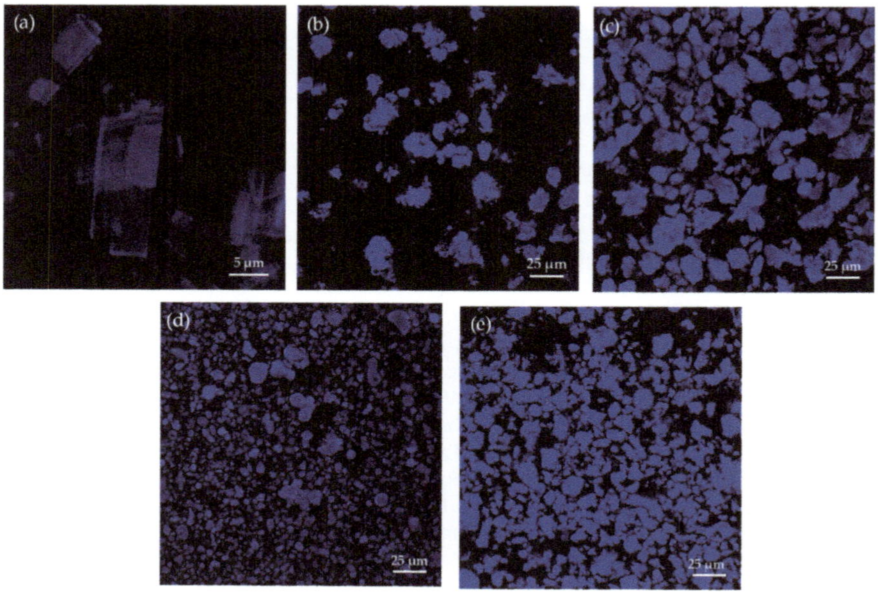

Figure 6. Confocal fluorescence imaging of: (**a**) CPT, (**b**) NP1 sample, (**c**) NP2 sample, (**d**) NP3 sample, (**e**) NP4 sample.

3.3. *CPT Release Study from the Nanosystems Composed of PAMAM Dendrimer/CPT Complex and Biodegradable Polymmer*

The in vitro release study of CPT was conducted for more than 400 h, utilizing phosphate buffer solutions at two distinct pH levels: 7.40 ± 0.05, which simulates physiological conditions found in the bloodstream, and 6.50 ± 0.05, representing the acidic environment characteristic of endosomes in cancer cells. This study aimed to assess stability and elucidate the CPT release characteristics from the developed nanosystems. The drug release profiles for the samples NP1, NP2, NP3, and NP4 are illustrated as a correlation between cumulative drug release and time (Figures 7 and 8). As it can be clearly seen in Figure 7, the drug release rate at a pH of 6.50 ± 0.05 reached a plateau after 120 h for NP4, 216 h for NP1 and NP2, and after 360 h for NP3. The highest drug release rate was observed for the samples NP3 and NP4 (78%), while the NP1 material released only 60% of the active substance. Figure 8 depicts the release rates at a pH of 7.40 ± 0.05. It can be observed that a plateau was achieved after 48 h for the samples NP1, NP2, and NP4, whereas sample NP3 reached its plateau after 168 h. The highest release rate was observed for the NP4 sample (91%), while the NP2 nanosystem demonstrated the lowest drug release rate (45%).

The findings from the two distinct release media are notably consistent, with the highest release rates recorded for the nanosystems obtained using PGACL (NP3 and NP4). This observation may be attributed to the presence of the GL units within the copolymeric chain. The degradation rates of GL copolymers are closely related to the GL composition, as these copolymers exhibit significant hydrophilicity, rendering them more susceptible to hydrolytic degradation [53].

To summarize these findings, it is important to highlight that coating the PAMAM dendrimer/CPT complex with a biodegradable polymer significantly influenced the drug release profile. The time-dependent mechanisms facilitated a gradual and controlled release of the drug from the formulated nanosystems. This phenomenon may be attributed to several factors, including the dissociation during dilution, the competitive displacement of the drug from the PAMAM dendrimer cavity by components of the release medium, the adsorption of the free drug onto the nanoparticle surface, and the diffusion of the free drug from the polymer chain structure [54].

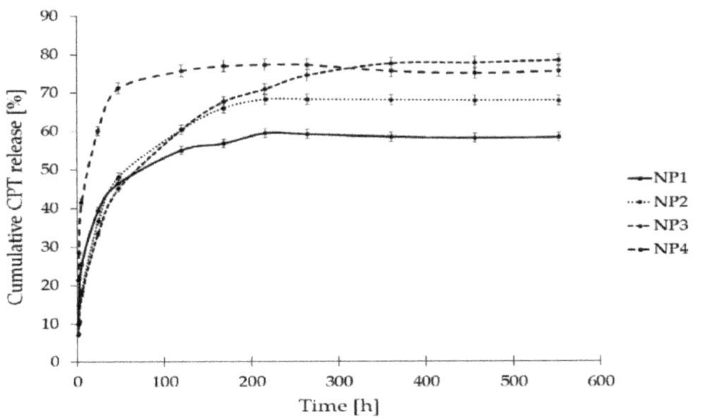

Figure 7. CPT release profiles from the developed nanosystems at pH 6.50 ± 0.05.

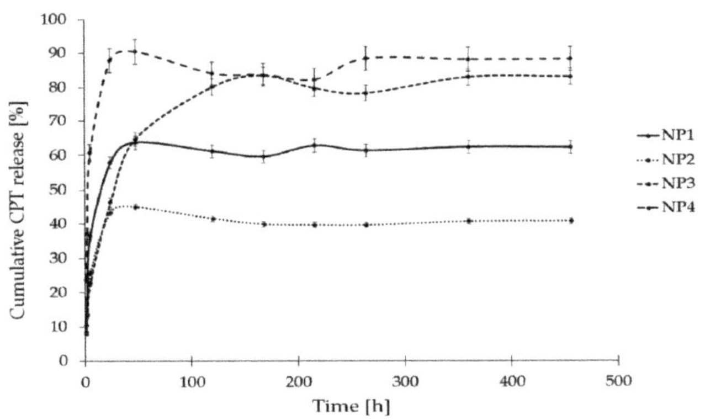

Figure 8. CPT release profiles from the developed nanosystems at pH 7.40 ± 0.05.

The release rates illustrated in Figures 7 and 8 include both the carboxylic form of CPT, which is pharmacologically inactive, and the lactone form, which is pharmacologically active. According to existing literature, these two forms exist in a state of equilibrium [55]. However, the percentage content of the lactone form of CPT is a critical factor to consider, especially in predicting tumor response. Given that physiological conditions facilitate the hydrolysis of the lactone ring, utilizing biodegradable polymers as a vehicle for CPT presents a viable solution to the issue of CPT instability. As can be seen in Figure S11 (Supplementary Materials), both forms of CPT were detected during the release studies conducted at pH 7.4 ± 0.05 (Figure S11a) and pH 6.5 ± 0.05 (Figure S11b). A comparative analysis of the lactone conformation percentage at pH 7.4 ± 0.05 reveals a notable increase in its content over the duration of incubation (Figure 9). This increase is probably attributable to the acidic degradation products of the polymer carriers present in the incubation environment, which effectively lower the pH and enhance the stability of the pharmacologically active form of CPT. A similar trend was observed in the release study conducted at pH 6.5 ± 0.05 (Figure 10). In all samples, the percentage of the lactone form of CPT was significantly higher than what has been reported in the existing literature [55]. Additionally, it is important to note that, in contrast to the findings of Liu and coworkers, who reported no observable conversion from lactone to carboxylate structures in CPT-loaded poly(ω-pentadecalactone-*co*-butylene-*co*-succinate) (PPBS) nanoparticles over a 24 h period [56], our study demonstrates a significant increase in the lactone form of CPT over a duration of 450 h. This increase is particularly pronounced at 6.50 ± 0.05, where all analyzed nanosystems exhibited a lactone form content exceeding 70%.

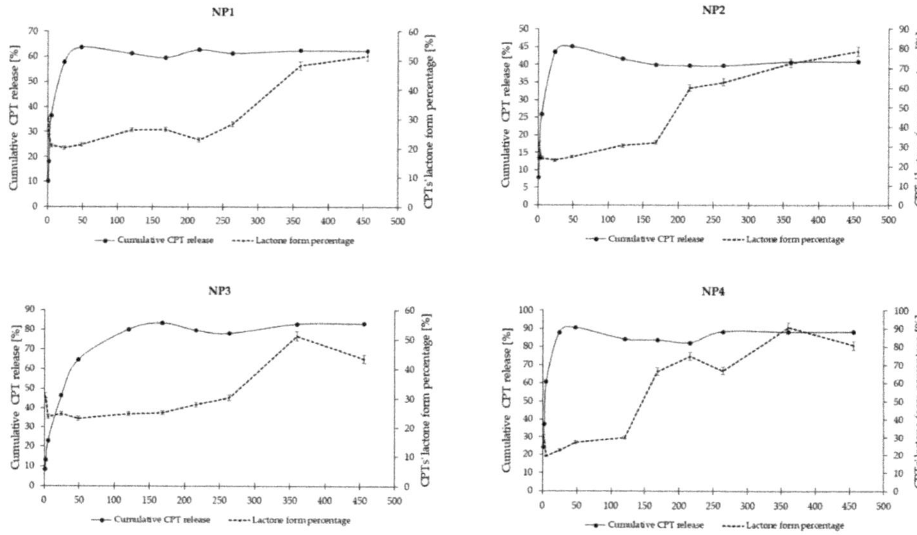

Figure 9. Correlation between cumulative CPT release and percentage of the lactone form of CPT at 7.40 ± 0.05.

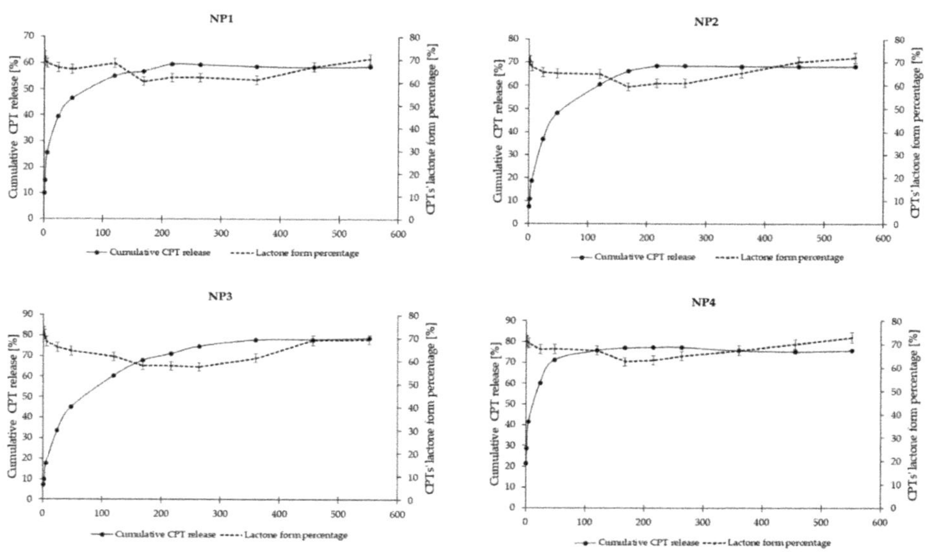

Figure 10. Correlation between cumulative CPT release and percentage of the lactone form of CPT at 6.50 ± 0.05.

Based on these findings, it can be concluded that the developed nanoparticulate systems enabled the stabilization of the pharmacologically active form of CPT and provided its protection against hydrolysis, even under physiological conditions.

In the next step, the data collected from the CPT release studies were analyzed using zero-order, first-order, Higuchi, and Korsmeyer–Peppas models to assess the kinetics and mechanism of CPT release from the developed nanosystems (Table 4).

Table 4. Analysis data of CPT release from obtained NPs.

Sample	pH	Zero-Order Model	First-Order Model	Higuchi Model	Kosmeyer-Peppas Model		Drug Transport Mechanism
		R^2	R^2	R^2	R^2	n	
NP1	7.4 ± 0.05	0.465	0.542	0.688	0.915	0.45	non-Fickian transport
NP2	7.4 ± 0.05	0.400	0.445	0.593	0.707	0.23	Fickian diffusion
NP3	7.4 ± 0.05	0.620	0.740	0.845	0.993	0.53	non-Fickian transport
NP4	7.4 ± 0.05	0.401	0.575	0.616	0.999	0.62	non-Fickian transport
NP1	6.5 ± 0.05	0.628	0.717	0.844	0.952	0.32	Fickian diffusion
NP2	6.5 ± 0.05	0.684	0.779	0.893	0.987	0.45	non-Fickian transport
NP3	6.5 ± 0.05	0.758	0.877	0.939	0.992	0.45	non-Fickian transport
NP4	6.5 ± 0.05	0.517	0.653	0.744	0.978	0.32	Fickian diffusion

The release kinetics of CPT at a pH of 7.4 ± 0.05 from the nanosystem NP3 conformed to a near-first-order model, as indicated by an R^2 value of 0.740. Additionally, drug release at a pH of 6.5 ± 0.05 from the samples NP1, NP2, and NP3 exhibited near-first-order kinetics, with R^2 values of 0.717, 0.779, and 0.877, respectively. It is also likely that CPT was released from the nanosystems NP1, NP2, and NP4 at pH 7.4 ± 0.05, as well as from NP4 at pH 6.5 ± 0.05, following first-order kinetics; however, this conclusion is made with caution due to the relatively low R^2 values ($R^2 < 0.7$). Analysis of the CPT release data using the Higuchi model indicated that CPT was released from the sample NP3 at pH 7.4 ± 0.05 and from all nanosystems at pH 6.5 ± 0.05 via a diffusion mechanism, as evidenced by R^2 values exceeding 0.7. Furthermore, the analysis of CPT release data from all nanosystems using the Korsmeyer–Peppas model suggested that the transport mechanism was either Fickian (n = 0.23–0.32, $R^2 > 0.7$) or non-Fickian (n = 0.45–0.62, $R^2 > 0.9$).

3.4. Molecular Modeling of the Nanosystems Composed of PAMAM Dendrimer/CPT Complex and Biodegradable Polymer

3.4.1. MODELS Preparation

Molecular simulations of dendrimer-drug complexes, while inherently challenging, provide valuable insights into the conformational flexibility of dendrimers and the atomic-level interactions that occur during the association of dendrimers with drugs. In our prior research, which detailed the molecular modeling of the PAMAM dendrimer/CPT complex [34], we established that the most stable configuration for the PAMAM dendrimer of generation 4.0 corresponds to a molar ratio of 1:3 for PAMAM dendrimer to CPT. This finding aligns with experimental data.

In our current study, we enhanced our model by incorporating the specific environments for each of the four types of prepared nanosystems. This development led to the creation of MODELS 1–4, which are detailed in the Materials and Methods section. Each of these models consists of a PAMAM dendrimer/CPT complex, featuring three CPT molecules for every PAMAM dendrimer of generation 4.0, all set within a polymer matrix that aligns with the experimental composition. It is important to highlight that, given the size of the experimentally obtained systems, which are several hundred nanometers, we conducted our calculations under periodic boundary conditions. This approach allows for a more accurate representation of the intramolecular forces that influence the structure and behavior of the system. The structures of MODELS 1–4 can be found in Figures 11–14.

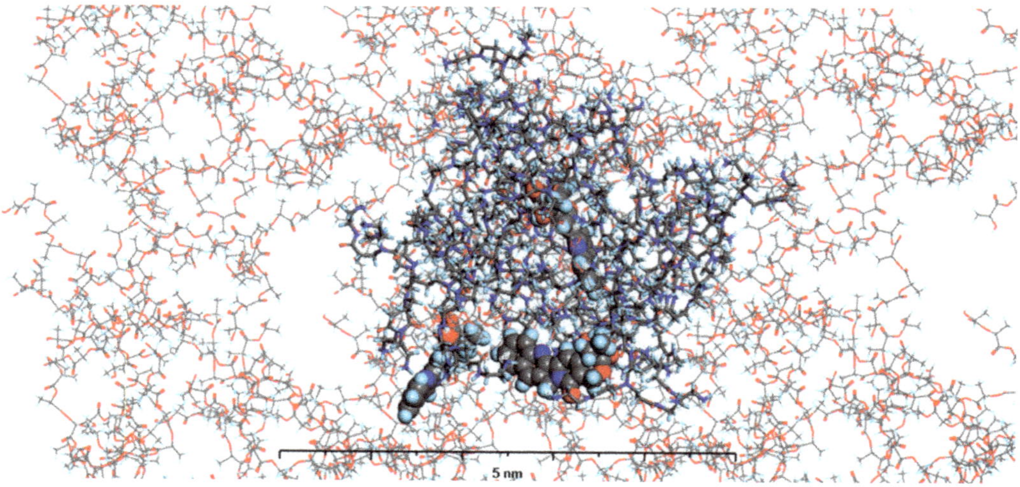

Figure 11. The structure of MODEL 1—PAMAM dendrimer generation 4.0 loaded with three molecules of CPT and surrounded by PLLA matrix. Atom coloring: Hydrogen—light blue, Nitrogen—dark blue, Carbon—grey, Oxygen—red. Rendering: the atoms and bonds of PLLA are rendered as sticks, the atoms of PAMAM dendrimer generation 4.0 are rendered as solid cylinders, CPT atoms are rendered as spheres with radii that are related to the van der Waals radii of its atoms.

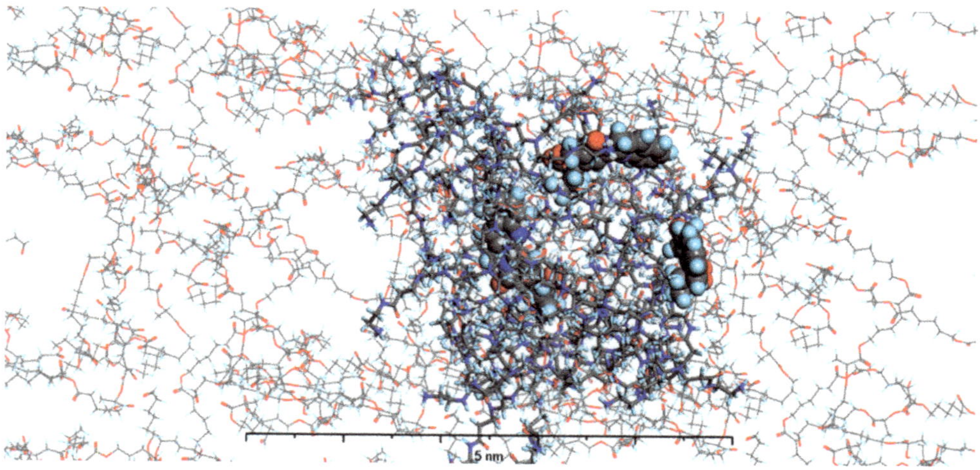

Figure 12. The structure of MODEL 2—PAMAM dendrimer generation 4.0 loaded with three molecules of CPT and surrounded by PLACL matrix. Atom coloring: Hydrogen—light blue, Nitrogen—dark blue, Carbon—grey, Oxygen—red. Rendering: the atoms and bonds of PLLA are rendered as sticks, the atoms of PAMAM dendrimer generation 4.0 are rendered as solid cylinders, CPT atoms are rendered as spheres with radii that are related to the van der Waals radii of its atoms.

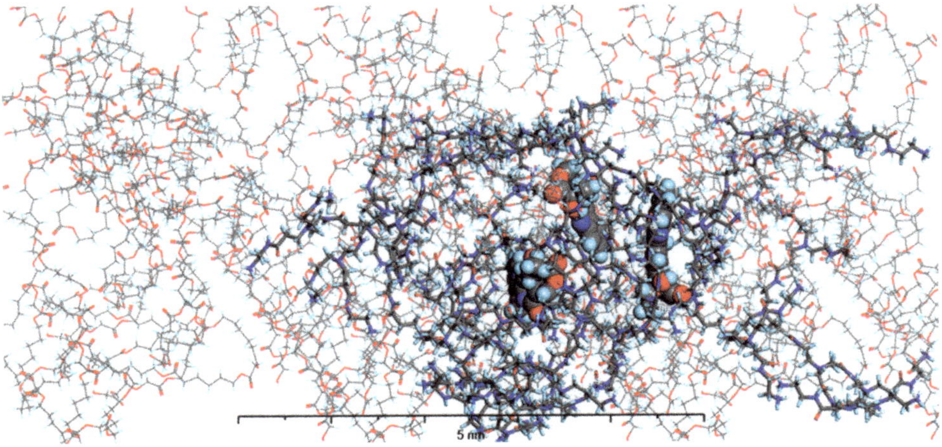

Figure 13. The structure of MODEL 3—PAMAM dendrimer generation 4.0 loaded with three molecules of CPT and surrounded by PGACL 85:15 (ε-CL:GL) matrix. Atom coloring: Hydrogen—light blue, Nitrogen—dark blue, Carbon—grey, Oxygen—red. Rendering: the atoms and bonds of PLLA are rendered as sticks, the atoms of PAMAM dendrimer generation 4.0 are rendered as solid cylinders, CPT atoms are rendered as spheres with radii that are related to the van der Waals radii of its atoms.

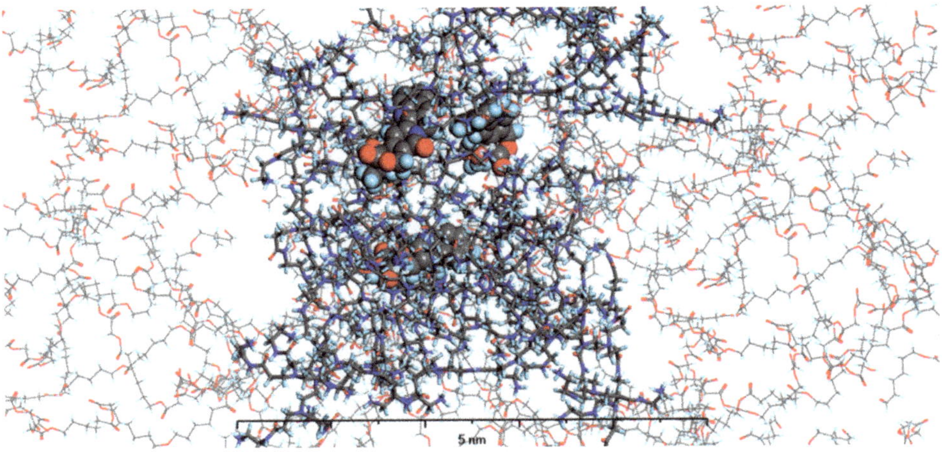

Figure 14. The structure of MODEL 4—PAMAM dendrimer generation 4.0 loaded with three molecules of CPT and surrounded by PGACL 90:10 (ε-CL:GL) matrix. Atom coloring: Hydrogen—light blue, Nitrogen—dark blue, Carbon—grey, Oxygen—red. Rendering: the atoms and bonds of PLLA are rendered as sticks, the atoms of PAMAM dendrimer generation 4.0 are rendered as solid cylinders, CPT atoms are rendered as spheres with radii that are related to the van der Waals radii of its atoms.

The structures presented exhibit similarities in the shape and size of the PAMAM dendrimer/CPT complex within the nanosystems, with the exception of MODEL 3. In this particular one, the PAMAM dendrimer structure is notably more branched and less compact, allowing the PGACL chains to easily interweave with the PAMAM dendrimer chains. This suggests that the interactions between the matrix components, PGACL and PAMAM dendrimer, are stronger in this nanosystem, resulting in reduced surface tension and enhanced miscibility. Furthermore, these interactions likely contribute to the aggregation observed in some nanosystems, as confirmed by the DLS graph analysis.

The structures of the MODELS align with the findings from the in vitro CPT release evaluation. MODELS 1 and 2, which feature a more compact arrangement of the PAMAM dendrimer/CPT components, exhibit a notably slower release of CPT in vitro. In contrast, MODELS 3 and 4 have a less dense structure, with copolymer molecules integrated even within the core of the PAMAM dendrimer. This structural difference accounts for the more efficient drug release observed in these two models, particularly at a pH of 7.4 ± 0.05. These insights suggest that the design of the optimized system may play a crucial role in determining drug release characteristics, especially when comparing multiple systems.

3.4.2. Molecular Dynamics (MD) Simulations

Based on the MD simulation results for the MODELS 1–4, chosen geometric features of the complexes were determined, including the mean gyration radius (R_g), solvent-accessible surface area (SASA), the radial distribution functions G(r), and root-mean-square deviation of atomic positions (RMSD).

Gyration radius (R_g) represents a measure of how much the polymer chains curl and their average dimensions. Opitz and Wagner used molecular dynamics simulations to study the molecular structure of PAMAM dendrimers and discovered that the gyration radius determined by the experiment was in good agreement with the simulation outcomes [57]. Also, in our previous work, we have successfully determined the R_g values using this computational approach [34]. The experimentally determined R_g of PAMAM dendrimer generation 4.0 at neutral pH was found to be 22.5 Å [58], while in this study the R_g for MODELS 1–4 PAMAM dendrimer/CPT complex were 20.4 Å, 21.0 Å; 24.5 Å, and 23.6 Å, respectively. The decrease of the R_g upon complexation, when compared with the free PAMAM dendrimer molecule, was observed in MODELS 1 and 2. This can be explained as resulting from the intermolecular forces (van der Waals, hydrogen bonds) existing between the host and guest (CPT) molecules that are located in the cavity of the PAMAM dendrimer. The expansion of PAMAM dendrimer dimensions observed in MODELS 4, and especially MODEL 3, results from the higher affinity of PAMAM dendrimer molecules towards the polymer matrix particles simulated in that model. Therefore, instead of existing in their spherical shape, the molecules of PAMAM dendrimer tend to increase their specific surface. It also explains the different behavior of nanosystems, observed in the dissolution studies. To confirm this observation, we have calculated the SASA for the nanosystems in each model.

To obtain the SASA, a probe radius of 1.4 Å was used as the van der Waals radius of a water molecule of 2.75 Å. The obtained results were 13,960.65, 14,969.37, 17,326.98 Å^2, and 16,414.81 Å^2 for the MODELS 1–4, respectively. These results are comparable to those obtained for PAMAM at pH = 7.0, namely 14,862.4 Å^2 [59]. Again, similar as for the R_g, the increase of SASA was observed for MODELS 3 and 4, which results from the more branched shape that the PAMAM dendrimer forms in these systems.

The radial distribution function (RDF) represents the features of the microstructure. This function is frequently employed to explore the structure and unique interactions of the condensed matter [60]. Its physical meaning relates to the ratio of the probability density of another atom at a distance from the center atom to the random distribution density. In the g(r)-r diagram (Figure 15), the chemical bonds and hydrogen bond interactions distances are mostly within 3.1 Å, and the non-bonding interactions such as Coulomb forces and van der Waals forces are primarily within 3.1–10.0 Å. The interactions greater than 10.0 Å are very weak. The radial distribution function, g(r), was calculated by averaging the distribution of interatomic vector lengths on a sphere of radius (r) and thickness (Δr). We used Δr = 0.1 Å with the radius, r, of the sphere varying in the range 1–20 Å. The interactions between PAMAM dendrimer and CPT molecules can be analyzed by means of RDFs that were created for each model (Figure 15). The highest peak exists slightly after 1.0 Å, indicating the presence of covalent bonds. Other peaks are visible in the region of 2.0 to 3.5 Å, which means that the H-bonds are formed between PAMAM dendrimer and CPT molecules. As there are not any peaks in the region above 5.0 Å, this indicates no major electrostatic interactions. Also, the RDFs were found to be similar, regardless of the studied model.

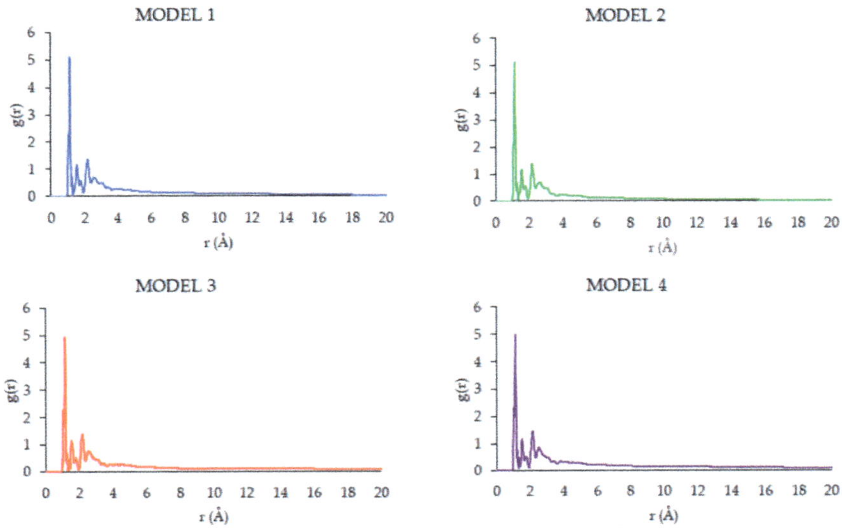

Figure 15. The RDFs between PAMAM and CPT molecules.

Figure 16 shows the root-mean-square deviation of atomic positions (RMSD) plots obtained for CPT in the studied models during the 100 ns MD simulations. RMSD analysis can indicate the dynamic stability of a molecule in a studied system; larger values of RMDS indicate more intense molecular motions and more efficient diffusion. All the models studied showed an increase in RMSD throughout the simulation time. However, the values reached after 100 ns depend on the model studied. The highest final RMSD was observed in MODEL 3, and the lowest in MODEL 1, 2.5 Å and 0.2 Å, respectively. This indicates that the polymer matrix has a major influence on the behavior of CPT in the nanosystem, which was also observed experimentally.

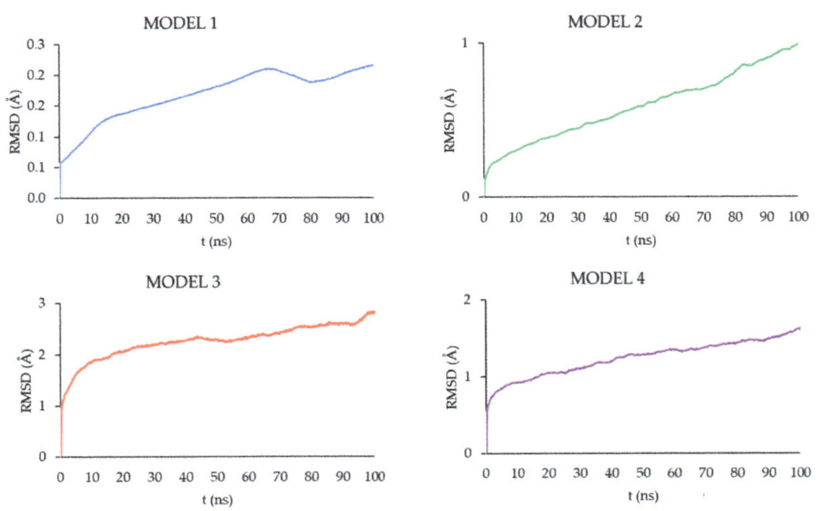

Figure 16. RMSD plots obtained for CPT in MODELS 1–4 during 100 ns MD simulation.

4. Conclusions

The development of DDSs has been influential in transforming innovative therapies into effective medical interventions. As the therapeutic environment has progressed, these systems and their underlying technologies have quickly evolved to accommodate the changing requirements of drug delivery. The physicochemical attributes of small molecules largely determine their delivery mechanisms, which in turn influence their bioavailability. Therefore, drug delivery strategies prioritize not only the improvement of solubility, but also the management of release profiles, the augmentation of therapeutic effects, and the customization of pharmacokinetic behaviors.

In line with this focus, our research concentrated on the development of forward-looking PAMAM dendrimer/biodegradable polymer nanosystems intended for the delivery of CPT. Despite the fact that this drug has been recognized as one of the most promising anticancer agents in recent years, challenges related to its physiological stability and solubility remain unresolved. Initially, four biodegradable homo- and copolymeric matrices were synthesized and extensively characterized, focusing on the microstructural aspects of their chains. The biological assessment conducted on these biodegradable materials, specifically hemolysis tests, revealed that all matrices exhibited hemolysis rates below 5%, thereby conforming to national safety standards for biological materials. Furthermore, fibroblasts exposed to the synthesized polymeric matrices demonstrated viability that was comparable and dependent on concentration. In the subsequent phase of our research, four nanosystems with diameters ranging from 110 to 406 nm and an entrapment efficiency of up to 27% were developed. These nanoparticulate systems were formulated from a PAMAM dendrimer/CPT complex, which was subsequently coated with an appropriate biodegradable matrix. Notably, confocal microscopy confirmed the successful entrapment of CPT within the PAMAM dendrimer cavity, as evidenced by the detection of fluorescence from the drug in all nanoparticulate systems. The research demonstrated that CPT was released from the engineered nanosystems in a sustained and controlled manner, exhibiting near-first-order and first-order kinetics without any burst release effect. Additionally, the biodegradable polymer matrices played a significant role in shaping the drug release profile. Notably, the nanoparticulate systems we have developed facilitated the stabilization of the pharmacologically active form of CPT, offering protection against hydrolysis even under physiological conditions. Through molecular modeling techniques, we constructed four MODELS, each comprising a PAMAM dendrimer/CPT complex with three CPT molecules associated with each generation 4.0 PAMAM dendrimer, all integrated within a polymer matrix that corresponds to the experimental setup. Our analysis revealed that the structures of the MODELS displayed similarities in the shape and size of the PAMAM dendrimer/CPT complex within the nanosystems, with MODEL 3 being an exception. In this particular model, the PAMAM dendrimer structure was significantly more branched and less compact, which facilitates the interweaving of PGACL matrix chains with the PAMAM dendrimer chains. This indicates that the interactions between the matrix components, PGACL and PAMAM dendrimer, were more robust in this nanosystem, leading to decreased surface tension and improved miscibility. The structural characteristics of the MODELS were consistent with the results obtained from the in vitro evaluation of CPT release.

In summary, we can assert that the nanoparticulate systems developed may serve as a novel platform for the delivery of significant hydrophobic anticancer drugs. Consequently, these nanomaterials hold great promise as delivery systems for cancer therapy, and further investigation of the in vivo behavior of these nanoparticulate materials is warranted in animal models.

Supplementary Materials: The following supporting information can be downloaded at: https://www.mdpi.com/article/10.3390/pharmaceutics16111482/s1, Figure S1: ^{1}H NMR spectrum of the synthesized PAMAM dendrimer/CPT complex, Figure S2: ^{1}H NMR spectrum of the PLLA (matrix M1), Figure S3: ^{13}C NMR spectrum of the PLLA (matrix M1), Figure S4: ^{1}H NMR spectrum of the PLACL 40:60 (matrix M2), Figure S5: ^{13}C NMR spectrum of the PLACL 40:60 (matrix M2), Figure S6: ^{1}H NMR spectrum of the PGACL (matrices M3 and M4), Figure S7: ^{13}C NMR spectrum of the PGACL (matrices M3 and M4), Figure S8: Expansion of the domain of interest in ^{13}C NMR spectrum of PLLA (matrix M1), Figure S9: Hemolytic activity of individual matrices. The graph depicts the level of hemolysis of RBC treated with increasing concentrations of the complex after 1 h of treatment. Statistical analysis using two-way ANOVA followed by the Bonferroni post-test revealed no significant differences ($p > 0.05$) between the obtained results, Figure S10: The viability of normal fibroblasts treated for 72 h with individual matrices at pH 7.4 ± 0.05 and 6.5 ± 0.05. The graphs depict differences in the susceptibility of cells to the complex. The MTS assay was used to determine the relative cell number. The results are given as mean ± SEM. Two-way ANOVA was used for statistical analysis, followed by Bonferroni post-tests. When the following conditions were met, the results were considered statistically significant: * $p < 0.05$; ** $p < 0.01$; *** $p < 0.005$, Figure S11: HPLC chromatograms of the CPT released in the lactone and carboxylic forms (a) pH = 7.4 ± 0.05; (b) pH = 6.5 ± 0.05.

Author Contributions: K.S.: methodology investigation, chemical research, formal analysis, and writing—original draft and editing; A.K.: analytical research—HPLC method; T.B.: analytical research—GPC method; A.B.-J.: analytical research—DLS method; A.L.: investigation, methodology, formal analysis—cell viability assay and hemolysis, and writing—original draft and editing; Ł.S.: investigation, formal analysis—molecular modeling, visualization, and writing—original draft and editing; M.G.: analytical research—confocal microscopy; M.S.: conceptualization, mathematical models investigation, formal analysis, and writing—original draft and editing; E.O.: conceptualization, supervision, methodology investigation, chemical research, formal analysis, and writing—original draft and editing. All authors have read and agreed to the published version of the manuscript.

Funding: This research received no external funding.

Institutional Review Board Statement: Not applicable.

Informed Consent Statement: Not applicable.

Data Availability Statement: The data presented in this study are available on request from the corresponding author.

Acknowledgments: The authors would like to thank Urszula Piotrowska for her suggestions on the preparation of the nanosystems.

Conflicts of Interest: The authors declare no conflict of interest.

References

1. Mazayen, Z.M.; Ghoneim, A.M.; Elbatanony, R.S.; Basalious, E.B.; Bendas, E.R. Pharmaceutical Nanotechnology: From the Bench to the Market. *Future J. Pharm. Sci.* **2022**, *8*, 12. [CrossRef] [PubMed]
2. Hadjidemetriou, M.; Al-Ahmady, Z.; Mazza, M.; Kostarelos, K. The Emergence of Nanopharmacy: From Biology to Nanotechnology and Drug Molecules to Nanodrugs. In *Pharmaceutical Nanotechnology: Innovation and Production*; John Wiley & Sons, Ltd.: Hoboken, NJ, USA, 2017; pp. 43–62. ISBN 978-3-527-80068-1.
3. Weissig, V.; Pettinger, T.; Murdock, N. Nanopharmaceuticals (Part 1): Products on the Market. *Int. J. Nanomed.* **2014**, *9*, 4357–4373. [CrossRef] [PubMed]
4. Afzal, O.; Altamimi, A.S.A.; Nadeem, M.S.; Alzarea, S.I.; Almalki, W.H.; Tariq, A.; Mubeen, B.; Murtaza, B.N.; Iftikhar, S.; Riaz, N.; et al. Nanoparticles in Drug Delivery: From History to Therapeutic Applications. *Nanomaterials* **2022**, *12*, 4494. [CrossRef] [PubMed]
5. Haag, R.; Kratz, F. Polymer Therapeutics: Concepts and Applications. *Angew. Chem. Int. Ed.* **2006**, *45*, 1198–1215. [CrossRef]
6. Silverstein, A.M. Paul Ehrlich's Passion: The Origins of His Receptor Immunology. *Cell. Immunol.* **1999**, *194*, 213–221. [CrossRef]
7. Allen, T.M.; Cullis, P.R. Drug Delivery Systems: Entering the Mainstream. *Science* **2004**, *303*, 1818–1822. [CrossRef]
8. Niemirowicz, K.; Car, H. Nanonośniki jako nowoczesne transportery w kontrolowanym dostarczaniu leków. *Chemik* **2012**, *66*, 868–881.
9. Mukherjee, C.; Varghese, D.; Krishna, J.S.; Boominathan, T.; Rakeshkumar, R.; Dineshkumar, S.; Rao, C.V.S.B.; Sivaramakrishna, A. Recent Advances in Biodegradable Polymers–Properties, Applications and Future Prospects. *Eur. Polym. J.* **2023**, *192*, 112068. [CrossRef]
10. Satchanska, G.; Davidova, S.; Petrov, P.D. Natural and Synthetic Polymers for Biomedical and Environmental Applications. *Polymers* **2024**, *16*, 1159. [CrossRef]
11. Chen, J. Design and Synthesis of Biomedical Polymer Materials. *Int. J. Mol. Sci.* **2024**, *25*, 5088. [CrossRef]

12. Deb, P.K.; Kokaz, S.F.; Abed, S.N.; Paradkar, A.; Tekade, R.K. Chapter 6—Pharmaceutical and Biomedical Applications of Polymers. In *Basic Fundamentals of Drug Delivery*; Tekade, R.K., Ed.; Advances in Pharmaceutical Product Development and Research; Academic Press: Cambridge, MA, USA, 2019; pp. 203–267. ISBN 978-0-12-817909-3.
13. Morsada, Z.; Hossain, M.M.; Islam, M.T.; Mobin, M.A.; Saha, S. Recent Progress in Biodegradable and Bioresorbable Materials: From Passive Implants to Active Electronics. *Appl. Mater. Today* **2021**, *25*, 101257. [CrossRef]
14. Nikzamir, M.; Hanifehpour, Y.; Akbarzadeh, A.; Panahi, Y. Applications of Dendrimers in Nanomedicine and Drug Delivery: A Review. *J. Inorg. Organomet. Polym. Mater.* **2021**, *31*, 2246–2261. [CrossRef]
15. Abdou, E.M. Pamam dendrimers as drug delivery carriers, benefits against risks. *Indo Am. J. Pharm. Sci.* **2017**, *4*, 1319–1332.
16. Cheng, Y.; Li, M.; Xu, T. Potential of Poly(Amidoamine) Dendrimers as Drug Carriers of Camptothecin Based on Encapsulation Studies. *Eur. J. Med. Chem.* **2008**, *43*, 1791–1795. [CrossRef] [PubMed]
17. Tripathy, S.; Das, M.K. Dendrimers and Their Applications as Novel Drug Delivery Carriers. *J. Appl. Pharm. Sci.* **2013**, *3*, 142–149.
18. Huang, D.; Wu, D. Biodegradable Dendrimers for Drug Delivery. *Mater. Sci. Eng. C* **2018**, *90*, 713–727. [CrossRef]
19. Siegel, R.L.; Giaquinto, A.N.; Jemal, A. Cancer Statistics, 2024. *CA Cancer J. Clin.* **2024**, *74*, 12–49. [CrossRef]
20. Wojciechowska, U.; Barańska, K.; Miklewska, M.; Didkowska, J.A. Cancer Incidence and Mortality in Poland in 2020. *Nowotw. J. Oncol.* **2023**, *73*, 129–145. [CrossRef]
21. Cegieła, U.; Janiec, W.; Folwarczna, J.; Janas, A.; Janiec, R.; Kaczmarczyk-Sedlak, I.; Londzin, P.; Nowińska, B.; Podwińska, E.; Pytlik, M.; et al. *Kompendium Farmakologii*; PZWL: Warszawa, Poland, 2021; ISBN 978-83-200-6052-2.
22. Strąg-Lemanowicz, A.; Leppert, W. Rola Onkologicznego Leczenia Systemowego u Pacjentów z Zaawansowaną Chorobą Nowotworową. *Palliat. Med. Pract.* **2014**, *8*, 11–22.
23. Ramadori, G.; Cameron, S. Effects of Systemic Chemotherapy on the Liver. *Ann. Hepatol.* **2010**, *9*, 133–143. [CrossRef]
24. Strzelecka, K.; Piotrowska, U.; Sobczak, M.; Oledzka, E. The Advancement of Biodegradable Polyesters as Delivery Systems for Camptothecin and Its Analogues—A Status Report. *Int. J. Mol. Sci.* **2023**, *24*, 1053. [CrossRef] [PubMed]
25. Ziomkowska, B.; Kruszewski, S.; Siuda, R.; Cyrankiewicz, M. Deactivation Rate of Camptothecin Determined by Factor Analysis of Steady-State Fluorescence and Absorption Spectra. *Opt. Appl.* **2006**, *36*, 137–146.
26. Pommier, Y. Topoisomerase I Inhibitors: Camptothecins and Beyond. *Nat. Rev. Cancer* **2006**, *6*, 789–802. [CrossRef] [PubMed]
27. Botella, P.; Rivero-Buceta, E.M. Safe Approaches for Camptothecin Delivery: Structural Analogues and Nanomedicines. *J. Controlled Release* **2017**, *247*, 28–54. [CrossRef] [PubMed]
28. Alshammari, M.K.; Alshehri, M.M.; Alshehri, A.M.; Alshlali, O.M.; Mahzari, A.M.; Almalki, H.H.; Kulaybi, O.Y.; Alghazwni, M.K.; Kamal, M.; Imran, M. Camptothecin Loaded Nano-Delivery Systems in the Cancer Therapeutic Domains: A Critical Examination of the Literature. *J. Drug Deliv. Sci. Technol.* **2023**, *79*, 104034. [CrossRef]
29. Min, K.H.; Park, K.; Kim, Y.-S.; Bae, S.M.; Lee, S.; Jo, H.G.; Park, R.-W.; Kim, I.-S.; Jeong, S.Y.; Kim, K.; et al. Hydrophobically Modified Glycol Chitosan Nanoparticles-Encapsulated Camptothecin Enhance the Drug Stability and Tumor Targeting in Cancer Therapy. *J. Control. Release* **2008**, *127*, 208–218. [CrossRef] [PubMed]
30. Watanabe, M.; Kawano, K.; Toma, K.; Hattori, Y.; Maitani, Y. In Vivo Antitumor Activity of Camptothecin Incorporated in Liposomes Formulated with an Artificial Lipid and Human Serum Albumin. *J. Control. Release* **2008**, *127*, 231–238. [CrossRef]
31. Kawano, K.; Watanabe, M.; Yamamoto, T.; Yokoyama, M.; Opanasopit, P.; Okano, T.; Maitani, Y. Enhanced Antitumor Effect of Camptothecin Loaded in Long-Circulating Polymeric Micelles. *J. Control. Release* **2006**, *112*, 329–332. [CrossRef]
32. Martins, S.M.; Sarmento, B.; Nunes, C.; Lúcio, M.; Reis, S.; Ferreira, D.C. Brain Targeting Effect of Camptothecin-Loaded Solid Lipid Nanoparticles in Rat after Intravenous Administration. *Eur. J. Pharm. Biopharm.* **2013**, *85*, 488–502. [CrossRef]
33. Kubiak, M. Dendrymery–fascynujące nanocząsteczki w zastosowaniu w medycynie. *Chemik* **2014**, *68*, 141–150.
34. Oledzka, E.; Paśnik, K.; Domańska, I.; Zielińska-Pisklak, M.; Piotrowska, U.; Sobczak, M.; Szeleszczuk, Ł.; Laskowska, A. Poly(Amidoamine) Dendrimer/Camptothecin Complex: From Synthesis to In Vitro Cancer Cell Line Studies. *Molecules* **2023**, *28*, 2696. [CrossRef] [PubMed]
35. Bero, M.; Kasperczyk, J.; Jedlinski, Z.J. Coordination Polymerization of Lactides, 1. Structure Determination of Obtained Polymers. *Makromol. Chem.* **1990**, *191*, 2287–2296. [CrossRef]
36. Kasperczyk, J.; Bero, M. Coordination Polymerization of Lactides, 2. Microstructure Determination of Poly[(L,L-Lactide)-co-(ε-Caprolactone)] with ^{13}C Nuclear Magnetic Resonance Spectroscopy. *Makromol. Chem.* **1991**, *192*, 1777–1787. [CrossRef]
37. Bero, M.; Czapla, B.; Dobrzyński, P.; Janeczek, H.; Kasperczyk, J. Copolymerization of Glycolide Andε-Caprolactone, 2. Random Copolymerization in the Presence of Tin Octoate. *Macromol. Chem. Phys.* **1999**, *200*, 911–916. [CrossRef]
38. Dash, S.; Murthy, P.; Nath, L.; Chowdhury, P. Kinetic Modeling on Drug Release from Controlled Drug Delivery Systems. *Acta Pol. Pharm.* **2010**, *67*, 217–223. [PubMed]
39. Singhvi, G.; Singh, M. Review: In Vitro Drug Release Characterization Models. *Int. J. Pharm. Stud. Res.* **2011**, *2*, 77–84.
40. Bialik, M.; Proc, J.; Zgadzaj, A.; Mulas, K.; Kuras, M.; Sobczak, M.; Oledzka, E. Development and Comprehensive Characteristics of Thermosensitive Liquid Suppositories of Metoprolol Based on Poly(Lactide-Co-Glycolide) Nanoparticles. *Int. J. Mol. Sci.* **2022**, *23*, 13743. [CrossRef]
41. Bialik, M.; Kurkowski, P.; Strzelecka, K.; Kuras, M.; Sobczak, M.; Mulas, K.; Zgadzaj, A.; Czerwińska, M.E.; Gniadek, M.; Oledzka, E. Dual-Controlled Delivery of Furosemide and Atenolol Using a Biodegradable Nanosystem for Antihypertensive Therapy. *J. Drug Deliv. Sci. Technol.* **2023**, *89*, 105006. [CrossRef]

42. Sæbø, I.P.; Bjørås, M.; Franzyk, H.; Helgesen, E.; Booth, J.A. Optimization of the Hemolysis Assay for the Assessment of Cytotoxicity. *Int. J. Mol. Sci.* **2023**, *24*, 2914. [CrossRef]
43. Otto, D.P.; Villiers, M.M. de All-atomistic Molecular Dynamics (AA-MD) Studies and Pharmacokinetic Performance of PAMAM-dendrimer-furosemide Delivery Systems. *Int. J. Pharm.* **2018**, *547*, 545–555. [CrossRef]
44. Sun, H.; Jin, Z.; Yang, C.; Akkermans, R.L.C.; Robertson, S.H.; Spenley, N.A.; Miller, S.; Todd, S.M. COMPASS II: Extended Coverage for Polymer and Drug-like Molecule Databases. *J. Mol. Model.* **2016**, *22*, 47. [CrossRef] [PubMed]
45. Wang, L.; Lv, C.; Liu, Z.; Zhang, N.; Zhou, W.; Wang, J. Study on the Mechanism of PAMAM(DETA as the Core) against Silica Scale. *J. Mol. Model.* **2021**, *27*, 304. [CrossRef] [PubMed]
46. Al Ameri, J.; Alsuraifi, A.; Curtis, A.; Hoskins, C. Effect of Poly(Allylamine) Molecular Weight on Drug Loading and Release Abilities of Nano-Aggregates for Potential in Cancer Nanomedicine. *J. Pharm. Sci.* **2020**, *109*, 3125–3133. [CrossRef] [PubMed]
47. Domańska, I.M.; Zgadzaj, A.; Kowalczyk, S.; Zalewska, A.; Oledzka, E.; Cieśla, K.; Plichta, A.; Sobczak, M. A Comprehensive Investigation of the Structural, Thermal, and Biological Properties of Fully Randomized Biomedical Polyesters Synthesized with a Nontoxic Bismuth(III) Catalyst. *Molecules* **2022**, *27*, 1139. [CrossRef]
48. Dobrovolskaia, M.A.; McNeil, S.E. Understanding the Correlation between in Vitro and in Vivo Immunotoxicity Tests for Nanomedicines. *J. Control. Release* **2013**, *172*, 456–466. [CrossRef]
49. Lu, S.; Duffin, R.; Poland, C.; Daly, P.; Murphy, F.; Drost, E.; MacNee, W.; Stone, V.; Donaldson, K. Efficacy of Simple Short-Term in Vitro Assays for Predicting the Potential of Metal Oxide Nanoparticles to Cause Pulmonary Inflammation. *Environ. Health Perspect.* **2009**, *117*, 241–247. [CrossRef]
50. Jeong, H.; Hwang, J.; Lee, H.; Hammond, P.T.; Choi, J.; Hong, J. In Vitro Blood Cell Viability Profiling of Polymers Used in Molecular Assembly. *Sci. Rep.* **2017**, *7*, 9481. [CrossRef]
51. Weiss, M.; Fan, J.; Claudel, M.; Sonntag, T.; Didier, P.; Ronzani, C.; Lebeau, L.; Pons, F. Density of Surface Charge Is a More Predictive Factor of the Toxicity of Cationic Carbon Nanoparticles than Zeta Potential. *J. Nanobiotechnol.* **2021**, *19*, 5. [CrossRef]
52. Li, F.; Jiang, T.; Li, Q.; Ling, X. Camptothecin (CPT) and Its Derivatives Are Known to Target Topoisomerase I (Top1) as Their Mechanism of Action: Did We Miss Something in CPT Analogue Molecular Targets for Treating Human Disease Such as Cancer? *Am. J. Cancer Res.* **2017**, *7*, 2350–2394.
53. Díaz-Celorio, E.; Franco, L.; Rodríguez-Galán, A.; Puiggalí, J. Study on the Hydrolytic Degradation of Glycolide/Trimethylene Carbonate Copolymers Having Different Microstructure and Composition. *Polym. Degrad. Stab.* **2013**, *98*, 133–143. [CrossRef]
54. Memişoğlu, E.; Bochot, A.; Özalp, M.; Şen, M.; Duchêne, D.; Hincal, A.A. Direct Formation of Nanospheres from Amphiphilic β-Cyclodextrin Inclusion Complexes. *Pharm. Res.* **2004**, *20*, 117–125. [CrossRef] [PubMed]
55. Fassberg, J.; Stella, V.J. A Kinetic and Mechanistic Study of the Hydrolysis of Camptothecin and Some Analogues. *J. Pharm. Sci.* **1992**, *81*, 676–684. [CrossRef] [PubMed]
56. Liu, J.; Jiang, Z.; Zhang, S.; Saltzman, W.M. Poly(ω-Pentadecalactone-Co-Butylene-Co-Succinate) Nanoparticles as Biodegradable Carriers for Camptothecin Delivery. *Biomaterials* **2009**, *30*, 5707–5719. [CrossRef] [PubMed]
57. Opitz, A.W.; Wagner, N.J. Structural Investigations of Poly(Amido Amine) Dendrimers in Methanol Using Molecular Dynamics. *J. Polym. Sci. Part B* **2006**, *44*, 3062–3077. [CrossRef]
58. Pourianazar, N.T.; Mutlu, P.; Gunduz, U. Bioapplications of Poly(Amidoamine) (PAMAM) Dendrimers in Nanomedicine. *J. Nanoparticle Res.* **2014**, *16*, 2342. [CrossRef]
59. Liu, Y.; Bryantsev, V.S.; Diallo, M.S.; Goddard III, W.A. PAMAM Dendrimers Undergo pH Responsive Conformational Changes without Swelling. *J. Am. Chem. Soc.* **2009**, *131*, 2798–2799. [CrossRef]
60. Canetta, E.; Maino, G. Molecular Dynamic Analysis of the Structure of Dendrimers. *Nucl. Instrum. Methods Phys. Res. Sect. B Beam Interact. Mater. At.* **2004**, *213*, 71–74. [CrossRef]

pharmaceutics

Article

Cationic Curcumin Nanocrystals Liposomes for Improved Oral Bioavailability: Formulation Development, Optimization, In Vitro and In Vivo Evaluation

Xiang Cheng [1], Xiaoran Han [1], Jia Si [1], Cong Dong [1], Zhongjuan Ji [1], Shicong Zhao [1], Xiangting Wu [1], Haiyan Li [2] and Xiangqun Jin [1,*]

[1] Department of Pharmacy, Jilin University, Changchun 130021, China; chengxiang22@mails.jlu.edu.cn (X.C.); hanxr22@mails.jlu.edu.cn (X.H.); jiasi23@mails.jlu.edu.cn (J.S.); jizj23@mails.jlu.edu.cn (Z.J.); dongcong23@mails.jlu.edu.cn (C.D.); sczhao@jlu.edu.cn (S.Z.); xiangting21@mails.jlu.edu.cn (X.W.)

[2] Department of Pharmacy, Changchun University of Chinese Medicine, Changchun 130021, China; hyl09@mails.jlu.edu.cn

* Correspondence: jinxq@jlu.edu.cn; Tel.: +86-138-4409-0377; Fax: +86-431-8561-9662

Abstract: Curcumin, a naturally occurring poorly water-soluble polyphenol with a broad spectrum, is a typical BCS IV drug. The objective of this study was to develop curcumin nanocrystals liposomes with the aim of improving bioavailability. In this study, we prepared cationic curcumin nanocrystals with a particle size of only 29.42 nm; such a phenomenal range of particle sizes is very rare. Moreover, we summarized and evaluated the parameters of the nanocrystal preparation process, including methods, formulations, etc., and the rules we concluded can be generalized to other nanocrystal preparation processes. To counteract the instability of the nanocrystals in the digestive tract, cationic curcumin nanocrystals were loaded into negatively charged liposomes through gravitational force between different charges. Unexpectedly, chitosan oligosaccharide was found to promote the self-assembly process of curcumin nanocrystal liposomes. In vitro and in vivo experiments demonstrated that chitosan-modified curcumin nanocrystal liposomes exhibited enhanced resistance to enzyme barriers, mucus barriers, and cellular barriers, resulting in a 5.4-fold increase in bioavailability compared to crude powder formulations. It can be concluded that cationic nanocrystals liposomes represent an appropriate novel strategy for improving the dissolution rate and bioavailability of poorly soluble natural products such as curcumin.

Keywords: curcumin; cationic nanocrystals; oral absorption; bioavailability enhancement; mucous barrier

1. Introduction

Curcumin (CUR), a primary constituent of turmeric, is commonly used as a spice in Indian cuisine [1]. Moreover, it finds widespread application in the food, medical, and healthcare industries. In recent decades, burgeoning interest in curcumin has led to extensive research, consistently showcasing its beneficial anti-inflammatory, antibacterial, hepatoprotective, antioxidant, and wound-healing properties [2–4]. Additionally, a growing body of clinical trials has affirmed CUR's efficacy in combatting various cancers, such as lung and colon cancer [5,6]. However, the low solubility, limited bioavailability, and instability of CUR's conjugated polyene structure in water pose substantial challenges to its utilization [7]. Hence, exploring its full potential through nanoformulation development is imperative.

Recent research in nanomedicine has concentrated on the design of smaller and more-stable particles and the optimization of their surface properties with a view to enhancing the therapeutic effects of drugs. Nonetheless, while most nanomedicines enhance drug bioavailability, their practical application is often hindered by their low drug-carrying capacity [8], typically less than 10%, necessitating significant carrier material usage to maintain the drug's nanostate, potentially leading to adverse effects. In contrast, drugs based on nanocrystals, with their nearly 100% drug loading capacity and robust plasticity, offer efficient therapeutic outcomes with only a minimal number of particles [9]. Consequently, an increasing number of drugs are being considered for delivery in the form of nanocrystals (NCs), including CUR, bioflavonoids [10], pomalidomide [11], paclitaxel [12,13], and berberine [14].

The techniques for producing nanosized crystalline particles can be categorized into top-down methods, such as milling and high-pressure homogenization, and bottom-up approaches like precipitation and self-assembly [15]. Each preparation method has its inherent advantages and disadvantages. For instance, high-pressure homogenization is universally applicable, enabling particle size reduction by adjusting the number of homogenizations and pressure [16]. Conversely, precipitation, while simple and cost-effective, necessitates the use of numerous solvents unavoidably. Moreover, a significant challenge with nanocrystalline drugs is poor stability, characterized by crystal aggregation, growth, and precipitation, which must be addressed. The most typical method by of achieving stable NCs involves adding stabilizers to the nanosuspension, preventing aggregation and sedimentation by enhancing the surface charge and electrostatic repulsion between the crystals. However, different stabilizers yield crystals with distinct shapes, surface charges, particle sizes, and stability—crucial factors in product evaluation.

Nanocrystals are formed by the stacking of π–π bonds between drug molecules and the interactions of van der Waals forces, hydrogen bonding, and other similar forces [12,17]. This state can only exist in a specific system in a relatively stable equilibrium. However, as soon as the nanocrystals enter the gastrointestinal tract, the blood, the abdominal cavity, and other environments, this equilibrium is broken. For example, Na^+ and Cl^- will break Van der Waals forces between molecules, which results in the nanocrystals aggregating into clusters in a short period of time and precipitating, thus losing the nano-properties of the drug. Although this method of drug delivery can still improve the oral bioavailability of BCS II and BCS IV drugs compared to the original powder, it is far from the desired effect in practice. Significantly, BCS II and BCS IV drugs encounter distinct challenges. Mere enhancement of drug dissolution does not address the issue of low bioavailability in BCS IV medications, attributed to P-glycoprotein (P-gp) exocytosis [18]. This necessitates the absorption of nanocrystals as complete entities to prevent premature dissolution during absorption. Furthermore, when nanocrystalline drugs are injected into the blood circulation, the clustered crystals will block the capillaries of the body, leading to end-circulation obstacles. Consequently, the initial challenge is to enhance the stability of nanocrystalline drugs. Xu, Z et al. demonstrated the stabilizing effect of rhodopsin nanocrystals by incorporating them into hydrogels [19]. Wang, Y et al. achieved a significant improvement in the oral bioavailability of etoposide by utilizing liposome-loaded etoposide nanocrystals [20]. Moreover, research suggests that cationic nanoparticles exhibit enhanced absorption by Caco-2 cells upon oral administration compared to anionic particles [21]. It is therefore anticipated that the development of cationic nanocrystalline liposomes will facilitate the delivery of orally administered drugs, overcoming the three major barriers that such drugs must overcome: (1) enzyme barrier; (2) mucus barrier; (3) cellular barrier.

In this study, we optimized the preparation process of CUR-NCs to produce cationic CUR-NCs with a size of 29.42 nm, while CUR-NCs prepared by peers are generally around 200 nm. Throughout NCs preparation, we delineated the general principles governing the influence of environmental and formulation factors on crystal size, conducting a series of investigations, including TEM, PXRD, and stability analyses, on the prepared NCs. In older to improve the stability of curcumin nanocrystals, we loaded cationic nanocrystals into anionic liposomes via the mutual attraction between different charges. Pharmacokinetic assessments, in vitro dissolution tests, and particle mucus diffusion experiments confirmed the superior absorption of cationic curcumin nanocrystals (CUR-NCs$^+$) compared to curcumin coarse powders (CUR-CCs), particularly highlighting the enhanced gastrointestinal mucosal penetration and oral absorption efficiency of CUR-NCs$^+$ over their anionic counterparts. Furthermore, following liposomal encapsulation, the capacity of

CUR-NCs+ to penetrate all three barriers was markedly enhanced, with a 5.4-fold increase in bioavailability compared to CUR-CCs.

2. Materials and Methods

2.1. Materials

CUR, domiphen bromide (DPB), NaOH, mannitol, lecithin from egg yolk pure, vitamin E-TPGS, pepsin, trypsin, coumarin 6, ethanol, chitosan oligosaccharide (Macklin Chemical Technology Co., Ltd., Shanghai, China); hydroxypropyl cellulose (HPMC), Sodium dodecyl sulphate (SDS), polyethylene glycol (PEG-1000), Plasdone K30 (PVP K30), sodium tylose (CMC-Na) (Tianjin Guangfu Fine Chemical Research Institute, Tianjin, China); polyvinyl alcohol (PVA), Benzalkonium Chloride (BZC) (Jiangxi Alpha Hi-tech Pharmaceutical Co., Ltd., Wuxi, China); hexadecyl trimethyl ammonium bromide (CTAB) (Beijing Mreda Technology Co., Ltd., Beijing, China); dimethyl sulfoxide (DMSO), methanol, acetone, and acetonitrile of chromatographic grade (BSZH Scientific Inc, Beijing, China). All reagents and chemicals used were of analytical or chromatographic grade. HT29-MTX-E12 (E12) cells, Caco-2 cell (Shanghai EK-Bioscience Biotechnology Co., Ltd., Shanghai, China). DMEM, DiI, DiO, Mucin from porcine stomach (Dalian Meilun Biotechnology Co., Ltd., Dalian, China).

2.2. Analysis Method

CUR was analyzed via HPLC. Chromatographic separation was achieved on Acchrom Tech s3000 with an Inert Sustain Swift C18 (250 mm, 4.6 mm, 5 μm) column using acetonitrile–4% acetic acid water 48:52 (v/v) as a mobile phase with a flow rate of 1 mL/min, detected at 430 nm [22].

2.3. Fabrication of Nanocrystals

This study assessed five common techniques for preparing NCs: milling (MIL); high-speed shearing (HSS); sonoprecipitation (SOP); freeze-drying (FRD); and sonoprecipitation combined with high-pressure homogenization (HPH).

In summary, HSS involves adding CUR-CCs to a high-speed shearing machine to yield smaller NCs. FRD entails dissolving CUR in DMSO, adding it to an aqueous solution with surfactant and freeze-drying protectant, rapidly solidifying it with liquid nitrogen, and lyophilizing to obtain the sample. HPH involves adding CUR-NCs (prepared via SOP) into a high-pressure homogenizer and homogenizing several times to achieve smaller NCs. SOP consists of dissolving CUR in DMSO, adding the solution to water with a surfactant under low-temperature ultrasound, centrifuging to remove the supernatant, and resuspending in water to obtain CUR-NCs.

This study optimized the preparation process of CUR-NCs by varying nearly ten parameters, using size, polydispersity index (PDI), and zeta potential as evaluation indicators.

Initially, different organic phases, including DMSO, acetone, ethanol, and 0.5 M NaOH, were tested by dissolving 0.2 g CUR in 20 mL of each, adding it in a 1:10 ratio to 0.25% PVP K30 solution at room temperature, and sonicating for 15 min to obtain the sample.

Subsequently, using the same parameters, nine surfactants were screened with DMSO as the organic phase to assess their impact on sample size and PDI.

Additionally, this study investigated the effects of temperature, ultrasonic time, phase ratio, and surfactant concentration on CUR-NCs size. The specific parameters are detailed in Table 1.

Table 1. Independent factors in the preparation of CUR-NCs.

Independent Variables	Level			
Temperature (°C)	0	20	40	60
Ultrasonic time (min)	0	5	10	15
Organic phase/aqueous phase (v/v)	1:10	1:20	1:40	1:100
Stabilizer concentration (% w/v)	0.15	0.10	0.05	0.025

Furthermore, the effects of drug concentration, scaling factor, sample preparation vessel, and centrifugal resuspension on CUR-NCs size and PDI were explored.

2.4. Fabrication of Liposome

The CUR-NCs@Lipo were prepared using the thin film hydration method [23]. Specifically, 300 mg of lecithin, 60 mg of cholesterol, and 40 mg of vitamin E-TPGS were dissolved in 40 mL of chloroform. The chloroform was removed via rotary evaporation, and the centrifugally resuspended CUR-NCs$^+$ were added. CUR-NCs@Lipo were then prepared by incubating the mixture at 4 °C on a shaker for 2 h, vortexing for 3 min, sonicating for 5 min, and filtering it through a 220 nm membrane. Subsequently, the particle size, PDI, and surface potential of CUR-NCs@Lipo were measured. Successful encapsulation was confirmed by observing a change in charge. CUR-NCs@Lipo were further combined with a 1% chitosan oligosaccharide solution in a 1:1 ratio to form CUR-NCs@Lipo-CS.

2.5. Characterization

2.5.1. Size, Zeta, and PDI

Size, zeta, and PDI were determined using a Malvern Nano-ZS instrument (Malvern Panalytical Ltd., Enigma Business Park, UK). Before each measurement, the samples underwent dilution with distilled water to achieve an optimal scattering intensity, followed by manual redispersion through shaking [24,25]. Triplicate samples were analyzed for size, PDI, and zeta potential, with each test conducted over ten repetitions at 4 °C.

2.5.2. Powder X-ray Diffraction (PXRD)

Add 5% lyoprotectant (mannitol) to the CUR-NCs, pre-freeze at −20 °C for 24 h, then freeze-dry for 60 h. The PXRD patterns of the CUR nanopowder were analyzed using Oxford Diffraction equipment (Oxford Diffraction Ltd., Abingdon, UK). Data were collected with Cu-Kα radiation at 40 kV voltage, with a scanning speed of 1°/min over a range from 5° to 90° [26].

2.5.3. Transmission Electron Microscope (TEM)

Position the copper grid, covered with a carbon support film, face up on a clean sealing film. Using a pipette, apply 5 µL of 0.75 mg/mL CUR-NCs$^+$, CUR-NCs$^-$, CUR-NCs@Lipo, and CUR-NCs@Lipo-CS onto the copper grid; allow it to stand for 10 min, then remove excess liquid with filter paper. Absorb any remaining liquid from the copper mesh. Next, use a pipette to apply 5 µL of 3% phosphotungstic acid dye (pH 7.0) onto the sealing film. Invert the copper mesh onto the phosphotungstic acid droplets and let it rest for 1 min. Absorb any excess liquid from the copper mesh with filter paper. Air-dry the grid at room temperature for 10 min before placing it in a transmission electron microscope (HT7800) for imaging and analysis [27].

Import the TEM images into ImageJ (2.14.0) software for analysis. Measure the size of no fewer than 200 particles, analyze the data obtained, and represent the size of CUR-NCs using the mean value (Z_D) [28]. Calculate the *PDI* of CUR-NCs according to Equation (1):

$$PDI = \left(\frac{Sigma}{Z_D}\right)^2, \tag{1}$$

where *sigma* is the standard deviation.

2.5.4. Saturated Solubility

In brief, excess CUR-CCs, CUR-NCs$^+$, and CUR-NCs$^-$ were added to distilled water, vortexed for 5 min, and agitated at 37 °C for 12 h on a shaking table. The resulting mixture was centrifuged at 14,000 rpm for 12 min, the supernatant was collected, filtered through a 220 nm microporous filter, and the concentration was analyzed via HPLC, with each step repeated three times.

2.5.5. In Vitro Release Analysis

Equal amounts of CUR-NCs$^+$, CUR-NCs$^-$, and CUR-CCs were dissolved in stimulated intestinal fluids (SIF), followed by dissolution analysis using a dissolution apparatus (RCZ-8A) (Tianjin Tianda Tianfa Technology Co., Ltd, Tianjing, China) [15]. The samples were subjected to agitation at 200 rpm and 37 °C. At intervals of 1, 2, 3, 5, 10, 15, 30, and 60 min, a 3 mL sample was withdrawn and centrifuged at 14,000 rpm and 4 °C for 15 min, and the supernatant was filtered through a 220 nm filter membrane. The concentration was determined using HPLC, with each step repeated three times.

2.5.6. Stability

CUR-NCs with high and low concentrations were prepared (2 mg/mL, 0.5 mg/mL) and stored in sealed containers at 4 °C and 25 °C for 2 h, 4 h, 8 h, 24 h, and 7 days. The size and PDI were measured [29].

The same concentration of CUR-NCs$^+$, CUR-NCs$^-$, and CUR-NCs@Lipo-CS (0.5 mg/mL) were added to stimulated gastric fluids (SGF) and SIF at 37 °C, and the size and PDI were measured after 0.5 h, 1 h, 2 h, and 12 h.

2.6. Bioavailability in SD Rats

Male Sprague-Dawley (SD) rats (200–220 g) were provided by SPF (Beijing) Biotechnology Co., Ltd. (Beijing, China). All animal experiments were performed following the approved guidelines of the use and care of animals established by Jilin University.

Twenty-four male adult rats were fasted for 12 h but did not abstain from taking water. They were then randomly divided into four groups (n = 6) and administered CUR-CCs, CUR-NCs$^+$, CUR-NCs@Lipo-CS, and CUR-NCs$^-$, respectively. The dosage administered was 200 mg/kg, and 0.3 mL of blood was collected from the orbit at 0.166, 0.333, 0.5, 1, 2, 4, 6, 8, 10, and 12 h post-administration into anticoagulant Eppendorf [30]. The blood samples were centrifuged at 14,000 rpm and 4 °C for 15 min. The supernatant was then mixed with twice the amount of methanol to precipitate proteins, vortexed for 3 min, and centrifuged again. The resulting supernatant was transferred to Eppendorf, freeze-dried, reconstituted with methanol, and analyzed using the HPLC method to determine drug content. The measurement conditions were consistent with the previous analysis. Pharmacokinetic data were processed using DAS2.0 software [31].

2.7. Multiple-Particle Tracking In Vitro

Coumarin 6-labeled CUR-NCs$^+$, CUR-NCs$^-$, and CUR-NCs@Lipo-CS were diluted 10 times and dispersed in 0.1% mucin solution for 5 min. We added 10 μL of the dispersion to 200 μL of 5% mucus and put 20 μL on a glass slide and covered it. Slides should be sealed with mounting fluid to avoid dehydration and convection. Each sample was imaged at various positions simultaneously for 20 s [32,33]. Following enhancement with contrast and sharpening using Photoshop, diffusion analysis was performed using the ParticleTracker plugin in ImageJ (2.14.0) [34]. The MSD and effective diffusivities (D_{eff}) were calculated using the following equations:

$$\text{MSD}_\tau = \left(x_{(t+\tau)} - x_t\right)^2 + \left(y_{(t+\tau)} - y_t\right)^2, \tag{2}$$

$$D_{\text{eff}} = \frac{\text{MSD}_\tau}{4\tau}, \tag{3}$$

where x and y represented the coordinates of the NPs, and τ is the time scale.

2.8. Cellular Uptake and Mechanisms

The conventional Caco-2 cell model was established, and CUR-NCs$^+$, CUR-NCs@Lipo-CS, and CUR-NCs$^-$ were introduced into the medium to reach a drug concentration of 100 μg/mL. Subsequent to drug administration, uptake was halted at 5 min, 10 min, 30 min, 1 h, and 2 h. After double PBS rinses, lysate was added, and samples were collected.

Curcumin content per unit protein was quantified through the bicinchoninic acid (BCA) assay and HPLC.

Given that chitosan oligosaccharide is predominantly adsorbed onto liposomes, we have prepared coumarin 6-labeled blanks of liposomes (Lipo-C6), with half of these modified with chitosan oligosaccharide (Lipo-C6-CS) and half left untreated. Lipo-C6-CS or Lipo-C6 was added to the culture medium of Caco-2/E12 cells (3:7). After 1 h, the medium was collected, and the cells were rinsed three times with PBS and detached using trypsin. The fluorescence intensity of the cells was measured using a BD LSR Fortessa flow cytometer. The fluorescence intensity of the medium collected, and the initial medium was assessed using Infinite 200 PRO (Tecan, Männedorf, Switzerland), with excitation at 450 nm and emission at 505 nm. The mucoadhesive properties were calculated according to Equation (4):

$$\text{Mucoadhesive properties }(\%) = 100 - \frac{OD(end) - OD(blank)}{OD(original) - OD(blank)} \times 100, \quad (4)$$

where *OD(end)* is the fluorescence intensity of the experimental groups, adding Lipo-C6-CS or Lipo-C6; *OD(original)* is the fluorescence intensity of the original medium with Lipo-C6-CS or Lipo-C6; and *OD(blank)* is the fluorescence intensity of pure medium.

For a deeper exploration of nanocrystal uptake mechanisms, Caco-2 cells were initially exposed to indomethacin, colchicine, quercetin, chlorpromazine, or an ice water bath. Subsequently, CUR-NCs$^+$, CUR-NCs$^-$, or CUR-NCs@Lipo-CS were introduced into the medium. Following a 1 h cellular uptake period, the curcumin content per unit protein was quantified using the BCA assay and HPLC.

2.9. Cell Cytotoxicity

The cytotoxicity of Caco-2 cells was assessed using the Cell Counting Kit-8 Assay. Cells were plated in 96-well plates at a density of 5×10^3 cells per well and cultured for 24 h. Following medium removal, cells were exposed to CUR-NCs$^+$, CUR-NCs$^-$, or CUR-NCs@Lipo-CS at concentrations of 0.1, 0.5, 1.0, 2.0, 5.0, 10, and 20 µg/mL for 24 h. Subsequently, cells were washed twice with PBS and incubated in 10% CCK-8 solution, shielded from light for 90 min. The absorbance was read at 450 nm using Infinite 200 PRO (Tecan, Switzerland). Cell viability was determined using Equation (5):

$$cell\ viability(\%) = \frac{OD(experiment) - OD(blank)}{OD(control) - OD(blank)} \times 100, \quad (5)$$

where *OD(experiment)* is the absorbance of the experimental groups, adding different forms of curcumin; *OD(control)* is the absorbance of the drug-free group containing only cells and medium; and *OD(blank)* is the absorbance of pure medium.

Similarly, the impact of inhibitors, CUR-NCs$^+$, CUR-NCs$^-$, and CUR-NCs@Lipo-CS, on cell viability at the designated experimental concentrations and time intervals was also examined.

2.10. Mucus Penetration

2.10.1. Fluorescent Labeling of Nanocrystals

To create FRET pairs, 0.1 mg each of DiI and DiO were combined with 20 mL of DMSO along with CUR. The CUR-NCs$^+$-FRET, CUR-NCs$^-$-FRET, and CUR-NCs-FRET@Lipo-C6-CS (liposomes labeled with coumarin-6) were synthesized following established protocols.

Furthermore, to establish the association between CUR-NCs-FRET and the FRET phenomenon, approximately 0.5 mL of CUR-NCs-FRET was introduced into 5.0 mL of either pure water or water containing 60% methanol. Subsequently, the emission spectra of the samples were promptly recorded using an RF-6000 Spectrofluorometer at an excitation wavelength of 458 nm.

2.10.2. 3D Mucus Penetration

To assess the interactions between CUR-NCs^{+}, CUR-NCs^{-}, and CUR-NCs@Lipo-CS with the mucus layer, Caco-2/E12 (7:3) cells were cultured on Transwell filter inserts (Corning) for 14–17 d. The medium was replaced by HBSS 30 min later, followed by replacing the upper HBSS with diluted CUR-NCs^{+}-FRET, CUR-NCs^{-}-FRET, and CUR-NCs-FRET@Lipo-C6-CS in the medium. The monolayers were then washed three times with HBSS, and the cells were stained with Hoechst 33342 (10 μg/mL) for 15 min at 37 °C. The cell layers supporting the membranes of the Transwell inserts were cut from the plastic support without fixation, mounted onto microscope slides, and covered with coverslips. The slides were immediately observed under a confocal microscope (LSCM, AXR(Ti2-E); Nikon, Tokyo, Japan). The sections were photographed using a laser confocal microscope in z-stack mode, and the results were reconstructed in 3D using NIS-Elements Viewer (5.21) software.

3. Results and Discussion

3.1. CUR-NCs Formulation Development and Optimization

3.1.1. Preparation Methods for Screening CUR-NCs

Numerous mainstream preparation methods exist for NCs. Figure 1A illustrates that NCs prepared via SOP exhibit significantly superior size and PDI compared to other groups. Specifically, the size range of NCs obtained through grinding is constrained by experimental conditions, leading to poor stability and susceptibility to agglomeration.

With the exception of FRD, the other four methods primarily utilize high shear forces from various sources to fragment crystals and reduce particle size. However, the limited shear force of the instruments in each method results in a theoretical minimum particle size. While repeated crushing may approach this limit and reduce PDI, it cannot further reduce particle size. Thus, we conclude that when the size of the NCs reaches the equipment's limit, prescription becomes the primary determinant of particle size.

In principle, the FRD inhibits NCs' aggregation and growth. As is known, in liquid dispersions, small particles dissolve more easily due to their larger specific surface area, resulting in increased drug concentration around them. This disrupts the dissolution balance, leading to continued drug crystallization and growth, with large particles as nuclei. Consequently, a smaller PDI indicates greater system stability. The FRD addresses this issue at its source, transitioning the system from an unstable liquid state to a stable solid state. However, this method has significant drawbacks: excess surfactant removal is impractical, and the product size becomes fixed upon NCs formation, allowing for size enhancement only through prescription optimization.

The microjet homogenizer utilized in this experiment lacks temperature control. Consequently, the high temperatures generated during operation cause NCs initially prepared via SOP to continue growing during homogenization, resulting in an increased NC size from 136.1 nm to 676.5 nm. The utilization of different instruments significantly contributes to the challenge of replicating the findings reported in the literature. While theoretically, higher shear forces in grinding and high-speed shearing yield smaller particles, in practice, nanoparticles smaller than 200 nm are challenging to achieve. The SOP, utilizing cavitation effects generated by ultrasound, applies large and uniform shear forces on CUR crystals, resulting in extremely uniform dispersion of prepared the NCs. Hence, this study ultimately selects the SOP.

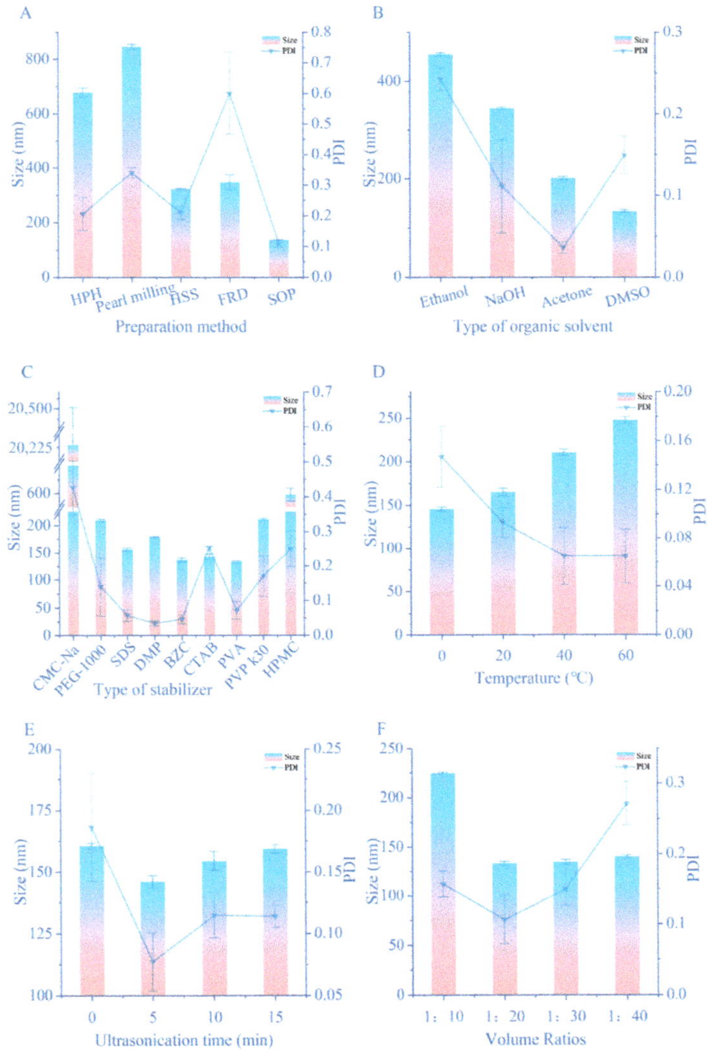

Figure 1. The effect of various parameters on size and PDI during nanocrystal preparation: (**A**) preparation method; (**B**) type of organic solvent; (**C**) type of stabilizer; (**D**) temperature; (**E**) ultrasonication time; (**F**) ratio of two phases. Data are means ± standard error of mean.

3.1.2. The Selection of the Organic Phase

Given our selection of the SOP method, the alternative organic solvent must exhibit a high diffusion coefficient in water to ensure rapid and uniform saturation of the drug in the solution, facilitating crystal precipitation [35]. As depicted in Figure 1B, crystals prepared using DMSO outperform those from acetone, ethanol, and sodium hydroxide solution groups in terms of size and PDI. Additionally, our experiments revealed that the acetone group yielded clusters after 24 h at 4 °C, a detrimental phenomenon. Furthermore, both the ethanol and NaOH groups exhibited varying degrees of agglomeration under the same conditions, whereas the DMSO group remained free from such issues. Moreover, given CUR's enhanced solubility in DMSO, the reliance on organic solvents in product formulation can be further reduced. Consequently, DMSO was chosen as the organic phase for NCs preparation.

3.1.3. Surfactant Selection

The choice of stabilizer not only determines the zeta potential of the final product but also dictates the complexity of subsequent formulation optimization and sets the lower limit for the size and PDI of the end product [36]. As depicted in Figure 1C, the SDS, PVP, PVA, CTAB, and BZC groups all demonstrated satisfactory performance. However, stability assessments revealed inadequacies in the SDS and CTAB groups, while the PVA group exhibited a smaller size compared to the PVP group. Consequently, BZC (a cationic surfactant) and PVA (an anionic surfactant) are earmarked for further use.

3.1.4. Surfactant Concentration

As illustrated in Figure 2A, increasing the surfactant concentration correlates with a reduction in product size; however, further escalation of surfactant concentration leads to an increase in PDI. This phenomenon arises from the dynamics of surfactant concentration relative to its critical micelle concentration (CMC). Below the CMC, the surfactant acts favorably by covering the NCs, thereby masking their hydrophobic layer—a beneficial effect. Conversely, exceeding the CMC results in the formation of free stabilizer micelles, contributing to the elevation of PDI [37]. Consequently, it is inferred that the optimal surfactant dosage is 0.05% (w/v).

In the preparation of the NCs, the most critical environmental factors are temperature, water-to-organic phase ratio, and ultrasonic time. The results are presented in Figure 1D–F. Notably, low temperature exhibits minimal impact on product size, underscoring why the size of prepared NCs increase following processing by a micro-jet homogenizer. A higher water phase ratio tends to reduce the size of CUR-NCs; however, indiscriminate escalation of this ratio does not consistently yield size reduction. The result obtained at a 1:20 ratio already represents the limit of NC size influenced by this factor. The presence and duration of ultrasound significantly affect NC size, but excessively prolonged ultrasound exposure should be avoided. The moment of crystallization is of significant importance with regard to the size of the nanocrystals. Ultrasound is an effective method of accelerating the homogeneous mixing of the organic phase with the mobile phase. Ultrasound induces bubble vibration and shear force, albeit with minimal impact on particle size and PDI in short durations due to energy dissipation. Consequently, the optimal conditions for NCs preparation are a water-to-organic phase ratio of 1:20 (v/v), a temperature of 4 °C, and ultrasonication for 5 min.

Minimizing the quantity of materials in the drug preparation process enhances its economic, safety, and environmental attributes. As previously concluded, a higher proportion of the water phase results in NCs approaching their size limit; however, this corresponds to reduced drug concentration, increased surfactant usage, and greater water volume for removal, presenting a drawback. To counter this, resuspending samples with the supernatant removed during centrifugal resuspension increases drug concentration while eliminating free active agents and residual organic solvents. Interestingly, multiple resuspension cycles have no effect on the final product's size and PDI, while CUR-NCs may be slightly affected by dissolved content in the solution, resulting in minor size reduction upon supernatant removal (Figure 2B,C). Moreover, factors such as drug concentration, amplification experiments, and sample preparation containers (Figure 2D–F) exhibit no significant impact on the final product's size and PDI. Nevertheless, if the conditions governing the prescription of the aforementioned factors are not optimized, the aforementioned every single factor may affect the experimental results. For instance, when CTAB was employed as a stabilizer in our experiments, the samples prepared were only able to yield nanocrystals of a small size if a conical flask was utilized and 20 mL of sample was prepared at a time. In addition, by observing the color of the sample, it is also easy to determine the size of the sample; the closer the color of the sample is to reddish brown (Figure 3C), the smaller the sample is; if the size of the sample is greater than 100, the color is closer to yellow (Figure 3C). After analyzing different nanocrystal preparation conditions, it was determined that the optimization challenge varies across parameters, impacting size and PDI in the following order: surfactant type > organic solvent type > ratio of two phases > temperature > surfactant dosage > ultrasonication time > others.

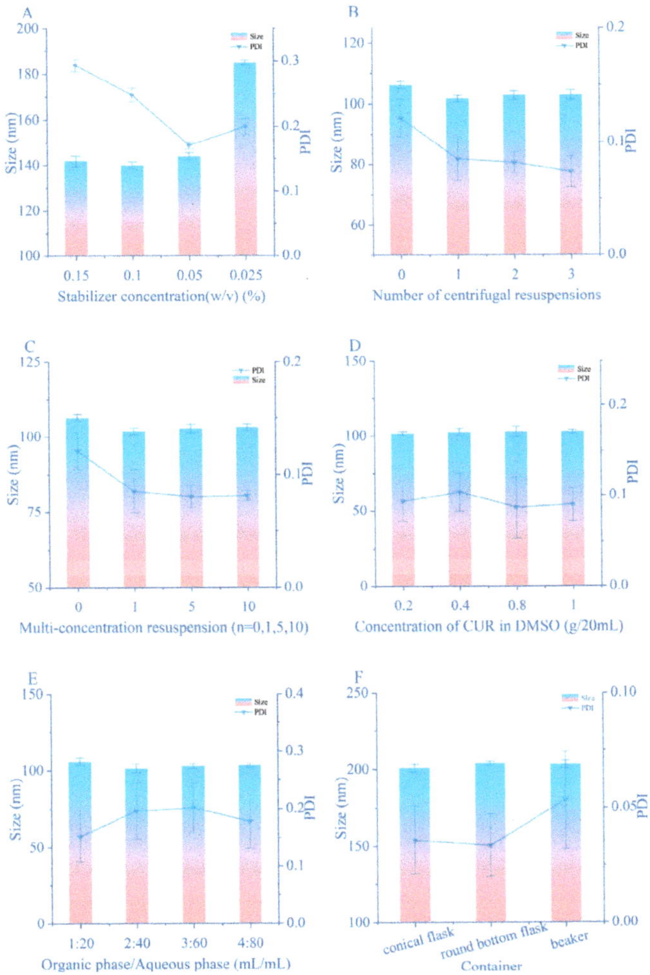

Figure 2. The effect of various parameters on size and PDI during nanocrystal preparation: (**A**) stabilizer concentration; (**B**) effect of multiple centrifugal resuspensions on particle size; (**C**) effect of centrifugal concentration on particle size; (**D**) effect of the concentration of the drug in the organic phase on the particle size; (**E**) effect of dose on particle size; (**F**) effect of experimental vessels on particle size. Representative images are presented. Data are means ± standard error of mean.

In summary, the optimal formulation for NCs is as follows: dissolve 1.0 g of CUR in 20 mL of DMSO, add 2 mL of this solution to 40 mL water with 0.05% (w/v) PVA or BZC, and ultrasonicate it at 4 °C for 5 min. This results in the final product with a size of 131.2 nm and a PDI of 0.093 for the PVA group, with a zeta potential of −4.52 mV, and a product with a size of 90.97 nm and a PDI of 0.105 for the BZC group, with a zeta potential of +54.6 mV.

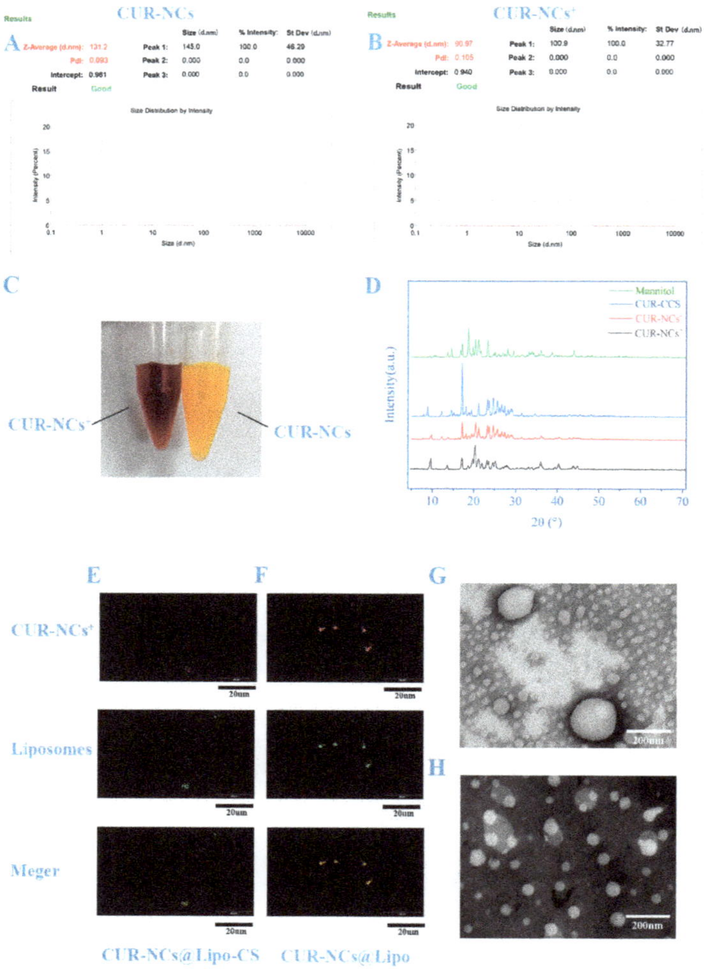

Figure 3. (**A**,**B**) Size and PDI of CUR-NCs$^+$ and CUR-NCs$^-$, measured via Malvern Nano-ZS. (**C**) Appearance of CUR-NCs$^+$ and CUR-NCs$^-$. (**D**) PXRD. (**E**,**F**) Laser scanning confocal fluorescence microscopy images of CUR-NCs@Lipo-CS and CUR-NCs@Lipo dissolved by water (scale bar is 20 µm). (**G**,**H**) TEM of CUR-NCs@Lipo and CUR-NCs@Lipo-CS. The number of liposomes represented in the images is indicative of the actual degree of encapsulation (concentrations of CUR-NCs@Lipo and CUR-NCs@Lipo-CS are same; scale bar is 200 nm). Representative images are presented.

3.2. PXRD

As shown in Figure 3C, the PXRD results show that CUR has characteristic absorption peaks at 17.14°, 20.52°, 21.24°, 23.18°, 24.56°, and 28.10°.The same characteristic peaks can be observed in the PXRD spectrum of CUR-NCs$^+$ and CUR-NCs$^-$. Therefore, it is believed that the crystal form of CUR did not change during the preparation of NCs.

3.3. TEM

Laser particle size analyzers utilize light scattering (diffraction) by particles to determine particle size. Essentially, when light encounters particles during propagation, some of it deviates from its original direction. The degree of deviation increases with smaller particle sizes and decreases with larger ones. While this method efficiently and straightforwardly measures particle size, errors become prominent when the size is <100 nm. Therefore, the precise particle size requires confirmation via scanning electron microscopy or transmission electron microscopy. The presence of a hydrated layer also results in larger measurements from the particle sizer than those observed in the electron micrographs. Figure 4 illustrates that the size of CUR-NCs$^+$ prepared according to the prescribed method is only 29.42 nm. Additionally, CUR-NCs$^-$, with a size of 92.20 nm, also exhibit commendable nano-properties.

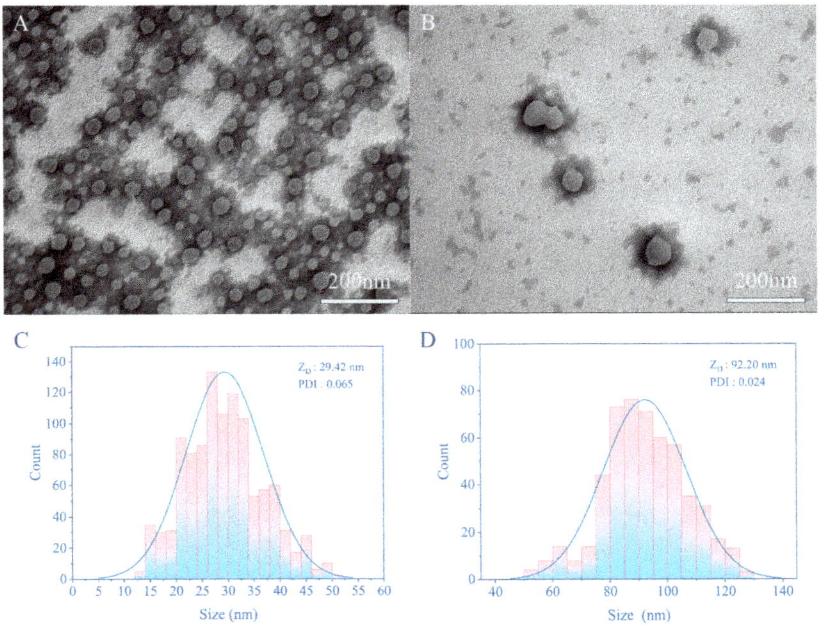

Figure 4. TEM images of CUR-NCs$^+$, CUR-NCs$^-$, and particle size distribution: (**A**,**C**) CUR-NCs$^+$; (**B**,**D**) CUR-NCs$^-$ (concentration of CUR-NCs$^+$ and CUR-NCs$^-$ are the same; scale bar is 200 nm). Representative images are presented.

3.4. Fabrication of Liposomes

The exceptional dissolution characteristics of nanocrystals have propelled their extensive integration into the development of BCS class-II drug models. However, BCS-IV drugs exhibit poor biomembrane permeability and susceptibility to P-gp. If nanocrystals can be efficiently internalized by cells while leveraging their potent drug-carrying capabilities, a substantial enhancement in the bioavailability of BCS class IV drugs is anticipated. Consequently, swift dissolution of nanocrystals is not envisaged during oral absorption. Encapsulation within liposomes serves a dual purpose: shielding nanocrystals from aggregation and expansion induced by diverse external factors like digestive fluids and mucous layers, while concurrently mitigating premature dissolution and enhancing overall bioavailability. The incorporation of E-TPGS into liposomes has demonstrated an inhibitory effect on P-gp, thereby further enhancing bioavailability.

Regarding the question of whether nanocrystals are encapsulated by liposomes, we disagree with the use of fluorescence colocalization, which often leads to false conclusions. In Figure 3E,F, we can clearly see that there is more fluorescence overlap in CUR-NCs@Lipo compared to CUR-NCs@Lipo-CS, which does not mean that the incorporation of oligochitosan ruptures the liposomes. Interestingly, during the preparation of CUR-NCs@Lipo, we found that CUR-NCs@Lipo-CS was positively charged and had a particle size of around 170 nm, whereas CUR-NCs@Lipo was negatively charged and had a particle size of around 200 nm. The addition of oligochitosan makes the particle size of the nanoparticles smaller, and there seems to be a high probability that the addition of oligochitosan caused this result; however, through the electron microscope image of CUR-NCs@Lipo (Figure 3G,H), we found that due to the interactions between the charges, the liposomes adsorbed a ring of nanocrystals at the periphery, resulting in the large size of the measured particle, whereas the addition of chitosan reversed the charge of the liposome, turning the attraction into mutual repulsion, and the liposome not wrapped around the nanocrystals shows its original size. Then, we found another interesting phenomenon from the electron micrographs, the encapsulation rate of liposomes increased after the addition of chitosan, and the number of liposomes encapsulated with nanocrystals increased significantly. This may be due to the fact that the inside of the liposome is still negatively charged, and the outside environment is positively charged, and this potential difference drives the nanocrystals to enter the liposome, resulting in a significant increase in the encapsulation rate.

3.5. *In Vitro Release*

Figure 5A shows the cumulative release curves of CUR-NCs$^+$, CUR-NCs$^-$, CUR-NCs@Lipo-CS, and CUR-CCs. It can be seen that CUR-CCs is insoluble in water and cannot be measured in water. Regardless of whether it is cationic or anionic, NCs can detect a large amount of CUR in the solution, but since the size of NCs$^+$ is smaller than that of NCs$^-$, according to the Noyes–Whitney equation:

$$\frac{dC}{dt} = kA(C_s - C_t), \tag{6}$$

where dC/dt is the dissolution rate, A is the surface area, k is a constant, C_s is the saturated solubility of the drug, and C_t is the drug concentration [38,39].

It is not difficult to find that the larger the specific surface area, the greater the dissolution rate of the drug, so CUR-NCs$^+$ has a higher release rate than CUR-NCs-. In addition, different surfactants have different solubilizing effects on drugs, making CUR-NCs$^+$ exhibit higher saturated solubility. At the same time, considering the influence of charge, we also prepared CUR-NCs without adding any surfactant. There is no doubt that this group of CUR-NCs has extremely poor stability and rapid polymerization. PDI > 0.7 and Zeta = −16.7 mV imply that CUR is naturally attracted to cationic surfactants, resulting in a better performance of CUR-NCs$^+$ than CUR-NCs$^-$ at the physical level, but we did not conduct similar experiments with other drugs to corroborate this idea. The slow and limited dissolution of CUR-NCs@Lipo-CS is a consequence of the protective effect of the liposome membrane on the nanocrystals. Since the size of the CUR-NCs is much smaller than the 220 nm pore size of the filter membrane, in order to increase the accuracy of the content determination, we removed the CUR-NCs suspended in the solution via centrifugation before the content measurement. We considered the measured concentration to be the true concentration of saturated solubility about CUR-NCs.

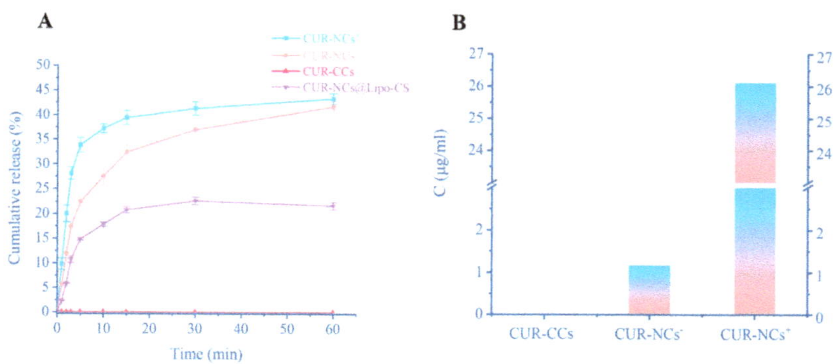

Figure 5. *Cont.*

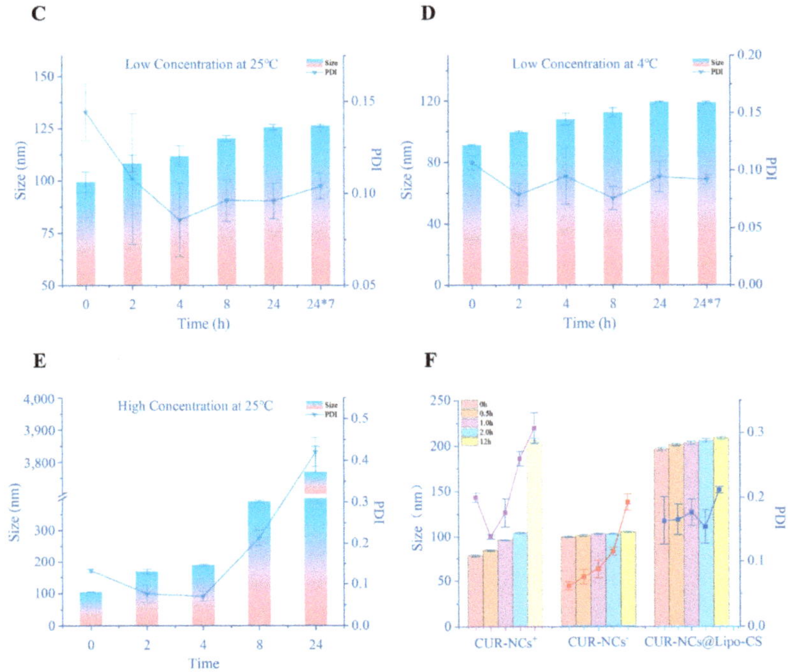

Figure 5. (**A**) Dissolution profile of CUR-NCs@Lipo-CS, CUR-NCs$^+$, CUR-NCs$^-$ and CUR-CCs (n = 3). (**B**) Saturation solubility of CUR-NCs$^+$ and CUR-NCs$^-$ (n = 3). (**C**) Stability of low-concentration nanocrystals at 25 °C (n = 3). (**D**) Stability of low-concentration nanocrystals at 4 °C (n = 3). (**E**) Stability of high-concentration nanocrystals at 25 °C (n = 3). (**F**) Stability of CUR-NCs$^+$, CUR-NCs$^-$ and CUR-NCs@Lipo-CS in Sif (n = 3). Representative images are presented. Data are means ± standard error of mean.

3.6. Stability Studies

Figure 5C is the change of size of CUR-NCs$^+$ at low concentration and room temperature, Figure 5D is the change of size of CUR-NCs$^+$ at low concentration and low temperature, and Figure 5E is the change of size of high-concentration CUR-NCs$^+$ at room temperature, as the time go by. Comparing C, D, and E, it can be seen that CUR-NCs$^+$ are sensitive to heat. The storage size of CUR-NCs$^+$ at room temperature was larger than that at low temperature. This phenomenon is more obvious in the high-concentration group. At the same time, we observed that when CUR-NCs$^+$ were still at the nanoscale, although the size increased slightly with time, it eventually stabilized, and the PDI continued to become smaller with time. It is not difficult to understand that small NCs dissolve and precipitate on large crystals, causing the size of the crystals to concentrate gradually; thus, the PDI decreases, and the system reaches a more stable state [40]. At the same time, due to the increase in concentration, the number of particles in the system increases and the entropy value increases, which means that the system is more unstable. In addition, the CUR-NCs in the high-concentration group are at room temperature. The increase in temperature further increases the entropy value, which leads to the CUR-NCs continuing to grow and aggregate, eventually losing their nanometer properties. After a week, all the crystals aggregate and sink to the bottom of the container. In general, although the high-concentration group is not as stable as the low-concentration group, the overall stability is still excellent during low-temperature storage, and the size change is minimal within a week. Therefore, it is believed that the stability of CUR-NCs prepared under this prescription condition is excellent.

The most apparent change in particle size is observed in CUR-NCs^{+}, while the change in particle size of CUR-NCs^{-} is less pronounced. However, the PDI of CUR-NCs^{-} has increased significantly and is still on an upward trajectory. In contrast, CUR-NCs@Lipo-CS exhibits minimal changes in both particle size and PDI, suggesting that CUR-NCs^{+}, which is rarely influenced by the enzyme and electrolytes in SIF under the protection of liposome, does not undergo aggregation.

3.7. Bioavailability

Using SD rats as the animal model, Figure 6A presents the drug–time curve after oral administration of each preparation. As shown in the results in Table 2, the C_{max} values of CUR-NCs@Lipo-CS, CUR-NCs^{+}, and CUR-NCs^{-} are 6.006, 3.098, and 2.251 times that of CUR-CCs. The AUG $_{(0–\infty)}$ values of CUR-NCs@Lipo-CS, CUR-NCs^{+}, and CUR-NCs^{-} are 5.427, 1.596. and 1.22 times that of CUR-CCs. These data all reflect that the nanocrystal delivery method has greatly improved the bioavailability of curcumin, among which CUR-NCs@Lipo-CS has the best effect.

Table 2. Pharmacokinetic parameters of oral CUR-NCs^{+}, CUR-NCs^{-}, CUR-CCs, and CUR-NCs@Lipo-CS.

Parameter	CUR-CCs (po)	CUR-NCs^{+} (po)	CUR-NCs^{-} (po)	CUR-NCs @Lipo-CS
T_{max} (h)	0.361 ± 0.068	0.361 ± 0.068	0.333	0.5
$t_{1/2}$ (h)	3.182 ± 1.096	3.534 ± 1.467	5.796 ± 2.727	2.384 ± 0.44
C_{max} (μg/L)	92.785 ± 37.442	287.493 ± 26.511	208.871 ± 51.702	557.311 ± 85.443
$AUC_{(0–t)}$ (μg·h/L)	189.899 ± 95.831	343.107 ± 81.295	233.062 ± 52.893	1030.536 ± 212.234
$AUC_{(0–\infty)}$ (μg/L·h)	209.477 ± 118.04	381.828 ± 99.082	305.729 ± 111.782	1047.894 ± 208.003

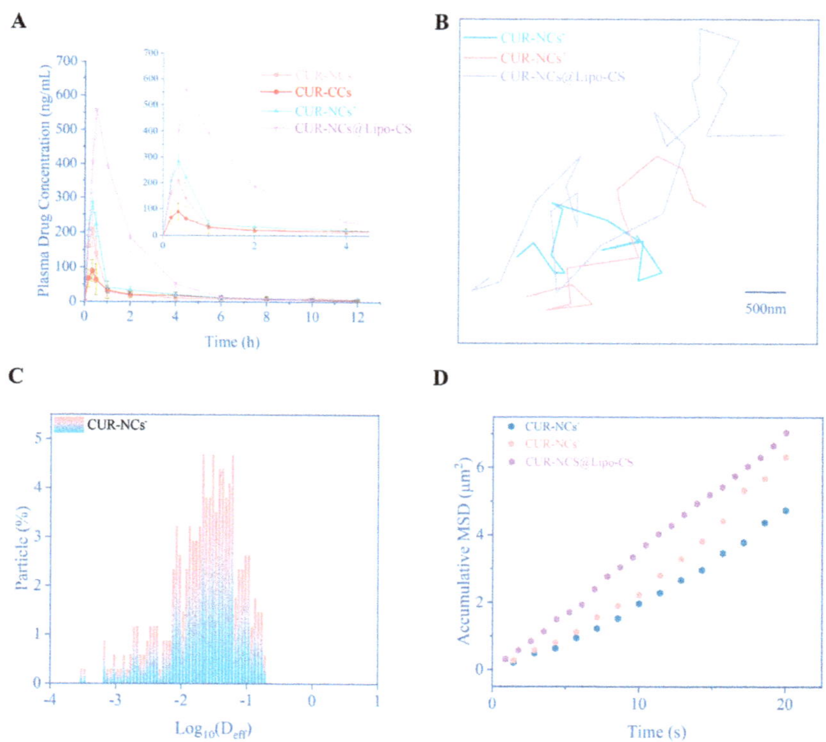

Figure 6. *Cont.*

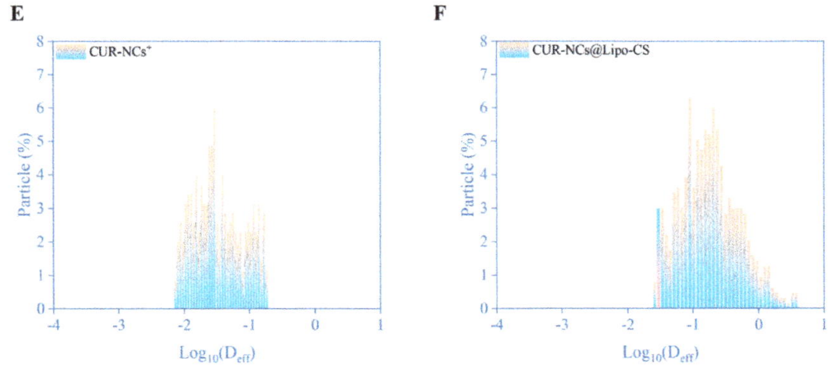

Figure 6. (**A**) Plasma concentration–time curves of oral CUR-NCs$^+$, CUR-NCs$^-$, CUR-CCs, and CUR-NCs@Lipo-CS (n = 6). (**B**) Mobility of CUR-NCs$^+$, CUR-NCs$^-$, and CUR-NCs@Lipo-CS at 37 °C. Representative trajectories of particle motion in 20 s. Scale bar is 500 nm. (**D**) MSD values as a function of time. (**C**,**E**,**F**) Distribution of the logarithms of individual particle effective diffusivities (D_{eff}) on a timescale of 20 s. Representative images are presented.

3.8. Multiple-Particle Tracking

The trajectory of CUR-NCs@Lipo-CS, CUR-NCs$^+$, and CUR-NCs$^-$ within the mucus layer is illustrated in Figure 6B. Notably, within the same scale, CUR-NCs@Lipo-CS exhibit a broader motion range, indicative of Brownian motion, suggesting superior mucus penetration compared to CUR-NCs$^+$ and CUR-NCs$^-$ [32,33]. Mean square displacement (MSD) was calculated on a 20 s time scale (Figure 6D), revealing that, on average, the MSD of CUR-NCs@Lipo-CS was approximately 1.46 times greater than that of CUR-NCs$^-$. Additionally, the effective diffusivity (D_{eff}) distribution shown in Figure 6C,E,F also shows that CUR-NCs@Lipo-CS have higher diffusivity. Thus, CUR-NCs@Lipo-CS are more adept at traversing the mucus barrier and accessing the upper cells of the small intestinal mucosa, consequently yielding enhanced bioavailability.

3.9. Cellular Uptake of CUR

3.9.1. Determination of Cellular Uptake of CUR

The utilization of Caco-2 as a model to mimic the uptake of CUR-NCs@Lipo-CS, CUR-NCs$^+$, and CUR-NCs$^-$ indicated a notably higher cellular uptake of CUR-NCs$^+$ at all time points compared to CUR-NCs@Lipo-CS and CUR-NCs$^-$ (Figure 7A). These results underscore the pivotal role of particle size in influencing nanocrystal uptake. The relatively diminished cellular uptake of CUR-NCs@Lipo-CS can be ascribed to the inherent constraints of the liposome membrane in releasing encapsulated CUR-NCs. Over time, the cellular uptake of CUR-NCs is modulated by P-gp, with transporter protein availability and energy determining the gradual accumulation of curcumin to an equilibrium state. In contrast, due to distinct transmembrane transport mechanisms and enhanced equilibrium solubility, CUR-NCs$^+$ with a smaller particle size did not reach equilibrium within 120 min. Furthermore, intracellular curcumin accumulation continued to rise gradually, elucidating the rationale behind the lowest observed IC50 value (Figure 7B,C). Despite the consistently lower cellular uptake of CUR-NCs@Lipo-CS compared to CUR-NCs, intracellular curcumin content increased steadily. This phenomenon contributes to the explanation for the smaller IC50 value of CUR-NCs@Lipo-CS.

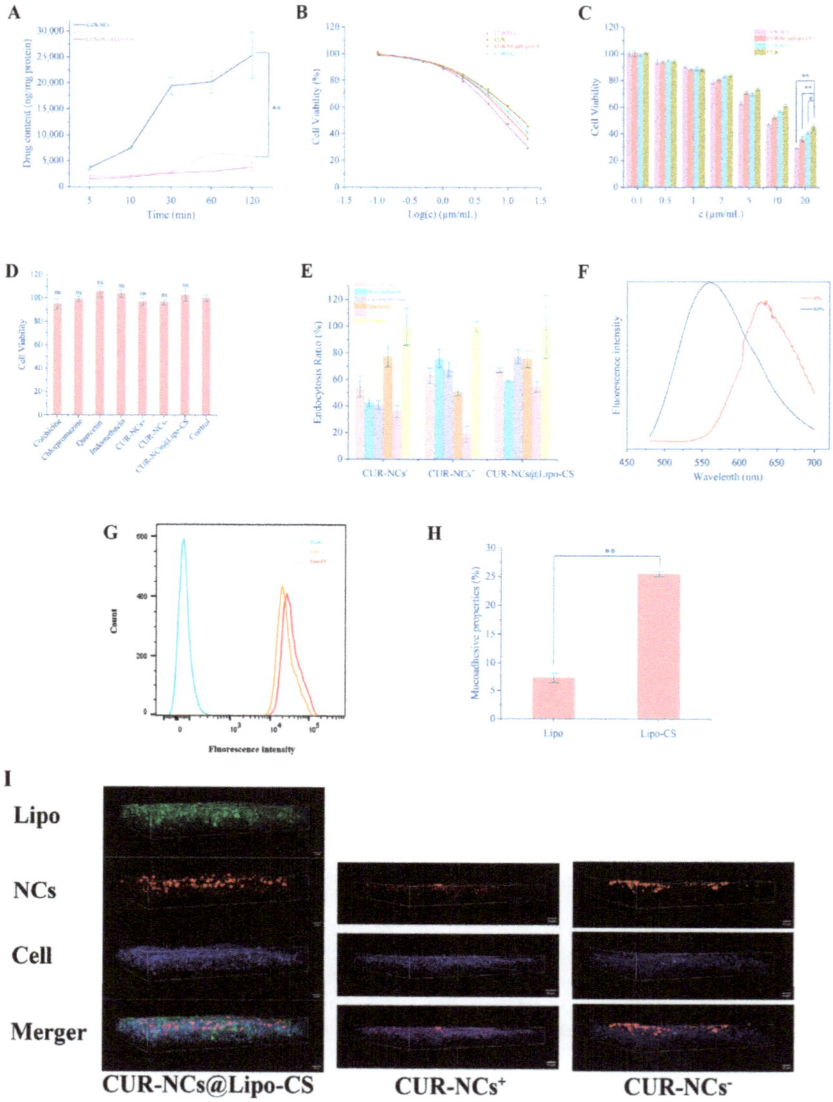

Figure 7. (**A**) Cellular uptake of CUR formulation on Caco-2 cells (n = 3 per group). (**B**) The IC50 value of Cur-LPs, Cur, and Cur-NCs in macrophages. (**C**) In vitro evaluation of Caco-2 cells' viability treated with CUR-NCs@Lipo-CS, Cur, Cur-NCs$^-$, and Cur-NCs$^+$ after 24 h (n = 3 per group). (**D**) In vitro cytotoxicity of endocytic inhibitors and CUR formulation based on Caco-2 cells (n = 3 per group). (**E**) Possible uptake mechanisms investigated via cellular uptake of CUR formulation (n = 3 per group). (**F**) Fluorescence emission spectra of ETO-NCs-FRET dissolved by water or methanol. (**G**) Flow cytometry analysis of cellular uptake and mean fluorescence intensities of Caco-2 cells incubated with coumarin 6-labeled Lipo-C6-CS and Lipo-C6. (**H**) Mucoadhesive properties of Lipo and Lipo-CS (n = 3 per group). (**I**) Uptake by mucus-containing E12/Caco-2 cells that simulated the multiple barriers of intestinal mucosa (scale bar is 20 μm). The proximity of the red component to the bottom indicates a heightened resistance of the nanocrystals to the cellular barrier. Representative images are presented. Data are means ± standard error of mean. ns, no significant difference; * $p < 0.05$ and ** $p < 0.01$ via one-way ANOVA and Bonferroni's test.

3.9.2. Mechanisms of Cellular Uptake of CUR

Chlorpromazine serves as an inhibitor of clathrin-mediated endocytosis, while indomethacin inhibits caveolae-mediated endocytosis. Colchicine acts as an inhibitor of macropinocytosis, and quercetin inhibits clathrin/caveolae-independent endocytosis [41]. A temperature of 4 °C primarily slows down cellular energy metabolism, thus impeding active transport. As depicted in Figure 7, the uptake of CUR-NCs@Lipo-CS, CUR-NCs$^+$, and CUR-NCs$^-$ is an energy-intensive process. Moreover, the data (Figure 7E) indicate that various inhibitors exert inhibitory effects on cellular uptake, suggesting the involvement of multiple uptake pathways. Non-grid- and non-nubbin-mediated endocytosis is the primary internalization mechanism for CUR-NCs$^+$, whereas nubbin-mediated endocytosis is the likely route for CUR-NCs@Lipo-CS. Cell viability experiments revealed that the addition of inhibitors, including CUR-NCs@Lipo-CS, CUR-NCs$^+$, and CUR-NCs$^-$, did not significantly impact cell viability throughout the experiments.

3.9.3. Fluorescence Properties

To determine if CUR-NCs are absorbed into cells as intact crystals with enhanced clarity, Dio and DiI were utilized together. The maximum emission wavelength shifted from 600 nm to 500 nm due to the transition of CUR-NCs-FRET from a colloidal to a solute state. This shift signifies the generation of the FRET signal solely within the CUR-NCs, vanishing upon crystal dissolution. Hence, the red fluorescence observed is emitted exclusively by the nanocrystals (Figure 7F).

3.9.4. Mucoadhesive Properties of Polycationic Chitosan Oligosaccharide

Chitosan, renowned for its exceptional hydrophilicity and positive charge, interacts favorably with the negative charge of the mucus layer, significantly prolonging drug residence time in the gastrointestinal tract when employed as a drug delivery carrier. To assess if the chitosan oligosaccharide utilized could elicit comparable effects in enhancing adhesion, mucoadhesive properties, and uptake of Lipo-C6-CS and Lipo-C6, investigations were conducted. As illustrated in Figure 7G,H, chitosan oligosaccharide proved effective in augmenting cell adhesion to liposomes; however, the improvement in cellular uptake was constrained.

3.9.5. Mucus Penetration on Caco-2/E12 Cells

Nonetheless, the existence of a mucus layer in the gastrointestinal tract hindered the accurate simulation of the authentic uptake by Caco-2 cells. Consequently, we opted to co-culture E12 cells with Caco-2 cells to replicate cellular uptake in the presence of the mucus layer. Figure 7I clearly demonstrates that CUR-NCs@Lipo-CS is more likely to penetrate the mucus layer and be taken up by cells than CUR-NCs$^+$ and CUR-NCs$^-$. Furthermore, the aggregation and deposition of CUR-NCs is reduced under the protection of liposomes. A considerable number of small particles traverse the cell layer. However, the cellular uptake of CUR-NCs$^+$ is still greater than that of CUR-NCs$^-$. Both CUR-NCs$^+$ and CUR-NCs$^-$ were primarily concentrated in the upper mucus layer of the cells and were predominantly aggregated, which is consistent with the previous experimental results.

4. Conclusions

In this study, the sonoprecipitation method was utilized to successfully synthesize cationic curcumin nanocrystal liposomes. The morphology of CUR-NCs@Lipo-CS was confirmed through a series of in vitro characterization experiments, validating the successful entrapment of nanocrystals within the lipid bilayer, enhanced by chitosan oligosaccharide. In vitro assays demonstrated a marked decrease in the rate and extent of CUR-NCs@Lipo-CS release from SIF in comparison to nanocrystals alone, highlighting the lipid bilayer's efficacy in impeding rapid core nanocrystal dissolution. Cell uptake studies indicated that CUR-NCs@Lipo-CS displayed superior mucus-penetrating capabilities, effectively mitigating the mucosal barrier's impact on nanocrystal absorption. These results emphasize the heightened potential for oral bioavailability of CUR-NCs@Lipo-CS in delivering BCS-IV drugs, affirming the success of pharmaceutical strategies in translating dissolution enhancement into comprehensive nanocrystal uptake within NCs-based oral BCS IV delivery systems.

Moreover, we recommend that our colleagues follow the sequence of screening the organic phase types, surfactant types, and ultrasound time and prepare nanocrystals of different drugs under low-temperature, high-water-ratio, and high-surfactant-concentration conditions in order to prepare the ideal nanocrystals.

Author Contributions: Software, X.C., X.H., C.D. and H.L.; Formal analysis, X.C., J.S., Z.J. and S.Z.; Investigation, X.C., X.W. and X.J.; Data curation, X.C.; Writing—original draft, X.C. All authors have read and agreed to the published version of the manuscript.

Funding: This research was supported by grants from the Jilin Province Science and Technology Development Plan Project (No. 20220401107YY).

Institutional Review Board Statement: This study was approved by Institutional Animal Care and Use Committee of Jilin University School of Pharmaceutical Science (No. 20230083).

Informed Consent Statement: Not applicable.

Data Availability Statement: Further inquiries can be directed to the corresponding authors.

Conflicts of Interest: The authors declare no conflicts of interest.

References

1. Li, X.; Zhu, R.; Jiang, H.; Yin, Q.; Gu, J.; Chen, J.; Ji, X.; Wu, X.; Fu, H.; Wang, H.; et al. Autophagy enhanced by curcumin ameliorates inflammation in atherogenesis via the TFEB-P300-BRD4 axis. *Acta Pharm. Sin. B* **2022**, *12*, 2280–2299. [CrossRef] [PubMed]
2. Pisano, M.; Pagnan, G.; Dettori, M.A.; Cossu, S.; Caffa, I.; Sassu, I.; Emionite, L.; Fabbri, D.; Cilli, M.; Pastorino, F.; et al. Enhanced anti-tumor activity of a new curcumin-related compound against melanoma and neuroblastoma cells. *Mol. Cancer* **2010**, *9*, 137. [CrossRef]
3. Kheradpezhouh, E.; Barritt, G.J.; Rychkov, G.Y. Curcumin inhibits activation of TRPM2 channels in rat hepatocytes. *Redox Biol.* **2016**, *7*, 1–7. [CrossRef] [PubMed]
4. Ran, C.; Xu, X.; Raymond, S.B.; Ferrara, B.J.; Neal, K.; Bacskai, B.J.; Medarova, Z.; Moore, A. Design, synthesis, and testing of difluoroboron-derivatized curcumins as near-infrared probes for in vivo detection of amyloid-beta deposits. *J. Am. Chem. Soc.* **2009**, *131*, 15257–15261. [CrossRef] [PubMed]
5. Zhang, T.; Chen, Y.; Ge, Y.; Hu, Y.; Li, M.; Jin, Y. Inhalation treatment of primary lung cancer using liposomal curcumin dry powder inhalers. *Acta Pharm. Sin. B* **2018**, *8*, 440–448. [CrossRef]
6. Zhong, D.; Zhang, D.; Chen, W.; He, J.; Ren, C.; Zhang, X.; Kong, N.; Tao, W.; Zhou, M. Orally deliverable strategy based on microalgal biomass for intestinal disease treatment. *Sci. Adv.* **2021**, *7*, eabi9265. [CrossRef]
7. Wang, Q.; Yu, W.; Li, Z.; Liu, B.; Hu, Y.; Chen, S.; de Vries, R.; Yuan, Y.; Erazo Quintero, L.E.; Hou, G.; et al. The stability and bioavailability of curcumin loaded α-lactalbumin nanocarriers formulated in functional dairy drink. *Food Hydrocoll.* **2022**, *131*, 107807. [CrossRef]
8. Alejo, T.; Uson, L.; Landa, G.; Prieto, M.; Yus Argón, C.; Garcia-Salinas, S.; de Miguel, R.; Rodríguez-Largo, A.; Irusta, S.; Sebastian, V.; et al. Nanogels with High Loading of Anesthetic Nanocrystals for Extended Duration of Sciatic Nerve Block. *ACS Appl. Mater. Interfaces* **2021**, *13*, 17220–17235. [CrossRef]
9. Hollis, C.P.; Weiss, H.L.; Leggas, M.; Evers, B.M.; Gemeinhart, R.A.; Li, T. Biodistribution and bioimaging studies of hybrid paclitaxel nanocrystals: Lessons learned of the EPR effect and image-guided drug delivery. *J. Control. Release* **2013**, *172*, 12–21. [CrossRef]
10. Pant, N.; Wairkar, S. Topical nanocrystals of bioflavonoids: A new technology platform for skin ailments. *Int. J. Pharm.* **2022**, *619*, 121707. [CrossRef]
11. Cristina Cardia, M.; Francesca Palmas, M.; Casula, L.; Pisanu, A.; Marceddu, S.; Valenti, D.; Sinico, C.; Pini, E.; Scerba, M.T.; Tweedie, D.; et al. Nanocrystals as an effective strategy to improve Pomalidomide bioavailability in rodent. *Int. J. Pharm.* **2022**, *625*, 122079. [CrossRef]
12. Huang, D.; Gui, J.; Chen, X.; Yu, R.; Gong, T.; Zhang, Z.; Fu, Y. Chondroitin Sulfate-Derived Paclitaxel Nanocrystal via π-π Stacking with Enhanced Stability and Tumor Targetability. *ACS Appl. Mater. Interfaces* **2022**, *14*, 51776–51789. [CrossRef] [PubMed]
13. Zhang, C.; Long, L.; Xiong, Y.; Wang, C.; Peng, C.; Yuan, Y.; Liu, Z.; Lin, Y.; Jia, Y.; Zhou, X.; et al. Facile Engineering of Indomethacin-Induced Paclitaxel Nanocrystal Aggregates as Carrier-Free Nanomedicine with Improved Synergetic Antitumor Activity. *ACS Appl. Mater. Interfaces* **2019**, *11*, 9872–9883. [CrossRef] [PubMed]

14. Xiong, W.; Sang, W.; Linghu, K.G.; Zhong, Z.F.; Cheang, W.S.; Li, J.; Hu, Y.J.; Yu, H.; Wang, Y.T. Dual-functional Brij-S20-modified nanocrystal formulation enhances the intestinal transport and oral bioavailability of berberine. *Int. J. Nanomed.* **2018**, *13*, 3781–3793. [CrossRef] [PubMed]
15. Pi, J.; Wang, S.; Li, W.; Kebebe, D.; Zhang, Y.; Zhang, B.; Qi, D.; Guo, P.; Li, N.; Liu, Z. A nano-cocrystal strategy to improve the dissolution rate and oral bioavailability of baicalein. *Asian J. Pharm. Sci.* **2019**, *14*, 154–164. [CrossRef]
16. He, H.; Lu, Y.; Qi, J.; Zhao, W.; Dong, X.; Wu, W. Biomimetic thiamine- and niacin-decorated liposomes for enhanced oral delivery of insulin. *Acta Pharm. Sin. B* **2018**, *8*, 97–105. [CrossRef]
17. Hong, S.; Wang, Y.; Park, S.Y.; Lee, H. Progressive fuzzy cation-π assembly of biological catecholamines. *Sci. Adv.* **2018**, *4*, eaat7457. [CrossRef]
18. Wang, Y.; Tan, X.; Fan, X.; Zhao, L.; Wang, S.; He, H.; Yin, T.; Zhang, Y.; Tang, X.; Jian, L.; et al. Current strategies for oral delivery of BCS IV drug nanocrystals: Challenges, solutions and future trends. *Expert. Opin. Drug Deliv.* **2021**, *18*, 1211–1228. [CrossRef]
19. Xu, Z.; Hou, Y.; Sun, J.; Zhu, L.; Zhang, Q.; Yao, W.; Fan, X.; Zhang, K.; Piao, J.G.; Wei, Y. Deoxycholic acid-chitosan coated liposomes combined with in situ colonic gel enhances renal fibrosis therapy of emodin. *Phytomedicine* **2022**, *101*, 154110. [CrossRef]
20. Wang, Y.; Wang, P.; Li, H.; Han, X.; Zhu, H.; Jin, X. Nanocrystal-Loaded Lipid Carriers for Improved Oral Absorption and Anticancer Efficacy of Etoposide: Formulation Development, Transport Mechanism, In Vitro and In Vivo Evaluation. *Mol. Pharm.* **2024**, *21*, 1170–1181. [CrossRef]
21. Ejazi, S.A.; Louisthelmy, R.; Maisel, K. Mechanisms of Nanoparticle Transport across Intestinal Tissue: An Oral Delivery Perspective. *ACS Nano* **2023**, *17*, 13044–13061. [CrossRef] [PubMed]
22. Li, G.; Yao, L.; Li, J.; Qin, X.; Qiu, Z.; Chen, W. Preparation of poly(lactide-co-glycolide) microspheres and evaluation of pharmacokinetics and tissue distribution of BDMC-PLGA-MS in rats. *Asian J. Pharm. Sci.* **2018**, *13*, 82–90. [CrossRef] [PubMed]
23. Zhang, L.; Zhu, Y.; Wei, X.; Chen, X.; Li, Y.; Zhu, Y.; Xia, J.; Huang, Y.; Huang, Y.; Wang, J.; et al. Nanoplateletsomes restrain metastatic tumor formation through decoy and active targeting in a preclinical mouse model. *Acta Pharm. Sin. B* **2022**, *12*, 3427–3447. [CrossRef] [PubMed]
24. Zhong, L.; Liu, Y.; Xu, L.; Li, Q.; Zhao, D.; Li, Z.; Zhang, H.; Zhang, H.; Kan, Q.; Sun, J.; et al. Exploring the relationship of hyaluronic acid molecular weight and active targeting efficiency for designing hyaluronic acid-modified nanoparticles. *Asian J. Pharm. Sci.* **2019**, *14*, 521–530. [CrossRef]
25. Zhang, J.; Sun, H.; Gao, C.; Wang, Y.; Cheng, X.; Yang, Y.; Gou, Q.; Lei, L.; Chen, Y.; Wang, X.; et al. Development of a chitosan-modified PLGA nanoparticle vaccine for protection against Escherichia coli K1 caused meningitis in mice. *J. Nanobiotechnol.* **2021**, *19*, 69. [CrossRef]
26. Dong, Y.; Wang, K.; Tan, Y.; Wang, Q.; Li, J.; Mark, H.; Zhang, S. Synthesis and Characterization of Pure Copper Nanostructures Using Wood Inherent Architecture as a Natural Template. *Nanoscale Res. Lett.* **2018**, *13*, 119. [CrossRef]
27. Chen, X.; Wan, Z.; Yang, L.; Song, S.; Fu, Z.; Tang, K.; Chen, L.; Song, Y. Exosomes derived from reparative M2-like macrophages prevent bone loss in murine periodontitis models via IL-10 mRNA. *J. Nanobiotechnol.* **2022**, *20*, 110. [CrossRef]
28. Liu, Y.; Luo, J.; Liu, Y.; Liu, W.; Yu, G.; Huang, Y.; Yang, Y.; Chen, X.; Chen, T. Brain-Targeted Biomimetic Nanodecoys with Neuroprotective Effects for Precise Therapy of Parkinson's Disease. *ACS Cent. Sci.* **2022**, *8*, 1336–1349. [CrossRef]
29. Bianchi, M.B.; Zhang, C.; Catlin, E.; Sandri, G.; Calderón, M.; Larrañeta, E.; Donnelly, R.F.; Picchio, M.L.; Paredes, A.J. Bioadhesive eutectogels supporting drug nanocrystals for long-acting delivery to mucosal tissues. *Mater. Today Bio* **2022**, *17*, 100471. [CrossRef]
30. Wang, Y.; Wang, S.; Xu, Y.; Wang, P.; Li, S.; Liu, L.; Liu, M.; Jin, X. Etoposide Amorphous Nanopowder for Improved Oral Bioavailability: Formulation Development, Optimization, in vitro and in vivo Evaluation. *Int. J. Nanomed.* **2020**, *15*, 7601–7613. [CrossRef]
31. Yang, S.; Liu, Z.; Wang, C.; Wen, S.; Meng, Q.; Huo, X.; Sun, H.; Ma, X.; Peng, J.; He, Z.; et al. Piperacillin enhances the inhibitory effect of tazobactam on β-lactamase through inhibition of organic anion transporter 1/3 in rats. *Asian J. Pharm. Sci.* **2019**, *14*, 677–686. [CrossRef]
32. Yang, Y.; Tian, F.; Nie, D.; Liu, Y.; Qian, K.; Yu, M.; Wang, A.; Zhang, Y.; Shi, X.; Gan, Y. Rapid transport of germ-mimetic nanoparticles with dual conformational polyethylene glycol chains in biological tissues. *Sci. Adv.* **2020**, *6*, eaay9937. [CrossRef] [PubMed]
33. Yu, M.; Song, W.; Tian, F.; Dai, Z.; Zhu, Q.; Ahmad, E.; Guo, S.; Zhu, C.; Zhong, H.; Yuan, Y.; et al. Temperature- and rigidity-mediated rapid transport of lipid nanovesicles in hydrogels. *Proc. Natl. Acad. Sci. USA* **2019**, *116*, 5362–5369. [CrossRef]
34. Bancaud, A.; Huet, S.; Daigle, N.; Mozziconacci, J.; Beaudouin, J.; Ellenberg, J. Molecular crowding affects diffusion and binding of nuclear proteins in heterochromatin and reveals the fractal organization of chromatin. *EMBO J.* **2009**, *28*, 3785–3798. [CrossRef] [PubMed]
35. Elmotasem, H.; Awad, G.E.A. A stepwise optimization strategy to formulate in situ gelling formulations comprising fluconazole-hydroxypropyl-beta-cyclodextrin complex loaded niosomal vesicles and Eudragit nanoparticles for enhanced antifungal activity and prolonged ocular delivery. *Asian J. Pharm. Sci.* **2020**, *15*, 617–636. [CrossRef] [PubMed]
36. Zhang, G.; Guan, H.; Li, J.; Li, M.; Sui, X.; Tian, B.; Dong, H.; Liu, B.; He, Z.; Li, N.; et al. Roles of effective stabilizers in improving oral bioavailability of naringenin nanocrystals: Maintenance of supersaturation generated upon dissolution by inhibition of drug dimerization. *Asian J. Pharm. Sci.* **2022**, *17*, 741–750. [CrossRef] [PubMed]
37. Patel, K.; Patil, A.; Mehta, M.; Gota, V.; Vavia, P. Oral delivery of paclitaxel nanocrystal (PNC) with a dual Pgp-CYP3A4 inhibitor: Preparation, characterization and antitumor activity. *Int. J. Pharm.* **2014**, *472*, 214–223. [CrossRef]

38. Ren, X.; Qi, J.; Wu, W.; Yin, Z.; Li, T.; Lu, Y. Development of carrier-free nanocrystals of poorly water-soluble drugs by exploring metastable zone of nucleation. *Acta Pharm. Sin. B* **2019**, *9*, 118–127. [CrossRef]
39. Ma, J.; Yang, Y.; Sun, Y.; Sun, J. Optimization, characterization and in vitro/vivo evaluation of azilsartan nanocrystals. *Asian J. Pharm. Sci.* **2017**, *12*, 344–352. [CrossRef]
40. Cheng, F.; Lian, L.; Li, L.; Rao, J.; Li, C.; Qi, T.; Zhang, Z.; Zhang, J.; Gao, Y. Hybrid Growth Modes of PbSe Nanocrystals with Oriented Attachment and Grain Boundary Migration. *Adv. Sci.* **2019**, *6*, 1802202. [CrossRef]
41. Qiu, L.; Ge, L.; Long, M.; Mao, J.; Ahmed, K.S.; Shan, X.; Zhang, H.; Qin, L.; Lv, G.; Chen, J. Redox-responsive biocompatible nanocarriers based on novel heparosan polysaccharides for intracellular anticancer drug delivery. *Asian J. Pharm. Sci.* **2020**, *15*, 83–94. [CrossRef] [PubMed]

pharmaceutics

Article

Iron-Reduced Graphene Oxide Core–Shell Micromotors Designed for Magnetic Guidance and Photothermal Therapy under Second Near-Infrared Light

Orlando Donoso-González [1,2], Ana L. Riveros [1,2], José F. Marco [3], Diego Venegas-Yazigi [4,5], Verónica Paredes-García [5,6], Camila F. Olguín [7], Cristina Mayorga-Lobos [2,8], Lorena Lobos-González [8,9], Felipe Franco-Campos [10], Joseph Wang [11], Marcelo J. Kogan [1,2], Soledad Bollo [1,2,12], Claudia Yañez [12,13,*] and Daniela F. Báez [2,7,*]

1 Departamento Química Farmacológica y Toxicológica, Facultad de Ciencias Químicas y Farmacéuticas, Universidad de Chile, Sergio Livingstone #1007, Independencia, Santiago 8380492, Chile; orlando.donoso@ug.uchile.cl (O.D.-G.); ana.riveros@ciq.uchile.cl (A.L.R.); mkogan@ciq.uchile.cl (M.J.K.); sbollo@ciq.uchile.cl (S.B.)
2 Advanced Center for Chronic Diseases (ACCDiS), Universidad de Chile, Sergio Livingstone #1007, Independencia, Santiago 8380492, Chile; cristina.mayorga@ug.uchile.cl
3 Instituto de Química Física Blas Cabrera, Consejo Superior de Investigaciones Científicas (CSIC), Serrano 119, 28006 Madrid, Spain; jfmarco@iqfr.csic.es
4 Departamento de Química de los Materiales, Facultad de Química y Biología, Universidad de Santiago de Chile, Libertador Bernardo O'Higgins #3363, Estación Central, Santiago 9170022, Chile; diego.venegas@usach.cl
5 Centro para el Desarrollo de La Nanociencia y la Nanotecnología (CEDENNA), Universidad de Santiago de Chile, Libertador Bernardo O'Higgins #3363, Estación Central, Santiago 9170022, Chile; vparedes@unab.cl
6 Departamento de Ciencias Químicas, Facultad de Ciencias Exactas, Universidad Andrés Bello, República 275, Santiago, Santiago 8370146, Chile
7 Escuela de Medicina, Universidad de Talca, Talca 3460000, Chile; camila.olguinc@usach.cl
8 Cellular Communication Laboratory, Center for Studies on Exercise, Metabolism and Cancer (CEMC), Institute of Biomedical Sciences (ICBM), Faculty of Medicine, University of Chile, Santiago 8380492, Chile; llobos@udd.cl
9 Center for Regenerative Medicine, Institute for Sciences and Innovation in Medicine, Facultad de Medicina, Clínica Alemana Universidad del Desarrollo, Santiago 7610658, Chile
10 Research Group in Alternative Methods for Determining Toxics Effects and Risk Assessment of Contaminants and Mixtures (RiskTox), Laboratory of Food Chemistry and Toxicology, Faculty of Pharmacy, University of Valencia, 46100 Valencia, Spain; felipe.franco@uv.es
11 Department of Nanoengineering, University of California San Diego, La Jolla, CA 92093, USA; josephwang@ucsd.edu
12 Centro de Investigación de Procesos Redox, CIPRex, Facultad de Ciencias Químicas y Farmacéuticas, Universidad de Chile, Sergio Livingstone #1007, Independencia, Santiago 8380492, Chile
13 Departamento de Química Orgánica y Fisicoquímica, Facultad de Ciencias Químicas y Farmacéuticas, Universidad de Chile, Sergio Livingstone #1007, Independencia, Santiago 8380492, Chile
* Correspondence: cyanez@ciq.uchile.cl (C.Y.); daniela.baez@utalca.cl (D.F.B.)

Abstract: Core–shell micro/nanomotors have garnered significant interest in biomedicine owing to their versatile task-performing capabilities. However, their effectiveness for photothermal therapy (PTT) still faces challenges because of their poor tumor accumulation, lower light-to-heat conversion, and due to the limited penetration of near-infrared (NIR) light. In this study, we present a novel core–shell micromotor that combines magnetic and photothermal properties. It is synthesized via the template-assisted electrodeposition of iron (Fe) and reduced graphene oxide (rGO) on a microtubular pore-shaped membrane. The resulting Fe-rGO micromotor consists of a core of oval-shaped zero-valent iron nanoparticles with large magnetization. At the same time, the outer layer has a uniform reduced graphene oxide (rGO) topography. Combined, these Fe-rGO core–shell micromotors respond to magnetic forces and near-infrared (NIR) light (1064 nm), achieving a remarkable photothermal conversion efficiency of 78% at a concentration of 434 μg mL^{-1}. They can also carry doxorubicin (DOX) and rapidly release it upon NIR irradiation. Additionally, preliminary results regarding the biocompatibility of these micromotors through in vitro tests on a 3D breast cancer model demonstrate low cytotoxicity and strong accumulation. These promising results suggest that such Fe-rGO core–shell micromotors could hold great potential for combined photothermal therapy.

Keywords: core–shell micromotors; magnetic guidance; photothermal effect; reduced graphene oxide; photothermal therapy; cancer

1. Introduction

Micro/nanomotors (MNM) are devices with the ability to generate autonomous movement through the conversion of several forms of stimulation, such as chemical reagents, light, ultrasound frequencies, and magnetic fields, among others [1–4]. To date, a large number of MNM with diverse morphologies and compositions have been geared toward biomedical and environmental applications [5–8]. In biomedicine, they have demonstrated outstanding performance in detecting or treating primary diseases such as cancer [9–13]. This ability is due to their continuous movement, which enhances their interaction with target molecules [14,15], facilitates drug delivery [16], improves the accumulation rate in complex biological environments [17], and enables penetration into tissues [18–21].

When designing and developing this kind of structure, it is necessary to select the driving stimuli, a crucial aspect when considering their introduction into the living body [6,22–24]. In this sense, magnetic motion has shown advantages compared to other kinds of stimuli, including external motion control, the possibility of tracking, the avoidance of fuel usage, as well as features like reconfigurability and recyclability [1,3,8,16,25–34]. Several efforts have been made to advance the operation of magnetic MNM in body fluids and whole organisms. Examples include hybrid micromotors using sperm flagellum to swim against flowing blood [35] or a magnetic stem cell spheroid that can interface with the human body navigating the bile duct [1]. However, this kind of biological component could make their clinical translation difficult. Among the simplest magnetic materials used for magnetic micromotors, nickel, iron, and their derivatives are the most reported [16,26,28]. However, iron and iron oxide-based materials are preferred because they present better biocompatibility instead of the potential negative effects that nickel can generate in animal and human bodies [36–41].

Photothermal therapy (PTT) is a noninvasive anticancer strategy that treats locally different types of tumors, promoted by materials known as photothermal agents (PTAs). These PTAs present the property of absorbing light and converting it into heat through different mechanisms [42]. The locally high temperature generates hyperthermia, leading to cancerous cell destruction, with minimum damage to normal tissue cells. Some nanomaterials, such as copper and gold nanoparticles [43,44] and some organic polymer nanoparticles [42,45,46], have been described as efficient heaters for photothermal therapy [25]. Notably, graphene-based nanomaterials like graphene oxide (GO) and reduced graphene oxide (rGO) [47,48] also share this essential property but also possess a large specific surface area, efficient adsorption properties, and a high absorption of light from the first and second NIR regions [49–51]. This aspect is essential since PTT triggered by light from the second NIR window (1000–1700 nm) has attracted significant attention [52] due to its ability to penetrate deeper into tissues. Also, there is the possibility of using a laser source with higher power intensities, causing negligible damage to the treated tissue. These properties make the therapy more effective when tumors are located deep within tissues.

Graphene-based micromotors have been previously developed as active systems to capture [31], transfer, and remove different kinds of analytes [53,54] and detect cancer biomarkers [32]. In these kinds of micromotors, the graphene component has been mostly used as the platform to support the recognition probe or to enhance the movement of light-driven micromotors [55,56]. However, their applicability as photothermal agents to treat cancer using hyperthermia has been little explored. Herein, the main purpose of this work was to develop a kind of micromotor to use as a magnetically guided photothermal agent. To that end, we carried out the micromotor preparation through the electrochemical template-assisted deposition method, placing rGO first to support the iron component and the loading of an anticancer drug. This arrangement resulted in a core–shell microtube with a core of iron nanoparticles and an outer layer of reduced graphene oxide (Fe-rGO). The exhaustive morphological characterization of Fe-rGO micromotors through scanning electron microscopy (SEM) confirmed the core–shell microtubular shape. The X-ray powder diffraction (XRD), X-ray photoelectron spectroscopy (XPS), and ^{57}Fe Mössbauer measurements demonstrated that the prepared Fe-rGO core–shell micromotors presented a soft ferromagnetic behavior attributed to the zero-valent iron nanoparticles in the core that allowed the controlled magnetic movement. The photothermal capacity of Fe-rGO micromotors, evaluated through irradiation with an 808 and 1064 nm NIR laser, confirmed in the first place that increased temperatures are obtained when using laser light from the second near-infrared window. Then, a high photothermal conversion efficiency, as well as the fast release of doxorubicin (DOX), was achieved under the application of NIR irradiation at 1064 nm. Additionally, preliminary viability assays on the MDA-MB-231 breast cancer cell line demonstrated that Fe-rGO micromotors presented no cytotoxicity for the three concentrations assessed. Moreover, strong accumulation was observed when Fe-rGO micromotors were magnetically stirred toward a 3D breast cancer tumoroids model.

2. Materials and Methods

2.1. Materials and Reagents

Our lab previously synthesized and characterized GO through a modified Hummer's method, and this reagent was dry-stored [50]. The alumina slurry was purchased from G. Busch & Cia. Ltd. (Valparaiso, Chile). Sulfuric acid (H_2SO_4) > 98%, MW: 98.08 g·mol^{-1}; sodium sulfate ($NaSO_4$) > 99.0%, MW: 142.04 g·mol^{-1}; iron chloride ($FeCl_2·4H_2O$) > 98%, MW: 198.81 g·mol^{-1}; ammonium chloride (NH_4Cl) > 99.995%, MW: 53.49 g mol^{-1}; iron sulfate ($FeSO_4·7H_2O$) > 99.5%, MW: 278.01 g·mol^{-1}; and potassium chloride (KCl) > 99.5%, MW: 74.56 g·mol^{-1} were purchased from Merck (Darmstadt, Germany). Cyclopore polycarbonate membranes (47 mm) with 5 μm tubular-shaped pore diameters (catalog No 7060-4710) were purchased from Whatman (Little Chalfont, UK). Methylene chloride (CH_2Cl_2) > 99.8%, MW: 84.93 g·mol^{-1}; isopropanol ($(CH_3)_2CHOH$) > 99.5%, MW: 60.10 g·mol^{-1}; ethanol (CH_3CH_2OH) > 99.2%, MW: 46.07 g·mol^{-1}; doxorubicin hydrochloride ($C_{27}H_{29}NO_{11}·HCl$) > 98%, MW: 579.98 g·mol^{-1}; and phosphate-buffered solution (PBS) tablets < 99% were obtained from Sigma Aldrich (Saint Louis, MO, USA). Ultrapure water was used to prepare all solutions.

2.2. Solutions

GO was prepared with 2.0 mg mL^{-1} in 20 mL of sulfuric acid (0.1 M) by ultrasonication for 15 min. Then, 0.014 g of Na_2SO_4 was added to the solution and manually stirred. The iron solution was prepared with 0.84 g of $FeCl_2·4H_2O$ in 20 mL of NH_4Cl (0.37 M), and then 5.0 g of $FeSO_4·7H_2O$ was added to the solution and manually shaken. This solution is freshly prepared when needed.

2.3. Preparation of Micromotors

The electrochemical synthesis of microtubes was conducted by an EmStat4s *HR* potentiostat (PalmSens, Houten, The Netherlands); a Pt wire and an Ag/AgCl (3 M KCl) electrode were used as auxiliary and reference electrodes, respectively. A polycarbonate membrane of double truncated cone pore in shape (5.0 μm diameter) was sputtered on one side with a gold film of 35 nm and used as a template and working electrode. The sputter was performed using Luxor^{Au} Sputter Coater equipment under air at room temperature.

First, the membrane was assembled into a customized Teflon cell where 30 mL of GO (0.1 mg mL^{-1}) solution was added to the cell and electrochemically reduced over the wall pores of the membrane at room temperature using cyclic voltammetry (CV, over +0.30 to −1.50 V, at 50 mV s^{-1}, for ten cycles). Subsequently, the iron component was electrodeposited over the surface of rGO by applying, amperometrically, a potential of −0.95 V at different times (900, 2000, and 2500 s) to reach a sufficient charge that allows the microtubular shape. The microtubes were released from the template membrane by polishing the gold layer through a mechanical polish with a 5.0 µm alumina slurry. Then, the membrane was dissolved three times in methylene chloride for 10 min by manual stirring. Then, the microtubes were collected by decantation. Afterward, successive washes with isopropanol followed by ethanol and ultrapure water (three times) were performed, with a 3 min centrifugation at 3835× g between each wash. All microtubes were stored in ultrapure water at 4 °C when not in use. The template preparation method resulted in reproducible micromotors.

2.4. Photothermal Conversion Efficiency of Micromotors

The photothermal conversion efficiency of 109, 217, and 434 µg mL^{-1} synthesized Fe-rGO micromotor solutions was determined in a closed dark chamber by using 808 nm (350 mW) and 1064 nm (200, 300, 350, 400 and 500 mW) lasers (Power Technology, New York, NY, USA), located 20 cm from the sample. The sample was placed in a 9 mm diameter and 28 mm length tube. The temperature increase was monitored using an infrared thermographic camera E8-XT—Handheld Infrared Camera (Teledyne FLIR, Wilsonville, OR, USA) with an accuracy of ±0.1 °C, located 20 cm from the sample. The temperature and thermography images were recorded every 60 s, during a total time interval of 20 m. Ultrapure water was irradiated as a solvent control.

2.5. Loading Doxorubicin on Micromotors

To load doxorubicin (DOX) onto Fe-rGO micromotors, 350 µL of 217 µg mL^{-1} Fe-rGO micromotors dispersed in ultrapure water were magnetized, followed by the removal of the supernatant. Subsequently, the supernatant was substituted with 350 µL of 10 µM of DOX in PBS at pH 7.4, which were then added to the Fe-rGO and stirred at 200 rpm for 24 h at room temperature, protected from light. Hereafter, the dispersion of Fe-rGO/DOX was magnetized, and the supernatant was collected and replaced with PBS 7.4. The DOX supernatant was quantitatively analyzed through a calibration curve using the Beer–Lambert law method. Accordingly, a series of standard stock DOX solutions ranging from 0.5 to 25 µM were prepared. Subsequently, the concentration of DOX was assessed by measuring absorbance at 490 nm, both before and after the interaction with the micromotors, using a Synergy Mx Microplate Reader SMA (Byotek, Winooski, VT, USA) equipped with a high-energy xenon flash lamp. The loading capacity of micromotors was then calculated using the following Equation (1):

$$Loading\ capacity\ (\%) : \frac{amount\ of\ \mathrm{DOX}\ loaded\ (\mu g)}{amount\ of\ micromotors\ (\mu g)} \times 100 \tag{1}$$

2.6. Micromotor Photothermal-Driven Release of Doxorubicin

The release of DOX was carried out at ambient temperatures. A 1064 nm laser with 500 mW of power intensity irradiated the Fe-rGO/DOX dispersion for 3, 5, 10, and 15 min. After irradiation, the dispersion was magnetized, and the supernatant was mixed with the same volume of a known concentration DOX solution for quantitative analysis before and after NIR laser irradiation. The concentration of DOX in the supernatant was determined by spectrophotometry, using the Beer–Lambert law method and the calibration curve previously constructed.

2.7. Cell Lines and Cell Culture

In general, for the cell culture and all biological evaluation, Fe-rGO micromotors were sterilized using 20 min exposure to ultraviolet light in a biosafety cabinet. Then, the micromotors were always loaded and handled under sterile conditions and in a cell culture cabinet. Human breast cancer cell line MDA-MB-231 was obtained from American Type

Culture Collection (ATCC, Manassas, VA, USA, HTB-26TM) and cultured in Dulbecco's Modified Eagle Medium (DMEM)/F12 medium (Gibco, Carlsbad, CA, USA) supplemented with 10% fetal bovine serum (FBS; Biological Industries, Kibbutz Beit-Haemek, Israel), 100 IU/mL penicillin, 0.1 mg/mL streptomycin and 0.05 mg/mL gentamicin (Gibco). The cells were cultured at 37 °C and 5% CO_2.

2.8. Cell Viability MTT Assay

Cell viability was assessed by using the 3-[4,5-dimethylthiazol-2-yl]-2,5diphenyl-tetrazolium bromide (MTT) (Promega, Fitchburg, WI, USA) assay. Briefly, MDA-MB-231 cells were seeded in pretreated 96-well plates at 3000 cells/well and allowed to attach at 37 °C and 5% CO2 for 24 h. Then, the medium was removed, and a fresh medium containing the treatment solutions was added and incubated. At 24, 48, and 72 h post-treatment, 20 μL/well of 5 mg ml^{-1} MTT was added and incubated for 2 h at 37 °C. Dimethyl sulfoxide (DMSO) was then added (150 μL/well) and incubated for 10 min at room temperature. Absorbance was measured at 570 nm in an Epoch microplate reader (Biotek, Winossky, VT, USA), and the cell viability was calculated compared to a nontreatment control as a live control. Statistical analysis was performed using GraphPad Prism V8.0.1. All the experimental data obtained using the MTT assay are expressed as means ± standard deviations and were analyzed using a non-parametric one-way ANOVA to calculate the significance level of the experimental data (n = 3). The differences were considered statistically significant at $p \leq 0.05$.

2.9. Tumoroid or 3D Model Formation Assay

MDA-MB-231 breast cancer cells were seeded on sterile 2% agar-covered plates (6-well plates), supplemented with mammary epithelial cell growth culture medium (at least 1.5 mL of MEGM™ (Lonza, Basel, Switzerland, cat. CC-3151) supplemented with EGF 25 ng/mL, hydrocortisone 0.5 g/mL, insulin 5 μg/mL (Lonza, cat. CC-4136) and bFGF 25 ng /mL (Invitrogen, Waltham, MA, USA, cat. PHG0026). Tumoroids (tumor spheroids or a 3D cancer model) were grown at 37 °C and 5% CO_2 for 14 days. The cell culture medium was not renewed during the 14 days of the experiment, and the formation of spheres was visually recorded by photography using the Micrometrics SE Premium 4.5.1 software in a Nikon Eclipse TS100 inverted microscope. After 14 days, the cell culture medium with the spheres was extracted from the well and passed through a 70 μm filter (BD Falcon, Franklin Lakes, NJ, USA, cat. 352350). The spheres retained on the filter were recovered and plated on a 12-well adhesion plate (Corning, Corning, NY, USA, cat. 3512).

2.10. Magnetic Motion

To magnetically operate the Fe-rGO-micromotors, a drop of 3 μL of the Fe-rGO micromotor solution, dispersed in ultrapure water or cellular medium (with or without tumoroids), was placed on a glass slide. Then, a magnetic field of 267 mT was applied by placing a small magnet away from the glass slide without changing the distances. By changing the direction of the magnet, the micromotors followed the orientation of the magnetic field. The motion of micromotors was registered using an inverted optical microscope (Olympus CKX41 equipped with a Nikon camera DS-Fi 2), and the Tracker AnalySIS 1.0 ® software was used for the tracking analysis.

2.11. Instruments and Characterization

Scanning electron microscopy (SEM) images and energy dispersive X-ray (EDX) analyses were obtained using a Field Emission-SEM Inspect F50, FEI.

X-ray powder diffraction (XRD) was performed with a Phillips diffractometer operated at 30 kV and 20 mA, working in the Bragg–Brentano configuration and using Cu Kα radiation.

XPS data were recorded using a PHOIBOS-150 hemispherical analyzer (Specs), Al Kα radiation, and a constant pass energy of 20 eV under a base pressure lower than

5×10^{-9} mbar. The binding energy scale was referenced to the main contribution to the C 1s spectrum, which was set at 284.6 eV.

^{57}Fe Mössbauer spectra were recorded at room temperature in the transmission mode using a conventional constant acceleration spectrometer and a ^{57}Co(Rh) source. The velocity scale was calibrated using a 6 μm thick iron metallic foil, and the chemical isomer shifts were referred to the centroid of the spectrum of α-Fe at room temperature.

The magnetic behavior of the samples was measured using a vibrating sample magnetometer (VSM) (Quantum Design, model PPMS Dynacool). The magnetic properties of the magnetic micromotors were obtained from dry samples by VSM. The magnetization measurements were obtained by applying a variable magnetic field of ±90 kOe at 298 K.

3. Results

3.1. Characterization of Fe-rGO Core-Shell Micromotors

The Fe-rGO core–shell micromotors were prepared through the electrochemical template-assisted method, using an electrically conductive membrane with tubular-shaped pores as a template. Following our previously reported method, the electrochemical deposition of graphene oxide was the first step in forming the microtube [32]. Supplementary Figure S1a shows the consecutive cyclic voltammograms for the reduction of GO. The first scan shows a large reduction peak at −0.88 V. The main reduction of GO, which occurs in this scan, was attributed to the reduction of oxygen moieties, such as ketones, hydroxyls, aldehydes, and carboxylic acids [50]. Then, the rGO layer supported the electrodeposition of the iron component. Supplementary Figure S1b illustrates the i-t curves obtained during the electrodeposition of iron under varying conditions: a potential pulse of −0.95 V vs. Ag/AgCl applied for 900 (blue curve), 2000 (red curve), or 2500 s (black curve). Despite the differences in deposition duration, consistent electrochemical behavior is observed initially across all three experimental settings. Initially, a decrease in current intensity was attributed to the nucleation process of iron nanoparticles [57], followed by subsequent growth until reaching a plateau, indicating a steady state over time. The associated charges for these conditions were approximately 46.5, 82.4, and 167 C, respectively. After finishing the synthesis process, the microtubes were released from the template by manually polishing and dissolving the membrane with a gradient of solvents. Finally, the microtubes were kept in ultrapure water until their use. The microtube morphology resulting from these conditions was subsequently assessed using scanning electron microscopy (SEM), as depicted in Supplementary Figure S2. Notably, when the potential pulse was applied for 900 and 2000 s to deposit iron, the structures lacked a microtubular form, with many appearing broken. This suggests that an extended electrodeposition time was necessary to achieve the microtubular shape. Specifically, a sufficient charge was attained at 2500 s of iron electrodeposition, facilitating the microtube formation and subsequent closure of the openings. These findings imply a dependence of the microtubular shape on the iron electrodeposition time, with 2500 s being the optimal timeframe in this study for achieving the desired microtubular morphology.

Figure 1a–c display representative SEM images providing different views of the Fe-rGO microtubes obtained. In Figure 1a, a distinct tubular morphology characterized by a uniform external topography can be observed. The external surface corresponds to the rGO layer, which appears thin and soft and constitutes the initial component electrodeposited in the synthesis process [32,54,58]. Figure 1b,c depict the lateral and zoomed views, revealing the internal structure of the Fe-rGO microtubes. In Figure 1c, oval-shaped nanoparticles are visible. These nanoparticles, which constitute the iron component, were consistently present in several microtubes, and their size ranged from approximately 80 to 120 nm (Supplementary Figure S3). The Fe-rGO microtubes displayed an average dimension of 14.9 ± 0.5 μm in length and 4.5 ± 0.03 μm in diameter. To further characterize the elemental composition of the Fe-rGO micromotors, SEM-EDX analysis was conducted in mapping mode. Figure 1d illustrates representative Fe-rGO SEM and EDX images, revealing a uniform distribution of iron (represented in yellow) from the core and carbon (represented in cyan) originating from the rGO throughout the microtube structure.

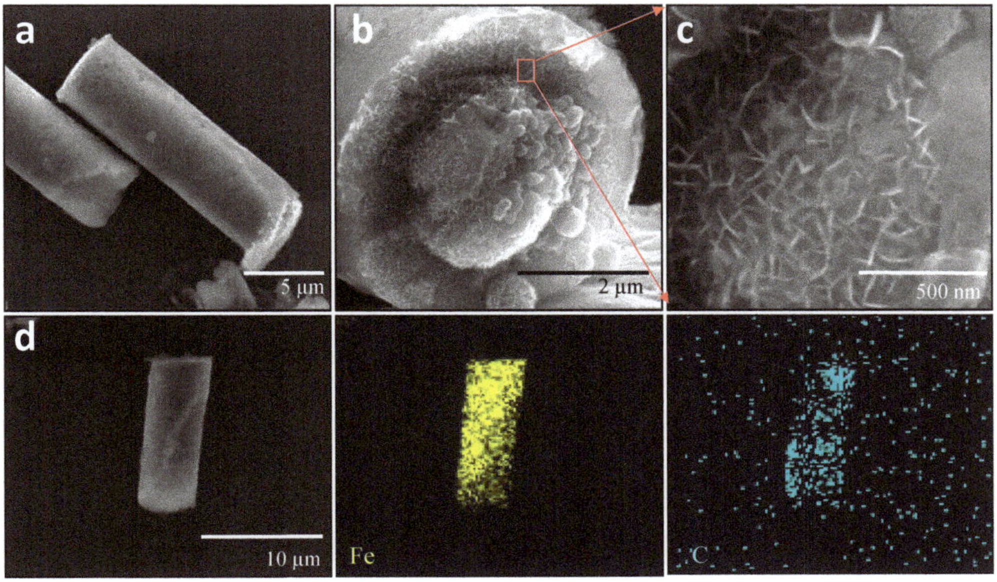

Figure 1. SEM images depicting the Fe-rGO micromotors from various perspectives. (**a**) The top view displays the surface morphology. (**b**) The lateral view provides a side profile (**c**) The red arrow and square denote the internal zoom view, revealing structural details. (**d**) SEM and corresponding EDX images of a Fe-rGO micromotor in mapping mode, showcasing the elemental distribution of iron (yellow) and carbon (cyan).

To determine the chemical composition of the micromotors and the iron oxidation state, the Fe-rGO micromotors were analyzed using X-ray photoelectron spectroscopy (XPS) and ^{57}Fe Mössbauer, respectively. The wide-scan XPS spectrum recorded from the Fe-rGO microtubes (Supplementary Materials) was mainly dominated by the photoemission and Auger carbon peaks, while no photoemission or Auger peaks corresponding to the iron species contained in the micromotors were observed. This suggests that the iron nanoparticles were wrapped within the rGO layer like in a core–shell configuration. Figure 2a shows the XPS C 1s spectrum. It was fitted to five different components located at 282.7 eV, 284.6 eV, 286.4 eV, 288.3 eV, and 290.8 eV, which we associate with the presence of sp^2 carbon, sp^3 C-C, C-O, C=O, and C π-π* satellites, respectively. The spectrum very much resembles what was recorded from electrochemically reduced GO [50]. Figure 2b shows the room temperature ^{57}Fe Mössbauer transmission spectra recorded from the Fe-rGO micromotors, showing two different contributions. The most intense one (green sextet), which accounts for 78% of the spectral area, has hyperfine parameters characteristic of α-Fe (isomer shift (δ) = 0.00 mms^{-1}, quadrupole shift (2ε) = 0.00 mms^{-1}, hyperfine magnetic field (H) = 33.0 T). The second contribution (magenta doublet), with a 22% of the spectral area, has hyperfine parameters (isomer shift (δ) = 0.38 mms^{-1}, quadrupole splitting (Δ) = 0.65 mms^{-1}), which are very similar to those shown by the Fe^{3+} oxyhydroxide goethite (α-FeOOH) in nanophasic form [59]. The results suggest that the micromotors are composed of an α-Fe core surrounded by a thin, nanometer-thick layer of goethite. The formation of the goethite results, most likely, from the surface oxidation of the α-Fe core, since it is well-known that nanophasic goethite is one of the corrosion products of iron under ambient conditions.

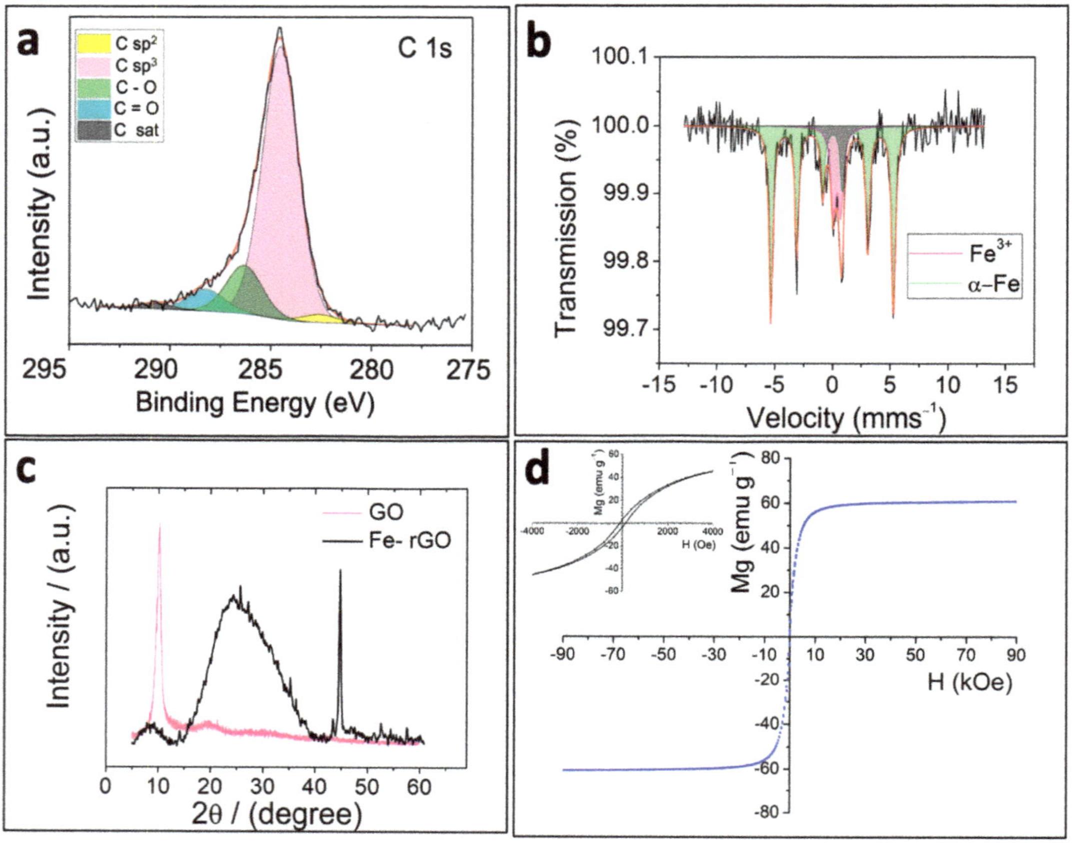

Figure 2. Characterization of Fe-rGO. (**a**) C1s XPS spectrum of Fe-rGO. (**b**) ^{57}Fe Mössbauer spectrum of Fe-rGO. (**c**) XRD patterns comparing GO (pink) and Fe-rGO (black). (**d**) Magnetic characterization of Fe-rGO at 300 K, with inset showing a zoom of the low-field range measurements.

In Figure 2c, the X-ray diffraction (XRD) pattern of Fe-rGO (black pattern) is presented, and for better comparison, the XRD pattern of GO (pink pattern) has been added. The first diffraction peak observed for Fe-rGO appears at around $2\theta = 8.9°$ with low intensity. This diffraction peak is characteristic of GO, presenting an intense signal at $2\theta = 10.1°$ (pink pattern) [50]. However, its presence implies that the reduction of GO has been incomplete. At the same time that this GO diffraction peak decreases, another prominent and broad diffraction peak appears at $2\theta = 24.6°$. This prominent peak is due to the interlayer spacing decreasing from rGO layers in an amorphous state during the reduction process. On the other hand, a sharp and intensive diffraction peak is observed at $2\theta = 44.8°$, characteristic of zero-valent iron [60] and consistent with the ^{57}Fe Mössbauer results.

Figure 2d shows the magnetic hysteresis of Fe-rGO obtained at room temperature between ±90 kOe, and the value of magnetization is given per unit of the total mass of the Fe-rGO micromotors sample. The inset is a zoom of the low-field range measurements. Fe-rGO is characterized by presenting a soft ferromagnetic behavior with H_C of 110 Oe (inset of Figure 2d). Remanent magnetization (M_r) and saturation magnetization (M_s) of 3 emu g^{-1} and 60 emu g^{-1}, respectively, were obtained for the Fe-rGO. The obtained values are lower than the reported by Krajewski et al., for α-Fe nanowires (Fe-NWs) and nanoparticles (Fe-NPs) [61]. In this work, the authors reported, for Fe-NWs, Hc, Mr, and Ms values of 300 Oe, 70 emu g^{-1}, and 164 emu g^{-1}, respectively, while, for Fe-NPs, Hc,

Mr, and Ms values of 360 Oe, 39 emu g^{-1}, and 153 emu g^{-1}, respectively, were obtained. Although the compared materials do not have the same composition, it is easy to note that, in any case, the as-synthesized α-Fe particles do not reach the saturation value of bulk iron (218 emu g^{-1}) [40]. Clearly, in the case of the Fe-rGO, the lower value obtained for Ms is a consequence of the matrix contribution. Considering this fact, a saturation value of 218 emu g^{-1} was taken as a reference to estimate the amount of magnetic material present in the as-synthesized composite. Then, 28% of magnetic material (α-Fe and α-FeOOH) is present in the Fe-rGO.

3.2. *In Vitro Photothermal Capacity of Fe-rGO Micromotors*

To investigate the possibility of using Fe-rGO micromotors as potential photothermal agents, it was crucial to assess whether the photothermal conversion relied on the laser wavelength employed. Therefore, we examined the temperature changes during 1200 s of NIR irradiation using a standard 808 nm laser source and a 1064 nm laser source seated at a power intensity of 350 mW to irradiate Fe-rGO samples of the same concentration. It can be seen in Figure 3a that, when using a 1064 nm laser source (represented by blue triangles), higher temperatures are obtained than when using an 808 nm laser source (represented by red circles), as expected. This temperature difference is evident from the beginning of the NIR irradiation, and even when the temperature rises, it stabilizes at approximately 400 s of NIR irradiation; this is higher when using the laser wavelength from the beginning of the second window. From that point until the end of the irradiation, the ΔT was around 3.2–4.0 °C of difference. Therefore, we selected the 1064 nm wavelength as the NIR laser source to irradiate Fe-rGO micromotors from this point onwards, mostly because longer wavelengths possess less energy per photon, allowing them to penetrate deeper into tissues, due to less light scattering by bio-interfaces, causing minimal damage [52].

Then, the photothermal performance of Fe-rGO micromotors was comprehensively evaluated, using the 1064 nm laser at varying power intensities and Fe-rGO sample concentrations. Figure 3b illustrates the temperature change over 1200 s NIR irradiation at four different power intensities, ranging from 200 to 500 mW, at the same sample concentration (434 µg mL^{-1}). It was evident that, as the laser power intensity increases, so does the temperature attained, suggesting a clear dependence on power intensity. Furthermore, the maximum temperature is reached between 400 and 500 s of NIR irradiation, followed by a steady state. This trend is observed regardless of the power intensity applied. Notably, when utilizing a laser power intensity of 500 mW, it is possible to obtain a ΔT of 30 °C within 7 min. Nevertheless, for the rendering of cancer cells, an equal or greater laser power intensity of 300 mW would be sufficient to cause hyperthermia after 6 min when using this system [62,63].

Figure 3c,d show the influence of the Fe-rGO micromotors on the temperature change during NIR irradiation. Figure 3c shows thermal images obtained in the absence (ultrapure water) and at a high concentration of Fe-rGO. The color of the tube containing the Fe-rGO micromotors rapidly changes when the system is exposed to NIR irradiation, due to the temperature increase. In contrast, when Fe-rGO is absent, the color scale is maintained. The temperature increase in the first case is mainly attributed to the light–heat conversion that the Fe-rGO micromotors undergo. In Figure 3d, we evaluated the Fe-rGO concentration vs. time of NIR irradiation. It can be observed that ultrapure water (green square curve) showed a non-significant increase in temperature even after 1200 s of NIR irradiation, as previously seen. In contrast, at 109, 217, and 434 µg mL^{-1} (pink, orange, and lilac curves, respectively) of Fe-rGO micromotors, there was a remarkable increase in the temperature change, demonstrating the enhanced photothermal effect of Fe-rGO. This temperature grows as the concentration grows, indicating a concentration dependence. The photothermal stability of Fe-rGO was also tested through four-cycle repeated heating (laser on) and cooling (laser off) measurements, without compromising the photothermal performance significantly, since the maximum steady-state temperature remained consistent without significant variations. This behavior indicates that Fe-rGO possesses good photothermal stability and can be reusable.

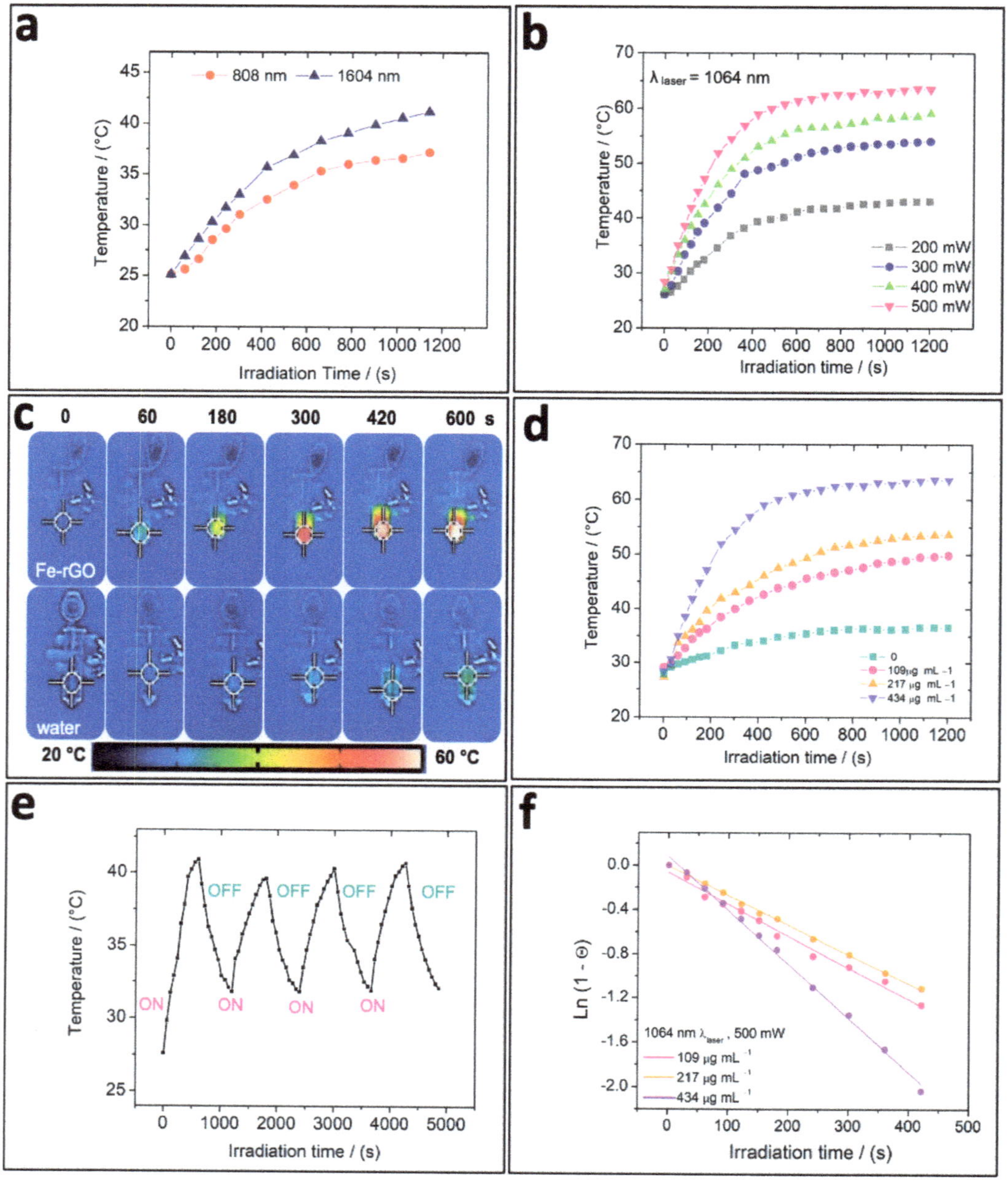

Figure 3. Photothermal performance of Fe-rGO micromotors dispersed in ultrapure water under laser irradiation. (**a**) Temperature change vs. irradiation time for two different laser wavelengths: 808 nm (red dotted curve) and 1064 nm (blue triangle curve). (**b**) Temperature change vs. irradiation time at various power intensities (200, 300, 400, and 500 mW). (**c**) Thermal images captured during NIR irradiation using a 1064 nm laser at 500 mW, showcasing the effect of Fe-rGO. (**d**) Photothermal heating curves at various concentrations of Fe-rGO. (**e**) Photothermal stability of Fe-rGO during 4 repeats of on/off NIR irradiation cycles. (**f**) Linear regression of Ln(1-θ) vs. time of 109 (pink), 217 (orange), and 434 μg mL^{-1}; data extracted from the temperature increase in the samples using a 1064 nm laser with a power intensity of 500 mW.

Photothermal conversion efficiency (η) is an important parameter to evaluate the photothermal capacity of different photothermal agents. It has been demonstrated that graphene-based nanomaterials exhibit excellent heat conductivity and, therefore, have been considered a great potential candidate for heat transfer and hyperthermia applications [48]. In addition, previous studies have shown that rGO presents better photothermal conversion than GO under the same experimental conditions [53,55,64–69]. To determine the photothermal conversion efficiency of Fe-rGO micromotors, we followed the method outlined by Liu and colleagues [70]. Figure 3f illustrates the linear regression of Ln (1-θ) vs. time for the three concentrations of Fe-rGO analyzed. This regression allows for the calculation of the time constant for heat transfer (τS), essential for determining the photothermal conversion efficiency (see the Supplementary Materials for the detailed calculation). Subsequently, we calculated the photothermal conversion efficiency (η) of the Fe-rGO micromotors to be 11.1%, 27%, and 78% for concentrations of 109, 217, and 434 μg mL^{-1}, respectively. This result demonstrates that Fe-rGO micromotors under 1064 nm laser irradiation can generate a high photothermal conversion efficiency and can be very suitable for photothermal applications.

3.3. Drug Loading and Release Triggered by NIR Irradiation

Hyperthermia can be combined with other therapeutic methods like chemotherapy through the use of different drugs. This combined therapy can synergize the cancer treatment because some tumor cells could remain viable after PTT, especially when tumors are in very deep tissues, as they may turn into a new tumor mass in the short term [71,72]. Here, doxorubicin (DOX), a conventional chemotherapeutic drug, was used as a model drug to investigate the release capacity from Fe-rGO micromotors under NIR irradiation, as schematized in Figure 4a. The DOX drug was initially adsorbed over the rGO surface, probably through π-π stacking and electrostatic interactions. In Figure 4b, we show the UV–Vis absorption of DOX in PBS 7.4 solution at different concentrations. Following the strong band at 490 nm, we constructed the standard curve (inset of Figure 4b), and a regression line was established to determine the DOX concentration. Figure 4c shows the absorbance of the DOX solution before and after the incubation reaction with Fe-rGO micromotors. Then, the loaded DOX concentration was quantified to be 0.69 μg mL^{-1} with a loading capacity of 0.3% (w/w). A higher loading capacity is expected due to the similar chemical composition between rGO and DOX, π–π aromatic rings, and electrostatic charges that facilitate direct adsorption. However, the low loading value could be attributed to the excess DOX used, the incubation's low stirring speed, and the reaction tube's vertical positioning. This vertical position likely caused the micromotors to settle, sterically hindering their interaction with the drug molecules. Therefore, by addressing these factors, the loading capacity should be enhanced.

As reported in previous studies, the photothermal effect can trigger the release of cancer drugs [47,49,73]. Consequently, we measured the DOX release under NIR irradiation at pH 7.4 to ensure that the release effect is mainly due to the photothermal effect. As shown in Figure 4d, the release rate was significantly higher upon NIR irradiation than without irradiation for identical study periods. Within 15 min, almost 82.3% of DOX was released from Fe-rGO micromotors, while, at the same time point, the Fe-rGO micromotors without irradiation had released only 28.6% of the adsorbed drug. Besides, at this point, the maximum photothermal effect had already been reached. Overall, considering that some drugs are responsive to pH, a lower pH could further improve the release of these from the Fe-rGO micromotor.

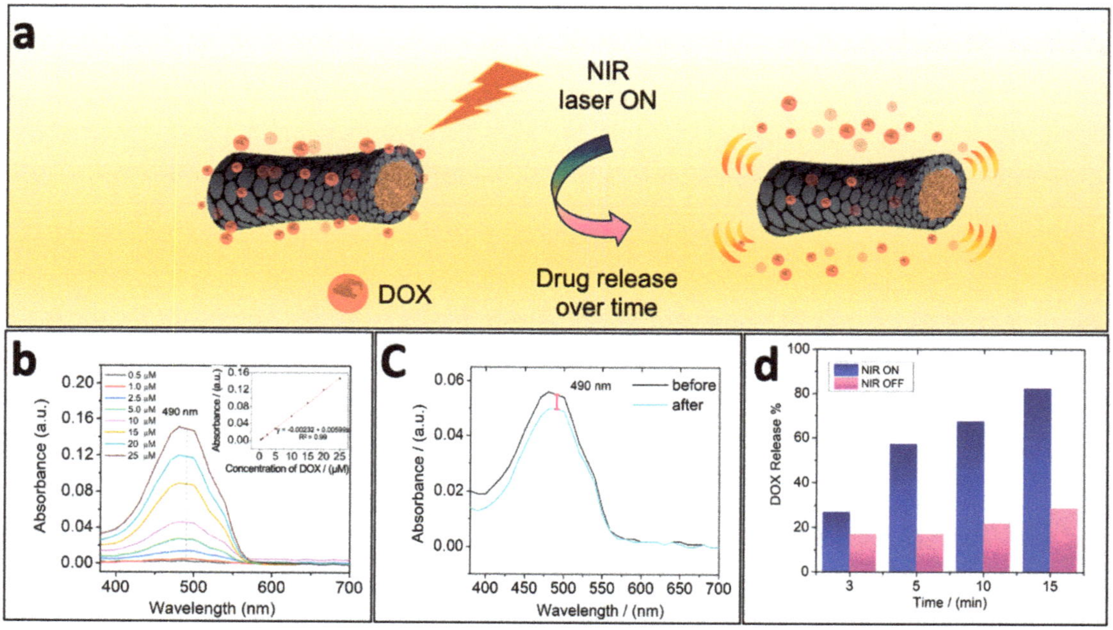

Figure 4. (**a**) Scheme of drug loading and release capacity from Fe-rGO micromotors under NIR irradiation. (**b**) UV–Vis absorption spectra of DOX at different concentrations and the linear relationship between the absorbance at 490 nm and the concentration of DOX (inset). (**c**) The absorbance of the DOX solution before (black curve) and after the incubation reaction (light blue curve) with Fe-rGO micromotors, pink bar shows the difference. (**d**) Effect of NIR irradiation (1064 nm) on DOX release from the Fe-rGO micromotors system.

3.4. Cytotoxicity of Fe-rGO Micromotors

The excellent photothermal properties of Fe-rGO micromotors prompted us to perform a preliminary assay of their cytotoxicity. The concentration-dependent effect of 22 μg mL^{-1}, 109 μg mL^{-1}, and 217 μg mL^{-1} of Fe-rGO micromotors on the cell viability was determined via a standard MTT assay on MDA-MB-231 breast cancer cells treated for 24 h, 48 h, and 72 h (Figure 5). As shown in Figure 5, mitochondrial metabolic activity, assessed using the MTT viability assay, showed no significant difference compared to the control in the concentration range and incubation times evaluated. Overall, the effects on the viability after treatment with Fe-rGO micromotors were not significant under the conditions studied. On the other hand, we evaluated the effects on cell viability in another cell line (SH-SY5Y cells), which are cells of neuronal origin. We did not observe changes in the cell morphology by optical microscopy images carried out with Fe-rGO micromotors at 109 μg mL^{-1} for 24 h (further details in the Supplementary Materials, Figure S6). Figure S6 shows that SH-SY5Y cells, with or without the addition of Fe-rGO micromotors, maintained their morphology and normal neuritic processes (projections between neuronal cells) in culture [74,75], indicating that they remained viable. Nevertheless, to complete the cytotoxicity study, cell viability assays in healthy cell lines should be carried out in the future.

In addition, tumoroids or three-dimensional (3D) cellular models have been extensively studied nowadays, as they are more accurate response models of tumors than 2-dimensional (2D) cell cultures [76–78]. Accordingly, Fe-rGO micromotors' response to the viability and morphological changes in MDA-MB-231 breast cancer cell tumoroids was studied. Figure 6 shows the optical microscopy images of one of the tests carried out after the exposition of different concentrations (22 μg mL^{-1}, 109 μg mL^{-1}, and 217 μg mL^{-1}) of

Fe-rGO micromotors with tumoroids for 96 h. Figure 6b shows a slight reduction, approximately 5%, in the effective area of the tumoroids when a concentration of 22 μg mL^{-1} was used. In contrast, Figure 6c presents a 55% decrease in the effective area when the Fe-rGO concentration increases at 109 μg mL^{-1}. Moreover, when the concentration of Fe-rGO micromotors was 217 μg mL^{-1}, a significant decrease of up to 91% in tumoroid size was observed, as shown in Figure 6d. Thus, high concentrations of Fe-rGO micromotors and prolonged exposure times can effectively trigger the disaggregation of tumoroids without additional stimuli.

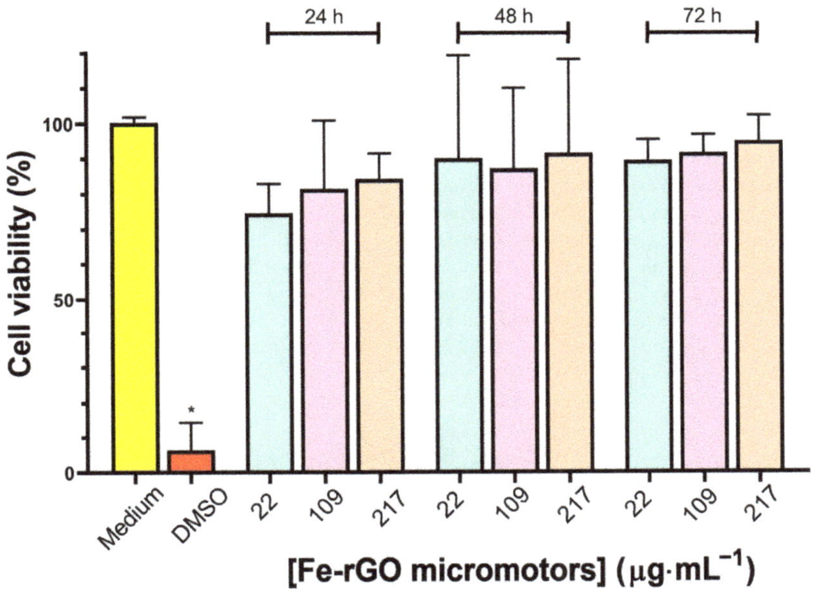

Figure 5. Cell viability assays based on mitochondrial metabolic activity in MDA-MB-231 breast cancer cells line at different concentrations of rGO-Fe micromotors for 24 h, 48 h, and 72 h (22 μg/mL^{-1}: green; 109 μg/mL^{-1}: violet; and 217 μg/mL^{-1}: orange). Data are shown as means ± standard deviation from three independent experiments, with each point performed in sextuplicate. Statistical analysis was performed using a non-parametric one-way ANOVA comparing all conditions with the medium control. (*) indicate statistical significance with $p < 0.05$.

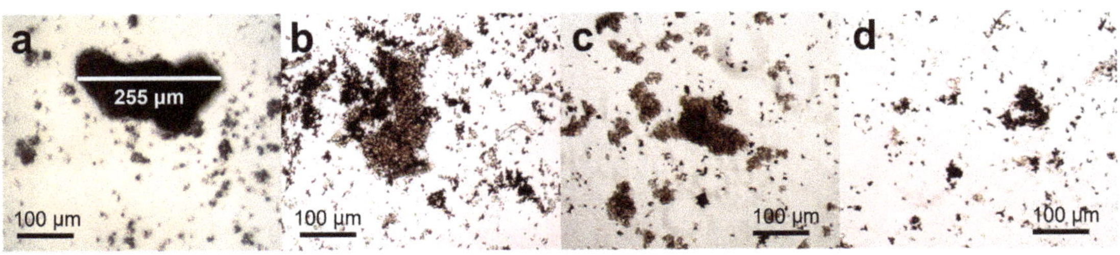

Figure 6. Representative and comparative images of 3D breast cancer model cells captured without micromotors (**a**) and with Fe-rGO micromotors for 96 h at different concentrations, namely (**b**) 22 μg mL^{-1}, (**c**) 109 μg mL^{-1}, and (**d**) 217 μg mL^{-1}. Scale bar: 100 μm.

3.5. Motion Analysis of Fe-rGO Micromotors

The magnetic motion of Fe-rGO micromotors was evaluated in ultrapure water (Video S1), cellular medium (Video S2), and breast cancer 3D model cells (Video S3). After dispersing the micromotors into the different kinds of media, the suspension was dripped onto a pre-cleaned glass slide, and then a magnet of 267 mT approached the glass slide. During the magnet's approach, the micromotors started to follow a unidirectional path toward the position of the magnet. The displacement per second calculated using this magnetic force in ultrapure water was 217 ± 49 μm. In contrast, in the cellular medium, the average displacement per second was considerably lower, reaching a distance traveled of 36 ± 20 μm. Once the magnet was removed, the micromotor motion stopped. Furthermore, regardless of the medium in which they were located, the micromotors tended to form a cluster when a magnetic force was applied. This can, therefore, cause their accumulation in a specific site.

The guided movement of Fe-rGO micromotors toward breast cancer 3D model cells was schematically illustrated in Figure 7a. Figure 7b shows images extracted every 10 s from the time-lapse Video S3 (Supplementary Materials). It can be seen at 10 s that a cluster formed of Fe-rGO micromotors guided toward the 3D breast cancer model was formed. Then, the cluster of Fe-rGO micromotors interacted with the tumoroid, resulting in their accumulation on the tumoroid surface. Once the Fe-rGO micromotors were coupled to the 3D model cell, this interaction was maintained over time, and their direction was dependent on the direction of the magnet. The intended direction of the micromotors is shown with a yellow arrow. Additionally, the movement did not cause any breakage between the 3D model cell and the micromotors. This strong interaction is advantageous since it allows the accumulation of the Fe-rGO micromotors, specifically on cancerous sites, to subsequently generate the photothermal effect and drug release under second NIR irradiation.

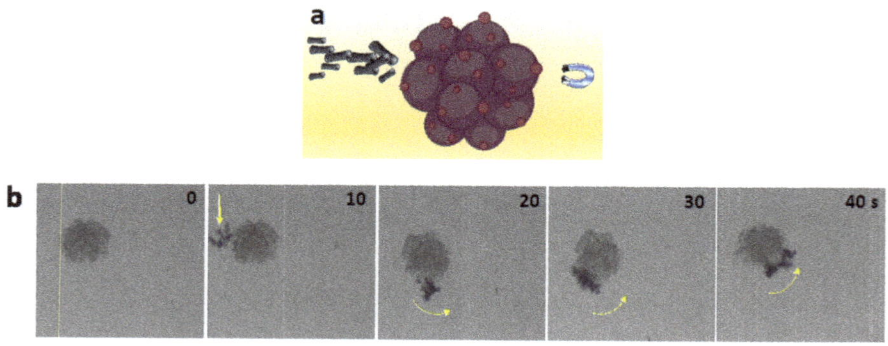

Figure 7. (**a**) Schematic illustration of the guided movement of Fe-rGO micromotors toward 3D cancer model cells. (**b**) Time-lapse images taken from magnetic navigation of Fe-rGO micromotors toward breast cancer 3D model cell (represented with a yellow vector) and corresponding tracking path every 10 s under the magnetic force of 267 mT (taken from Video S3, Supplementary Materials).

4. Conclusions

In conclusion, we have developed a magnetic microtubular core–shell micromotor with magnetic and photothermal functionality in this study, serving as a promising secondary NIR photothermal agent. The shell, composed of rGO, exhibits strong light absorption in the second NIR region, enhancing the photothermal effect. Meanwhile, the core, consisting of zero-valent iron nanoparticles, facilitates guided movement and enables the accumulation of these micromotors on a 3D breast cancer model cell. Comparing the effects of irradiation at different wavelengths, we found superior temperature changes in the Fe-rGO dispersion when irradiated at 1064 nm compared to 808 nm, demonstrating the advantages of irradiating with laser light from the second NIR window. Additionally, we noted that the photothermal response of Fe-rGO micromotors was dependent on laser intensity and concentration. An excellent parameter for evaluating photothermal agents is the photothermal conversion efficiency. Here, we found a remarkable photothermal conversion efficiency of

78% at a Fe-rGO concentration of 434 μg mL^{-1}. Furthermore, the rGO shell also allowed the loading of the chemotherapeutic drug doxorubicin, which can be rapidly released upon NIR irradiation. Finally, preliminary results from in vitro tests on a 3D breast cancer model showed low cytotoxicity and strong accumulation of these micromotors guided by magnetic motion. These promising findings suggest that Fe-rGO core–shell micromotors are viable candidates with significant potential for enhancing cancer treatment through combined photothermal therapy. The results presented have established the groundwork to continue with future work, exploring the photothermal effect of this system on 3D or in vivo models.

Supplementary Materials: The following supporting information can be downloaded at: https://www.mdpi.com/article/10.3390/pharmaceutics16070856/s1. Figure S1: electrochemical synthesis, Figure S2: SEM images of Fe-rGO micromotors from different experimental conditions, Figure S3: SEM images of rGO-Fe microtubes obtained, Figure S4: UV/vis absorbance spectra of rGO-Fe, Figure S5: schematic illustration of the photothermal measurement equipment, Figure S6: analyses of Fe-rGO micromotors effect in SH-SY5Y cells, Table S1: calculated parameters: τS, hS, and photothermal transduction efficiency (η), as well as temperature increment (Tincr.), Video S1: magnetic motion of Fe-rGO micromotors in water under magnetic force, Video S2: magnetic motion of Fe-rGO microtubular motors in a cellular medium, Video S3: magnetic motion of Fe-rGO microtubular motors approaching the 3D tumor model cell.

Author Contributions: Conceptualization, D.F.B.; methodology, D.F.B.; Validation, A.L.R., J.F.M., D.V.-Y., V.P.-G., L.L.-G., J.W., M.J.K., S.B., C.Y. and D.F.B.; formal analysis, O.D.-G., A.L.R., J.F.M., D.V.-Y., V.P.-G., C.F.O., C.M.-L., L.L.-G., F.F.-C., J.W., M.J.K., S.B., C.Y. and D.F.B.; investigation, O.D.-G., C.F.O. and D.F.B.; resources, J.F.M., D.V.-Y., V.P.-G., L.L.-G., F.F.-C., J.W., S.B., M.J.K. and D.F.B.; data curation, O.D.-G., J.F.M., D.V.-Y., V.P.-G., C.F.O., C.M.-L., L.L.-G., F.F.-C., M.J.K., S.B., C.Y. and D.F.B.; writing—original draft preparation, O.D.-G. and D.F.B.; writing—review and editing, O.D.-G., A.L.R., J.F.M., D.V.-Y., V.P.-G., C.F.O., C.M.-L., L.L.-G., F.F.-C., J.W., M.J.K., S.B., C.Y. and D.F.B.; visualization, D.F.B.; supervision, D.F.B.; project management, D.F.B.; funding acquisition, M.J.K., S.B. and D.F.B. All authors discussed the results and commented on the manuscript. All authors have read and agreed to the published version of the manuscript.

Funding: D.F.B. received funding from ANID-FONDECYT number 11200416, ANID-FOVI220173, ANID-FONDEQUIP EQM 170141, and EQM 130086. O.D.-G. received funding from ANID Post-doctoral FONDECYT number 3240075; F.C.F. received funding from CIGRIS/2021/073 scholarship; L.L.-G. received funding from FONDECYT number 1211223; M.J.K. received funding from FONDE-CYT number 1211482, Anillo ACT 210068, FONDEQUIP EQM170111. D.F.B., L.L.-G. and M.J.K. received funding from ANID-FONDAP ACCDiS 15130011 and Apoyo 1523A0008.

Institutional Review Board Statement: Not applicable.

Informed Consent Statement: Not applicable.

Data Availability Statement: The raw data supporting the conclusions of this article will be made available by the authors on request.

Conflicts of Interest: The authors declare no conflicts of interest.

References

1. Zhou, H.; Mayorga-Martinez, C.C.; Pané, S.; Zhang, L.; Pumera, M. Magnetically Driven Micro and Nanorobots. *Chem. Rev.* **2021**, *121*, 4999–5041. [CrossRef]
2. Wang, B.; Chan, K.F.; Yuan, K.; Wang, Q.; Xia, X.; Yang, L.; Ko, H.; Wang, Y.X.J.; Sung, J.J.Y.; Chiu, P.W.Y.; et al. Endoscopy-Assisted Magnetic Navigation of Biohybrid Soft Microrobots with Rapid Endoluminal Delivery and Imaging. *Sci. Robot.* **2021**, *6*, eabd2813. [CrossRef]
3. Venugopalan, P.L.; Ghosh, A. Investigating the Dynamics of the Magnetic Micromotors in Human Blood. *Langmuir* **2021**, *37*, 289–296. [CrossRef]
4. Latiyan, S.; Suneet, K.; Jain, S. Magneto-conducting Multifunctional Janus Microbots for Intracellular Delivery of Biomolecules. *J. Tissue Eng. Regen. Med.* **2021**, *15*, 625–633. [CrossRef]
5. Wang, Q.; Yang, S.; Zhang, L. Untethered Micro/Nanorobots for Remote Sensing: Toward Intelligent Platform. *Nano-Micro Lett.* **2024**, *16*, 40. [CrossRef]

6. Li, H.; Peng, F.; Yan, X.; Mao, C.; Ma, X.; Wilson, D.A.; He, Q.; Tu, Y. Medical Micro- and Nanomotors in the Body. *Acta Pharm. Sin. B* **2023**, *13*, 517–541. [CrossRef]
7. Zhang, F.; Mundaca-Uribe, R.; Askarinam, N.; Li, Z.; Gao, W.; Zhang, L.; Wang, J. Biomembrane-Functionalized Micromotors: Biocompatible Active Devices for Diverse Biomedical Applications. *Adv. Mater.* **2022**, *34*, 2107177. [CrossRef]
8. Peng, X.; Urso, M.; Kolackova, M.; Huska, D.; Pumera, M. Biohybrid Magnetically Driven Microrobots for Sustainable Removal of Micro/Nanoplastics from the Aquatic Environment. *Adv. Funct. Mater.* **2023**, *34*, 2307477. [CrossRef]
9. Chen, B.; Sun, H.; Zhang, J.; Xu, J.; Song, Z.; Zhan, G.; Bai, X.; Feng, L. Cell-Based Micro/Nano-Robots for Biomedical Applications: A Review. *Small* **2024**, *20*, e2304607. [CrossRef]
10. Wang, J.; Dong, R.; Wu, H.; Cai, Y.; Ren, B. A Review on Artificial Micro/Nanomotors for Cancer-Targeted Delivery, Diagnosis, and Therapy. *Nano-Micro Lett.* **2020**, *12*, 11. [CrossRef]
11. Yuan, K.; Jiang, Z.; Jurado-Sánchez, B.; Escarpa, A. Nano/Micromotors for Diagnosis and Therapy of Cancer and Infectious Diseases. *Chem.-Eur. J.* **2020**, *26*, 2309–2326. [CrossRef]
12. Rastmanesh, A.; Tavakkoli Yaraki, M.; Wu, J.; Wang, Z.; Ghoderao, P.; Gao, Y.; Tan, Y.N. Bioinspired Micro/Nanomotors towards a Self-Propelled Noninvasive Diagnosis and Treatment of Cancer. *Mol. Syst. Des. Eng.* **2021**, *6*, 566–593. [CrossRef]
13. Wang, W.; Zhou, C. A Journey of Nanomotors for Targeted Cancer Therapy: Principles, Challenges, and a Critical Review of the State-of-the-Art. *Adv. Healthc. Mater.* **2021**, *10*, e2001236. [CrossRef] [PubMed]
14. Chen, Q.; Guo, W.; Fang, D.; Li, T.; Chen, L.; Mao, C.; Wan, M.; Shen, J. Mg-Based Micromotors for Efficient Electrochemical Detection of Circulating Tumor Cells. *Sens. Actuators B Chem.* **2023**, *390*, 133933. [CrossRef]
15. Gao, W.; de Ávila, B.E.-F.; Zhang, L.; Wang, J. Targeting and Isolation of Cancer Cells Using Micro/Nanomotors. *Adv. Drug Deliv. Rev.* **2018**, *125*, 94–101. [CrossRef]
16. Hou, K.; Zhang, Y.; Bao, M.; Xin, C.; Wei, Z.; Lin, G.; Wang, Z. A Multifunctional Magnetic Red Blood Cell-Mimetic Micromotor for Drug Delivery and Image-Guided Therapy. *ACS Appl. Mater. Interfaces* **2022**, *14*, 3825–3837. [CrossRef]
17. Li, Z.; Fu, S.; Li, H.; Chen, B.; Xie, D.; Fu, D.; Feng, Y.; Gao, C.; Liu, S.; Wilson, D.A.; et al. Light-Driven Micromotor Swarm Induced in-Situ Polymerization and Synergistic Photothermal Therapy. *Chem. Eng. J.* **2023**, *468*, 143393. [CrossRef]
18. Gao, C.; Feng, Y.; Wilson, D.A.; Tu, Y.; Peng, F. Micro-Nano Motors with Taxis Behavior: Principles, Designs, and Biomedical Applications. *Small* **2022**, *18*, e2106263. [CrossRef]
19. Zhang, X.; Chen, G.; Cai, L.; Fan, L.; Zhao, Y. Dip-Printed Microneedle Motors for Oral Macromolecule Delivery. *Research* **2022**, *2022*, 9797482. [CrossRef]
20. Maric, T.; Adamakis, V.; Zhang, Z.; Milián-Guimerá, C.; Thamdrup, L.H.E.; Stamate, E.; Ghavami, M.; Boisen, A. Microscopic Cascading Devices for Boosting Mucus Penetration in Oral Drug Delivery—Micromotors Nesting Inside Microcontainers. *Small* **2023**, *19*, e2206330. [CrossRef]
21. Lopez-Ramirez, M.A.; Soto, F.; Wang, C.; Rueda, R.; Shukla, S.; Silva-Lopez, C.; Kupor, D.; McBride, D.A.; Pokorski, J.K.; Nourhani, A.; et al. Built-In Active Microneedle Patch with Enhanced Autonomous Drug Delivery. *Adv. Mater.* **2020**, *32*, e1905740. [CrossRef]
22. Gordón, J.; Arruza, L.; Ibáñez, M.D.; Moreno-Guzmán, M.; López, M.Á.; Escarpa, A. On the Move-Sensitive Fluorescent Aptassay on Board Catalytic Micromotors for the Determination of Interleukin-6 in Ultra-Low Serum Volumes for Neonatal Sepsis Diagnostics. *ACS Sens.* **2022**, *7*, 3144–3152. [CrossRef]
23. Esteban-Fernández de Ávila, B.; Angell, C.; Soto, F.; Lopez-Ramirez, M.A.; Báez, D.F.; Xie, S.; Wang, J.; Chen, Y. Acoustically Propelled Nanomotors for Intracellular siRNA Delivery. *ACS Nano* **2016**, *10*, 4997–5005. [CrossRef]
24. Gao, C.; Wang, Y.; Ye, Z.; Lin, Z.; Ma, X.; He, Q. Biomedical Micro-/Nanomotors: From Overcoming Biological Barriers to In Vivo Imaging. *Adv. Mater.* **2021**, *33*, 2000512. [CrossRef]
25. Van de Walle, A.; Figuerola, A.; Espinosa, A.; Abou-Hassan, A.; Estrader, M.; Wilhelm, C. Emergence of Magnetic Nanoparticles in Photothermal and Ferroptotic Therapies. *Mater. Horiz.* **2023**, *10*, 4757–4775. [CrossRef]
26. Villa, K.; Krejčová, L.; Novotný, F.; Heger, Z.; Sofer, Z.; Pumera, M. Cooperative Multifunctional Self-Propelled Paramagnetic Microrobots with Chemical Handles for Cell Manipulation and Drug Delivery. *Adv. Funct. Mater.* **2018**, *28*, e1804343. [CrossRef]
27. Wang, Y.; Liu, Y.; Li, Y.; Xu, D.; Pan, X.; Chen, Y.; Zhou, D.; Wang, B.; Feng, H.; Ma, X. Magnetic Nanomotor-Based Maneuverable SERS Probe. *Research* **2020**, *2020*, 7962024. [CrossRef]
28. Qin, F.; Wu, J.; Fu, D.; Feng, Y.; Gao, C.; Xie, D.; Fu, S.; Liu, S.; Wilson, D.A.; Peng, F. Magnetically Driven Helical Hydrogel Micromotor for Tumor DNA Detection. *Appl. Mater. Today* **2022**, *27*, 101456. [CrossRef]
29. Vyskočil, J.; Mayorga-Martinez, C.C.; Jablonská, E.; Novotný, F.; Ruml, T.; Pumera, M. Cancer Cells Microsurgery via Asymmetric Bent Surface Au/Ag/Ni Microrobotic Scalpels through a Transversal Rotating Magnetic Field. *ACS Nano* **2020**, *14*, 8247–8256. [CrossRef]
30. Sun, M.; Fan, X.; Meng, X.; Song, J.; Chen, W.; Sun, L.; Xie, H. Magnetic Biohybrid Micromotors with High Maneuverability for Efficient Drug Loading and Targeted Drug Delivery. *Nanoscale* **2019**, *11*, 18382–18392. [CrossRef]
31. Molinero-Fernández, Á.; Jodra, A.; Moreno-Guzmán, M.; López, M.Á.; Escarpa, A. Magnetic Reduced Graphene Oxide/Nickel/Platinum Nanoparticles Micromotors for Mycotoxin Analysis. *Chem.-Eur. J.* **2018**, *24*, 7172–7176. [CrossRef] [PubMed]

32. Báez, D.F.; Ramos, G.; Corvalán, A.; Cordero, M.L.; Bollo, S.; Kogan, M.J. Effects of Preparation on Catalytic, Magnetic and Hybrid Micromotors on Their Functional Features and Application in Gastric Cancer Biomarker Detection. *Sens. Actuators B Chem.* **2020**, *310*, 127843. [CrossRef]
33. Schwarz, L.; Medina-Sanchez, M.; Schmidt, O.G. Magnetic Micromotors for Resilient and Reversible Cargo Transport in and between Microfluidic Environments. In Proceedings of the 2019 International Conference on Manipulation, Automation and Robotics at Small Scales (MARSS), Helsinki, Finland, 1–5 July 2019; pp. 1–5. [CrossRef]
34. Yang, L.; Chen, X.; Wang, L.; Hu, Z.; Xin, C.; Hippler, M.; Zhu, W.; Hu, Y.; Li, J.; Wang, Y.; et al. Targeted Single-Cell Therapeutics with Magnetic Tubular Micromotor by One-Step Exposure of Structured Femtosecond Optical Vortices. *Adv. Funct. Mater.* **2019**, *29*, e1905745. [CrossRef]
35. Xu, H.; Medina-Sánchez, M.; Maitz, M.F.; Werner, C.; Schmidt, O.G. Sperm Micromotors for Cargo Delivery through Flowing Blood. *ACS Nano* **2020**, *14*, 2982–2993. [CrossRef] [PubMed]
36. More, S.L.; Kovochich, M.; Lyons-Darden, T.; Taylor, M.; Schulte, A.M.; Madl, A.K. Review and Evaluation of the Potential Health Effects of Oxidic Nickel Nanoparticles. *Nanomaterials* **2021**, *11*, 642. [CrossRef] [PubMed]
37. Katsnelson, B.A.; Minigaliyeva, I.A.; Panov, V.G.; Privalova, L.I.; Varaksin, A.N.; Gurvich, V.B.; Sutunkova, M.P.; Shur, V.Y.; Shishkina, E.V.; Valamina, I.E.; et al. Some Patterns of Metallic Nanoparticles' Combined Subchronic Toxicity as Exemplified by a Combination of Nickel and Manganese Oxide Nanoparticles. *Food Chem. Toxicol.* **2015**, *86*, 351–364. [CrossRef] [PubMed]
38. Begum, W.; Rai, S.; Banerjee, S.; Bhattacharjee, S.; Mondal, M.H.; Bhattarai, A.; Saha, B. A Comprehensive Review on the Sources, Essentiality and Toxicological Profile of Nickel. *RSC Adv.* **2022**, *12*, 9139–9153. [CrossRef]
39. Farzin, A.; Etesami, S.A.; Quint, J.; Memic, A.; Tamayol, A. Magnetic Nanoparticles in Cancer Therapy and Diagnosis. *Adv. Healthc. Mater.* **2020**, *9*, 1901058. [CrossRef] [PubMed]
40. Huber, D.L. Synthesis, Properties, and Applications of Iron Nanoparticles. *Small* **2005**, *1*, 482–501. [CrossRef]
41. Wu, Y.; Kong, L. Advance on Toxicity of Metal Nickel Nanoparticles. *Environ. Geochem. Health* **2020**, *42*, 2277–2286. [CrossRef]
42. Cui, X.; Ruan, Q.; Zhuo, X.; Xia, X.; Hu, J.; Fu, R.; Li, Y.; Wang, J.; Xu, H. Photothermal Nanomaterials: A Powerful Light-to-Heat Converter. *Chem. Rev.* **2023**, *123*, 6891–6952. [CrossRef]
43. Bolaños, K.; Sánchez-Navarro, M.; Giralt, E.; Acosta, G.; Albericio, F.; Kogan, M.J.; Araya, E. NIR and Glutathione Trigger the Surface Release of Methotrexate Linked by Diels-Alder Adducts to Anisotropic Gold Nanoparticles. *Mater. Sci. Eng. C* **2021**, *131*, 112512. [CrossRef]
44. Dheyab, M.A.; Aziz, A.A.; Khaniabadi, P.M.; Jameel, M.S.; Oladzadabbasabadi, N.; Rahman, A.A.; Braim, F.S.; Mehrdel, B. Gold Nanoparticles-Based Photothermal Therapy for Breast Cancer. *Photodiagnosis Photodyn. Ther.* **2023**, *42*, 103312. [CrossRef]
45. Wei, W.; Zhang, X.; Zhang, S.; Wei, G.; Su, Z. Biomedical and Bioactive Engineered Nanomaterials for Targeted Tumor Photothermal Therapy: A Review. *Mater. Sci. Eng. C* **2019**, *104*, 109891. [CrossRef]
46. Duan, S.; Hu, Y.; Zhao, Y.; Tang, K.; Zhang, Z.; Liu, Z.; Wang, Y.; Guo, H.; Miao, Y.; Du, H.; et al. Nanomaterials for Photothermal Cancer Therapy. *RSC Adv.* **2023**, *13*, 14443–14460. [CrossRef]
47. Li, X.; Wang, Y.; Liu, T.; Zhang, Y.; Wang, C.; Xie, B. Ultrasmall Graphene Oxide for Combination of Enhanced Chemotherapy and Photothermal Therapy of Breast Cancer. *Colloids Surf. B Biointerfaces* **2023**, *225*, 113288. [CrossRef]
48. Báez, D.F. Graphene-Based Nanomaterials for Photothermal Therapy in Cancer Treatment. *Pharmaceutics* **2023**, *15*, 2286. [CrossRef]
49. Hao, L.; Song, H.; Zhan, Z.; Lv, Y. Multifunctional Reduced Graphene Oxide-Based Nanoplatform for Synergistic Targeted Chemo-Photothermal Therapy. *ACS Appl. Bio Mater.* **2020**, *3*, 5213–5222. [CrossRef]
50. Báez, D.; Pardo, H.; Laborda, I.; Marco, J.; Yáñez, C.; Bollo, S. Reduced Graphene Oxides: Influence of the Reduction Method on the Electrocatalytic Effect towards Nucleic Acid Oxidation. *Nanomaterials* **2017**, *7*, 168. [CrossRef]
51. Sahu, A.; Choi, W.I.; Lee, J.H.; Tae, G. Graphene Oxide Mediated Delivery of Methylene Blue for Combined Photodynamic and Photothermal Therapy. *Biomaterials* **2013**, *34*, 6239–6248. [CrossRef]
52. Xu, C.; Pu, K. Second Near-Infrared Photothermal Materials for Combinational Nanotheranostics. *Chem. Soc. Rev.* **2021**, *50*, 1111–1137. [CrossRef]
53. Esteban-Fernández de Ávila, B.; Lopez-Ramirez, M.A.; Báez, D.F.; Jodra, A.; Singh, V.V.; Kaufmann, K.; Wang, J. Aptamer-Modified Graphene-Based Catalytic Micromotors: Off–On Fluorescent Detection of Ricin. *ACS Sens.* **2016**, *1*, 217–221. [CrossRef]
54. Vilela, D.; Parmar, J.; Zeng, Y.; Zhao, Y.; Sanchez, S. Graphene Based Microbots for Toxic Heavy Metal Removal and Recovery from Water. *Nano Lett.* **2016**, *16*, 2860–2866. [CrossRef]
55. Yang, Q.; Xu, H.; Wen, H.; Zhao, H.; Liu, X.; Cai, Y.; Wang, H.; Dong, R. Graphene Oxide Induced Enhancement of Light-Driven Micromotor with Biocompatible Fuels. *Appl. Mater. Today* **2021**, *22*, 100943. [CrossRef]
56. Zhou, X.; Li, Z.; Tan, L.; Zhang, Y.; Jiao, Y. Near-Infrared Light-Steered Graphene Aerogel Micromotor with High Speed and Precise Navigation for Active Transport and Microassembly. *ACS Appl. Mater. Interfaces* **2020**, *12*, 23134–23144. [CrossRef]
57. Palomar-Pardavé, M.; Mostany, J.; Muñoz-Rizo, R.; Botello, L.E.; Aldana-González, J.; Arce-Estrada, E.M.; de Oca-Yemha, M.G.M.; Ramírez-Silva, M.T.; Romo, M.R. Electrochemical Study and Physicochemical Characterization of Iron Nanoparticles Electrodeposited onto HOPG from Fe(III) Ions Dissolved in the Choline Chloride-Urea Deep Eutectic Solvent. *J. Electroanal. Chem.* **2019**, *851*, 113453. [CrossRef]
58. Martín, A.; Jurado-Sánchez, B.; Escarpa, A.; Wang, J. Template Electrosynthesis of High-Performance Graphene Microengines. *Small* **2015**, *11*, 3568–3574. [CrossRef]
59. Yoshida, Y.; Langouche, G. *Mössbauer Spectroscopy*; Springuer: Berlin/Heidelberg, Germany, 2013; ISBN 978-3-642-32219-8.

60. Ordoukhanian, J.; Karami, H.; Nezhadali, A. One Step Paired Electrochemical Synthesis of Iron and Iron Oxide Nanoparticles. *Mater. Sci.-Pol.* **2016**, *34*, 655–658. [CrossRef]
61. Krajewski, M.; Lin, W.S.; Lin, H.M.; Brzozka, K.; Lewinska, S.; Nedelko, N.; Slawska-Waniewska, A.; Borysiuk, J.; Wasik, D. Structural and Magnetic Properties of Iron Nanowires and Iron Nanoparticles Fabricated through a Reduction Reaction. *Beilstein J. Nanotechnol.* **2015**, *6*, 1652–1660. [CrossRef]
62. Chu, Y.; Xu, X.-Q.; Wang, Y. Ultradeep Photothermal Therapy Strategies. *J. Phys. Chem. Lett.* **2022**, *13*, 9564–9572. [CrossRef]
63. Liu, P.; Ye, M.; Wu, Y.; Wu, L.; Lan, K.; Wu, Z. Hyperthermia Combined with Immune Checkpoint Inhibitor Therapy: Synergistic Sensitization and Clinical Outcomes. *Cancer Med.* **2023**, *12*, 3201–3221. [CrossRef] [PubMed]
64. Choi, H.; Lee, G.H.; Kim, K.S.; Hahn, S.K. Light-Guided Nanomotor Systems for Autonomous Photothermal Cancer Therapy. *ACS Appl. Mater. Interfaces* **2018**, *10*, 2338–2346. [CrossRef]
65. Cheon, Y.A.; Bae, J.H.; Chung, B.G. Reduced Graphene Oxide Nanosheet for Chemo-Photothermal Therapy. *Langmuir* **2016**, *32*, 2731–2736. [CrossRef] [PubMed]
66. Yang, K.; Wan, J.; Zhang, S.; Tian, B.; Zhang, Y.; Liu, Z. The Influence of Surface Chemistry and Size of Nanoscale Graphene Oxide on Photothermal Therapy of Cancer Using Ultra-Low Laser Power. *Biomaterials* **2012**, *33*, 2206–2214. [CrossRef] [PubMed]
67. Robinson, J.T.; Tabakman, S.M.; Liang, Y.; Wang, H.; Sanchez Casalongue, H.; Vinh, D.; Dai, H. Ultrasmall Reduced Graphene Oxide with High Near-Infrared Absorbance for Photothermal Therapy. *J. Am. Chem. Soc.* **2011**, *133*, 6825–6831. [CrossRef] [PubMed]
68. Tan, S.; Wu, X.; Xing, Y.; Lilak, S.; Wu, M.; Zhao, J.X. Enhanced Synergetic Antibacterial Activity by a Reduce Graphene Oxide/Ag Nanocomposite through the Photothermal Effect. *Colloids Surf. B Biointerfaces* **2020**, *185*, 110616. [CrossRef]
69. Dong, Y.; Wang, L.; Wang, J.; Wang, S.; Wang, Y.; Jin, D.; Chen, P.; Du, W.; Zhang, L.; Liu, B.F. Graphene-Based Helical Micromotors Constructed by "Microscale Liquid Rope-Coil Effect" with Microfluidics. *ACS Nano* **2020**, *14*, 16600–16613. [CrossRef]
70. Liu, W.; Zhang, X.; Zhou, L.; Shang, L.; Su, Z. Reduced Graphene Oxide (rGO) Hybridized Hydrogel as a near-Infrared (NIR)/pH Dual-Responsive Platform for Combined Chemo-Photothermal Therapy. *J. Colloid Interface Sci.* **2019**, *536*, 160–170. [CrossRef] [PubMed]
71. Beniwal, N.; Verma, A.; Putta, C.L.; Rengan, A.K. Recent Trends in Bio-Nanomaterials and Non-Invasive Combinatorial Approaches of Photothermal Therapy against Cancer. *Nanotheranostics* **2024**, *8*, 219–238. [CrossRef]
72. Li, Z.; Chen, Y.; Yang, Y.; Yu, Y.; Zhang, Y.; Zhu, D.; Yu, X.; Ouyang, X.; Xie, Z.; Zhao, Y.; et al. Recent Advances in Nanomaterials-Based Chemo-Photothermal Combination Therapy for Improving Cancer Treatment. *Front. Bioeng. Biotechnol.* **2019**, *7*, 293. [CrossRef]
73. Yang, J.; Sun, Z.; Dou, Q.; Hui, S.; Zhang, P.; Liu, R.; Wang, D.; Jiang, S. NIR-Light-Responsive Chemo-Photothermal Hydrogel System with Controlled DOX Release and Photothermal Effect for Cancer Therapy. *Colloids Surf. Physicochem. Eng. Asp.* **2023**, *667*, 131407. [CrossRef]
74. Kovalevich, J.; Langford, D. Considerations for the Use of SH-SY5Y Neuroblastoma Cells in Neurobiology. In *Neuronal Cell Culture*; Amini, S., White, M.K., Eds.; Methods in Molecular Biology; Humana Press: Totowa, NJ, USA, 2013; Volume 1078, pp. 9–21, ISBN 978-1-62703-639-9.
75. Lopez-Suarez, L.; Awabdh, S.A.; Coumoul, X.; Chauvet, C. The SH-SY5Y Human Neuroblastoma Cell Line, a Relevant in Vitro Cell Model for Investigating Neurotoxicology in Human: Focus on Organic Pollutants. *NeuroToxicology* **2022**, *92*, 131–155. [CrossRef]
76. Eguchi, T.; Sheta, M.; Fujii, M.; Calderwood, S.K. Cancer Extracellular Vesicles, Tumoroid Models, and Tumor Microenvironment. *Semin. Cancer Biol.* **2022**, *86*, 112–126. [CrossRef] [PubMed]
77. Pape, J.; Emberton, M.; Cheema, U. 3D Cancer Models: The Need for a Complex Stroma, Compartmentalization and Stiffness. *Front. Bioeng. Biotechnol.* **2021**, *9*, 660502. [CrossRef] [PubMed]
78. Durán-Jara, E.; Del Campo, M.; Gutiérrez, V.; Wichmann, I.; Trigo, C.; Ezquer, M.; Lobos-González, L. Lactadherin Immunoblockade in Small Extracellular Vesicles Inhibits sEV-Mediated Increase of pro-Metastatic Capacities. *Biol. Res.* **2024**, *57*, 1. [CrossRef] [PubMed]

pharmaceutics

MDPI

Article

Transferrin-Bearing, Zein-Based Hybrid Lipid Nanoparticles for Drug and Gene Delivery to Prostate Cancer Cells

Khadeejah Maeyouf [1], Intouch Sakpakdeejaroen [1,2], Sukrut Somani [1], Jitkasem Meewan [1], Hawraa Ali-Jerman [1], Partha Laskar [1,3], Margaret Mullin [4], Graeme MacKenzie [1], Rothwelle J. Tate [1] and Christine Dufès [1,*]

1 Strathclyde Institute of Pharmacy and Biomedical Sciences, University of Strathclyde, Glasgow G4 0RE, UK; khadeejah.maeyouf.2018@uni.strath.ac.uk (K.M.); intouch@tu.ac.th (I.S.); sukrut.somani@outlook.com (S.S.); jitkasem.meewan@strath.ac.uk (J.M.); hawraa-f-r-m-ali@strath.ac.uk (H.A.-J.); plaskar@gitam.edu (P.L.); graeme.mackenzie@strath.ac.uk (G.M.); r.j.tate@strath.ac.uk (R.J.T.)
2 Faculty of Medicine, Thammasat University, Klong Nueng, Klong Luang, Pathumthani 12121, Thailand
3 Department of Chemistry, School of Science, Gandhi Institute of Technology and Management, Visakhapatnam 530045, Andhra Pradesh, India
4 Glasgow Imaging Facility, College of Medical, Veterinary and Life Sciences, University of Glasgow, Glasgow G12 8QQ, UK; margaret.mullin@glasgow.ac.uk
* Correspondence: c.dufes@strath.ac.uk; Tel.: +44-141-548-3796

Abstract: Gene therapy holds great promise for treating prostate cancer unresponsive to conventional therapies. However, the lack of delivery systems that can transport therapeutic DNA and drugs while targeting tumors without harming healthy tissues presents a significant challenge. This study aimed to explore the potential of novel hybrid lipid nanoparticles, composed of biocompatible zein and conjugated to the cancer-targeting ligand transferrin. These nanoparticles were designed to entrap the anti-cancer drug docetaxel and carry plasmid DNA, with the objective of improving the delivery of therapeutic payloads to prostate cancer cells, thereby enhancing their anti-proliferative efficacy and gene expression levels. These transferrin-bearing, zein-based hybrid lipid nanoparticles efficiently entrapped docetaxel, leading to increased uptake by PC-3 and LNCaP cancer cells and significantly enhancing anti-proliferative efficacy at docetaxel concentrations exceeding 1 μg/mL. Furthermore, they demonstrated proficient DNA condensation, exceeding 80% at polymer–DNA weight ratios of 1500:1 and 2000:1. This resulted in increased gene expression across all tested cell lines, with the highest transfection levels up to 11-fold higher than those observed with controls, in LNCaP cells. These novel transferrin-bearing, zein-based hybrid lipid nanoparticles therefore exhibit promising potential as drug and gene delivery systems for prostate cancer therapy.

Keywords: zein-based hybrid lipid nanoparticles; transferrin; tumor targeting; delivery system; cancer therapy; prostate cancer

1. Introduction

Prostate cancer, the second leading cause of cancer-related deaths in men, claims the lives of over 300,000 patients worldwide per year. Its incidence has continued to rise over the last two decades [1–4]. While treatments like cryoablation, chemotherapy, radiotherapy, and radical prostatectomy can be efficacious against localized tumors, there is still no effective treatment for patients with recurrent or metastatic disease [5]. Consequently, there is an urgent need for new therapeutic approaches to address the needs of these patients.

Among novel experimental strategies, gene therapy holds great promise for the treatment of prostate cancer. However, its practical application is currently hindered by the lack of suitable delivery systems capable of transporting therapeutic DNA and drugs while specifically targeting tumors, without causing adverse effects on healthy tissues [6].

To address this challenge, we hypothesize that the use of hybrid lipid nanoparticles composed of biocompatible and biodegradable zein and conjugated to transferrin (whose receptors are overexpressed on prostate cancer cells [7–9]) would be able to entrap the hydrophobic anti-cancer drug docetaxel and carry plasmid DNA. It is expected that these nanoparticles would enhance the delivery of therapeutic payloads to prostate cancer cells, consequently increasing their anti-proliferative efficacy and gene expression levels.

Zein, a hydrophobic and biodegradable protein extracted from corn, has received approval from the US Food and Drug Administration as generally regarded as safe (GRAS) for various applications in food, pharmaceutical, and biomedical industries [10–13]. Due to its amphiphilic molecular structure, zein exhibits solubility in 50–90% (v/v) aqueous ethanol, but its composition, comprising more than 50% lipophilic amino acids, renders it insoluble in water. Additionally, its high glutamine content makes it insoluble in absolute alcohol [14]. By taking advantage of its different solubilities in ethanol and water, zein has demonstrated significant potential as a carrier system for the delivery of nutraceuticals, drugs, and DNA [15–18]. Furthermore, the modification of zein through conjugation with poly(ethylene glycol) (PEG) has been shown to introduce a steric shielding of the carrier system [19], therefore decreasing any potential opsonization and providing a sustained release of the entrapped drug [20–23].

The drug selected to be entrapped within the zein-based hybrid lipid nanoparticles, docetaxel, is a semi-synthetic analogue of paclitaxel used as an anti-neoplastic therapy for the treatment of prostate tumors. It was approved by both the FDA and the European Medicines Agency in 2004 as afirst-line treatment for advanced prostate cancer [24]. Due to its bulky polycyclic structure [25], docetaxel is insoluble in water. It exerts its therapeutic effect by hyper-stabilizing the protein structure of microtubules, inhibiting their disassembly through binding to the beta-tubulin subunit. This leads to the persistence of microtubule structure, a loss of cytoskeleton flexibility, cell cycle arrest, and ultimately, cell death. Docetaxel is employed as a first-line treatment option for prostate cancer, either as a single agent or in combination with estramustine for androgen-independent prostate cancer. However, due to its high lipophilicity, which adversely impacts its pharmacokinetic profile, commercially available docetaxel formulations incorporate the surfactant Tween® 80 to enhance its solubility, physicochemical properties, and its cell membrane permeability [26]. Furthermore, docetaxel is associated with various adverse effects, including high toxicity, low sensitivity, and the potential development of resistance, thereby limiting its therapeutic efficacy [24,27]. It is therefore important to entrap this drug within a delivery system that would deliver it specifically to its site of action.

The objectives of this study were therefore to synthesize and characterize transferrin-bearing, zein-based hybrid lipid nanoparticles, to evaluate their ability to entrap docetaxel and complex a plasmid DNA, and to assess their cellular uptake, transfection, and anti-proliferative efficacy on prostate cancer cells.

2. Materials and Methods

2.1. Reagents and Cell Lines

Yellow zein, human holo-transferrin (Tf), cupric sulphate (pentahydrate), 2-iminothiolane hydrochloride (Traut's reagent), 2-nitrophenyl-β-D-galactopyranoside (ONPG), docetaxel *purum* (≥97.0%), Vivaspin® 6 centrifuge tubes with a molecular weight cut-off (MWCO) of 5000 and 100,000 Daltons, and all the chemicals not mentioned below were obtained from Sigma-Aldrich (Poole, UK). 1,2-distearoyl-sn-glycero-3-phosphoethanolamine-N-[maleimide (polyethylene glycol)-2000] (DSPE-PEG2K-MAL) was purchased from Jenkem Technology (Plano, TX, USA). 1,2-distearoyl-sn-glycero-3-phosphoethanolamine-N-(carbonyl methoxypolyethylene-glycol 2000), sodium salt (DSPE-PEG2K) was obtained from NOF Corporation (Tokyo, Japan). The expression plasmid encoding β-galactosidase (pCMVsport β-galactosidase) was obtained from Invitrogen (Paisley, UK) and was purified using an Endotoxin-free Giga Plasmid Kit (Qiagen, Hilden, Germany). Bioware® androgen-irresponsive PC-3M-luc-C6 human prostate adenocarcinoma that expresses the firefly luciferase was purchased from Caliper Life Sciences (Hopkinton, MA, USA), while the androgen-irresponsive DU145 and androgen-sensitive LNCaP prostate cancer cell lines came from the European Collection of Cell Cultures (Salisbury, UK). Roswell Park Memorial Institute 1640 (RPMI) cell culture medium, Quant-iT® PicoGreen® dsDNA reagent, fetal bovine serum (FBS), sodium pyruvate, L-glutamine, N-2-hydroxyethylpiperazine-N-2-ethane sulfonic acid (HEPES), penicillin-streptomycin, TrypLE® Express, and Tubulin Tracker® Green (Oregon Green® 488 Taxol, bis-acetate) were purchased from Life Technologies (Paisley, UK). Passive lysis 5× buffer was obtained from Promega (Southampton, UK). Vectashield® mounting medium containing 4′,6-diamidino-2-phenylindole (DAPI) came from Vector Laboratories (Peterborough, UK).

2.2. Evaluation of the Concentration of Ethanol Needed to Dissolve Zein

To assess the solubility of zein in ethanol, 2 mL of ethanol (50, 60, 70, 80, and 90%) was added to 20 mg of zein and thorough mixing ensued to yield a transparent, yellow solution. The subsequent nanoparticle preparation was performed by employing the specific ethanol concentration at which zein demonstrated complete dissolution.

2.3. Preparation and Optimization of Zein-Based Hybrid Lipid Nanoparticles Entrapping Coumarin

2.3.1. Comparison of One-Step Nanoprecipitation and Coacervation Methods

Zein-based hybrid lipid nanoparticles entrapping coumarin-6 were prepared by using both one-step nanoprecipitation and coacervation methods.

Initially, the nanoparticles were prepared through the nanoprecipitation method, using the ethanol concentration (80%) that enabled complete zein dissolution.

The other experimental parameters were first fixed: the weight ratio of lipid 1,2-distearoyl-sn-glycero-3-phosphoethanolamine-N-[maleimide (polyethylene glycol)-2000] (DSPE-PEG2K-MAL) to zein at 1:5 (w/w), the volume ratio of water to ethanol at 2:1 (v/v), the zein concentration of 10 mg/mL in the organic solvent, and the theoretical drug loading at 0.5% of zein weight.

To initiate the process, DSPE-PEG2K-MAL (6 mg) was dispersed in 6 mL of Milli-Q ultrapure water (15.0 MΩ·cm) at 65 °C with continuous shaking at 700 rpm for 1 h. Subsequently, a solution of coumarin-6 (150 µg in 75 µL DMSO) was added to the zein solution (30 mg in 3 mL ethanol (80%)). The resulting mixture was then introduced dropwise into the lipid phase and stirred for 15 min at 25 °C, allowing for the formation of homogenous nanoparticles. The resulting nanoparticles were collected by centrifugation conducted at 8000 rpm (14,000× g) for 20 min at 20 °C, using a Hermle® Z323K centrifuge (Wehingen, Germany). The collected nanoparticles underwent a washing step with 1 mL of ultrapure water to remove any unentrapped coumarin-6. After washing, the nanoparticles were centrifuged once more under the same conditions. Subsequently, the nanoparticles were resuspended in 1 mL of ultrapure water and stored at 4 °C. Control zein-based hybrid lipid nanoparticles entrapping coumarin-6 were prepared using an identical protocol, with the exception that DSPE-PEG2K-MAL was replaced with DSPE-PEG2K as the lipid component.

In the coacervation method, aqueous and organic solutions were prepared following the same procedures as outlined in the nanoprecipitation method. However, the sequence of addition was reversed. Specifically, the aqueous solution (consisting of lipid dispersed in water) was added dropwise into the organic solution (comprising zein dissolved in ethanol). This addition was carried out under identical conditions as those employed in the nanoprecipitation method.

2.3.2. Variation in Water–Ethanol Volume Ratios

Zein-based hybrid lipid nanoparticles entrapping coumarin-6 were prepared via the nanoprecipitation method. Various volume ratios of water–ethanol (2:1, 3:1, 4:1, and 5:1) corresponding to 6, 9, 12, 15 mL of ultrapure water were used. Meanwhile, the lipid–zein weight ratio was maintained at 1:5, the zein concentration in the organic solution was set at 10 mg/mL, and the loading of coumarin-6 was fixed at 0.5% of the zein weight. DSPE-PEG2K-MAL (6 mg) was dispersed through stirring at 65 °C for 1 h in 6, 9, 12, and

15 mL of ultrapure water. Subsequently, a solution of coumarin-6 (150 µg in 75 µL DMSO) was added to the zein solution (30 mg in 3 mL ethanol (80%)). The nanoparticles were then generated, collected, and stored as described above.

2.3.3. Use of Probe Sonication

The nanoparticles were prepared as described above, with the inclusion of an extra step involving probe sonication (sonication for 3 × 2 min at 21% amplitude using a Vibra-Cell® probe sonicator (Sonics, Newtown, CT, USA)). Following this, the nanoparticles were gathered through centrifugation.

2.3.4. Addition of One-Hour Incubation before Centrifugation

The nanoparticles were prepared as described above, with the addition of a one-hour incubation period following the dropwise addition of the organic solution to the aqueous solution at 25 °C, prior to the centrifugation step.

2.3.5. Variation in Lipid–Zein Weight Ratios

Three distinct weight ratios of lipid–zein were used: 1:4, 1:5, and 1:6. The water–ethanol volume ratio was held at 2:1, with a constant zein amount of 30 mg and a zein concentration of 10 mg/mL in the organic solvent. Various lipid amounts (5, 6, and 7.5 mg) were dispersed in 6 mL of ultrapure water. The zein solution was prepared and added to the lipid dispersion as described above, after which probe sonication was carried out for three cycles of two minutes each. Subsequently, the nanoparticles were gathered via centrifugation, in accordance with the method described above.

2.3.6. Variation in the Amount of Zein

Nanoparticles were prepared using three amounts of zein: 30, 40, and 50 mg. The drug loading remained constant at 0.5% of the zein weight, with the zein concentration in the organic solvent set at 10 mg/mL. The water–ethanol ratio was maintained at 2:1, while the lipid–zein ratio was fixed at 1:5. Lipids (6, 8, and 10 mg) were dispersed in 6, 8, and 10 mL of ultrapure water as described above. For the incorporation of coumarin-6, solutions containing 150 µg in 75, 100, and 125 µL of DMSO were introduced to zein solutions containing 30, 40, and 50 mg of zein in 3, 4, and 5 mL of 80% ethanol, respectively. The zein solutions were then added dropwise to the aqueous solutions as described above.

2.3.7. Variation in Drug Amount Related to Zein Weight

Nanoparticle formulations were prepared by using two distinct percentages of coumarin-6 relative to the zein weight. Specifically, coumarin-6 was loaded at two ratios (0.1 and 0.5% of the zein weight), while maintaining a fixed zein amount of 40 mg. The lipid to zein weight ratio was set at 1:5, and the volume ratio of water to ethanol was maintained at 2:1. Lipids (8 mg) were dispersed in 8 mL of ultrapure water through stirring for a duration of 1 h within the temperature range of 60–65 °C. Subsequently, 40 µg of coumarin-6 in 20 µL DMSO (for a 0.1% loading of zein weight) and 200 µg of coumarin-6 in 100 µL DMSO (for a 0.5% loading of zein weight) was added to 40 mg of zein dissolved in 4 mL of 80% ethanol. Zein solutions were subsequently added dropwise into the lipid solution as described above.

The amount of coumarin-6 entrapped within the nanoparticles was measured through spectrofluorimetry, using an Agilent Varian Cary Eclipse® spectrofluorometer (Agilent Technologies, Santa Clara, CA, USA). The excitation wavelength (λ_{exc}) was set at 463 nm, while the emission wavelength (λ_{em}) was set at 510 nm, with a slit width of 5 nm. The results were expressed as a percentage of entrapment efficiency.

2.4. Preparation of Transferrin-Bearing Zein-Based Hybrid Lipid Nanoparticles Encapsulating Docetaxel

Zein nanoparticles entrapping docetaxel were prepared through the nanoprecipitation method as refined based on the optimization using coumarin-6. Briefly, DSPE-PEG2K-MAL (8 mg) was dispersed in 8 mL of ultrapure water by shaking at 700 rpm at 60–65 °C for a duration of 1 h. A solution of docetaxel (200 μg in DMSO) was added to the zein solution (40 mg in 4 mL of 80% ethanol). The organic phase, consisting of zein dissolved in ethanol, was added dropwise into the aqueous phase, where lipid was dispersed in water, and mixed through stirring at 25 °C for 15 min. Following this, the mixture underwent an additional 15 min of stirring to enhance uniformity before undergoing probe sonication for three cycles of two minutes each. The nanoparticles were then subjected to centrifugation at 14,000× *g* for a duration of 20 min at 20 °C, using an Avanti® J-E centrifuge (Beckman Coulter, London, UK). To remove unentrapped docetaxel, the nanoparticles were subjected to a wash step using 2 mL of ultrapure water, followed by another round of centrifugation under identical conditions. Ultimately, the nanoparticles had their final volume adjusted to 1 mL with ultrapure water and were stored at 4 °C. The amount of docetaxel in the nanoparticles was determined through spectrophotometry (λ_{max}: 312 nm), using an Agilent Varian Cary® 50 UV-Vis spectrophotometer (Agilent Technologies, Santa Clara, CA, USA). The results were expressed as percentage of entrapment efficiency.

Transferrin was conjugated to the nanoparticles through the thiol–maleimide 'click' reaction method described by Hermanson [28]. Initially, 10 mg of transferrin dissolved in 1 mL of 50 mM sodium phosphate buffer containing 0.15 M sodium chloride (pH 8) was reacted with a 10-fold molar excess of Traut's reagent (2-iminothiolane hydrochloride) (85 μL of Traut's reagent, 2 mg/mL in deionized water) under moderate stirring at 25 °C for a duration of 2 h. The resultant thiolated Tf was then isolated from the unreacted reagent through centrifugation at 9500 rpm (10,500× *g*) for 15 min at 20 °C (Hermle® Z323K centrifuge, Wehingen, Germany), using Vivaspin® 6 centrifuge tubes with a molecular weight cut-off of 5000 Daltons (Sartorius Ltd., Epsom, UK). It was immediately conjugated to 1 mL of nanoparticles prepared as described above while under continuous stirring at 25 °C for 1 h. Any residual unreacted Tf was subsequently removed from the hybrid lipid nanoparticles by centrifugation at 7500 rpm (6600× *g*) for 15 min at 20 °C, using Vivaspin® 6 centrifuge tubes with a molecular weight cut-off of 100,000 Daltons.

Parallelly, control nanoparticles underwent purification through the same centrifugation method as described above, using Vivaspin® 6 centrifuge tubes with a molecular weight cut-off of 5000 Daltons. Post purification, their final volume was adjusted to 1 mL using ultrapure water and they were then stored at 4 °C.

The amount of transferrin conjugated to the nanoparticles was determined by the Lowry assay [29], using a previously established protocol [30].

The morphology of transferrin-bearing and control zein-based hybrid lipid nanoparticles was visualized through transmission electron microscopy. Initially, formvar/carbon-coated copper grids (400 mesh) were subjected to glow discharge. Subsequently, a 3–5 μL droplet of each sample, previously diluted to a 1:10 ratio with deionized water, was deposited onto the hydrophilic support film and left to air-dry overnight. The dried samples were then subjected to imaging using a Jeol JEM-1200EX® transmission electron microscope (Jeol, Peabody, MA, USA), operating at an accelerating voltage of 80 kV and equipped with a Gatan 794 MultiScan® camera (Gatan, Pleasanton, CA, USA).

The size and zeta potential of Tf-bearing and control zein-based hybrid lipid nanoparticles entrapping docetaxel were measured using photon correlation spectroscopy and laser Doppler electrophoresis, using a Zetasizer Nano-ZS® (Malvern Instruments Ltd., Malvern, UK). All samples were appropriately diluted to a 1:50 ratio in ultrapure water. The diluted samples were then brought to a final volume of 1 mL to fall within the analytical measurement range before being transferred into disposable cuvettes and folded capillary cells for size and zeta potential measurement, respectively. The experiment was performed in quadruplicate.

2.5. Stability of the Formulations

The stability of Tf-conjugated and control zein-based hybrid lipid nanoparticles entrapping docetaxel, along with the blank nanoparticles, was assessed through a systematic process. All samples were securely sealed in tightly closed tubes, shielded from light, and then stored under controlled conditions at 4 °C over a span of 4 weeks. To monitor the stability, the size and zeta potential of the nanoparticles were, respectively, measured using the Zetasizer Nano-ZS®, as described above. Measurements were conducted on Days 0, 7, 14, 21, and 28 to gauge any changes over time. The amount of docetaxel retained within the formulations was quantified via spectrophotometry.

2.6. Drug Release

The release profile of docetaxel was assessed using a dialysis technique at various pH conditions (5.5, 6.5, and 7.4), simulating the acidic endosomal pH of cancer cells, the extracellular environment pH of tumors, and the physiological pH found in normal tissue and blood, respectively. To do so, docetaxel either formulated as Tf-bearing, control zein-based hybrid lipid nanoparticles, or in solution (500 µg of docetaxel in 2.5 mL distilled water) was placed into a SnakeSkin® dialysis tube with a molecular weight cut-off of 7000 Da (ThermoFisher Scientific, Waltham, MA, USA) and was dialyzed against 100 mL of phosphate buffer (pHs 5.5, 6.5, and 7.4) at 37 °C under gentle stirring. Throughout the experiment, aliquots of 1 mL of the dialysate were withdrawn in triplicate at specific time intervals (30 min, then every hour for the initial six hours (1, 2, 3, 4, 5, and 6 h), then every 2 h for the next 6 h (8, 10, and 12 h), and 24 h. For each sample, the withdrawn volume was replenished with 3 mL of fresh buffer, maintaining a consistent buffer volume of 100 mL. The amount of docetaxel in the formulations was quantified through spectrophotometry using an Agilent Varian Cary® 50 UV-Vis spectrophotometer set at an absorption wavelength of 312 nm. The results were expressed as a percentage cumulative drug release.

2.7. In Vitro Studies

2.7.1. Cellular Uptake

Flow cytometry was employed as a method for quantifying the fluorescence intensity of docetaxel that was internalized by the cancer cells. To this end, PC3-Luc, DU145, and LNCaP cells were initially seeded at a density of 1×10^6 cells/well in 6-well plates and cultured at a temperature of 37 °C for a period of 24 h. Following the removal of the culture medium, the cells were treated with fluorescein-labelled docetaxel (12 µg/well), which was either entrapped within Tf-bearing or control zein-based hybrid lipid nanoparticles or in solution, for an additional 15 h at a temperature of 37 °C. Following the incubation period, the cells were subjected to thorough washing, involving 3 washes with cold PBS (2 mL). Subsequently, they were detached from the plates using TrypLE® Express (250 µL). The trypsinization reaction was then stopped by adding 500 µL of fetal bovine serum (FBS) (1% in PBS) to the cell suspension. The mean fluorescence intensity (MFI) of the drug taken up by the cells was measured through using Attune® NxT Acoustic Focusing cytometer (Thermo Fisher Scientific, Waltham, MA, USA), with Attune® NxT Auto Sampler software version 3.1.2 (Thermo Fisher Scientific, Waltham, MA, USA), using a FITC filter (Exc_{max}: 494 nm/Em_{max}: 520 nm). Thirty thousand cells (gated events) were counted and analyzed for each sample.

The cellular uptake of fluorescein-labelled docetaxel entrapped within transferrin-bearing and control zein-based hybrid lipid nanoparticles, or in solution, was also qualitatively assessed through confocal microscopy. PC3-Luc, DU145, and LNCaP cells were initially seeded at a density of 2×10^5 cells per well on coverslips in 6-well plates. Subsequently, the cells were incubated for a period of 24 h at a temperature of 37 °C, in a humid atmosphere containing 5% CO_2. The culture medium was then removed, and the cells were exposed to fluorescein-labelled docetaxel (12 µg/well), formulated either as Tf-bearing or control zein-based hybrid lipid nanoparticles, or as a solution, for 15 h. Following incubation with the respective treatments, the cells were washed three times with 3 mL of phosphate-buffered saline (PBS), before being fixed with 2 mL methanol for a duration of 10 min at a temperature of 20 °C. After staining the cell nuclei with Vectashield® mounting medium containing 4′,6-diamidino-2-phenylindole (DAPI) for 2 h, the imaging of cells was executed using a Leica TCS SP5® confocal microscope (Wetzlar, Germany). DAPI (which stained the cell nuclei) was excited using a 405 nm laser line, with an emission bandwidth ranging from 400 to 480 nm. On the other hand, fluorescein-labeled docetaxel was excited using a 494 nm laser line, with an emission bandwidth spanning from 510 to 530 nm.

2.7.2. Mechanisms of Cellular Uptake

To determine the underlying mechanisms governing the cellular uptake of docetaxel, PC3-Luc cells were seeded in six-well plates at a density of 1×10^6 cells/well and grown for 24 h. They were then pre-treated with the endocytosis inhibitors transferrin (50 µM), chlorpromazine (20 µg/mL), filipin (5 µg/mL), colchicine (40 µg/mL), and poly-L-lysine (40 µg/mL) at 37 °C for 30 min. Afterwards, the treatments were replaced with co-incubation of fluorescein-labelled docetaxel (12 µg per well) entrapped in Tf-bearing nanoparticles and each inhibitor at identical concentrations (except chlorpromazine, which was added at a concentration of 5 µg/mL) for an additional 15 h incubation at 37 °C. The cells then underwent processing for flow cytometry and confocal analysis as described above.

2.7.3. Anti-Proliferative Efficacy

The anti-proliferative efficacy of docetaxel entrapped in targeted and control zein-based hybrid lipid nanoparticles as well as in solution, was assessed through a MTT assay on PC3-Luc, DU145, and LNCaP prostate cancer cells. To do so, cells were seeded at a density of 2000 cells/well in 96-well plates and incubated for a period of 72 h at a temperature of 37 °C, in a humid atmosphere containing 5% CO_2. Afterward, the cells were treated with various concentrations of docetaxel (ranging from 0.00001 to 30 µg/mL), either entrapped in Tf-bearing or control zein-based hybrid lipid nanoparticles or in solution. After 72 h treatment, 50 µL of MTT solution (0.5% *w*/*v* in PBS) was added to each well and incubated with the cells for 4 h. The solution was then replaced with 200 µL of dimethyl sulfoxide (DMSO) to dissolve the purple formazan product generated by viable cells. Triton X-100 (0.1% *w*/*v* in PBS) and fresh medium were used as positive and negative control, respectively. Three independent experiments for each formulation, with $n = 5$ for each concentration level, were conducted. The optical density of the formazan solution was measured at an absorbance at 570 nm using a Multiskan Ascent® microplate reader (Thermo Labsystems, Beverly, MA, USA). Percentage absorbance values were used to construct dose–response curves. These curves were fitted to determine the IC_{50} values, which represent the concentration of docetaxel that results in a 50% reduction in cell viability.

2.8. Evaluation of the Potential Use of Tf-Bearing Zein-Based Hybrid Lipid Nanoparticles for Gene Therapy

2.8.1. Evaluation of DNA Condensation

The ability of Tf-bearing and control zein-based hybrid lipid nanoparticles to complex DNA was assessed through a PicoGreen® assay. PicoGreen® solution was prepared by following the protocol provided by the supplier. PicoGreen® reagent was diluted 200-fold in Tris-EDTA (TE) buffer (10 mM Tris, 1 mM EDTA, adjusted to pH 7.5) on the day of the experiment, in a plastic container to shield it from light. Nanoparticles formulated as Tf-bearing or control zein-based hybrid lipid nanoparticles were prepared as described above. HCL (0.1 M) was added to the nanoparticles to make them positively charged (zeta potentials of 20 and 26 mV for Tf-bearing and control nanoparticles, respectively, at a pH~4). Briefly, 1 mL of PicoGreen® solution was added to 1 mL of nanoparticles–DNA complex at various polymer–DNA weight ratios (2000:1, 1500:1, 1000:1, 500:1, 250:1, 100:1, 50:1, 20:1, 10:1, 5:1, 2:1, 1:1, 0.5:1). The intensity of PicoGreen® fluorescence was immediately measured by spectrofluorimetry (λ_{exc}: 480 nm, λ_{em}: 520 nm). The DNA concentration was maintained at a consistent level of 10 μg/mL throughout the experiment. Fluorescence measurements were conducted at multiple time points (0, 30 min, 1 h, 2 h, 4 h, 6 h, 24 h) with $n = 4$ to monitor the interaction between the nanoparticles and DNA.

DNA condensation was also assessed using a gel retardation assay. Tf-bearing and control zein-based hybrid lipid nanoparticles complexed with DNA were prepared as outlined above. After mixing with the loading buffer (2 μL), the resulting samples (15 μL) were loaded onto a 1× Tris-Borate-EDTA (TBE) (89 mM Tris base, 89 mM boric acid, 2 mM Na_2-EDTA, pH 8.3) buffered 0.8% (*w*/*v*) agarose gel containing ethidium bromide (0.4 μg/mL), with 1×TBE as a running buffer and Bioline HyperLadder® 1 kb as a DNA size marker. Electrophoresis was conducted at a constant voltage of 50 V for a duration of 1 h. The gel was then visualized under UV light, allowing for the observation of the migration of DNA bands.

2.8.2. Measurement of the Size and Zeta Potential of the Complexes

The size and zeta potential of Tf-bearing and control zein-based hybrid lipid nanoparticles–DNA complexes in TE buffer were measured for various polymers–DNA weight ratios ranging from 50:1 to 2000:1, by photon correlation spectroscopy and laser Doppler electrophoresis, using a Malvern Zetasizer Nano-ZS® (Malvern Instruments Ltd., Malvern, UK). The DNA concentration was maintained at a constant level of 10 μg/mL throughout the experiment. The experiment was conducted in quadruplicate.

2.8.3. Gene Expression

A transfection assay was performed to assess the expression of the plasmid DNA encoding β-galactosidase complexed to Tf-bearing and control zein-based hybrid lipid nanoparticles, in PC3-Luc, DU145, and LNCaP prostate cancer cells. The cells were seeded in quintuplicate at a density of 2000 cells/well in 96-well plates and incubated for 72 h at 37 °C in a humid atmosphere with 5% CO_2. They were then treated with Tf-bearing nanoparticles complexed to plasmid DNA, at six polymers–DNA weight ratios (2000:1, 1500:1, 1000:1, 500:1, 250:1, 100:1). Three independent experiments were conducted. Polyethylenimine (PEI) and generation 3-diaminobutyric polypropylenimine (DAB) dendrimer complexed to DNA (at a polymer–DNA weight ratio of 5:1 for both complexes) were used as positive controls, while naked DNA served as a negative control. The plasmid DNA concentration was maintained at a consistent level of 1 μg per well throughout the entire experiment. After 72 h treatment, the cells were lysed with 1× passive lysis buffer (PLB) (50 μL/well) for 20 min at 37 °C. The cell lysates were then analyzed for β-galactosidase expression by adding 50 μL of 2× assay buffer (sodium phosphate buffer 200 mM; magnesium chloride 0.5 M; β-mercaptoethanol 50 mM; pH 7.3) containing ONPG solution (1.33 mg/mL in 2× assay buffer) to each well containing the lysates. The plates were then incubated for 2 h in the dark at 37 °C before reading the absorbance of each well at 405 nm using a Multiskan Ascent® microplate reader (Thermo Labsystems, Beverly, MA, USA).

2.9. Statistical Analysis

The results were expressed as means ± standard error of the mean (S.E.M). Statistical significance was assessed by one-way analysis of variance (ANOVA), and Tukey's multiple comparison post-test (Minitab® software version 20.0, State College, PE, USA). Differences were considered statistically significant for p values lower than 0.05.

3. Results

3.1. Evaluation of the Concentration of Ethanol Needed to Dissolve Zein

Zein exhibited complete solubility in ethanol concentrations of 70%, 80%, and 90%, resulting in a distinct, pale-yellow solution. Conversely, its solubility was reduced in 50% and 60% ethanol solutions. Zein remained insoluble in absolute ethanol. Based on this finding, the experiments in this study were then conducted by utilizing zein that had been dissolved in ethanol solutions of 70%, 80%, or 90%. This approach aligns with the findings of Paraman and Lamsal [31], as well as Shukla and Cheryan [10], who previously reported the solubility of α-zein in aqueous ethanol concentrations ranging from 60% to 95%.

3.2. Preparation and Optimization of Zein-Based Hybrid Lipid Nanoparticles Entrapping Coumarin-6

3.2.1. Comparison of One-Step Nanoprecipitation and Coacervation Methods

Zein-based hybrid lipid nanoparticles were successfully prepared using the nanoprecipitation method with various concentrations of ethanol. They exhibited sizes of 140.3 ± 0.8 nm, 146.6 ± 0.9 nm, and 160.5 ± 1.2 nm for formulations prepared with 70%, 80%, and 90% ethanol in the organic phase, respectively (Table 1). The polydispersity index revealed a narrow size distribution across all these formulations, with values consistently below 0.2 (0.06 ± 0.02, 0.08 ± 0.01, and 0.07 ± 0.01 for the nanoparticles prepared with 70%, 80% and 90% ethanol, respectively). The nanoparticles exhibited a negative charge, with zeta potential values of −29.5 ± 0.5 mV, −30.4 ± 0.8 mV, and −30.5 ± 1.0 mV when prepared using 70%, 80%, and 90% ethanol samples, respectively. These findings collectively indicated robust formulation stability, with a combination of a slightly lower zeta potential and size lower than 150 nm for the formulation prepared with 80% ethanol in the organic phase. Consequently, an ethanol concentration of 80% was selected for nanoparticle preparation.

Table 1. Optimization of zein-based hybrid lipid nanoparticles. Values in green indicate the best results obtained.

	Size (nm)	Polydispersity Index (PDI)	Zeta Potential (mV)	Entrapment Efficiency (%)
Ethanol concentration (%)				
70	140.3 ± 0.8	0.06 ± 0.02	−29.5 ± 0.5	
80	146.6 ± 0.9	0.08 ± 0.01	−30.4 ± 0.8	
90	160.5 ±1.2	0.07 ± 0.01	−30.5 ± 1.0	
Preparation method				
Nanoprecipitation	205.7 ± 9.4	0.35 ± 0.06	−24.6 ± 0.8	74.8 ± 1.1
Coacervation	572.6 ± 37.5	0.19 ± 0.053	−21.2 ± 0.5	76.4 ± 2.8
Water: ethanol ratio (*v*/*v*)				
2:1	224.3 ± 28.0	0.27 ± 0.06	−21.8 ± 1.0	94.1 ± 2.7
3:1	217.1 ± 69.2	0.40 ± 0.06	−23.2 ± 0.8	51.9 ± 0.9
4:1	408 ± 73.1	0.67 ± 0.07	−23.1 ± 1.2	37.7 ± 3.0
5:1	178.9 ± 24.2	0.58 ± 0.09	−21.6 ± 0.9	32.0 ± 1.6
Use of probe sonication	236.4 ± 20.1	0.14 ± 0.05	−23.5 ± 3.4	
One-hour incubation	260.2 ± 3.1	0.38 ± 0.07	−20.9 ± 1.5	
Lipid: zein ratio (*w*/*w*)				
1:4	231.1 ± 3.4	0.17 ± 0.02	− 17.2 ± 0.7	87.9 ± 2.7
1:5	236.4 ± 20.1	0.14 ± 0.05	−23.5 ± 3.4	94.1 ± 2.7
1:6	224.8 ± 7.9	0.15 ± 0.03	−20.1 ± 0.7	89.9 ± 3.3
Zein amount (mg)				
30	236.4 ± 20.1	0.14 ± 0.05	−23.5 ± 3.4	80 ± 1.9
40	215.9 ± 6.8	0.16 ± 0.04	−18.4 ± 0.5	92.0 ± 0.9
50	225.3 ± 6.2	0.15 ± 0.01	−16.6 ± 0.0	83.7 ± 1.8
Amount of drug added related to zein weight (%)				
0.1	201.2 ± 6.7	0.11 ± 0.02	−17.2 ± 0.8	10.0 ± 0.2
0.5	215.9 ± 6.8	0.16 ± 0.04	−18.4 ± 0.5	92.0 ± 0.9

Hybrid lipid nanoparticles entrapping coumarin-6 as a fluorescent hydrophobic drug model were effectively prepared via both nanoprecipitation and coacervation methods. Through the nanoprecipitation approach, they exhibited a small size (205.7 ± 9.4 nm), coupled with a narrow size distribution (with a PDI of 0.35 ± 0.06) and an inherent negative charge (zeta potential of −24.6 ± 0.8 mV). Impressively, they were able to entrap 74.8 ± 1.1% (equivalent to 112.2 μg) of coumarin-6 (Table 1).

The nanoparticles generated via the coacervation method entrapped a non-statistically different percentage of coumarin-6 (76.4 ± 2.8%, corresponding to 114.6 μg) and displayed a slightly higher negative zeta potential (−21.2 ± 0.5 mV), but exhibited a substantially larger size (572.6 ± 37.5 nm), higher than the cut-off size (400 nm) crucial for extravasation into tumor tissue [32,33]. As a result, the nanoprecipitation method was selected for subsequent optimization.

3.2.2. Variation in Water–Ethanol Volume Ratios

Zein-based hybrid lipid nanoparticles entrapping coumarin-6 were prepared using four distinct water–ethanol volume ratios (2:1, 3:1, 4:1, and 5:1) (Table 1). Their size was relatively close when using water–ethanol ratios of 2:1 and 3:1 (224.3 ± 28.0 nm and 217.1 ± 69.2 nm, respectively), slightly smaller at a ratio of 5:1 (178.9 ± 24.2 nm), but much larger (408.0 ± 73.1 nm) at a ratio of 4:1. Their PDI values exhibited an upward trend as the water–ethanol volume ratio increased from 2:1 to 4:1 (0.25 ± 0.06, 0.40 ± 0.06, and 0.67 ± 0.07 from 2:1 to 4:1, respectively). Their zeta potentials spanned a range from −21 to −23 mV (−21.8 ± 1.0 mV, −23.2 ± 0.8 mV, −23.1 ± 1.2 mV, and −21.6 ± 0.9 mV for the water–ethanol volume ratios 2:1 to 5:1, respectively). Conversely, the percentage of drug entrapment in the nanoparticles widely differed. Optimal entrapment (94.1 ± 2.7%) was achieved at a 2:1 ratio. Contrastingly, the three other ratios yielded notably diminished drug entrapment (51.9 ± 0.9%, 37.7 ± 3.0%, and 32.0 ± 1.6% for ratios 3:1 to 5:1, respectively). A water–ethanol volume ratio of 2:1 was thus selected for further studies.

3.2.3. Use of Probe Sonication

Nanoparticles prepared through probe sonication showcased a size that was non-statistically different when compared to those prepared without probe sonication (236.4 ± 2.0 nm) (Table 1). Their negative zeta potential remained similar (−23.5 ± 3.4 mV). However, their size distribution was narrower (PDI of 0.14 ± 0.05). The subsequent nanoparticle preparation therefore included probe sonication in further experiments.

3.2.4. Addition of One-Hour Incubation before Centrifugation

Incorporating a one-hour incubation period prior to centrifugation yielded nanoparticles characterized by an increased size (260.2 ± 3.1 nm), with a marginally broader size distribution (with a PDI of 0.38 ± 0.07) (Table 1). Their zeta potential exhibited no statistically significant variation (−20.9 ± 1.5 mV). Consequently, this supplementary step was subsequently omitted from the nanoparticle preparation process in subsequent experiments.

3.2.5. Variation in Lipid–Zein Weight Ratios

Three lipid–zein weight ratios (1:4, 1:5, and 1:6) were employed for the formulation of zein-based hybrid lipid nanoparticles entrapping coumarin-6 (Table 1). The nanoparticle sizes exhibited similarity (231.1 ± 3.4 nm, 236.4 ± 2.0 nm, and 224.8 ± 7.9 nm for 1:4, 1:5, and 1:6 ratios, respectively), with low PDI values (0.17 ± 0.02, 0.14 ± 0.05, and 0.15 ± 0.03 for 1:4, 1:5, and 1:6 ratios, respectively). Their zeta potentials demonstrated a negative charge (−17.2 ± 0.7 mV, −23.5 ± 3.4 mV, and −20.1 ± 0.7 mV for ratios 1:4 to 1:6, respectively), with the highest level of stability observed at a 1:5 ratio. Drawing from these findings, the 1:5 ratio was selected for nanoparticle preparation in subsequent experiments.

3.2.6. Variation in the Amount of Zein

Three amounts of zein (30, 40, and 50 mg) were used in nanoparticle preparation. The resultant nanoparticles consistently displayed sizes below 240 nm, with the smallest size achieved utilizing 40 mg of zein (236.4 ± 2.0 nm, 215.9 ± 6.8 nm, and 225.3 ± 6.2 nm for 30, 40, and 50 mg of zein, respectively) (Table 1). The nanoparticles showcased a very narrow size distribution, reflected by PDI values below 0.2 (0.14 ± 0.05, 0.16 ± 0.04, and 0.15 ± 0.01 when using 30, 40, and 50 mg of zein, respectively). Their zeta potential increased with increasing amounts of zein (ranging from −23.5 ± 3.4 mV to −16.6 ± 0.0 mV for 30 and 50 mg of zein, respectively). The percentage of coumarin-6 entrapment within the nanoparticles was very high (80.0 ± 1.9% and 83.7 ± 1.8% for 30 and 50 mg of zein weight), with the highest (92.0 ± 0.9%) achieved when using 40 mg zein. Considering these findings, a 40 mg amount of zein was therefore selected for subsequent experiments, due to the smallest resultant particle size and the highest percentage of drug entrapment.

3.2.7. Variation in Drug Amount Related to Zein Weight

Nanoparticles entrapping coumarin-6 were prepared by employing two distinct percentages of coumarin amount (0.1 and 0.5%) relative to the zein weight.

Notably, the nanoparticles formulated with a drug amount of 0.1% of zein weight displayed a reduced size of 201.2 ± 6.7 nm, compared with the nanoparticles prepared with 0.5% of coumarin to zein weight (215.9 ± 6.8 nm). However, their zeta potential was similar (−17.2 ± 0.8 mV and −18.4 ± 0.5 mV for 0.1% and 0.5% of the drug amount added, respectively) (Table 1). Both formulations exhibited narrow size distributions (with PDIs lower than 0.2 for both cases). However, a significant contrast emerged in terms of drug entrapment, with a mere 10.0 ± 0.2% of the drug being entrapped in the 0.1% coumarin-6 formulation, as opposed to the substantially higher drug entrapment (92.0 ± 0.9%) achieved with the 0.5% coumarin-6 formulation. In light of these observations, a coumarin amount of 0.5% relative to zein weight was selected for subsequent experiments.

The optimized formulation of zein-based hybrid lipid nanoparticles entrapping coumarin-6 was therefore prepared using the nanoprecipitation method, coupled with probe sonication. This optimal formulation encompassed key parameters, including a zein weight of 40 mg, a water–ethanol volume ratio of 2:1, and a lipid–zein weight ratio of 1:5. Additionally, the formulation incorporated a 0.5% drug content relative to the zein weight, achieved by adding 100 µL from a 2 mg/mL stock of coumarin-6.

3.3. *Preparation of Transferrin-Bearing Zein-Based Hybrid Lipid Nanoparticles Encapsulating Docetaxel*

Transferrin-bearing zein-based hybrid lipid nanoparticles entrapping docetaxel were successfully prepared. TEM images revealed that they had a spherical shape (Figure 1).

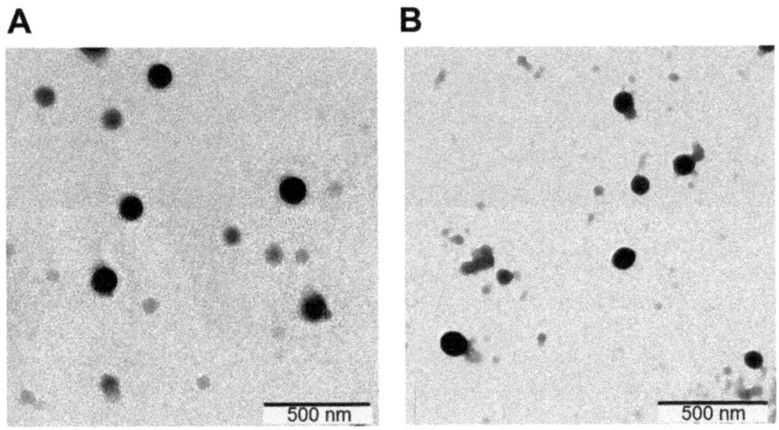

Figure 1. TEM pictures of (**A**) transferrin-bearing and (**B**) control zein-based hybrid lipid nanoparticles.

The entrapment efficiency of docetaxel within the nanoparticles was relatively high, respectively, 59.6 ± 2.1% and 67.7 ± 1.8% of docetaxel for Tf-bearing and control nanoparticles (equivalent to 119.2 ± 1.7 mg and 135.4 ± 1.2 µg of docetaxel, respectively).

Tf was conjugated to the nanoparticles at the substantial level of 66.9 ± 0.8% of the initial Tf (equivalent to 6.7 ± 0.5 mg of Tf per mL of nanoparticles).

The conjugation of Tf to the surface of the nanoparticles led to an increase in the hydrodynamic size of the targeted nanoparticles (344.2 ± 15.9 nm, with a PDI of 0.24 ± 0.03). In contrast, the size of control nanoparticles was notably smaller, measuring 182.0 ± 2.5 nm with a PDI of 0.12 ± 0.02. It also marginally decreased the net surface charge of Tf-bearing nanoparticles (−28.9 ± 0.5 mV), relative to the control formulation (−23.3 ± 1.4 mV).

3.4. Stability of the Formulations

Transferrin-bearing and control zein-based hybrid lipid nanoparticles entrapping docetaxel were found to be stable when stored at 4 °C for a duration of 4 weeks. They displayed a slight increase in size and polydispersity index over the course of 28 days (from 271.6 ± 6.1 nm (PDI: 0.25 ± 0.02) on Day 0 to 342.2 ± 1.4 nm (PDI: 0.33 ± 0.03) on Day 28 for Tf-bearing formulations; from 272.8 ± 5.7 nm (PDI: 0.18 ± 0.02) on Day 0 to 334.1 ± 10.8 nm (PDI: 0.22 ± 0.02) on Day 28 for control formulations) (Figure 2A,B).

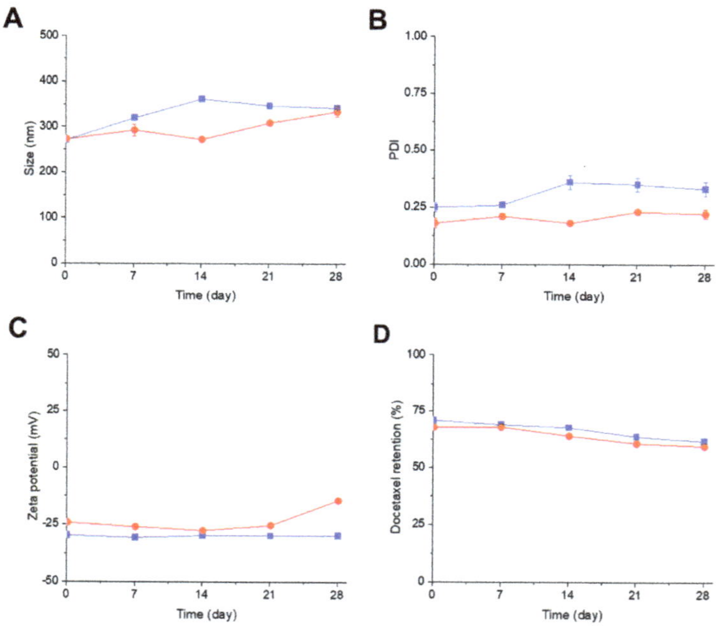

Figure 2. Size (**A**), polydispersity index (**B**), zeta potential (**C**), and drug retention (**D**) of Tf-bearing (■, blue) and control (•, red) zein-based hybrid lipid nanoparticles entrapping docetaxel after storage at 4 °C for 4 weeks (n = 4) (error bars smaller than symbols when not visible).

The zeta potential of the targeted formulation remained stable throughout the entire experiment (−29.8 ± 0.3 mV on Day 0 and −29.9 ± 0.6 mV on Day 28), in contrast to control nanoparticles, which displayed an increase in zeta potential (from −24.4 ± 0.0 mV on Day 0 to −14.4 ± 0.6 mV on Day 28) (Figure 2C).

In terms of drug leakage, the percentage of drug retention, although gradually decreasing, remained notably high over the 4-week period (reducing from 70.9 ± 1.0% on Day 0 to 61.6 ± 0.9% on Day 28 for targeted nanoparticles, and from 67.7 ± 0.8 on Day 0 to 59.5 ± 0.4% on Day 28 for control nanoparticles) (Figure 2D).

3.5. Drug Release

The Tf-bearing and control zein-based hybrid lipid nanoparticles consistently demonstrated sustained drug release profiles across pH levels of 5.5, 6.5, and 7.4, following an initial burst release phase. Notably, the drug released from the solution exhibited rapid diffusion through the dialysis membrane, resulting in complete release within 8 h (Figure 3).

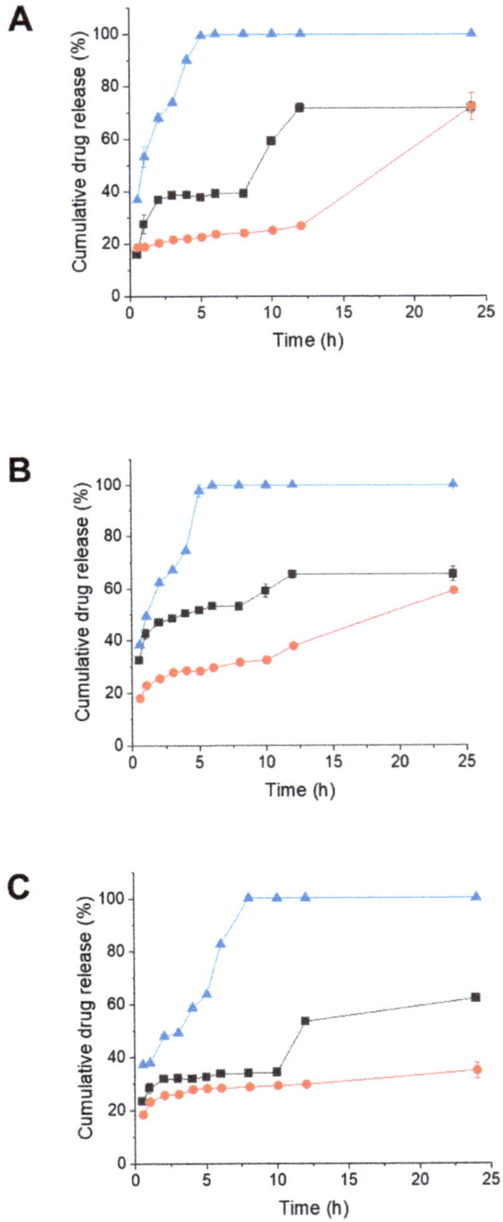

Figure 3. Drug release profile of docetaxel entrapped in Tf-bearing (■, black), control zein-based hybrid lipid nanoparticles (•, red), or in solution (▲, blue) in phosphate buffers at pH 5.5 (**A**), 6.5 (**B**), and 7.4 (**C**) over 24 h ($n = 3$) (error bars smaller than symbols when not visible).

At pH 5.5, transferrin-bearing nanoparticles exhibited a gradual initial release of docetaxel, with 40% of the maximum release occurring within the first 8 h (Figure 3A). Subsequently, the drug release then increased, reaching its highest percentage (72%) at 12 h. In comparison, control nanoparticles displayed a slower drug release within the first 12 h (peaking at 26.9% of docetaxel released), followed by a sharp surge in release to match the levels of the Tf-bearing formulation (72% of the drug released at 24 h). Conversely, docetaxel in solution was fully released from the dialysis tubing within 5 h (Figure 3A).

At pH 6.5, transferrin-bearing nanoparticles led to a faster drug release than at pH 5.5, with 53% of the drug released within the initial 8 h and reaching 65% at 12 h (Figure 3B). In contrast, control nanoparticles exhibited a slower drug release profile compared to transferrin-bearing nanoparticles (with only 59.3% of the drug released at 24 h), while docetaxel in solution reached complete release within 6 h. The cumulative drug release percentages for both transferrin-bearing and control nanoparticles were lower than those observed at pH 5.5 (Figure 3B).

At pH 7.4, transferrin-bearing nanoparticles resulted in an even more restrained drug release compared to pH 5.5 and 6.5. Over the initial 10 h, the drug exhibited a gradual release (34% released) to reach its highest percentage of 62.1% at 24 h (Figure 3C). Control nanoparticles displayed a similarly limited drug release, with only 34.9% of the drug released within 24 h. In contrast, docetaxel in solution attained complete release in 7 h.

Overall, the highest cumulative drug release percentages were observed at pH 5.5 for both transferrin-bearing and control nanoparticles (Figure 3).

3.6. *In Vitro Studies*

3.6.1. Cellular Uptake

The entrapment of docetaxel in Tf-bearing zein-based hybrid lipid nanoparticles significantly increased the drug uptake by both PC-3 and LNCaP cancer cell lines compared to control nanoparticles and drug solution (Figure 4).

In PC3-Luc cells, the drug uptake was higher than that of the control nanoparticles and the drug solution by 1.8-fold and 1.2-fold, respectively (13,880 ± 221 a.u for Tf-bearing nanoparticles, 7366 ± 520 a.u for control nanoparticles, and 11,239 ± 532 a.u. for the drug solution) (Figure 4A).

In contrast, within DU145 cells, the treatment with docetaxel solution yielded the highest cellular uptake, exhibiting a mean fluorescence intensity of 146 ± 11.67 a.u., in contrast to 88 ± 7.57 a.u. and 103.3 ± 8.9 a.u. for docetaxel entrapped in targeted and non-targeted nanoparticles, respectively (Figure 4B).

In the case of LNCaP cells, the conjugation of transferrin to the nanoparticles notably enhanced the cellular uptake of fluorescein-labelled docetaxel, leading to a 1.3-fold increase in mean fluorescence intensity (3740 ± 16 a.u.) compared to control nanoparticles (with a mean fluorescence intensity of 2783 ± 64 a.u.) (Figure 4C). Conversely, the uptake of docetaxel solution was comparatively the lowest, with a mean fluorescence intensity of 2504 ± 56 a.u.

These findings correlated well with the observations made through confocal microscopy.

In PC-3-Luc cells, the treatment with transferrin-bearing zein-based hybrid lipid nanoparticles yielded a notably higher cellular uptake of docetaxel, contrasting against the uptake seen with control nanoparticles (Figure 5A). The fluorescence intensity associated with cellular uptake following drug solution treatment also appeared substantial.

For DU145 cells, the most pronounced fluorescence intensity was observed in cells treated with docetaxel in solution, followed by cells treated with control zein-based hybrid lipid nanoparticles, with transferrin-bearing nanoparticles entrapping fluorescein-labelled docetaxel displaying comparatively lower fluorescence intensity (Figure 5B).

Within LNCaP cells, the peak fluorescence intensity was observed in cells treated with docetaxel entrapped within the targeted delivery system. This was followed by cells treated with docetaxel entrapped within the control delivery system (Figure 5C).

Throughout these treatments, fluorescein-labelled docetaxel showcased distribution within the cell cytoplasm, with no observable co-localization within the nucleus.

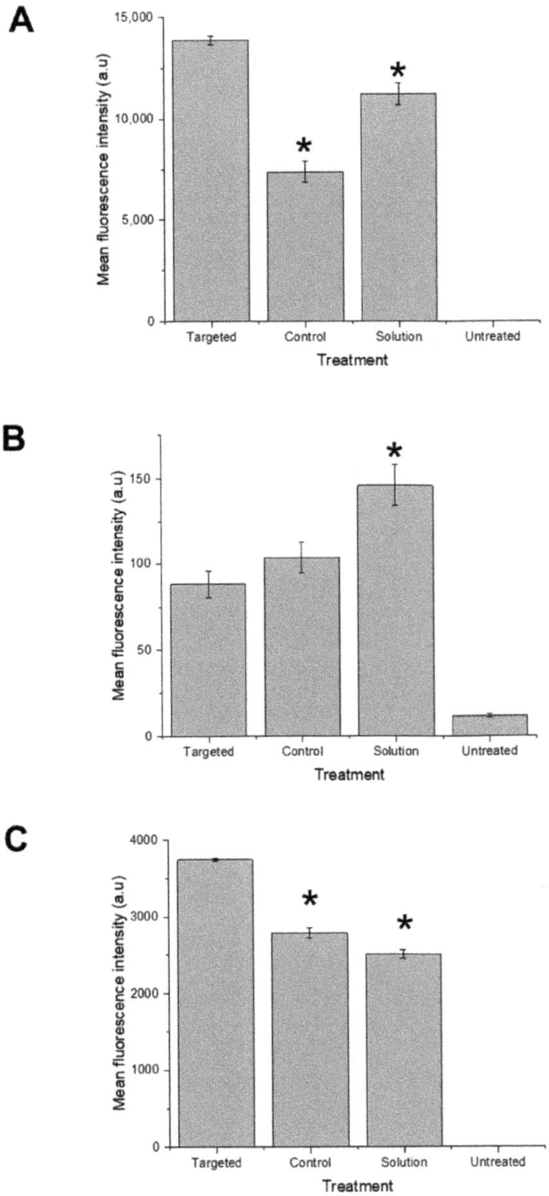

Figure 4. Quantification of the cellular uptake of fluorescein-labelled docetaxel entrapped in Tf-bearing and control zein-based hybrid lipid nanoparticles or as solution in PC3-Luc (**A**), DU145 (**B**), and LNCaP (**C**) cells (a.u.: arbitrary units) (*: $p < 0.05$ vs. Tf-bearing zein-based hybrid lipid nanoparticles). Results represent mean ± SEM of 3 independent experiments.

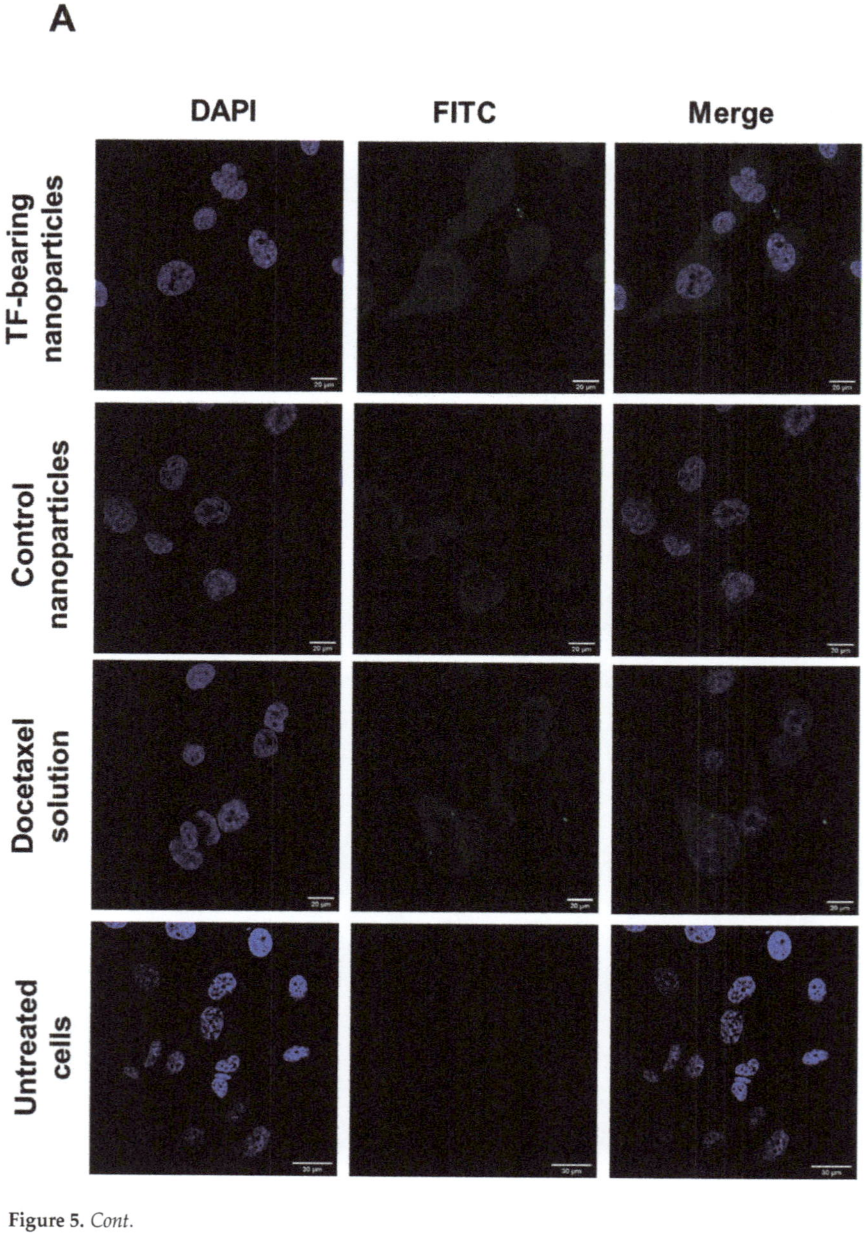

Figure 5. *Cont.*

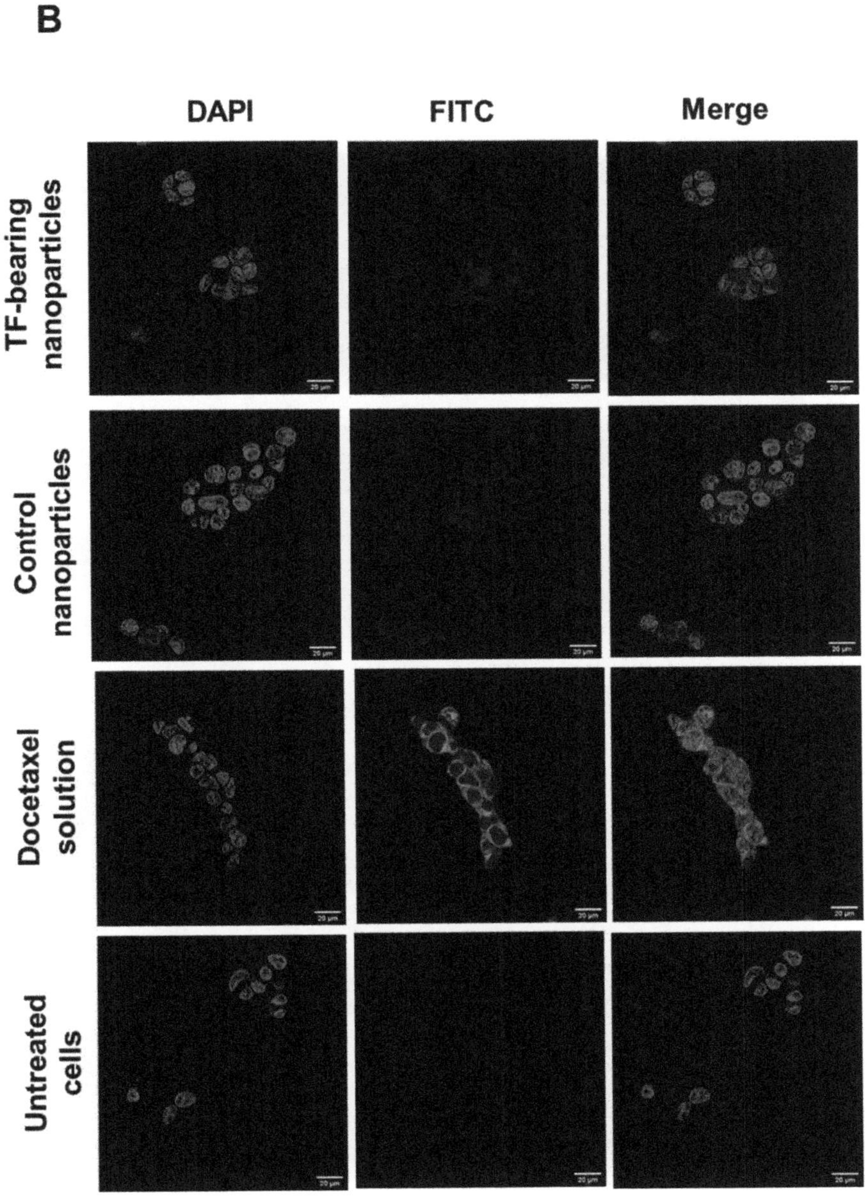

Figure 5. *Cont.*

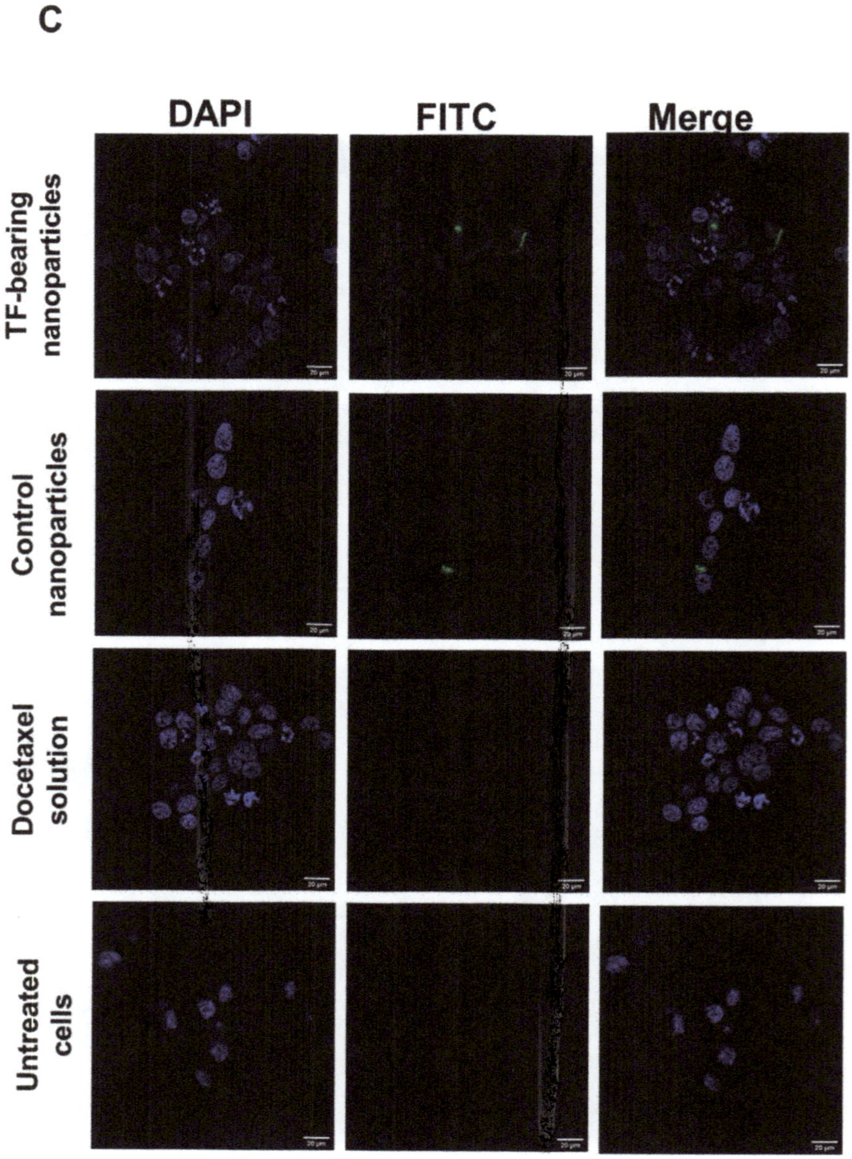

Figure 5. Confocal microscopy images of the cellular uptake of fluorescein-labelled docetaxel (at a concentration of 12 μg/well) entrapped in transferrin-bearing and control zein-based hybrid lipid nanoparticles as well as in solution, after incubation for 15 h with PC3-Luc (**A**), DU145 (**B**), and LNCaP cells (**C**). Blue: nuclei stained with DAPI (excitation: 405 nm laser line, bandwidth: 400–480 nm), green: fluorescein-labelled docetaxel (excitation: 494 nm laser line, bandwidth: 510–530 nm) (bar size: 20 μm).

3.6.2. Mechanisms of Cellular Uptake

The uptake of docetaxel entrapped within transferrin-bearing zein-based hybrid lipid nanoparticles was significantly decreased by both filipin and colchicine, resulting in cellular uptake inhibitions of 92.0% and 92.4%, respectively. These outcomes suggest that the primary mechanism of internalization involves caveolae-mediated endocytosis and macropinocytosis (Figure 6).

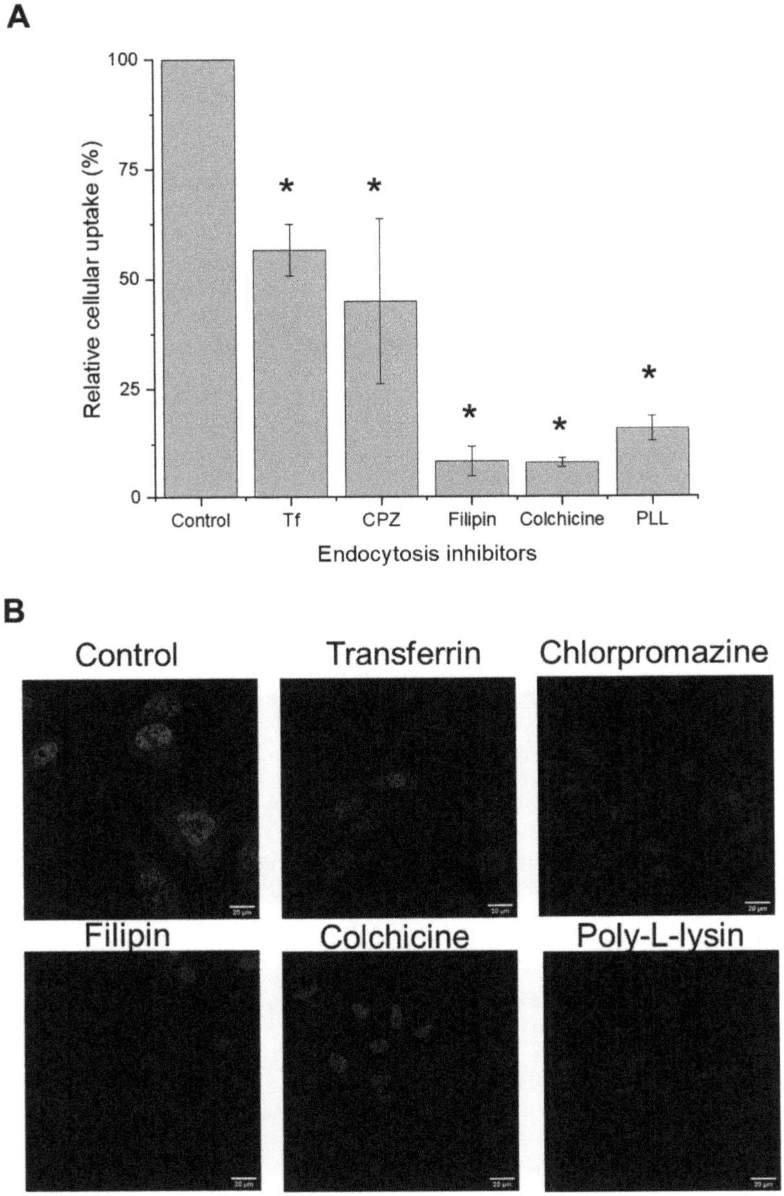

Figure 6. Relative cellular uptake of fluorescein-labelled docetaxel entrapped in Tf-bearing zein-based hybrid lipid nanoparticles by PC3-Luc cells in the presence of endocytosis inhibitors, using flow cytometry (**A**) and confocal microscopy (**B**) (*: $p < 0.05$ vs. no inhibitor). Results represent mean ± SEM of 3 repeats.

Pre-treatment of the cells with PLL, which acts as an uptake inhibitor for cationic delivery systems, resulted in a notable 84.5% reduction in cellular uptake, thus demonstrating the influence of nanoparticle charges on the internalization of docetaxel entrapped within transferrin-bearing nanoparticles.

In addition, the nanoparticles uptake was partially inhibited by free transferrin and chlorpromazine (with inhibitions of 45 and 59%, respectively), suggesting that this delivery system was also internalized through transferrin receptors and clathrin-mediated endocytosis (Figure 6A). Confocal microscopy imaging of cellular uptake mechanisms yielded similar trends (Figure 6B).

3.6.3. Anti-Proliferative Efficacy

In PC3-Luc cells, treatment of the cells with docetaxel entrapped within transferrin-bearing zein-based hybrid lipid nanoparticles resulted in a significant increase in anti-proliferative efficacy compared to docetaxel solution, when using docetaxel concentrations exceeding 1 μg/mL (Figure 7A). Both Tf-bearing and control formulations showcased similar anti-proliferative efficacy. At a drug concentration of 30 μg/mL, the percentages of cell viability were 31.0 ± 2.1% and 31.8 ± 1.9% for Tf-bearing and control formulations, respectively, whereas treatment with docetaxel solution yielded a higher cell viability of 45.9 ± 1.9%.

In DU145 cells, the conjugation of Tf to the nanoparticles led to a significantly enhanced antiproliferative efficacy at drug concentrations of 0.1, 1, and 10 μg/mL, although the most potent formulation at these concentrations remained docetaxel solution (Figure 7B). At the highest drug concentration tested (30 μg/mL), the cell viability was 10.3 ± 0.4% and 9.6 ± 0.3% following treatment with Tf-bearing and control nanoparticles, which was about 3-fold higher than that resulting from docetaxel solution treatment (3.6 ± 0.2%).

In LNCaP cells, docetaxel nanoparticle formulations at drug concentrations of 1 μg/mL and above demonstrated increased anti-proliferative efficacy when compared to the drug solution, with the highest efficacy observed following treatment with the control nanoparticles (Figure 7C). At the highest tested docetaxel concentration (30 μg/mL), the percentages of cell viability were 12.0 ± 0.7%, 4.6 ± 0.3%, and 16.3 ± 1.9% for cells treated with docetaxel entrapped in Tf-bearing, control zein-based hybrid lipid nanoparticles, and docetaxel in solution, respectively.

The anti-proliferative efficacy of docetaxel entrapped within transferrin-bearing zein-based hybrid lipid nanoparticles exhibited a ranking order of higher efficacy in DU145 cells, followed by LNCaP cells, and then PC3 cells, with respective reductions in cell viability of 89.7%, 88%, and 70%.

Docetaxel entrapped within Tf-bearing lipid nanoparticles exhibited notably higher anti-proliferative efficacy in comparison to control nanoparticles when evaluated on DU145 and LNCaP cells (IC_{50}: 0.02 ± 0.01 μg/mL vs. 1.96 ± 0.54 μg/mL for Tf-bearing and control formulations in DU145 cells; 0.02 ± 0.00 μg/mL vs. 0.05 ± 0.01 μg/mL for Tf-bearing and control formulations in LNCaP cells). However, despite these enhancements, docetaxel solution continued to demonstrate the utmost anti-proliferative efficacy across all three cell lines, displaying its most minimal IC_{50} of $0.0006 \pm 8 \times 10^{-4}$ μg/mL in PC3 cells (Table 2).

Table 2. Anti-proliferative efficacy of docetaxel entrapped in Tf-bearing and control zein-based hybrid lipid nanoparticles, or in solution, in PC3-Luc, DU145, and LNCaP cells. Results are expressed as mean ± S.E.M (n = 15).

IC_{50} (μg/mL) (mean ± S.E.M.)			
	Formulations		
Cell Line	**Tf-bearing LNP**	**Control LNP**	**Docetaxel Solution**
PC3-Luc	0.25 ± 0.04	0.08 ± 0.02	$0.0006 \pm 8 \times 10^{-4}$
DU145	0.02 ± 0.01	1.96 ± 0.54	0.0045 ± 0.0009
LNCaP	0.02 ± 0.00	0.05 ± 0.01	0.0023 ± 0.0014

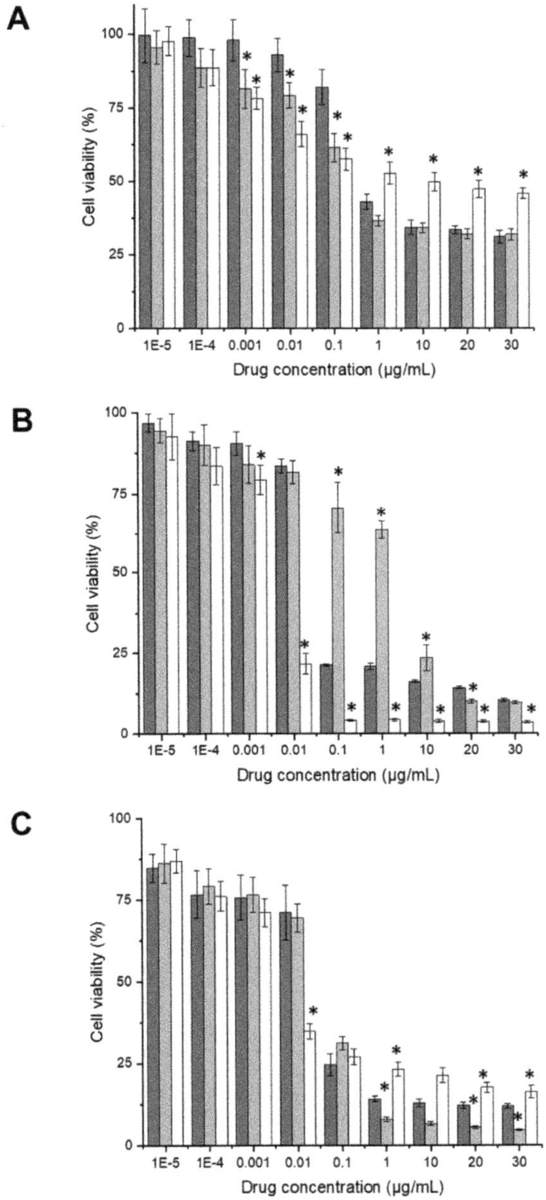

Figure 7. Anti-proliferative efficacy of docetaxel entrapped in Tf-bearing zein-based hybrid lipid nanoparticles (dark grey), control lipid nanoparticles (grey), or in solution (white), on PC3-Luc (**A**), DU145 (**B**), and LNCaP (**C**) cells (*: $p < 0.05$ vs. the drug concentration leading to the highest cell viability) ($n = 15$).

3.7. Evaluation of the Potential Use of Tf-Bearing Zein-Based Hybrid Lipid Nanoparticles for Gene Therapy

3.7.1. Evaluation of DNA Condensation

Tf-bearing zein-based hybrid lipid nanoparticles effectively condensed over 80% of DNA at polymer–DNA weight ratios of 1500:1 and 2000:1, showcasing condensation capabilities of 83% and 84%, respectively (Figure 8A). This DNA condensation occurred instantly and exhibited stability for a minimum of 24 h. As the polymer–DNA weight ratios decreased, the level of DNA condensation also decreased. At lower polymer–DNA weight ratios of 500:1 and 1000:1, it dropped to 49% and 60%, respectively. At even lower ratios ranging from 250:1 to 50:1, DNA complexation was notably limited, ranging from 29% to 10%.

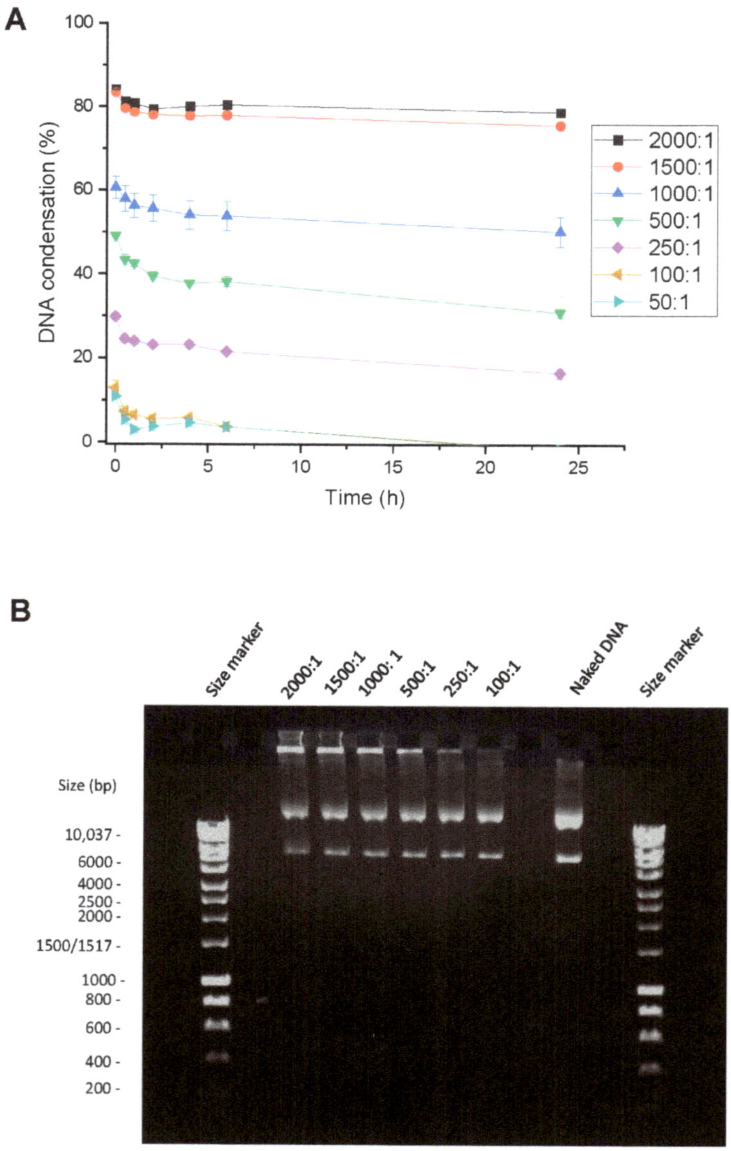

Figure 8. DNA condensation to Tf-bearing zein-based hybrid lipid nanoparticles at various polymer–DNA ratios, using PicoGreen® assay (**A**) (n = 4) and gel retardation assay (**B**) (error bars smaller than symbols when not visible).

A gel retardation assay confirmed the complete and partial condensation of DNA by Tf-bearing zein-based hybrid lipid nanoparticles (Figure 8B). At polymer–DNA weight ratios of 1500:1 and 2000:1, DNA was predominantly condensed by Tf-bearing zein-based hybrid lipid nanoparticles, effectively inhibiting the intercalation of ethidium bromide with DNA. Consequently, minimal DNA was visually discernible at these ratios. Conversely, at polymer–DNA ratios of 250:1 and 100:1, DNA underwent partial condensation by transferrin-bearing nanoparticles. This allowed for ethidium bromide to intercalate with DNA, resulting in a prominent band indicative of free DNA at these two ratios.

3.7.2. Measurement of the Size and Zeta Potential of the Complexes

Transferrin-bearing zein-based hybrid nanoparticles complexed with DNA consistently displayed an average size of less than 600 nm across all polymer–DNA weight ratios investigated (Figure 9A). Their size increased with increasing weight ratios used (Figure 9A), spanning from 456.7 ± 3.0 nm at a polymer–DNA weight ratio of 50:1 to 583.1 ± 48.8 nm at a ratio of 2000:1.

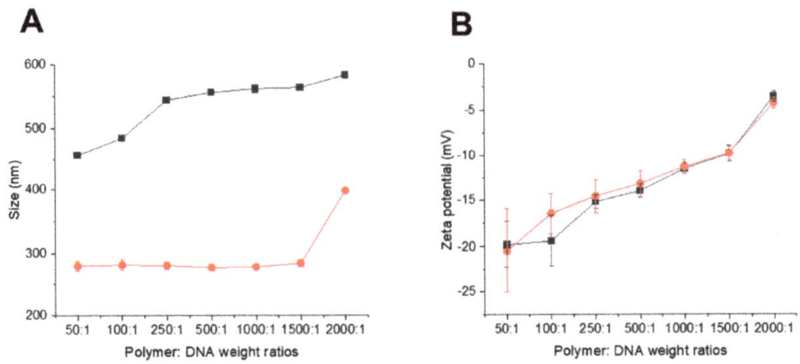

Figure 9. Size (**A**) and zeta potential (**B**) of transferrin-bearing zein-based hybrid lipid nanoparticles (black, ■) and control zein-based hybrid lipid nanoparticles (red, •) complexed with DNA at various polymer–DNA weight ratios. Results are expressed as mean ± SEM (n = 4) (error bars smaller than symbols when not visible).

Conversely, the size of control zein-based hybrid nanoparticles complexed with DNA remained stable within the range from 50:1 to 1500:1 ratios, measuring between 279.2 ± 8.1 nm and 283.5 ± 6.6 nm. It increased at the higher polymer–DNA ratio of 2000:1, reaching 397.7 ± 0.5 nm (Figure 9A).

Both transferrin-bearing and control zein-based hybrid nanoparticles complexed with DNA were bearing a negative surface charge, which increased with increasing polymer–DNA ratios (from −19.8 ± 2.5 mV DNA at a weight ratio of 50:1 to −3.5 ± 0.5 mV at a weight ratio of 2000:1 for the transferrin-bearing complex; from −20.5 ± 4.5 mV to −4.2 ± 0.5 mV at 50:1 and 2000:1 ratios for the control complex (Figure 9B).

3.7.3. Gene Expression

Transferrin-bearing zein-based hybrid lipid nanoparticles complexed to a plasmid DNA encoding β-galactosidase exhibited increased gene expression at optimal polymer–DNA ratios across the three tested cell lines, in comparison to DAB–DNA and PEI–DNA complexes (Figure 10). The highest level of transfection was achieved at polymer–DNA weight ratios of 2000:1 for all three cell lines (11.19 ± 0.48 mU/mL in PC3-Luc cells, 8.71 ± 0.37 mU/mL in DU145 cells, and 12.23 ± 0.29 mU/mL in LNCaP cells). This result marked a substantial increase of 1.7-fold, 6.7-fold, and 11.4-fold when compared to DAB–DNA in PC3-Luc, DU145, and LNCaP cells; and 6.5-fold, 8.3-fold, and 11.9-fold in comparison to PEI–DNA in the corresponding cell lines. Notably, the highest transfection efficacy was observed in LNCaP cells, followed by PC-3-Luc cells.

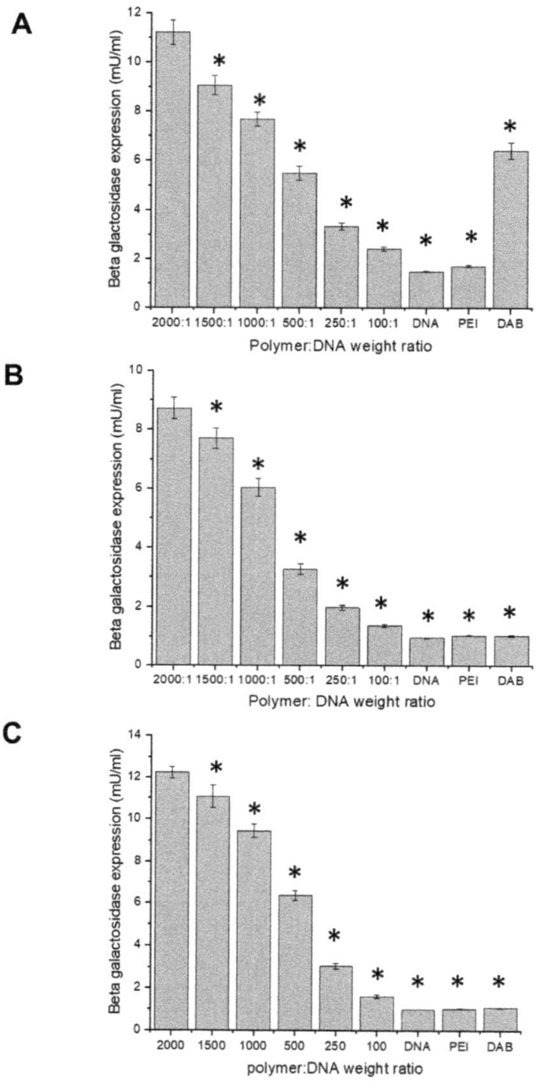

Figure 10. Gene expression efficacy of transferrin-bearing zein-based hybrid lipid nanoparticles in PC3-Luc (**A**), DU145 (**B**), and LNCaP cells (**C**). Results are expressed as mean ± SEM ($n = 15$), using DAB–DNA and PEI–DNA as positive controls (*: $p < 0.05$ vs. the polymer–DNA ratio leading to the highest transfection).

In PC3-luc cells, the three highest ratios of transferrin-bearing zein-based hybrid lipid nanoparticles complexed to a plasmid DNA led to an increased gene expression relative to DAB–DNA. Furthermore, all the tested ratios of this formulation resulted in increased transfection compared to PEI–DNA (Figure 10A). Similarly, in DU145 and LNCaP cells, the transferrin-bearing complex at all ratios led to an increased gene expression compared to PEI–DNA and DAB–DNA (Figure 10B,C).

4. Discussion

The potential application of nanomedicines in cancer therapy is currently hindered by the limitations in existing delivery systems. These systems often fail to achieve precise targeting, leading to adverse effects on healthy tissues [34]. Additionally, they struggle to encapsulate hydrophobic anti-cancer drugs, which constitute over 40% of emerging pharmaceuticals [35], and effectively transport therapeutic nucleic acids. Furthermore, the complexity of their manufacturing methods imposes further restrictions on their practical application [36].

To address these challenges, we hypothesize that hybrid lipid nanoparticles made of biocompatible and biodegradable zein and conjugated to transferrin (whose receptors are overexpressed on cancer cells), able to entrap the hydrophobic anti-cancer drug docetaxel and carry plasmid DNA, would enhance the delivery of the therapeutic payloads to prostate cancer cells and increase their anti-proliferative efficacy and gene expression levels.

In this study, coumarin-6 was entrapped within zein-based hybrid lipid nanoparticles. Zein, a hydrophobic and biodegradable protein extracted from corn, was used to form the polymeric core of these hybrid nanoparticles. The core effectively entrapped coumarin-6, while a lipid monolayer composed of DSPE-PEG2K-MAL surrounded it. This lipid layer served multiple functions, including conferring a stealth effect and facilitating surface modification [37–39].

The lipid nanoparticles were successfully prepared using nanoprecipitation, where the zein dissolved in ethanol was mixed with the lipid dispersed in water to allow for self-assembling. Mixing these two solutions caused a decrease in the concentration of the organic solvent (ethanol) within the dissolved zein solution. This reduction triggered processes such as desolvation, phase separation, and ultimately, the formation of nanoparticles. In addition, the one-step nanoprecipitation method exhibited distinct advantages over alternative techniques for nanoparticle generation, such as the two-step nanoprecipitation method. This one-step approach consumed less time and energy. Due to its efficiency, it has gained widespread popularity for encapsulating various drugs [40,41].

Among the various formulations investigated, zein-based hybrid lipid nanoparticles entrapping coumarin-6 (used as a fluorescent lipophilic drug model) prepared using the nanoprecipitation method, coupled with probe sonication, formulated with a zein weight of 40 mg, a water–ethanol volume ratio of 2:1, and a lipid–zein weight ratio of 1:5, and incorporating a 0.5% drug content relative to the zein weight, yielded optimal results. They were found to exhibit a compact particle size (215.9 $\pm$ 6.8 nm), with a low PDI (0.16 $\pm$ 0.04). Additionally, they displayed a negative zeta potential (-18.4 ± 0.5 mV), while maintaining a high entrapment of coumarin-6 (92.0 $\pm$ 0.9%). These hybrid lipid nanoparticles had a size smaller than the critical threshold for extravasation (which has been determined to be around 400 nm for most tumors [33]) and therefore have the required properties to access the cancer cells and deliver the entrapped drug. Moreover, the negative charge they carried further contributed to their efficacy. This negative charge would diminish the likelihood of electrostatic interactions with negatively charged cell membranes, therefore reducing any non-specific uptake by non-cancerous cells [42].

The optimal formulation of zein-based hybrid lipid nanoparticles was obtained when using a low water to organic solvent volume ratio of 2:1, which resulted in a small particle size while concurrently maintaining a high entrapment of coumarin-6 (exceeding 90%). Increasing the volume ratio of water to organic solvent caused a significant decrease in the entrapment efficiency of coumarin-6, as the drug exhibits poor solubility similarly to our findings when optimizing transferrin-targeted PEGylated nanoparticles entrapping the hydrophobic plumbagin [43].

Low lipid to zein weight ratios were needed to achieve an optimal formulation of zein-based hybrid lipid nanoparticles to ensure that the surface of the zein core was enveloped by the lipids [44]. When employing high lipid to zein weight ratios, the surplus of DSPE-PEG2K-MAL lipids would have the potential to spontaneously form liposomes. This outcome would lead to a noticeable increase in the overall hydrodynamic size of the nanoparticles and a subsequent reduction in their zeta potential value.

The specific arrangements of PEG chains at varying grafting densities could also influence the size of the delivery system [45,46]. When present at a low density (10–30 mol%), the PEG chains adopted a mushroom-like conformation which had a limited effect on the size and zeta potential of the particles. In contrast, higher grafting densities prompted the PEG chains to stretch and form a brush-like structure, leading to an increase in the size and zeta potential of the particles.

Subsequently, the zein-based hybrid lipid nanoparticles were then conjugated with transferrin using the thiol–maleimide 'click' reaction, a commonly used thiol-based bioconjugation technique for conjugating antibodies, proteins, or peptides to delivery systems. Its popularity stems from its compatibility with aqueous environments, swift reaction kinetics (without necessitating heat or catalysts), and high selectivity [47]. Traut's reagent (2-iminothiolane) was used as a cross-linking agent to produce a thiolated form of Tf by thiolation of the amino group present within the transferrin, which could subsequently interact with the thiol-reactive maleimide group. As a result of this procedure, the conjugation process was successful, with a yield of 66.9 ± 0.8% of the initial Tf being effectively conjugated. While no existing literature detailing the formulation of a transferrin-bearing zein-based delivery system was found for comparative purposes, our results aligned with prior findings from our research group. This consistency was observed across various delivery systems previously explored by our group in the context of Tf conjugation [9].

The conjugation of transferrin to the surface of nanoparticles led to a noticeable increase in the mean diameter of the nanoparticles when compared with control nanoparticles, due to the substantial molecular weight of transferrin (ranging from 70,000 to 80,000 Daltons) [48]. Nonetheless, it is essential to note that both the transferrin-bearing and control nanoparticles maintained sizes that remained beneath the threshold necessary for extravasation through the tumor tissue vessels (approximately 400 nm for solid tumors).

Transferrin-bearing hybrid lipid nanoparticles exhibited negative surface charges, attributed to the presence of transferrin itself (with a zeta potential of −28.9 ± 0.5 mV). These negative charges, in conjunction with the PEGylation of the formulation, would effectively prevent the opsonization of the nanoparticles by serum proteins, therefore avoiding a rapid clearance by the mononuclear phagocytic system and extending their circulation time within the bloodstream [49,50]. Furthermore, the transferrin-bearing hybrid lipid nanoparticles could be classified as moderately stable colloidal systems, as their zeta potential value falls within the range from −20 to −30 mV [51].

The entrapment efficiency of docetaxel within the nanoparticles was relatively high, respectively, at 59.6 ± 2.1% and 67.7 ± 1.8% of docetaxel for Tf-bearing and control nanoparticles (equivalent to 119.2 ± 1.7 mg and 135.4 ± 1.2 μg of docetaxel, respectively). This was slightly higher than that reported when entrapping docetaxel within zein nanoparticles coated by a green tea polyphenols/iron coordination complex (45.0 ± 3.1%) [52]. However, it remained below the levels observed when employing glucose-bearing zein nanoparticles (85.23 ± 3.15%) [53], folate-conjugated zein/soy lecithin/carboxymethyl chitosan core−shell nanoparticles (86.75 ± 1.61%) [54], or chondroitin sulfate-hybridized zein nanoparticles (64.2 ± 1.9%) [55]. We were unable to find any existing publications detailing the entrapment efficiency of docetaxel within hybrid lipid nanoparticles for the purpose of comparison with our findings. Moreover, when stored at 4 °C over a span of 4 weeks, the transferrin-bearing hybrid lipid nanoparticles demonstrated minimal alterations in size and drug leakage. This stability over time and under these storage conditions is an encouraging indicator of the robustness of the formulation.

Transferrin-bearing hybrid lipid nanoparticles displayed a sustained release profile of docetaxel, likely attributed to the diffusion of the drug entrapped within the zein core through water-filled pores. This diffusion-based mechanism of release is a widely recognized phenomenon in polymer-based nanoparticles [56].

It was initially anticipated that the Tf-bearing nanoparticles would exhibit a comparatively slower drug release when compared with the control formulation. This expectation arose from the hypothesis that the conjugated transferrin might hinder the diffusion of the drug out of the zein core. However, that was not the case in this study. The observed release profile was consistent with findings from other studies involving chondroitin sulfate-hybridized zein nanoparticles, folate-conjugated zein/soy lecithin/carboxymethyl chitosan core−shell nanoparticles, and glucose-bearing zein nanoparticles. In all these cases, approximately 60% of the drug was released within a 24 h timeframe [53–55]. This similarity suggests a common release pattern among these formulations.

The cellular uptake studies revealed a significant increase in drug uptake upon the conjugation of transferrin to zein-based hybrid lipid nanoparticles, particularly in comparison with the control formulation and the drug solution on PC-3 and LNCaP cancer cell lines. These findings were in accordance with earlier research conducted by Guo and colleagues. In their study, the use of transferrin as a targeting ligand on lipid-coated PLGA nanoparticles entrapping doxorubicin led to a substantial 2.8-fold improvement in cellular uptake of doxorubicin compared to non-targeted nanoparticles in A549 cells [57]. Similar findings were also reported by Zheng and colleagues, who demonstrated that transferrin-conjugated lipid-coated PLGA nanoparticles entrapping calcein exhibited more effective uptake by SKBR-3 breast cancer cells than their non-targeted counterparts [58]. Furthermore, the presence of transferrin has been shown to impede the efflux of delivery systems from within cells, resulting in increased retention of drugs within the cells [59]. The cellular uptake of docetaxel within the targeted nanoparticles displayed the lowest rates in DU145 cells compared with the two other cell lines. This variation was attributed to the lower expression of transferrin receptors on DU145 cells, as documented by Deng and colleagues [60].

The uptake of docetaxel entrapped within transferrin-bearing zein-based hybrid lipid nanoparticles was predominantly hindered by both filipin and colchicine. Filipin, known as a pinocytosis inhibitor, blocks the caveolae-mediated process, which is a form of clathrin-independent endocytosis [61]. Colchicine has previously been shown to inhibit macropinocytosis, a non-specific process used to internalize particles and fluids [62]. These findings collectively propose that the principal mode of internalization for transferrin-bearing zein-based hybrid lipid nanoparticles encompasses two pathways: caveolae-mediated endocytosis, which is essential for Tf receptor-mediated endocytosis, and macropinocytosis.

The entrapment of docetaxel within transferrin-bearing zein-based hybrid lipid nanoparticles led to a significant increase in anti-proliferative efficacy when compared to docetaxel solution, at high docetaxel concentrations exceeding 1 μg/mL, in PC-3 cells. This could be attributed to the enhanced cellular uptake facilitated by the targeted formulation. However, in DU145 cells, the most potent formulation at high drug concentrations remained the docetaxel solution, aligning with the higher cellular uptake observed for this formulation. Intriguingly, the highest anti-proliferative efficacy emerged from the treatment with control nanoparticles in LNCaP cells. Prior research has already highlighted the capability of various zein-based delivery systems to improve the anti-proliferative efficacy of docetaxel. For example, the IC_{50} values of docetaxel solution and chondroitin sulfate-hybridized zein nanoparticles were reported as 170.7 ± 7.5 and 61.2 ± 10.4 ng/mL after 72 h of incubation in PC-3 cells. This can be partly attributed to the enhanced cellular uptake efficiency of the zein nanoparticles [55]. Similarly, in another study, the anti-proliferative efficacy induced by folate-conjugated zein/soy lecithin/carboxymethyl chitosan core−shell nanoparticles surpassed that of docetaxel solution, especially at higher drug concentrations, in both MCF-7 and SKOV-3 cells [54].

The potential application of Tf-bearing zein-based hybrid lipid nanoparticles for gene therapy was also examined. These nanoparticles exhibited effective DNA condensation, achieving over 80% condensation levels at polymer–DNA weight ratios of 1500:1 and 2000:1. This DNA condensation remained stable for a minimum of 24 h. While various studies have demonstrated that zein-based delivery systems can condense DNA, quantification of the condensation level has not always been provided. For instance, zein/sodium alginate nanocomposites have been shown to condense DNA using electrophoresis [63]. In another investigation, the DNA condensation by zein-oligochitosan-modified zein was shown to increase with an increasing amount of vector. Moreover, no degradation of plasmid DNA was observed for this polyplex [64].

Interestingly, the size of transferrin-bearing zein-based hybrid nanoparticles complexed with DNA was surprisingly high, consistently ranging from 400 nm to 590 nm. This was observed even at high polymer–DNA ratios of 2000:1 and 1500:1 that led to high DNA condensation. This was unexpected, particularly given that the size of control nanoparticles remained stable and below 400 nm after DNA complexation, and will require further investigation for clarification.

Furthermore, transferrin-bearing hybrid lipid nanoparticles complexed with DNA were bearing negative surface charges, closely resembling those observed with the Tf-bearing formulation entrapping docetaxel.

Despite the observed challenges related to nanoparticle size, and in line with outcomes of DNA condensation observed at the various ratios, transferrin-bearing zein-based hybrid lipid nanoparticles complexed to a plasmid DNA encoding β-galactosidase exhibited increased gene expression at optimal polymer–DNA ratios across the three tested cell lines, in comparison to DAB–DNA and PEI–DNA complexes. The highest level of transfection was achieved at a polymer–DNA weight ratio of 2000:1, which correlated with the highest degree of DNA condensation. It was up to 11-fold higher than that observed with DAB-DNA and PEI-DNA in LNCaP cells. This remarkable improvement surpassed the findings with zein/sodium alginate nanocomposites compared to PEI-DNA transfection [63]. Similarly, Kumari and colleagues reported that increasing the weight ratio could significantly enhance cell transfection efficiency for zein-oligochitosan polyplexes [64]. This polyplex exhibited superior gene transfection levels compared to TOOLSmooth-Fect and 293EZ-FECT transfection reagents. However, differences in cell lines and positive controls used in the two studies prevent direct comparison of the outcomes.

5. Conclusions

In this study, hybrid lipid nanoparticles composed of biocompatible and biodegradable zein, and conjugated to transferrin, were successfully prepared using the nanoprecipitation method. They effectively entrapped the hydrophobic drug docetaxel and demonstrated sustained release over a 24 h period, Notably, they exhibited a cumulative drug release of 72% at pH 5.5, mimicking the acidic endosomal pH of cancer cells. Furthermore, they exhibited enhanced cellular uptake of the drug, with an increase of up to 1.8-fold compared with the control formulation and the drug solution on PC-3 and LNCaP cancer cell lines. This heightened uptake was facilitated through mechanisms including caveolae-mediated endocytosis, which is an essential process for transferrin receptor-mediated endocytosis, and macropinocytosis. Treatment of PC-3 cells with these nanoparticles yielded a substantial increase in anti-proliferative efficacy when compared to docetaxel solution, at high docetaxel concentrations exceeding 1 μg/mL.

In addition, the targeted delivery system demonstrated the ability to condense DNA effectively, achieving condensation rates exceeding 80% at polymer–DNA weight ratios of 1500:1 and 2000:1. This led to an increased gene expression at optimal polymer–DNA ratios across all the three tested cell lines, in comparison to DA–DNA and PEI–DNA complexes. The highest level of transfection was up to 11-fold higher than that observed with DAB-DNA and PEI-DNA in LNCaP cells.

These novel transferrin-bearing zein-based hybrid lipid nanoparticles therefore hold promising prospects as a novel approach for prostate cancer treatment and warrant further investigation to assess the combination of docetaxel and plasmid DNA for cancer therapy.

Author Contributions: Author Contributions: Conceptualization, K.M., S.S. and C.D.; methodology, K.M., I.S., S.S., J.M., H.A.-J., P.L., M.M., G.M., R.J.T. and C.D; validation, K.M., I.S., S.S., J.M., H.A.-J., P.L., M.M., G.M., R.J.T. and C.D.; formal analysis, K.M., I.S., S.S., J.M., H.A.-J., P.L., M.M., G.M., R.J.T. and C.D.; investigation, K.M., I.S., S.S., J.M., H.A.-J., P.L., M.M., G.M., R.J.T. and C.D.; writing—original draft preparation, K.M.; writing—review and editing, K.M. and C.D.; supervision, C.D.; project administration, C.D.; funding acquisition, K.M. and C.D. All authors have read and agreed to the published version of the manuscript.

Funding: K.M. is in receipt of a PhD studentship from the Libyan Government (Libya). I.S. is in receipt of a Thammasat University Scholarship [scholarship number TU_9708] (Thailand). H.A.J. is in receipt of a PhD studentship from Kuwait University (Kuwait). S.S. and P.L. are respectively funded by research grants from The Dunhill Medical Trust [grant number R463/0216] and Worldwide Cancer Research [grant number 16-1303].

Institutional Review Board Statement: Not applicable.

Informed Consent Statement: Not applicable.

Data Availability Statement: The data that support the findings of this study are available from the corresponding author, [CD], upon request.

Conflicts of Interest: The authors declare no conflict of interest.

References

1. Rawla, P. Epidemiology of Prostate Cancer. *World J. Oncol.* **2019**, *10*, 63–89. [CrossRef] [PubMed]
2. Sung, H.; Ferlay, J.; Siegel, R.L.; Laversanne, M.; Soerjomataram, I.; Jemal, A.; Bray, F. Global Cancer Statistics 2020: GLOBOCAN, Estimates of Incidence and Mortality Worldwide for 36 Cancers in 185 Countries. *CA Cancer J. Clin.* **2021**, *71*, 209–249. [CrossRef] [PubMed]
3. Wang, L.; Lu, B.; He, M.; Wang, Y.; Wang, Z.; Du, L. Prostate Cancer Incidence and Mortality: Global Status and Temporal Trends in 89 Countries From 2000 to 2019. *Front. Public Health* **2022**, *10*, 811044–811062. [CrossRef] [PubMed]
4. Siegel, R.L.; Miller, D.M.; Wagle, N.S.; Jemal, A. Cancer statistics 2023. *CA Cancer J. Clin.* **2023**, *73*, 17–48. [CrossRef] [PubMed]
5. Zhao, J.; Guercio, B.J.; Sahasrabudhe, D. Current Trends in Chemotherapy in the Treatment of Metastatic Prostate Cancer. *Cancers* **2023**, *15*, 3969–3988. [CrossRef] [PubMed]
6. Luo, D.; Saltzman, W.M. Synthetic DNA delivery systems. *Nat. Biotechnol.* **2000**, *18*, 33–37. [CrossRef] [PubMed]
7. Daniels, T.R.; Bernabeu, E.; Rodríguez, J.A.; Patel, S.; Kozman, M.; Chiappetta, D.A.; Holler, E.; Ljubimova, J.Y.; Helguera, G.; Penichet, M.L. Transferrin receptors and the targeted delivery of therapeutic agents against cancer. *Biochim. Biophys. Acta.* **2012**, *1820*, 291–317. [CrossRef] [PubMed]
8. Dufès, C.; Al Robaian, M.; Somani, S. Transferrin and the transferrin receptor for the targeted delivery of therapeutic agents to the brain and cancer cells. *Ther. Deliv.* **2013**, *4*, 629–640. [CrossRef]
9. Al Robaian, M.; Chiam, K.Y.; Blatchford, D.R.; Dufès, C. Therapeutic efficacy of intravenously administered transferrin-conjugated dendriplexes encoding TNF-α, TRAIL and interleukin-12 on prostate carcinomas. *Nanomedicine* **2014**, *9*, 421–434. [CrossRef]
10. Shukla, R.; Cheryan, M. Zein: The industrial protein from corn. *Ind. Crop. Prod.* **2001**, *13*, 171–192. [CrossRef]
11. Lawton, J.W. Zein: A History of Processing and Use. *Cereal Chem.* **2002**, *79*, 1–18. [CrossRef]
12. Lin, T.; Lu, C.; Zhu, L.; Lu, T. The Biodegradation of Zein In Vitro and In Vivo and its Application in Implants. *AAPS PharmSciTech* **2011**, *12*, 172–176. [CrossRef] [PubMed]
13. Paliwal, R.; Palakurthi, S. Zein in controlled drug delivery and tissue engineering. *J. Control. Release* **2014**, *189*, 108–122. [CrossRef] [PubMed]
14. Gianazza, E.; Viglienghi, V.; Righetti, P.G.; Salamini, F.; Soave, C. Amino acid composition of zein molecular components. *Phytochemistry* **1977**, *16*, 315–317. [CrossRef]
15. Parris, N.; Cooke, P.H.; Hicks, K.B. Encapsulation of Essential Oils in Zein Nanospherical Particles. *J. Agric. Food Chem.* **2005**, *53*, 4788–4792. [CrossRef] [PubMed]
16. Regier, M.C.; Taylor, J.D.; Borcyk, T.; Yang, Y.; Pannier, A.K. Fabrication and characterization of DNA-loaded zein nanospheres. *J. Nanobiotechnol.* **2012**, *10*, 44–57. [CrossRef] [PubMed]
17. Dong, F.; Dong, X.; Zhou, L.; Xiao, H.; Ho, P.Y.; Wong, M.S.; Wang, Y. Doxorubicin-loaded biodegradable self-assembly zein nanoparticle and its anti-cancer effect: Preparation, *in vitro* evaluation, and cellular uptake. *Colloids Surf. B. Biointerfaces* **2016**, *140*, 324–331. [CrossRef]
18. Thapa, R.K.; Nguyen, H.T.; Jeong, J.H.; Shin, B.S.; Ku, S.K.; Choi, H.G.; Yong, C.S.; Kim, J.O. Synergistic anticancer activity of combined histone deacytylase and proteasomal inhibitor-loaded zein nanoparticles in metastatic prostate cancers. *Nanomed. NBM.* **2017**, *13*, 885–896. [CrossRef]
19. Wen, P.; Ke, W.; Dirisala, A.; Toh, K.; Tanaka, M.; Li, J. Stealth and pseudo-stealth nanocarriers. *Adv. Drug Deliv. Rev.* **2023**, *198*, 114895. [CrossRef]
20. Podaralla, S.; Averineni, R.; Alqahtani, M.; Perumal, O. Synthesis of Novel Biodegradable Methoxy Poly(ethylene glycol)–Zein Micelles for Effective Delivery of Curcumin. *Mol. Pharm.* **2012**, *9*, 2778–2786. [CrossRef]
21. Song, R.; Zhou, Y.; Li, Y.; Yang, Z.; Li, F.; Huang, Q.; Shi, T.; Zhang, G. Preparation and characterization of mPEG-g-α-zein biohybrid micelles as a nano-carrier. *J. Appl. Polym. Sci.* **2015**, *132*, 1–6. [CrossRef]
22. Meewan, J.; Somani, S.; Laskar, P.; Irving, C.; Mullin, M.; Woods, S.; Roberts, C.W.; Alzahrani, A.R.; Ferro, V.A.; McGill, S.; et al. Limited impact of the protein corona on the cellular uptake of PEGylated zein micelles by melanoma cancer cells. *Pharmaceutics* **2022**, *14*, 439. [CrossRef] [PubMed]

23. Meewan, J.; Somani, S.; Almowalad, J.; Laskar, P.; Mullin, M.; MacKenzie, G.; Khadke, S.; Perrie, Y.; Dufès, C. Preparation of zein-based nanoparticles: Nanoprecipitation versus microfluidic-assisted manufacture, effects of PEGylation on nanoparticle characteristics and cellular uptake by melanoma cells. *Int. J. Nanomed.* **2022**, *17*, 2809–2822. [CrossRef]
24. Fernandes, M.A.; Eloy, J.O.; Luiz, M.T.; Junior, S.L.R.; Borges, J.C.; Fuente, L.R.; Luis, C.O.; Marchetti, J.M.; Santos-Martinez, M.J.; Chorilli, M. Transferrin-functionalized liposomes for docetaxel delivery to prostate cancer cells. *Colloids Surf. A Physicochem. Eng.* **2021**, *611*, 125806. [CrossRef]
25. Mia, Y.; Liua, Y.; Feng, S.-S. Formulation of Docetaxel by folic acid-conjugated d-α-tocopheryl polyethyleneglycol succinate 2000 (Vitamin E TPGS2k) micelles for targeted and synergistic chemotherapy. *Biomaterials* **2011**, *32*, 4058–4066. [CrossRef] [PubMed]
26. Tan, Q.; Liu, X.; Fu, X.; Li, Q.; Dou, J.; Zhai, G. Current development in nanoformulations of docetaxel. *Expert. Opin. Drug Deliv.* **2012**, *9*, 975–990. [CrossRef] [PubMed]
27. Chen, J.; Wu, Z.; Ding, W.; Xiao, C.; Zhang, Y.; Gao, S.; Gao, Y.; Cai, W. SREBP1 siRNA enhance the docetaxel effect based on a bone-cancer dual-targeting biomimetic nanosystem against bone metastatic castration-resistant prostate cancer. *Theranostics* **2020**, *10*, 1619–1632. [CrossRef]
28. Hermanson, G.T. Dendrimers and Dendrons. In *Bioconjugate Techniques*, 3rd ed.; Elsevier Inc.: London, UK, 2013; pp. 351–387.
29. Lowry, O.H.; Rosebrough, N.J.; Farr, A.L.; Randall, R.J. Protein measurement with the Folin phenol reagent. *J. Biol. Chem.* **1951**, *193*, 265–275. [CrossRef]
30. Dufès, C.; Schätzlein, A.G.; Tetley, L.; Gray, A.I.; Watson, D.G.; Olivier, J.C.; Couet, W.; Uchegbu, I.F. Niosomes and Polymeric Chitosan Based Vesicles Bearing Transferrin and Glucose Ligands for Drug Targeting. *Pharm. Res.* **2000**, *17*, 1250–1258. [CrossRef]
31. Paraman, I.; Lamsal, B.P. Recovery and characterization of α-zein from corn fermentation coproducts. *J. Agric. Food Chem.* **2011**, *59*, 3071–3077. [CrossRef]
32. Maeda, H. The tumor blood vessel as an ideal target for macromolecular anticancer agents. *J. Control. Release* **1992**, *19*, 315–324. [CrossRef]
33. Maeda, H.; Wu, J.; Sawa, T.; Matsumura, Y.; Hori, K. Tumor vascular permeability and the EPR effect in macromolecular therapeutics: A review. *J. Control. Release* **2000**, *65*, 271–284. [CrossRef] [PubMed]
34. Li, J.; Kataoka, K. Chemo-physical Strategies to Advance the in Vivo Functionality of Targeted Nanomedicine: The Next Generation. *J. Am. Chem. Soc.* **2021**, *143*, 538–559. [CrossRef] [PubMed]
35. Loftsson, T.; Brewster, M.E. Pharmaceutical applications of cyclodextrins: Basic science and product development. *J. Pharm. Pharmacol.* **2010**, *62*, 1607–1621. [CrossRef] [PubMed]
36. Hua, S.; de Matos, M.B.C.; Metselaar, J.M.; Storm, G. Current trends and challenges in the clinical translation of nanoparticulate nanomedicines: Pathways for translational development and commercialization. *Front. Pharmacol.* **2018**, *9*, 790–804. [CrossRef] [PubMed]
37. Čeh, B.; Winterhalter, M.; Frederik, P.M.; Vallner, J.J.; Lasic, D.D. Stealth®liposomes: From theory to product. *Adv. Drug Deliv. Rev.* **1997**, *24*, 165–177.
38. Barenholz, Y. Doxil®—The first FDA-approved nano-drug: Lessons learned. *J. Control. Release* **2012**, *160*, 117–134. [CrossRef] [PubMed]
39. Sharma, S.; Parmar, A.; Kori, S.; Sandhir, R. PLGA-based nanoparticles: A new paradigm in biomedical applications. *TrAC Trends Anal. Chem.* **2016**, *80*, 30–40. [CrossRef]
40. Suzuki, T.; Sato, E.; Matsuda, T.; Tada, H.; Unno, K.; Kato, T. Preparation of zein microspheres conjugated with antitumor drugs available for selective cancer chemotherapy and development of a simple colorimetric determination of drugs in microspheres. *Chem. Pharm. Bull.* **1989**, *37*, 1051–1054. [CrossRef]
41. Liu, X.; Sun, Q.; Wang, H.; Zhang, L.; Wang, J. Microspheres of corn protein, zein for an invermectin drug delivery system. *Biomaterials* **2005**, *26*, 109–115. [CrossRef]
42. Qian, Z.M.; Li, H.; Sun, H.; Ho, K. Targeted drug delivery via the transferrin receptor-mediated endocytosis pathway. *Pharmacol. Rev.* **2002**, *54*, 561–587. [CrossRef] [PubMed]
43. Sakpakdeejaroen, I.; Somani, S.; Laskar, P.; Irving, C.; Mullin, M.; Dufès, C. Anti-tumor activity of intravenously administered plumbagin entrapped in targeted nanoparticles. *J. Biomed. Nanotechnol.* **2020**, *16*, 85–100. [CrossRef] [PubMed]
44. Zhang, L.; Chan, J.M.; Gu, F.X.; Rhee, J.W.; Wang, A.Z.; Radovic-Moreno, A.F.; Alexis, F.; Langer, R.; Farokhzad, O.C. Self-Assembled Lipid–Polymer Hybrid Nanoparticles: A Robust Drug Delivery Platform. *ACS Nano* **2008**, *2*, 1696–1702. [CrossRef] [PubMed]
45. Zhan, X.; Tran, K.K.; Shen, H. Effect of the poly(ethylene glycol) (PEG) density on the access and uptake of particles by antigen-presenting cells (APCs) after subcutaneous administration. *Mol. Pharm.* **2012**, *9*, 3442–3451. [CrossRef] [PubMed]
46. Zhang, S.; Tang, C.; Yin, C. Effects of poly(ethylene glycol) grafting density on the tumor targeting efficacy of nanoparticles with ligand modification. *Drug Deliv.* **2015**, *22*, 182–190. [CrossRef] [PubMed]
47. Stenzel, M.H. Bioconjugation Using Thiols: Old Chemistry Rediscovered to Connect Polymers with Nature's Building Blocks. *ACS Macro Lett.* **2013**, *2*, 14–18. [CrossRef] [PubMed]
48. Yuan, F.; Dellian, M.; Fukumura, D.; Leunig, M.; Berk, D.A.; Torchilin, V.P.; Jain, R.K. Vascular permeability in a human tumor xenograft: Molecular size dependence and cutoff size. *Cancer Res.* **1995**, *55*, 3752–3756.
49. Ernsting, M.J.; Murakami, M.; Roy, A.; Li, S.D. Factors Controlling the Pharmacokinetics, Biodistribution and Intratumoral Penetration of Nanoparticles. *J. Control. Release* **2013**, *172*, 782–794. [CrossRef]

50. Blanco, E.; Shen, H.; Ferrari, M. Principles of nanoparticle design for overcoming biological barriers to drug delivery. *Nat. Biotechnol.* **2015**, *33*, 941–951. [CrossRef]
51. Bhattacharjee, S. DLS and zeta potential—What they are and what they are not? *J. Control. Release* **2016**, *235*, 337–351. [CrossRef]
52. Yu, X.; Han, N.; Dong, Z.; Dang, Y.; Zhang, Q.; Hu, W.; Wang, C.; Du, S.; Lu, Y. Combined Chemo−Immuno−Photothermal Therapy for Effective Cancer Treatment via an All-in-One and One-for-All Nanoplatform. *ACS Appl. Mater. Interfaces* **2022**, *14*, 42988–43009. [CrossRef] [PubMed]
53. Xing, Y.; Li, X.; Cui, W.; Xue, M.; Quan, Y.; Guo, X. Glucose-Modified Zein Nanoparticles Enhance Oral Delivery of Docetaxel. *Pharmaceutics* **2022**, *14*, 1361–1375. [CrossRef] [PubMed]
54. Wu, Z.; Li, J.; Zhang, X.; Li, Y.; Wei, D.; Tang, L.; Deng, S.; Liu, G. Rational Fabrication of Folate-Conjugated Zein/Soy Lecithin/Carboxymethyl Chitosan Core−Shell Nanoparticles for Delivery of Docetaxel. *ACS Omega* **2022**, *7*, 13371–13381. [CrossRef] [PubMed]
55. Lee, H.S.; Kang, N.W.; Kim, H.; Kim, D.H.; Chae, J.W.; Lee, W.; Song, G.Y.; Cho, C.W.; Kim, D.D.; Lee, J.Y. Chondroitin sulfate-hybridized zein nanoparticles for tumor-targeted delivery of docetaxel. *Carbohydr. Polym.* **2021**, *253*, 117187–117200. [CrossRef] [PubMed]
56. Fredenberg, S.; Wahlgren, M.; Reslow, M.; Axelsson, A. The mechanisms of drug release in poly(lactic-co-glycolic acid)-based drug delivery systems—A review. *Int. J. Pharm.* **2011**, *415*, 34–52. [CrossRef] [PubMed]
57. Guo, L.; Zhang, H.; Wang, F.; Liu, P.; Wang, Y.; Xia, G.; Liu, R.; Li, X.; Yin, H.; Jiang, H.; et al. Targeted multidrug-resistance reversal in tumor based on PEG-PLL-PLGA polymer nano drug delivery system. *Int. J. Nanomed.* **2015**, *10*, 4535–4547.
58. Zheng, Y.; Yu, B.; Weecharangsan, W.; Piao, L.; Darby, M.; Mao, Y.; Koynova, R.; Yang, X.; Li, H.; Xu, S.; et al. Transferrin-conjugated lipid-coated PLGA nanoparticles for targeted delivery of aromatase inhibitor 7α-APTADD to breast cancer cells. *Int. J. Pharm.* **2010**, *390*, 234–241. [CrossRef] [PubMed]
59. Sutradhar, K.B.; Amin, M.L. Nanotechnology in Cancer Drug Delivery and Selective Targeting. *ISRN Nanotechnol.* **2014**, *2014*, 1–12. [CrossRef]
60. Deng, Z.; Manz, D.H.; Torti, S.V.; Torti, F.M. Iron-responsive element-binding protein 2 plays an essential role in regulating prostate cancer cell growth. *Oncotarget* **2017**, *8*, 82231–82243. [CrossRef]
61. Gao, H.; Yang, Z.; Zhang, S.; Cao, S.; Shen, S.; Pang, Z.; Jiang, X. Ligand modified nanoparticles increases cell uptake, alters endocytosis and elevates glioma distribution and internalization. *Sci. Rep.* **2013**, *3*, 2534–2542. [CrossRef]
62. Oh, N.; Park, J.H. Endocytosis and exocytosis of nanoparticles in mammalian cells. *Int. J. Nanomed.* **2014**, *9*, 51–63.
63. Chen, Y.; Liu, C.; Yang, Z.; Sun, Y.; Chen, X.; Liu, L. Fabrication of zein-based hydrophilic nanoparticles for efficient gene delivery by layer-by-layer assembly. *Int. J. Biol. Macromol.* **2022**, *217*, 381–397. [CrossRef]
64. Kumari, M.; Liu, C.H.; Wu, W.C. Protein moiety in oligochitosan modified vector regulates internalization mechanism and gene delivery: Polyplex characterization, intracellular trafficking and transfection. *Carbohydr. Polym.* **2018**, *202*, 143–156. [CrossRef]

pharmaceutics

Review

Exploiting Pharma 4.0 Technologies in the Non-Biological Complex Drugs Manufacturing: Innovations and Implications

Vera Malheiro [1], Joana Duarte [1], Francisco Veiga [1,2] and Filipa Mascarenhas-Melo [1,2,3,*]

1 Drug Development and Technology Laboratory, Faculty of Pharmacy, University of Coimbra, Pólo das Ciências da Saúde, Azinhaga de Santa Comba, 3000-548 Coimbra, Portugal; veracatarina.am13@gmail.com (V.M.); joanainesduarte@hotmail.com (J.D.); fveiga@ff.uc.pt (F.V.)
2 LAQV, REQUIMTE, Department of Pharmaceutical Technology, Faculty of Pharmacy, University of Coimbra, Pólo das Ciências da Saúde, Azinhaga de Santa Comba, 3000-548 Coimbra, Portugal
3 Higher School of Health, Polytechnic Institute of Guarda, Rua da Cadeia, 6300-307 Guarda, Portugal
* Correspondence: filipamelo@ff.uc.pt; Tel.: +351-239-488-400; Fax: +351-239-488-503

Abstract: The pharmaceutical industry has entered an era of transformation with the emergence of Pharma 4.0, which leverages cutting-edge technologies in manufacturing processes. These hold tremendous potential for enhancing the overall efficiency, safety, and quality of non-biological complex drugs (NBCDs), a category of pharmaceutical products that pose unique challenges due to their intricate composition and complex manufacturing requirements. This review attempts to provide insight into the application of select Pharma 4.0 technologies, namely machine learning, in silico modeling, and 3D printing, in the manufacturing process of NBCDs. Specifically, it reviews the impact of these tools on NBCDs such as liposomes, polymeric micelles, glatiramer acetate, iron carbohydrate complexes, and nanocrystals. It also addresses regulatory challenges associated with the implementation of these technologies and presents potential future perspectives, highlighting the incorporation of digital twins in this field of research as it seems to be a very promising approach, namely for the optimization of NBCDs manufacturing processes.

Keywords: Pharma 4.0; non-biological complex drugs; three-dimensional (3D) printing; digital twins; in silico modeling; machine learning

1. Introduction

It is widely recognized that bringing a new pharmaceutical drug to the market is a complex, lengthy, and costly process associated with high uncertainty. This process is known as drug development and encompasses various stages, including preclinical research, drug design and production, regulatory filling, clinical trials in humans, obtaining regulatory approval, and the subsequent steps of manufacturing and marketing [1]. Throughout the years, the pharmaceutical industry has undergone significant changes and advancements, progressing from Pharma 1.0 to Pharma 4.0, and more recently reaching the era of Pharma 5.0. Even though Pharma 4.0 is a relatively recent development, the truth is that certain pharmaceuticals are already venturing into the 5.0 era [2].

During Pharma 1.0, the processing of materials derived from minerals, animals, and plants underwent a significant transformation. The use of basic hand-operated tools gave way to the introduction of commercial-scale equipment capable of crushing, blending, milling, and pressing a larger quantity of medicines. In fact, certain key machines developed during the Pharma 1.0 era continue to be widely used in the present day, showcasing their durability and effectiveness [3]. Subsequently, electricity and early electronic machines ushered in a new era in the evolution of the pharmaceutical industry. This phase witnessed the integration of digital tools into various aspects of pharmaceutical research, development, manufacturing, and distribution [4]. For the pharmaceutical sector, this technological incorporation marked a significant milestone because it allowed for a more data-driven and patient-centric approach, besides providing a larger-scale production and more efficient quality control. However, these process controls were far from perfect, since they were confined to pre-determined and static settings, which only allowed for the monitoring of process performance and passive control strategies [3]. The third industrial revolution was enabled by the emergence of computers and communication technologies, including networked computing, the internet, and wireless communications [4]. This development resulted in increased automation of both processes and equipment, fostering the implementation of continuous manufacturing and enhanced active control. This revolution, known as Pharma 3.0, enabled the adoption of advanced control strategies, elevating product and process quality and reducing the need for human operators. This decrease in reliance on human operators also streamlined the tracking of parameters and production metrics. Although some industries are well into Industry 3.0, the pharmaceutical industry is still very much transitioning into it [3]. Pharma 3.0 also brought the implementation of advanced process analytical technology (PAT), which provides real-time data on process and product quality. It also enhanced quality-by-design (QbD) processes, which focus on controlling product quality within specific parameters [3]. While Pharma 3.0 already enables a much-improved understanding of how to capture, analyze, and secure large amounts of data in pharmaceutical manufacturing, there is still room for further technological advancements to achieve the full potential of PAT and QbD [5]. Later on, with the appearance of artificial intelligence (AI), cloud computing, machine learning (ML), big data analytics, in silico modeling, 3D printing, and other advanced manufacturing technologies, the manufacturing process was actualized, forcing the emergence of another industrial revolution, known as Pharma 4.0 [6]. These advanced manufacturing technologies empower autonomous and self-organizing systems capable of operating independently without human intervention [3].

In the pharmaceutical sector, the fourth industrial revolution allowed for a shift in the paradigm of formulation development [7]. The potential to integrate diverse data sources facilitates the connection of both external and internal information, establishing a comprehensive network. In the context of pharmaceutical manufacturing, this integration entails merging external data, including patient experiences, market demands, supplier inventories, and public health emergencies, with internal data encompassing energy and resource management, modeling and simulation results, and laboratory data. This fusion enables unparalleled real-time responsiveness, monitoring, control, and predictive capabilities [3].

In an ever-evolving marketplace characterized by a fast-changing and smartly integrated supply chain, coupled with more active participation of patients in their healthcare decision-making, pharmaceutical companies face an urgent imperative to maintain their competitive advantage. In this setting, the key factor that sets businesses apart is their ability to meet the expectation of Pharma 4.0, which, despite being a complex process to implement, provides enhanced resources for ensuring product safety compliance, safeguarding the supply chain, and fostering pharmaceutical development [6]. This concept of Pharma 4.0 is closely linked to artificial intelligence (AI), a technology-based system involving various advanced tools and networks that can mimic human intelligence [3]. It possesses systems and software with the ability to interpret and learn from the input data, enabling them to autonomously make decisions in order to achieve specific objectives [8]. AI plays a crucial role in Pharma 4.0 by enabling smart, data-driven decision-making and optimization throughout the entire pharmaceutical value chain [9].

Non-biological complex drugs (NBCDs) are complex, often comprising intricate structures and diverse components [10]. Therefore, traditional quality control methods may not fully capture the complexities of these drugs. Pharma 4.0 techniques can offer real-time monitoring and predictive quality control, allowing for more effective detection of deviations and potential issues. Besides, since NBCD manufacturing involves handling a vast amount of data from multiple stages of the production process, these innovative technologies can leverage this data to support data-driven decision-making, enabling manufacturers to identify patterns, trends, and correlations that may impact product quality, stability, and reproducibility [11]. In this sense, this manuscript presents a view on the application of select Pharma 4.0 technologies, namely machine learning, in silico modeling, and 3D printing, for enhancing the overall efficiency, safety, and quality of non-biological complex drugs (NBCDs), a category of pharmaceutical products that pose unique challenges due to their intricate composition and complex manufacturing requirements.

However, it is important to keep in mind that to attain Pharma 4.0, while embracing cutting-edge manufacturing technologies, it is also important to simultaneously overcome regulatory obstacles [12]. In this context, this review not only addresses these regulatory challenges but also explores potential future perspectives, notably the incorporation of Digital Twins in the development and manufacturing of non-biological complex drugs (NBCDs).

2. Emerging Tools of Pharma 4.0

The following sections of this review will highlight and describe emerging tools of Pharma 4.0, such as additive manufacturing (3D printing), in silico modeling, and machine learning, which are represented in Figure 1.

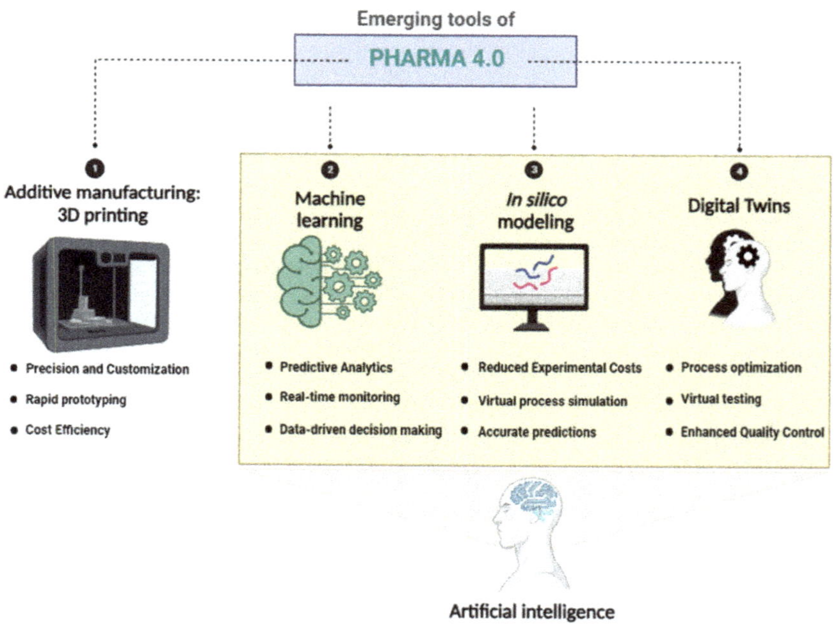

Figure 1. Emerging tools of Pharma 4.0 and their main advantages in drug manufacturing.

2.1. *Additive Manufacturing: Three-Dimensional (3D) Printing*

Additive manufacturing encompasses all manufacturing techniques that involve the sequential addition of material to build a 3D object. Typically, a digital representation of the desired object is created using computer-aided design software; subsequently, the product is produced using one or more additive technologies [13].

3D printing, as an additive manufacturing technique, holds immense potential within the pharmaceutical sector. It consists of the layer-by-layer creation of 3D objects based on digital designs and holds promise for the development of versatile release models. These models aim to address clinical needs and facilitate patient-centric treatment, including personalized dosing tailored to specific disease states or patient populations [14]. The classification of 3D printing techniques can be simplified into three main categories:

printing-based inkjet systems, nozzle-based deposition systems, and laser-based writing systems [15].

Spritam® (levetiracetam), an epilepsy medication developed by Aprecia Pharmaceuticals, was the first 3D-printed pharmaceutical to receive approval from the Food and Drug Administration (FDA) [16]. It utilizes a unique 3D printing technology called ZipDose®, which allows for the production of a highly porous tablet that dissolves rapidly in a small amount of liquid. This orodispersible tablet, characterized by its porous and soluble matrix composition, demonstrated similar pharmacological efficacy comparable to conventional tablets. On the other hand, this tablet exhibited a significant solubilization time improvement, indicative of faster dissolution [15]. It is worth noting that the approval of Spritam® as a 3D-printed pharmaceutical by the FDA was a significant milestone in the field of pharmaceutical manufacturing, as it demonstrated the potential of 3D printing technology in the production of unique drug formulations and opened up possibilities for personalized medicine [16].

Extensive research has been dedicated to advancing the use of 3D printing techniques in pharmaceutical manufacturing. As these endeavors progress, additive manufacturing technology has not only demonstrated its potential for creating personalized medications tailored to individual patients but has also emerged as a viable option for large-scale manufacturing, thanks to its ability to generate dosage forms with unique performance characteristics, which would be difficult to achieve via traditional methods [17].

Advancements in the Pharmaceutical Industry Offered by 3D Printing Technology

In the pharmaceutical industry, 3D printing offers the benefit of creating products with sophisticated external shapes. In fact, this technique was employed to produce orally disintegrating printlets specifically tailored for individuals with visual impairment. These printlets were meticulously designed with Braille and Moon patterns on their surfaces, allowing patients to identify medications even when removed from their original packaging. This approach shows the potential to enhance accessibility and independence for visually impaired patients in managing their medication regimens, thereby reducing potential errors [18].

3D printing has also demonstrated unprecedented potential in controlling drug release and influencing drugs' pharmacokinetic profiles. In fact, the use of 3D printing techniques was leveraged to produce multiparticulates, known as miniprintlets, loaded with paracetamol, which exhibited prolonged drug release patterns, offering a novel approach to drug delivery with remarkable flexibility and control over release properties. By adjusting parameters such as dimensions and matrix composition, the therapeutic effect can be finely tuned, enabling the production of multi-drug systems. Furthermore, the possibility of creating miniprintlets containing two drugs, namely paracetamol and ibuprofen, was also investigated. A miniprintlet utilizing different polymers was created, so that one drug was released immediately and the second was sustained over an extended period [19].

Another promising advantage of 3D-printing is the ability to delay drug release, reaching even the colon in the gastrointestinal (GI) tract. This advancement holds tremendous potential as a breakthrough for the treatment of inflammatory bowel diseases [17,20].

For its numerous advantages, this technology has been employed to manufacture an extensive range of pharmaceutical products. These includes printlets (3D printed tablets), capsules, subcutaneous implants, and transdermal microneedles, among other innovative drug delivery devices [14,21,22].

2.2. *In Silico Modeling*

In silico modeling refers to the use of computational methods and computer simulations to study and analyze complex systems, typically in the fields of science, engineering, and medicine [23].

This approach involves creating virtual representations or models of real-world systems, based on mathematical algorithms, statistical techniques, and biological or physical principles. By simulating the behavior of these models, researchers can gain insights into underlying mechanisms, predict outcomes, and test hypotheses without the need for costly or time-consuming physical experiments [24].

In the pharmaceutical sector, in silico modeling is used to predict the behavior of drug molecules, their interactions with biological targets, and their potential efficacy and safety profiles [25]. From this context arises the term "in silico trials", which refers to the application of computer modeling and simulation to assess the safety and effectiveness of medicinal products, including drugs, medical devices, diagnostic products, and advanced therapy medicinal products [23].

Over the years, numerous reviews have described how in silico methods can be used for predicting the absorption, distribution, metabolism, excretion, and toxicity (ADME/TOX) of different drugs [26]. This plays a crucial role in assisting decision-making, since it is not possible to experimentally test all possible combinations of drug interactions [27]. By simulating the behavior of substances in silico, researchers can quickly identify compounds with unfavorable ADME/TOX profiles and prioritize those with higher chances of success for further experimental evaluation, thus saving time and resources and reducing the risk of costly failures in later stages of drug development [26].

This technique also provides a mechanistic insight into the underlying processes and interactions involved in ADME/TOX because it can simulate the behavior of substances at the molecular level, allowing researchers to understand the interactions between transporters, enzymes, receptors, and other factors influencing ADME/TOX properties. Such information can help in understanding the mechanisms of action, potential toxicities, and the design of safer and more effective drugs [28].

In addition, in silico models can also be employed to study complex biological systems, such as cellular processes and signaling pathways. These models can help unravel the underlying mechanisms governing these systems and aid in the understanding of diseases, as well as the development of therapeutic interventions [29,30].

As an illustrative example of the applicability of in silico modeling in the pharmaceutical field, one can consider the design of these models to predict and comprehend the mechanism of action of the human ether-a-go-go-related gene (hERG) blockers. This is relevant because the hERG gene encodes a crucial ion channel in the heart, namely he hERG potassium channel, which plays a crucial role in regulating the electrical activity of this organ. Certain drugs may inadvertently block the hERG channel, leading to a drug-induced QT prolongation, which can result in a potentially life-threatening heart rhythm disturbance called Torsade de Pointes. Therefore, understanding and predicting the effects of potential hERG blockers through in silico methods are vital in drug development and safety assessment [31].

2.3. Machine Learning (ML)

ML is an artificial intelligence-based technology that focuses on constructing computational models by training them with a set of data. It enables machines to automatically analyze and interpret complex patterns and data, improving their performance in making predictions or decisions. For instance, ML might predict the stability of a specific drug formulation by considering data from a range of previous experiments that investigated formulation stability [32].

Machine learning algorithms identify patterns, anomalies, and potential risks, enabling proactive quality management and enhancing accuracy, efficiency, and compliance, while ensuring high product standards, regulatory compliance, and patient safety [9]. In fact, by automating inspection processes, analyzing data for defects and deviations, and predicting quality outcomes, this AI technology is revolutionizing quality control and assurance processes.

This technology can be broadly categorized into three types: supervised learning, unsupervised learning, and reinforcement learning [33]. In the first one, the algorithm is supplied with training data that includes both recorded observations and their corresponding labels. With this information, the algorithm constructs a model that can predict the appropriate output label for new observations [34]. Unsupervised learning, on the other hand, deals with unlabeled data, where the algorithm aims to discover hidden patterns or structures in the data without any predefined labels. Basically, the model learns to cluster similar data points or find relationships between the variables [35]. Finally, reinforcement learning involves a learning approach that relies on the use of rewards to categorize inputs as "good" or "bad" data, based on their interaction with the surrounding environment. Through this process, the algorithm learns to optimize its actions to maximize positive outcomes and minimize negative ones [36].

The initial applications of machine learning in drug formulation date back to the 1990s when neural networks (NNs) were employed to forecast properties related to immediate-release oral tablets. This involved the preparation and assessment of a diverse array of tablet formulations and the training of the neural network with the acquired data, enabling the prediction of different outcomes such as disintegration time, dissolution rate, and friability. These early experiments marked the pioneering use of machine learning techniques in optimizing drug formulation processes [32].

In fact, regarding the machine learning domain, these neural networks remain the most used technique. However, when dealing with a small amount of data, this can be prone to overfitting due to the high complexity and risk of learning noise in the limited dataset. In such cases, alternative machine learning methods such as support vector machines (SVMs) and random forests can be more suitable choices.

SVMs represent a category of learning machines rooted in statistical learning theory. The fundamental concept behind employing SVMs for pattern classification can be summarized as follows. Initially, input vectors are mapped into a feature space, which can be of higher dimension, achieved via either linear or non-linear transformations. Subsequently, within this feature space, the objective is to identify an optimal linear division. This involves constructing a hyper-plane capable of effectively separating two classes with minimal error and maximal margin. The SVMs' training process consistently strives for a globally optimized solution while preventing overfitting, rendering them proficient in managing a large number of features [37].

The random forest algorithm is a well-established machine learning technique which operates by creating decision trees using random subsets of the provided dataset. These trees are divided into nodes, which serve as decision points where the algorithm categorizes the given sample. As the data are processed, each decision tree generated by the algorithm makes an individual prediction, which is then compared against those of other trees. The final prediction is then determined based on the majority vote of the individual decision trees. This approach is particularly useful in handling small datasets effectively [38].

Nowadays, the application of ML in the healthcare sector allows for improved cancer diagnosis, the discovery of new antifibrotic and antibiotic molecules, and the development of self-driving laboratories. It also allows for the prediction of the products of certain chemical reactions and, consequently, the optimization of these reactions [32].

2.4. Digital Twins

In the pharmaceutical industry, digital twins can have several uses and take different forms and as such are being increasingly adopted to improve efficiency, productivity, and quality control of drug manufacturing processes. For instance, researchers have developed computer simulations to create digital twins of dissolution apparatuses, namely USP II, and tablets to mimic their behavior realistically. By using these digital twins, they could investigate drug release profiles and shear rates that act on the tablet, under different paddle speeds, in both USP II and biorelevant colon models. The objective was to understand how the USP II could be operated to achieve more realistic hydrodynamic conditions that resemble the conditions in the human colon in vivo. To ensure accuracy and relevance in the simulations, the behavior of the tablet and the motility patterns within the colon are derived from experimental data and in vivo observations, respectively. Based on their findings, the researchers recommend using an "on–off" operating mode in the USP II rather than a constant paddle speed. This "on–off" mode generates shear rate peaks, which better reflect the in vivo conditions of the human colon. This change in operating mode can help achieve more realistic simulation results, providing deeper insights into the tablet's disintegration and drug release processes in colon-targeted solid dosage forms [39].

These digital twins were also employed as a digital representation of the continuous manufacturing process for pharmaceuticals. This allows for the prediction of critical process parameters (such as those in the feeders, blender, and tablet press) and critical quality attributes (tablet composition, weight, thickness, and hardness) throughout the manufacturing process. This means that pharmaceutical companies can study the steady-state operation of the process within the design space; examine the impact of different operating conditions, materials, and process parameters; and understand dynamic response to disturbances or variations in the process [40].

In addition, researchers have developed a new and innovative concept called a "neural network–intelligent digital twin" to describe, predict, and optimize the outcomes of the manufacturing process of solidified nanosuspensions. The authors integrated the artificial neural network into the digital twin development process in a stepwise manner. The steps included data sampling, model deployment, and curve fitting. This means that the NN was trained using a dataset containing information about the manufacturing process, where the network´s architecture and parameters were optimized (curve fitting) to effectively represent the behavior of the process. One of the primary roles of the ANN within the digital twin is to augment the amount of available data. Since training a neural network typically requires a significant amount of data, the ANN generates additional simulated data points to further calibrate and validate the model. In the process, the digital twin can be fine-tuned to better represent the real-world manufacturing process, without the need for extensive physical experiments, while reducing uncertainties in the model´s predictions. Overall, this research introduces a sophisticated approach that combines NN technology and digital twin concepts to improve the understanding, prediction, and optimization of the manufacturing process for solidified nanosuspensions. This has the potential to lead to more efficient and cost-effective manufacturing processes in the pharmaceutical sector [41].

Another—and very recent—example of the applications of digital twins is the use of this technology, enabled by process analytical technology (PAT) approaches, to improve various aspects of the SARS–COVID-19 vaccine manufacturing process, such as capacity multiplication, reduction of out-of-specification batch failures, personnel training, efficient operation, optimal utilization of resources, and faster product release. Specifically, the focus is on messenger ribonucleic acid (mRNA) vaccine processing and the potential use of digital twins to address bottlenecks and optimize the process. Researchers have suggested creating a digital twin of the entire process which would convert plasmid deoxyribonucleic acid (pDNA) into mRNA. By combining digital twins with PAT, the vaccine production process can be enhanced, rendering it more efficient, and manufacturing capacity can be multiplied without compromising production quality and efficiency. In addition, researchers also believe that digital twins can also be used as a training tool for personnel to become qualified in operating the manufacturing process effectively and efficiently. The technology additionally facilitates the optimization of the utilization of scarce buffers and chemicals. This in turn leads to better resource management in the manufacturing process and a faster product release, enabling vaccines to be swiftly distributed to meet global demand [42].

In general, digital twins allow for enhanced drug formulation development, reduced reliance on costly experiments, and improved drug performance assessment. They enable pharmaceutical companies to move towards more data-driven and agile manufacturing processes, leading to better products and reduced costs. However, despite their potential benefits, the pharmaceutical industry has not fully embraced the use of digital twins in their operations [41].

3. Non-Biological Complex Drugs (NBCDs)

NBCDs are defined as medicinal products that are not derived from living organisms but are entirely synthesized via a fully synthetic process. They are also characterized by an active substance comprising multiple structures that cannot be entirely isolated, quantified, characterized, or fully described using physicochemical analytical methods [43].

NBCDs are closely related to nanoparticles, and some examples include fat emulsions, liposomes, polymeric micelles, iron-carbohydrate complexes, dendrimers, swelling cross-linked polymers, and glatiramoids, among others. Sometimes, low molecular weight heparins, dry powder inhalers, ocular/intravenous emulsions, and dermal patches are seen as NBCDs as well [11]. Figure 2 illustrates the NBCDs that are within the scope of this manuscript.

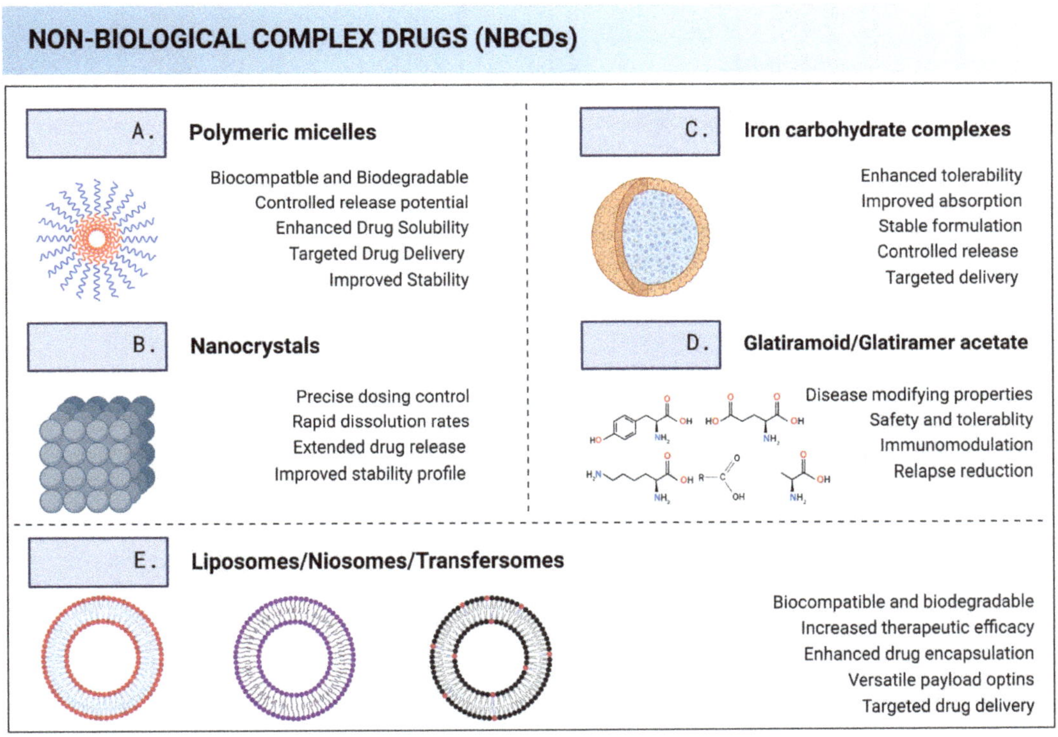

Figure 2. Illustrative depiction of non-biological complex drugs (NBCDs) and descriptions of their main technological advantages.

In a conference that took place in Budapest (October 2014), Dr. De Vlieger listed a few key attributes for an NBCD [1]: (1) it consists of a multitude of closely related structures; (2) the entire complex is the active pharmaceutical ingredient; (3) the properties cannot be fully characterized via physicochemical analysis; and (4) a robust and well-controlled manufacturing process is key to reproducing the product.

Regarding NBCDs, one of their major challenges lies in the characterization process, specifically in evaluating batch-to-batch similarity and assessing the impact of manufacturing process variations. This sensitivity to manufacturing changes can give rise to challenges in ensuring reproducibility when produced by different manufactures. A noteworthy example of this occurred with follow-on products for iron sucrose complexes, where reports indicated that patient safety was compromised by switching patients to a follow-on product [44]. The complex nature of NBCDs may arise from various factors. For instance, the complexity may stem from the active substance itself, as seen with glatiramer acetate, or it may arise from the formulation, as observed with liposomes [10].

All of above explain why NBCDs fall under a distinct regulatory framework compared to small molecule drugs [45].

Much like biologics, the quality of NBCD products is intricately linked to a robust and meticulously controlled manufacturing process. This poses challenges for generic drug developers aiming to replicate NBCD products once the market exclusivity of the originator product has expired. Unlike biologics, which benefit from a well-established biosimilar pathway, NBCDs lack recognition as a distinct category of medicines. Consequently, a formal regulatory pathway for their approval has yet to be defined. Presently, a "case-by-case" approach is employed to regulate NBCD follow-on products in the EU. Additionally, NBCDs may undergo a non-centralized authorization procedure, decentralizing regulatory approval to competent national authorities. However, this decentralized approach can introduce heterogeneity in the regulatory assessment of NBCD follow-on products across the EU, potentially leading to varied outcomes and, in some instances, raising concerns related to safety and efficacy. For that reason, given the regulatory uncertainty still surrounding these products, we can only infer that by incorporating Pharma 4.0 tools, a more standardized and data-driven approach can be applied to the development and manufacturing of NBCDs. For example, the implementation of real-time monitoring systems, guided by Pharma 4.0 principles, enhances our understanding of critical manufacturing parameters for complex NBCDs, ensuring consistency in product attributes essential for establishing pharmaceutical equivalence. Data analytics tools analyze vast datasets, enabling trend identification and maintenance of product attributes. In silico modeling capabilities of Pharma 4.0 optimize NBCD formulation design, predicting and assessing variations to ensure bioequivalence. Machine learning algorithms enable adaptive control strategies during NBCD manufacturing, dynamically responding to variations and contributing to bioequivalence maintenance, particularly in the absence of a consistent regulatory framework. Aligning with the QbD principles of Pharma 4.0, a systematic QbD approach addresses factors affecting bioequivalence, providing a structured framework for regulatory assessments. In totality, Pharma 4.0 tools offer comprehensive solutions to bridge the current regulatory gap associated with NBCDs, promoting consistency and efficacy in their evaluation and approval processes. Moreover, the conventional generic approach, centered on establishing pharmaceutical equivalence and bioequivalence, has been instrumental in introducing numerous safe and effective alternatives to innovative medicines. Nevertheless, this approach has primarily been employed for products that can be thoroughly characterized. In the case of more intricate molecules characterized by inherent complexities and challenges in characterization, such NBCDs demonstrating bioequivalence may benefit from the exploration of alternative methodologies [46,47]. However, given the criticality of this issue, more research, more evidence and discussion are needed around it.

3.1. Polymeric Micelles

Polymeric micelles are nanoscale particles (sizes ranging between 20 and 200 nm) that consist of a hydrophobic core, serving as a reservoir for poorly soluble active pharmaceutical ingredients (APIs), and a hydrophilic shell that offers colloidal stability and limits protein adsorption and opsonization, leading to extended circulation times [48]. Since the physicochemical properties and the in vivo distribution, safety, and efficacy of the final product are highly dependent on the chosen polymer chemistry and manufacturing process, this explains why polymeric micelles are classified as NBCDs [49]. Despite the challenges associated with them, these structures hold great promise in drug manufacturing and delivery, as they offer several advantages which make them attractive for various therapeutic applications [48]. By encapsulating hydrophobic drugs in their core, these structures provide increased solubility and stability, facilitating their delivery to target sites. [49]. Simultaneously, these nanocarriers also have shown improved therapeutic outcomes when compared to the free drug [50]. In addition, the biocompatibility of many polymers used in micelle formulation makes them well tolerated by the body, reducing the risk of adverse reactions [48]. Moreover, by modifying the surface properties of the micelles, these can be engineered to selectively accumulate at specific disease sites, taking advantage of the enhanced permeability and retention effect of tumor tissues or inflamed regions [51].

More recently, researchers have been studying combinations of two or more polymers in order to assemble polymeric mixed micelles [52]. The underlying concept is to combine polymers with complementary characteristics to enhance drug encapsulation, stability, and targeted delivery. Overall, this is a direct and convenient approach to improve the physical stability and enhance the drug-loading capacities of conventional polymeric micelles for drug delivery [53].

3.2. *Liposomes*

Liposomes are colloidal and spherical vesicles composed of lipid molecules, primarily phospholipids, which have a hydrophilic head and hydrophobic tails, allowing them to form, in an aqueous environment, a closed bilayered structure [54]. They are classified according to their size, which can go from 0.025 µm (very small liposomes) to several µm (large liposomes), and their number of double layers [55]. The formulation of these structures involves the dispersion of the lipid molecules in an aqueous phase to form the vesicles. This can be carried out via mechanical methods (microfluidization, extrusion), replacement of organic solvents via aqueous media methods (ethanol injection, reverse phase evaporation), and detergent removal methods [54]. These structures have been studied in several pharmaceutical studies as drug delivery systems due to their remarkable capacity to encapsulate molecules with varying solubilities, namely that hydrophilic molecules can be accommodated in the internal core, hydrophobic molecules within the lipid bilayer, and amphiphilic molecules at the water/lipid bilayer interface. Moreover, their exceptional biocompatibility, biodegradability, lack of toxicity, and non-immunogenic nature further enhance their potential as an excellent therapeutic options [56].

Liposomes offer a host of additional benefits, including the capability to carry substantial drug loads, the capacity for self-assembly, and the versatility to modify a wide range of physicochemical and biophysical properties, thereby allowing for precise control over their biological characteristics [54]. It is therefore clear that liposomes are incredibly versatile structures that find applications across diverse fields. In fact, they can be found as a therapeutic option for cancer [57] as well for the treatment of skin conditions such as hyperpigmentation, among many others [58].

Over the years, diverse delivery systems based on liposomes have been developed, such as niosomes, transfersomes, ethosomes, and dendrossomes, of which we highlight the first two.

3.2.1. Niosomes

Niosomes were initially developed for the cosmetic industry but have now a wide range of applications in the pharmaceutical field [59]. They consist of biodegradable and biocompatible vesicles composed of nonionic surfactants and, sometimes, cholesterol or its derivatives [60]. These structures allow us to overcome some limitations associated with liposomes, since they are not only more cost-effective and easier to prepare but also demonstrate a higher encapsulation efficiency [61]. This explains why niosomes have garnered significant attention in numerous studies for diverse applications, including for several types of cancers and fungal infections [62].

3.2.2. Transfersomes

Transfersomes are specialized lipid-based nanocarriers composed of phospholipids and edge-active agents. These systems possess exceptional deformability and flexibility, allowing them to squeeze through the narrow pores of the stratum corneum [59]. This characteristic enables efficient transdermal drug delivery, offering a non-invasive alternative for systemic drug administration [63]. Transfersomes have garnered significant attention due to their potential to enhance drug absorption, minimize side effects, and improve patient compliance [64,65].

3.3. Glatiramoid/Glatiramer Acetate (GA)

Glatiramer acetate (GA), also known as Copolymer-1 or Cop-1, is a heterogeneous mixture of synthetic polypeptides, comprising L-alanine, L-lysine, L-glutamic acid, and L-tyrosine [66]. Its discovery took place in the late 1960s, when researchers were investigating the immunological properties of synthetic amino acid polymers in the quest for a synthetic antigen capable of inducing experimental autoimmune encephalomyelitis (EAE), the most commonly used model for studying multiple sclerosis (MS) [67]. In the US and Europe, GA has been approved as a disease-modifying treatment (DMT) for patients with relapsing forms of MS, a chronic inflammatory disease of the central nervous system (CNS) that starts as an autoimmune reaction leading to acute CNS inflammation, along with the disruption of myelin, ensheathing axons, and axonal damage [67].

Despite not being completely random, the amino acid sequences are not completely conserved from batch to batch, even when the process is tightly controlled. Therefore, the quality of these substances heavily relies on the precision of the manufacturing process [66].

GA falls under the category of NBCDs not only due to its intricate structure and variable composition, but also because fully characterizing and analyzing its molecular structure is exceptionally challenging compared to traditional small-molecule drugs [66,68].

3.4. Iron Carbohydrate Complexes Drugs

Iron carbohydrate complexes drugs are effective iron replacement agents for iron deficiency anemia treatment [69]. This is an area of great interest because it is the most common micronutrient deficiency worldwide [70].

Oral iron supplements in the form of ferrous iron may not be the perfect therapeutic approach due to their association with gastrointestinal intolerance, prolonged iron store repletion time, and impaired iron absorption. As a way to overcome these problems, intravenous iron–carbohydrate complexes appear to be an alternative approach that can lead to higher hemoglobin levels as well as faster replenishment of the body's iron stores [71].

These structures consist of colloidal formulations composed of an iron core and a complex carbohydrate coating with an average particle size at the nanoscale. Different formulations differ in terms of the iron core size, carbohydrate shell coating material, and hydrodynamic size of the product. The stability of iron–carbohydrate complexes and the rate at which iron is released from the matrices vary among different products [72]. Furthermore, it is crucial to have a comprehensive knowledge of the physicochemical characteristics of the various intravenous iron–carbohydrate complexes to improve the safety and efficacy of the currently available products as well as for the formulation of new iron preparations in the future [69].

3.5. Nanocrystals

Nanocrystals are carrier-free drug particles with sizes in the nanometer range and crystalline characteristics [73]. Thanks to high drug loading, nanocrystals guarantee efficient drug delivery to cells or tissues and maintain potent therapeutic concentrations to achieve the desired pharmacological effect. Consequently, these transporters have become very attractive treatment options for various types of diseases [74].

This technology of nanocrystallization offers a very promising and effective way to deal with the low solubility and poor bio-availability of poorly soluble drugs because, due to their nanosize, they allow for increased dissolution pressure and a higher dissolution rate [73]. To produce nanocrystals, several methods have been implemented and they can be divided into three main categories: top-down (nanonization), bottom-up (crystal growth or nucleation), and combination techniques [75].

Capitalizing on the aforementioned advantages, these NBCDs have found application across various disease categories, such as in cancer therapy, inflammatory diseases (due to their capacity to improve on the physicochemical properties of Biopharmaceutics Classification System (BCS) class II drugs), and in the prevention of preterm birth (as progesterone is a BCS class IV drug, with poor solubility and very low permeability, which renders therapeutics difficult), among many other purposes [74,76].

4. Applying Pharma 4.0 Tools in the Production of Non-Biological Complex Drugs

4.1. Additive Manufacturing: 3D Printing

4.1.1. Polymeric Micelles

3D printing has exhibited promising results in the manufacturing of diverse drug delivery systems, such as polymeric micelles. In a recent investigation, chitosan-based polymeric micelles containing camptothecin (CPT) were integrated into 3D printing systems and coated with an enteric layer. This approach aimed to safeguard the nanosystems from the harsh conditions of the gastrointestinal tract [77]. The manufacturing process involved the use of a bioprinter that combines fused deposition modeling (FDM)—a widely used 3D printing method that involves melting and extruding filament materials layer by layer—and injection volume filling (IVF)—a technique that enables the incorporation of solutions or dispersions at room temperature into the extruded scaffold [77,78]. The internal structure of the printfills is depicted in Figure 3A. The in vitro drug release profile showed that both printfills containing the free drug and those with micelles effectively managed drug release. Consequently, there was no drug release from the printfills within the initial 2-h period at pH 1.2. However, when pH changed to 6.8, the retarding polymer began to dissolve, permitting the entry of water (Figure 3B). Researchers also concluded that both polymeric micelles and the free drug present in the dissolution media did not exhibit any cytotoxic effects on Caco-2 cells, a colorectal cancer cell line. In fact, these cells showed an increase in metabolic activity of up to 100%, which could be attributed to the presence of simulated gastrointestinal fluids (Figure 3C). Furthermore, as illustrated in Figure 3D, the permeability of CPT from the micelles was observed to be higher than that of the free drug in both Caco-2 standard model (a) and a 3D intestinal model (b), with significant differences becoming evident during the final incubation periods. In the 3D model, CPT permeability reached approximately 27%, representing an enhancement compared to the standard model´s permeability of 20%. This heightened permeability in the 3D model aligns more closely with the in vivo human intestine, reflecting a drug permeability that is more akin to real-world conditions. The experiment also demonstrated consistent transepithelial electrical resistance (TEER) maintenance for both micelles and the free drug, reflecting the monolayer integrity and consequently suggesting that the tested formulation is safe. Besides, the apparent permeability coefficients exhibited notable disparities between the micelles and the free drug. In the 3D model, the apparent permeability coefficients of CPT from the micelles indicate a significant increase in CPT permeability and, consequently, bio-availability. On the other hand, the free drug maintained an apparent permeability coefficient that was similar in both models, signifying that the drug´s permeability was nearly half that of the micellar drug, specifically within the context of the 3D model (Figure 3D(c)). Furthermore, to ensure the structural integrity of the membrane following the permeability experiment, hematoxylin, and eosin (H&AND) staining was conducted for both models and under all conditions (Figure 3E). This staining process employed two dyes: hematoxylin, a basic dye, and eosin, an acidic dye. Hematoxylin imparts a purple hue to acidic structures, such as the nucleus, while eosin imparts a pink color to basic structures, such as the cytoplasm and extracellular matrix. Considering this staining mechanism, Figure 3E presents a consistent monolayer in both models, which underscores the preservation of cellular membrane integrity. These observations indicate that the membrane remained intact and well-formed throughout and following the permeability assay. Overall, this study's findings showed that the printfills were able to keep the micelles intact until they reached the intestinal pH, increasing the CPT intestinal absorption and, consequently, its oral availability. Furthermore, the combination of 3D printing and nanotechnology holds considerable potential for the targeted release of polymeric micelles in the colon. This advancement can enhance the absorption of drugs in the intestines while safeguarding them from degradation as they go through the gastrointestinal tract [77].

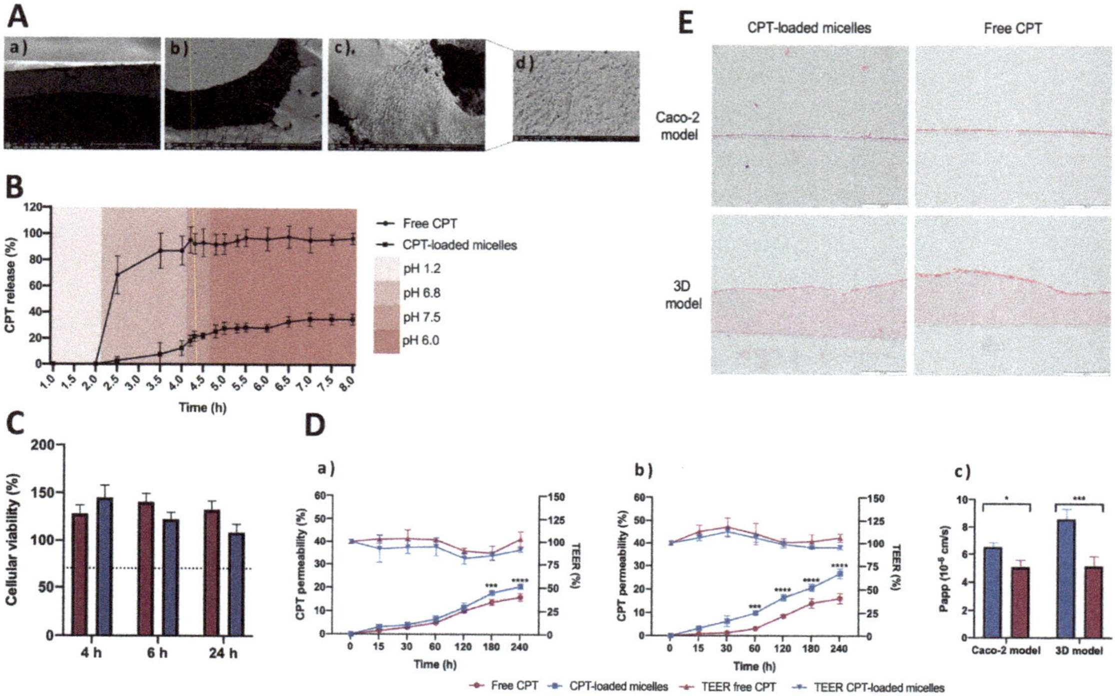

Figure 3. (**A**) Images obtained via scanning electron microscopy of (**a**) top layer of Eudragit in the printfills, (**b**) CPT crystals within the printfills, (**c**) micelles loaded with CPT inside of the printfills, and (**d**) magnified polymeric micelles inside the printfills. (**B**) Cumulative release of CPT from the printfills in simulated gastrointestinal fluids. The release of CPT-loaded micelles is depicted with squares, while the release of free CPT is indicated with circles. (**C**) The cell viability of the dissolution medium sourced from the printfills containing CPT-loaded micelles (depicted as blue columns) and free CPT (illustrated with pink columns) was assessed following 4, 6, and 24 h of incubation with Caco-2 cells. (**D**) Intestinal permeability and respective TEER values of CPT across a standard Caco-2 cell model (**a**) and across a 3D intestinal model (**b**) and apparent permeability coefficients of CPT-loaded micelles (blue) and free CPT (pink) in both Caco-2 monoculture model and the 3D model (**c**), where * $p < 0.05$, *** $p < 0.001$ and **** $p < 0.0001$ (**E**) H&AND staining to assess cellular integrity following exposure to the dissolution medium containing CPT-loaded micelles and free CPT during permeability assay. The cytoplasm was stained pink, while the nucleus was stained purple. The transwell membrane, positioned just beneath the cellular monolayer, remains transparent [77]. **CPT**: camptothecin; **H&AND**: hematoxylin, and eosin; **TEER**: transepithelial electrical resistance.

In another study, researchers focused on creating a bio-ink suitable for 3D printing a hydrogel implant with controlled drug release capability. To achieve this, simvastatin was loaded into polymeric micelles composed of polylactide/poly (ethylene glycol) triblock copolymers (PLA-PEG-PLA). These micelles were then incorporated into hydrogels via a photo-cross-linking 3D printing process. The resulting simvastatin-loaded triple-network hydrogel demonstrated remarkably long-term drug release for over 14 weeks, consistently maintaining a therapeutic concentration. These findings indicate that these micelles hold great promise as a bio-ink material, providing long-term hydrogel stability, biodegradability, and sustained delivery of hydrophobic drugs, such as simvastatin [79].

4.1.2. Liposomes/Niosomes

Due to their numerous benefits, liposomes have garnered significant attention, especially in the fields of cancer treatment and vaccinology. However, their development remains a challenge, making it crucial to seek out innovative approaches that enable fast, safe, and consistent production with high-level batch-to-batch reliability [80].

In an experimental study, researchers used 3D printing technology to create a 3D-printed niosomal hydrogel (3DP-NH) containing cryptotanshinome (CPT) as a topical delivery system for acne therapy. To formulate the CPT-loaded niosomal hydrogel, the CPT-loaded niosomes were carefully added, drop by drop, into the hydrogel. Subsequently, the resulting mixture was printed using an extrusion-based 3D printer to produce a 3D-printed CPT-loaded niosomal hydrogel (3DP-CPT-NH) with a specific drug dosage, shape, and size. The findings were that the 3DP-CPT-NH exhibited a significant anti-acne effect without causing any skin irritation [81].

Another investigation was conducted, combining microfluidic technology (MF) and 3D printing, leading to the formulation of "diamond-shaped" devices designed for the production of liposomes loaded with lysozyme as a model drug. Computer-aided design software was used to design microfluidic devices with diverse geometries, which were then printed using high-resolution digital light processing (DLP)—3DP. Stability tests confirmed the consistency of the developed formulations, and an encapsulation efficacy study showed positive results. Overall, this study showcased the effectiveness of combining MF and 3DP, highlighting the potential for synergistic growth in this field [80].

4.1.3. Nanocrystals

In the pharmaceutical field, 3D printing has also been making an impact in the manufacturing of nanocrystals, allowing for more precise control over drug dosage and release profiles [82]. For instance, additive manufacturing has been used to encapsulate nanocrystals within polymeric matrices, creating drug-loaded filaments or tablets, and improving the solubility and bio-availability of poorly soluble drugs. The precise control over the placement of nanocrystals in the printed structure allows for enhanced drug delivery and therapeutic efficacy. In fact, a recent study aimed to develop fast-dissolving oral polymeric film formulations loaded with indomethacin nanocrystals using 3D printing technology, and the outcomes demonstrated that this offers a promising approach for enhancing solubility in immediate-release formulations [83].

Another experiment focused on the development of an in situ forming robust injectable and 3D printable hydrogel based on cellulose nanocrystals. The results demonstrated that the hydrogels exhibited excellent injectability and maintained their shape fidelity without the need for additional cross-linking steps. The interlayer bonding between the printed layers was strong, resulting in the formation of sTable 3D structures, even up to 10 layers [84].

Additive manufacturing also allows for the creation of personalized drug delivery systems by incorporating nanocrystals. For instance, researchers have used 3D printing to fabricate patient-specific tablets containing nanocrystals of poorly soluble drugs. This enables customized dosages and controlled release profiles to be tailored to individual patient needs. In the first-ever study that included nanocrystals within 3D-printed tablets, albendazole nanocrystals were successfully incorporated into tablets, achieving a concentration of up to 50% *w*/*w*, which is not typically attainable with conventional tablets. Moreover, the printlet formulation with nanocrystals exhibited superior efficacy in improving drug dissolution in HCL 0.1N when compared to nanocrystals in hard gelatin capsules. The nanocrystals exhibited consistent particle size, crystallinity, and chemical stability both before and after 180 days of storage. Overall, the findings demonstrated the promising pharmaceutical potential of combining 3D printing and nanocrystals for the development of stable, fast-release, oral solid dosage forms of poorly soluble drugs. This experiment employed propylene glycol as a carrier and demonstrated that this technique holds promise for printing objects utilizing various types of nanocrystals embedded in low-melting-temperature polymers [85].

4.2. *In Silico Modeling*

4.2.1. Polymeric Micelles

A recent study focused on developing a novel technology called MeltDrops, which used hot-melt extrusion (HME) for continuous manufacturing of in situ gelling systems (ISGS) known to prolong the retention time and improve the bio-availability of ophthalmic drugs. This is relevant because the traditional manufacturing of ISGS has been challenging and costly, hindering their industrial scale-up and clinical implementation. However, MeltDrops technology offers a one-step extrusion process to develop these systems (Figure 4A), which overcomes the limitations of batch manufacturing. Based on in silico modeling, researchers employed a molecular dynamics (MD) simulation to analyze the difference in physical properties of two types of MeltDrops—loaded with timolol maleate (TIM) or dorzolamide hydrochloride (DRZ)—under two different temperature conditions, 300 K (room temperature) and 308 K (physiological temperature) (Figure 4B). These simulations offered evidence of heightened interactions among drug, polymer, and water molecules at a higher temperature (308 K), suggesting the formation of ISGS with desired properties, including a solution–gel transition at physiological temperatures. Researchers also concluded that the in vitro drug release from MeltDrops technology demonstrated sustained and controlled release behavior, while marketed eyedrops showed complete drug release in less than 30 min (Figure 4C). Besides, the results demonstrated a percentage decrease in intraocular pressure (IOP) following the administration of MeltDrops and marketed eyedrops, highlighting the superior IOP-reducing potential of MeltDrops compared to conventional options (Figure 4D). Finally, a HET-CAM test was conducted in order to evaluate the potential ocular irritancy of MeltDrops. The results showed no signs of irritation, indicating that they are safe and well tolerated for ocular use [86].

Previously, a continuous manufacturing technique that utilizes a coaxial turbulent jet in co-flow was established for the production of paclitaxel-loaded polymeric micelles. More recently, researchers have employed coarse-grained molecular dynamics simulations to gain deeper insights into the impact of material attributes (specifically, the drug-polymer ratio and ethanol concentration) and process parameters (such as temperature) on the self-assembly process of polymeric micelles. Additionally, these simulations provided molecular-level information on micelle instability. The findings demonstrated a clear correlation between the micelle shape and drug encapsulation. As the paclitaxel content increased, the micelles transformed from spherical to ellipsoidal structures. From the simulation data, researchers were able to identify the critical aggregation number, which represents the minimum number of polymer and drug molecules required for this shape transition. Moreover, this investigation indicated that larger micellar size and reduced solvent accessibility contributed to the enhanced structural stability of the micelles. Additionally, researchers conducted an evaluation of the micellar dissociation free energy using steered molecular dynamics simulations across various temperatures and ethanol concentrations. The simulations showed that higher ethanol levels and temperatures led to micellar destabilization, resulting in a more significant release of paclitaxel. This increased drug release was attributed to the solvation of the hydrophobic core, promoting micellar swelling and reducing hydrophobic interactions, ultimately leading to a loosely packed micellar structure. In general, the computational predictions provided valuable insights into the micelle self-assembly process, morphological changes, drug release, and thermodynamic instability and showed excellent agreement with experimental results, underscoring its efficacy in studying the impact of material attributes and process parameters on the polymeric micelle formulation during continuous processing [87].

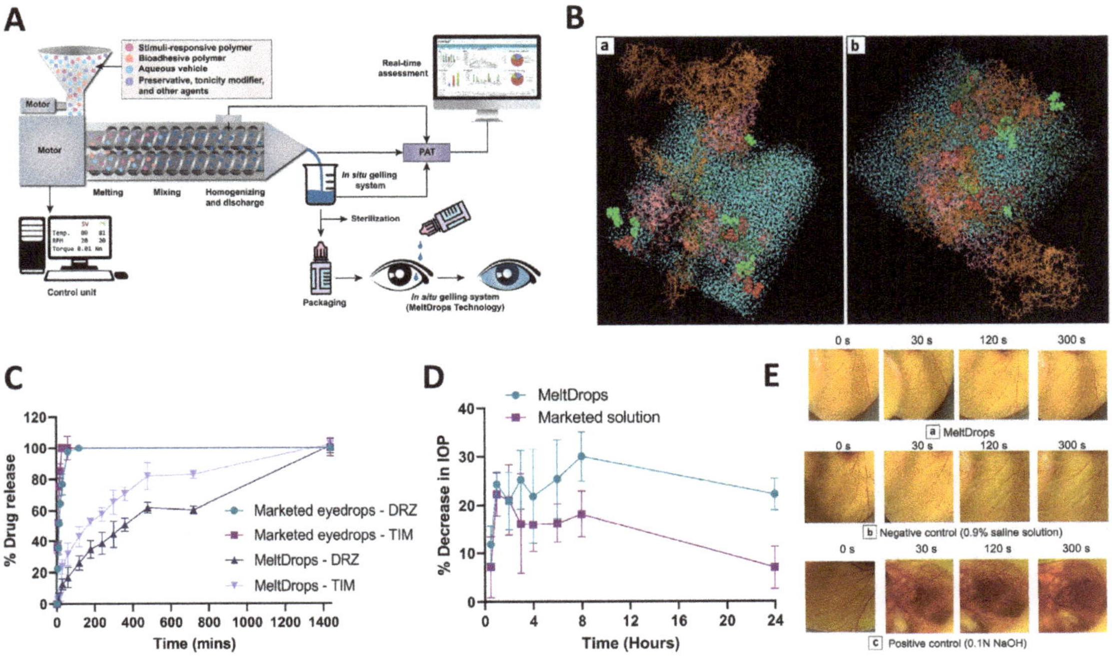

Figure 4. (**A**) Schematic depiction of the ISGS manufacturing process via MeltDrops technology. (**B**) Molecular interactions forming between the components of the formulation at two different temperatures: 300 K (**a**) and 308 K (**b**): Green CPK model = TIM; Red = DRZ; Blue = Sodium chloride; Yellow = Benzalkonium chloride; Pink = HPMC; Orange = Poloxamer 407; Green wire model = Poloxamer 188; Blue = water. (**C**) Cumulative release of timolol maleate (TIM) and dorzolamide hydrochloride (DRZ) over time from both MeltDrops and commercially available solutions. (**D**) Percentage decrease in IOP following the administration of MeltDrops and commercially available eyedrops. (**E**) HET-CAM test results after the application of (**a**) MeltDrops with no signs of irritation, (**b**) 0.9% *w*/*v* saline solutions, also showing no signs of irritation, and (**c**) 0.1 N Sodium hydroxide solution, revealing features such as vascular lysis, coagulation, and hemorrhage [86]. **DRZ**: dorzolamide hydrochloride; **IOP**: intraocular pressure; **ISGS**: in situ gelling system; **TIM**: timolol maleate.

In another study, researchers used coarse-grained molecular dynamics simulations to investigate the behavior of a specific type of block copolymer called poly (ethylene oxide)-poly (propylene oxide)-poly (ethylene oxide) (PEO-PPO-PEO), commonly known as pluronics or poloxamers. They studied the effect of polymer and surfactant concentration on the morphology of these block copolymers and ionic surfactants, namely sodium dodecyl sulfate (SDS), in aqueous solutions. The results showed that when pluronics and SDS are present together in the solution, they tend to form mixed micelles and that the shape of those micelles depends on the relative concentrations of pluronics and SDS in the solution. The core of the mixed micelles consists of PPO chains from the pluronics, the alkyl tail of SDS, and some water molecules. The surrounding shell is composed of PEO chains, water molecules, and the sulfate headgroups of the SDS. Notably, with an increasing amount of added SDS, the observed morphology of the mixed micelles undergoes a transition from spherical to wormlike–cylindrical geometry. Overall, the molecular insights gained from studying the co-assembly of an ionic surfactant and an amphiphilic triblock copolymer in aqueous media have potential applications in various complex fluid mixtures. However, the accuracy of the results relies on the coarse-grained force field used, which can be improved with more computationally expensive atomistic simulations for quantitative comparisons with experimental data [88].

4.2.2. Liposomes/Transfersomes

In silico modeling has been employed in the manufacturing of liposomes because it allows researchers to simulate and predict the behavior of these structures, such as their stability, size, composition, drug encapsulation efficiency, and release kinetics. Furthermore, these models can help to optimize the manufacturing process, predict the performance of liposomal formulations, and guide experimental design [89].

In a recent study, the authors constructed computational models to identify active pharmaceutical ingredients (APIs) that can achieve the desired high concentrations in nano-liposomes via remote loading. The models aimed to predict the suitability of APIs for nano-liposomal delivery by considering fixed main experimental conditions, such as liposome lipid composition and size. The researchers also added a prediction of drug leakage from the nano-liposomes during storage, which is crucial for ensuring the development of pharmaceutically viable nano-drugs. More so, by using "load and leak" models, this group screened two large molecular databases to identify candidates' APIs for delivery by nano-liposomes. Through the screening process, the researchers identified 667 molecules that showed positive results in both the loading and leakage models, indicating high-loading and stable characteristics. Among these molecules, 318 received high scores in both properties and, notably 67 of them are FDA-approved drugs [90]. These findings underscore the significance of computational modeling in optimizing liposomal formulations. By narrowing the search to molecules exhibiting high-loading and stability characteristics, researchers can concentrate their efforts on candidates with a higher likelihood of success. This approach facilitates efficient use of time, resources, and cost savings compared to traditional trial-and-error methods.

These computational approaches can—and should—be combined with experimental studies because it allows for a better understanding of the mechanisms that are being investigated. Computational modeling not only aids in explaining experimental results, but has also the potential to guide and inspire new directions for experimental research in the development of liposomal drug delivery systems [91].

In a study that aimed to develop active targeting liposomes to deliver anticancer agents to the treatment of hepatocellular carcinoma, computational modeling was used to gain insight into the structure and behavior of the intended targeted liposomal drug delivery systems within the bloodstream. This research showcases the complementary nature of these simulations alongside experimental research, often offering valuable mechanistic context [92].

Another example of the predictive power of in silico modeling in the pharmaceutical industry is an investigation that explored the use of thermosensitive liposomes (TSL) for targeted drug delivery to tumors. The researchers created a three-dimensional computer model to simulate the delivery of the TSL-encapsulated doxorubicin to mouse tumors. To do so, a mouse hind limb was scanned using a 3D scanner, and the resulting geometry was imported into finite element modeling software. A virtual tumor was added to the model, and the authors simulated the heating process using a surface probe. In addition to the heat transfer model, the researchers also developed a drug delivery model that simulates the kinetics of drug release. It is important to mention that the computed model was validated by performing experimental studies using gel phantoms and in vivo fluorescence imaging studies in mice with lung tumor xenografts. By comparing the results of the computer model with the experimental studies, the researchers can assess the accuracy of the model. The results showed that in silico modeling accurately reproduces the temperature profile observed in the phantom experiments and that the drug delivery profile simulated by the model also aligns with the results of the in vivo studies. Overall, it demonstrates the feasibility of using a computer model to accurately simulate drug delivery in preclinical studies [89].

To investigate the distribution of three drugs with different polarities (5-fluorouracil, ligustrazine, and osthole) within liposomes and transfersomes, researchers conducted a study using molecular dynamics simulation. To understand the drug distribution, these authors employed the radial distribution function—which calculates the probability of finding a drug molecule at a specific distance from a reference drug molecule within the vesicle—and the potential of mean force—which describes the potential energy between a drug molecule and the surrounding lipid molecules, indicating the strength of their interactions. By using these measures, the authors were able to characterize the distribution of drugs within the lipid vesicles. The results highlight the potential of molecular simulation technology in understanding the characteristics of lipid vesicles and their interactions with drugs [93].

4.2.3. Nanocrystals

A study aimed to develop and evaluate an advanced in silico modeling for understanding the pharmacokinetics of Foscan®, a formulation containing temoporfin that has received approval for palliative photodynamic therapy of squamous cell carcinoma of the head and neck. The researchers conducted precipitation experiments in the presence of biorelevant media, thereby simulating conditions akin to those encountered in the human body. This approach aimed to observe the behavior of Foscan® under these physiologically relevant circumstances. When introduced in these media, the drug underwent a process of precipitation, forming nanocrystals. Moreover, nanoparticle tracking analysis was employed to investigate these nanocrystals, providing the means to measure their size and analyze the distribution of these structures within the sample. Incorporating the data from these precipitation experiments and nanoparticle tracking analysis, the model predicted how nanocrystals of Foscan® were formed, their size distribution, and how they interacted with biological fluids in the body. This information could help them explain and predict the Foscan® pharmacokinetics more accurately, as nanocrystals can significantly impact how a drug is absorbed, distributed, and eliminated [94].

In another study, to evaluate the impact of polymers in the production of stable dexibuprofen (Dexi) nanocrystals with improved therapeutic potential, researchers combined in silico modeling techniques (namely AutoDockVina, Marven Sketch, and Maestro) with experimental studies. The results provided molecular insight into the mechanisms of binding of the optimal polymers to the surface of Dexi nanocrystals, showing that the combination of hydroxypropyl methylcellulose (HPMC)-polyvinyl pyrrolidone (PVP) and HPMC-Eudragit (EUD) was the most effective in stabilizing Dexi nanocrystals. Overall, the combination of computational modeling with experimental studies allows researchers to save time and resources by focusing on the most promising polymer combinations, thereby expediting the drug development process. Additionally, this integrated approach provides a deeper understanding of the molecular mechanisms underlying the stabilization of nanocrystals, helping researchers make more informed decisions in their pursuit of developing better pharmaceutical formulations [95].

4.3. Machine Learning

4.3.1. Polymeric Micelles

Machine learning algorithms can be utilized to predict various properties and behaviors of polymeric micelles. For example, models can be trained using data on polymer structure, composition, molecular weight, and other relevant parameters, along with experimental outcomes such as micelle size, stability, drug loading, and release profiles. These models can then be used to predict the behavior of new polymeric systems, guiding the design and selection of optimal micellar formulations [96].

Researchers used an artificial neural network (ANN) to create a model for the release of a chemotherapeutic drug—doxorubicin—from polymeric micelles (specifically Pluronic P105) under two different ultrasound frequencies. Although the exact number of samples used in the study was not explicitly mentioned, the model was trained using experimentally obtained input–output data concerning the release of doxorubicin from the micelles. The developed ANN model was then employed to optimize the application of ultrasound in order to achieve the desired drug release at the tumor site. The ANN method accurately predicted the release behavior and demonstrated maximum prediction errors of 0.002 and 0.001 at ultrasound frequencies of 20 and 70 kHz, respectively. The results demonstrate the successful design and testing of a controller capable of adjusting ultrasound frequency, intensity, and pulse length to maintain a constant release of Dox, potentially enhancing targeted drug delivery to tumor sites [97].

4.3.2. Liposomes/Niosomes

By analyzing large datasets of liposomal properties and characteristics, machine learning models can identify patterns and correlations between various liposome components (lipids and encapsulated substances, among others) and their properties (size, stability, drug release profile). This information can guide the selection of optimal liposome compositions and improve formulation success rates [98]. In addition, ML models can also be trained on existing data to predict important liposomes properties, which may include encapsulation efficiency, drug release kinetics, stability under different conditions, and targeting capabilities. By utilizing historical data and relevant features, machine learning algorithms can provide valuable insights and predictions, enabling more efficient and targeted liposome development [99].

In fact, there are some trials applying machine learning for liposome formulation optimization or prediction. For instance, one study proposed a machine learning framework to address the challenges associated with optimizing the drug entrapment efficiency of niosomal vesicles, showing that these algorithms allow for the synthesis of niosomal systems with optimal entrapment efficiency at a lower cost and time (Kashani-Asadi-Jafari et al., 2022). In another study, scientists built an artificial neural network (ANN) and advanced machine learning model to optimize the percentage of cytarabine entrapped in the liposome, showing that the ANN provided more accurate prediction formulations when compared with the multiple regression analysis method [100]. An ANN model was also developed to predict the size and polydispersity index of liposomes made of DOPC (1,2 Dioleoyl-sn-glycero-3-phosphocholine), cholesterol, and DSPE-PEG 2000 1,2 Distearoyl-sn-glycero-3-phosphoethanolamine-N [amino (polyethylene glycol)-2000] (ammonium salt)) using a microfluidic system. The results demonstrated that microfluidic-based preparation techniques assisted by computational tools can accelerate the development and clinical translation of nano-based pharmaceutical products [101].

Recently, machine learning has been combined with molecular descriptors, which are a set of quantitative values or features that represent various properties of a molecule's structure, composition, and behavior. These are used to encode complex chemical information into numerical data, which can then be used as input for various computational analysis and machine learning models. Fundamentally, ML models leverage patterns within data to predict the properties of novel molecules, eliminating the need for physical synthesis or testing [98,102]. To illustrate this, an ANN was constructed to develop computational models focused on optimizing a continuous liposome manufacturing system. In this system, the liposomes were generated using a co-axial turbulent jet within a co-flow technology. This means that two phases were used—an ethanol phase with lipids and an aqueous phase—to create liposomes of uniform sizes. The ANN was used to optimize this manufacturing process and so, it took various input parameters known as critical material attributes (CMAs) and critical process parameters (CPPs). CMAs include characteristics of the raw materials, such as the length of the hydrocarbon tail in lipids, the percentage of cholesterol, and the type of buffer used. CPPs include process conditions, such as solvent temperature and flow rate. The ANN's purpose was to predict critical quality attributes (CQAs) of the liposomes. In this study, the CQAs were the particle size and polydispersity index (PDI), which indicate how uniform the liposome sizes are. Thus, two types of ANN architectures were evaluated, namely a multiple-input–multiple-output (MIMO) model—which takes multiple inputs and produces multiple outputs—and a multiple-input–single-output (MISO) model—which takes multiple inputs but produces a single output (Figure 5A). The study found that the MISO architecture outperformed the MIMO architecture in terms of accuracy for the task at hand. Apart from the ANN model, a graphical user interface was also created to help end-users perform interactive simulated risk analysis and visualize the predictions made by the ANN model (Figure 5B). Evaluations demonstrated that the developed graphical user interface yields accurate predictions for both liposome particle size and PDI as long as the chosen inputs fall within the scope of the studied conditions during the initial ANN training. These predictions have the potential to contribute to the formulation of a control strategy designed to mitigate the impact of process disturbances on liposome particle size. Utilizing the five input features mentioned earlier, an ANN was trained with the primary goal of minimizing the mean relative error (MRE), which was successfully achieved at a level below 5%. It was notably a very low error for predicting particle size, as is evident from the comparison between the target and predicted values presented in Figure 5C. However, the prediction accuracy for PDI was notably inadequate, as indicated by the results displayed in Figure 5D. Basically, despite the successful predictions for particle size, the model encountered challenges in accurately forecasting PDI values. To mitigate the training error, researchers introduced molecular descriptors as supplementary inputs to the ANN. These were obtained using PaDEL-Descriptor software and helped the ANN understand the characteristics of the raw materials. A combination of CMAs, CPPs, and molecular descriptors was used to train the MISO ANN model and allowed for the reduction of errors during both training and testing, indicating improved model performance (Figure 5E). Overall, via a combination of critical material attributes, process parameters, and molecular descriptors, this study improved the accuracy of predicting the quality attributes of liposomes [103].

In another study, ML techniques were used to create prediction models capable of individually predicting crucial parameters of liposomes, such as size, PDI, zeta potential, and encapsulation efficiency. To validate the predictive prowess of these models, liposome formulations were created for two distinct compounds: naproxen (NAP) and palmatine HCL (PAL), representing insoluble and water-soluble molecules, respectively. In order to evaluate the significance of drug properties in liposome behavior, further investigation into the molecular interactions and behaviors of NAP and PAL within liposomes was undertaken via coarse-grained molecular dynamics simulations. Figure 6A(a,a1) depict the initial configurations of the two systems, of which ten underwent dynamic simulations lasting 1 microsecond. Snapshots captured during the modeling process are illustrated in Figure 6A(b,b1), while the ultimate structures of the respective liposomes are displayed in Figure 6A(c,c1). Additionally, the size distribution was assessed, and the structures of the liposomes containing NAP and PAL were characterized using transmission electron microscopy, showcased in Figure 6A(d1,d2). These simulations demonstrated that NAP molecules tend to integrate into the lipid layer, while a majority of PAL molecules aggregate within the inner aqueous phase of the liposome. The marked disparity in the physical states of NAP and PAL underlines the pivotal role of drug properties in formulating liposomes. Additionally, formulation attributes were ranked to offer significant insights for designing effective formulations. Given that logS (logarithm of a compound's aqueous solubility), molecular complexity (an assessment of the intricacy of a structure), and XLogP3 (represent a predictive estimation of the octanol–water partition coefficient, determined via a specific algorithm) of the drug molecules held significant influence over encapsulation efficiency, their correlation was illustrated using a heatmap, depicted in Figure 6B. This heatmap employed color visualization in a two-dimensional format to depict the data relationship effectively. Basically, drug molecules with certain properties, such as a logS value between −3 and −6, a molecular complexity between 500 and 1000, and a XLogP3 value greater than or equal to 2, are considered a priority for formulating liposomes with better encapsulation. Finally, in Figure 6C, it is possible to observe a congruence between predicted and experimental outcomes, which serves as confirmation of the ML model's satisfactory accuracy. In summary, the researchers established comprehensive prediction models for anticipating liposome formulations, and the influences of key factors were dissected by combining ML techniques with molecular modeling. The study successfully validates the availability and rationality of these intelligent prediction systems, offering promising applications for the future development of liposome formulations [98].

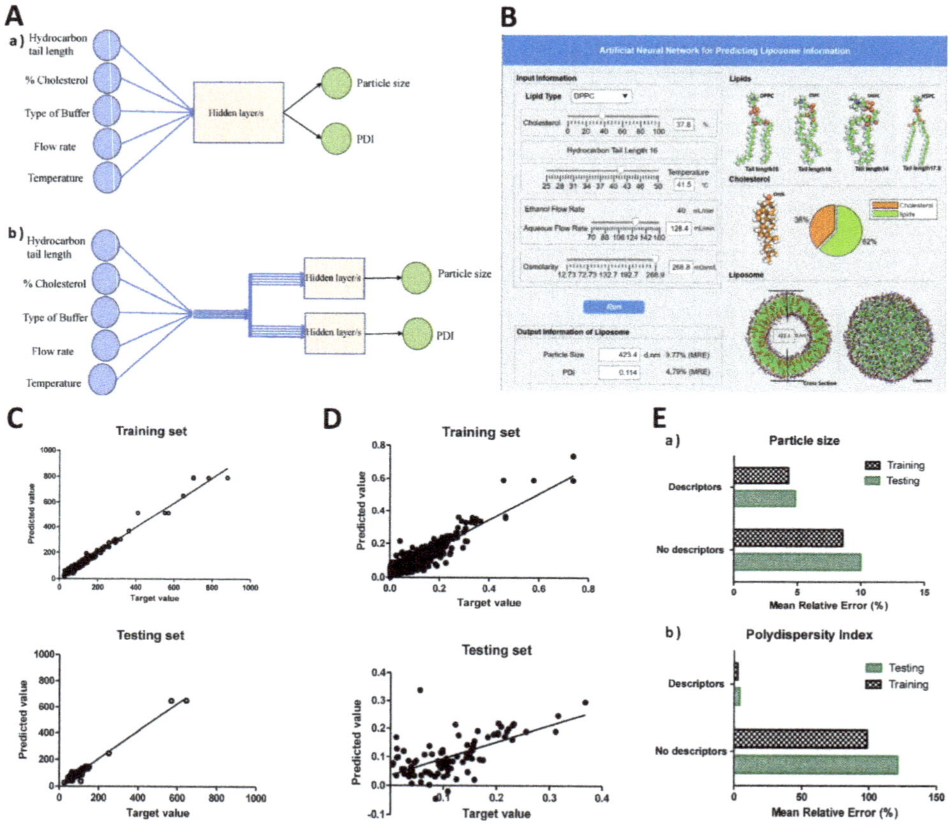

Figure 5. (**A**) Comparative illustration of MIMO model (**a**) and MISO model (**b**). (**B**) Graphical user interface of the ANN for liposome particle size and PDI prediction in continuous liposome manufacturing. (**C**) Comparison of predicted vs. target values for liposome particle size in the training and testing sets, without molecular descriptors. (**D**) Comparison of predicted vs. target values for liposome PDI in the training and testing sets, without molecular descriptors. (**E**) Evaluation of MRE with and without incorporating molecular descriptors in the ANN input: (**a**) particle size and (**b**) PDI [103]. **ANN**: artificial neural network; **MIMO**: multiple-input–multiple-output; **MISO**: multiple-input–single-output; **PDI**: polydispersity index; **MRE**: mean relative error.

Based on all of that, it is safe to say that machine learning plays a valuable role in the development of liposomes by assisting in formulation design, predicting liposome properties, optimizing drug loading and release, analyzing characterization data, and optimizing manufacturing processes. By leveraging machine learning techniques, researchers can expedite the development and improve the performance of liposomal formulations for drug delivery and other biomedical applications [104].

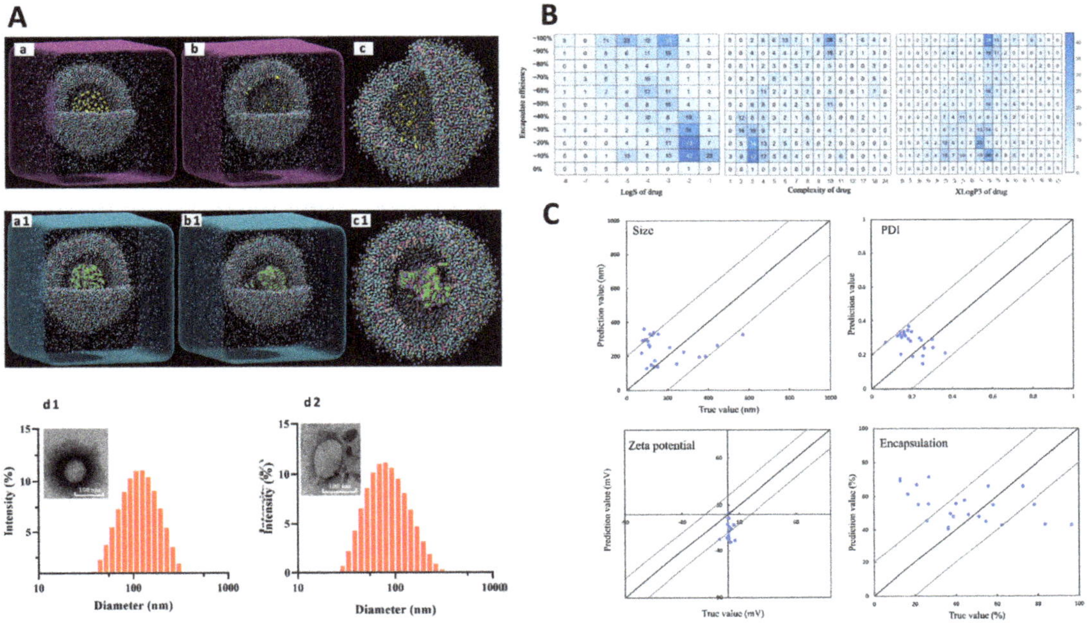

Figure 6. (**A**) Snapshots captured during 1 microsecond of molecular dynamics simulations, alongside the experimental size distribution of NAP liposomes (**a–c**,**d1**) and PAL liposomes (**a1–c1**,**d2**). (**B**) Heat map assessment illustrating the connection between logS, molecular complexity, and XLogP3 of the drug with encapsulation within liposomes. The numerical values within each matrix indicate the frequency of encapsulation occurrences corresponding to each specific property. (**C**) A scatter plot displaying the comparison between experimental and predicted values for size, PDI, zeta potential, and encapsulation [98]. **NAP**: naproxen; **PAL**: palmatine HCL; **PDI**: polydispersity index.

4.3.3. Nanocrystals

Machine learning techniques have been increasingly employed in the field of nanocrystal development. For instance, they can be trained to predict the properties of nanocrystals by using data from a variety of sources, including experimental measurements, theoretical calculations, and molecular descriptors. These predictive models can assist in the design and selection of nanocrystals with desired properties, saving time and resources by reducing the need for extensive experimental testing. In fact, to address this issue, researchers collected data on nanocrystal size (910 data points) and polymer dispersity index (341 data points) using three different preparation methods—ball wet milling (BWM), high-pressure homogenization (HPH), and antisolvent precipitation (ASP)—in order to construct prediction models [105].

The results indicated that the machine learning performed well in predicting those properties for BWM and HPH methods but showed relatively poor predictions for the ASP method. Figure 7A displays scatter plots comparing the predicted values, generated by the machine learning model, with the experimental values of nanocrystals sizes within BWM, HPM, and ASP size dataset subsets. Within the BWM subsets, the predicted values closely matched the experimental values in the size range of 0–500 nm. Nevertheless, for data points outside of this range, particularly those exceeding 500 nm, predicted values displayed significant disparities from the experimental values, especially in the validation and test datasets. The findings suggest that the constructed learning model exhibits superior predictive accuracy for data points falling within the 0–500 nm range, particularly where the data density is higher in the BWM size dataset. It is evident that the uneven distribution of data within the dataset significantly influences the model's construction and predictive performance. On the other hand, due to the limited availability of input data within the size range of 500 to 1000 nm, learning algorithms struggled to discern the underlying data patterns, leading to less accurate predictions. The scatter plots for the HPH and ASP subsets showed comparable results, with predicted values closely aligning with experimental values in regions where data density was higher [105].

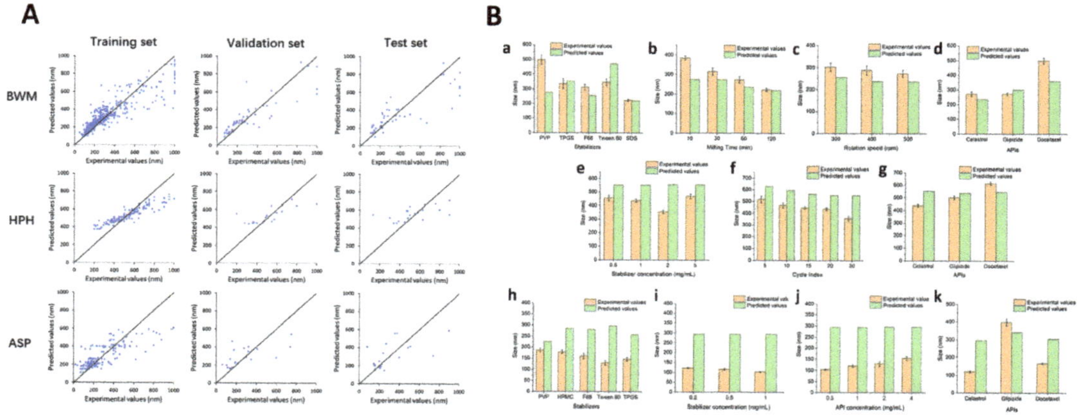

Figure 7. (**A**) Scatter plots comparing the predicted values obtained from the machine learning algorithm with the experimental values for nanocrystal size on the training, validation, and test subsets within the BWM, HPH, and ASP size datasets. (**B**) Contrasts in the predicted values generated by the algorithm with the actual sizes of nanocrystals prepared with BWM (**a–d**), HPH (**e–g**), and ASP (**h–k**) [105]. **ASP**: antisolvent precipitation; **BWM**: ball wet milling; **HPH**: high-pressure homogenization.

Figure 8A, on the other hand, displays scatter plots comparing the predicted values to the experimental values of PDI data. The machine learning algorithm performed admirably in predicting this property values within the BWM and HPH subsets, as indicated by the close alignment of data points with the black line. Despite the relatively small datasets with only 133 and 119 data points in the BWM and HPH PDI datasets, respectively, the algorithm still demonstrated accurate predictions, likely due to the concentrated data distribution. Conversely, in the ASP subsets, the predictive performance in the training set was notably less accurate. This could be attributed to the smaller volume of data and the lower data quality within these subsets [105].

The researchers speculated that the poor prediction for the ASP method might be due to the lower quality of data resulting from the poor reproducibility and instability of nanocrystals prepared using this method. It was also found that the majority of commercialized nanocrystals products were manufactured using BWM and HPH approaches. ML helped rank the factors influencing nanocrystal properties, indicating that milling time, cycle index, and stabilizer concentration were crucial factors for the nanocrystals prepared by BWM, HPH, and ASP methods, respectively. The accuracy of these predictions was further confirmed by experiments with newly prepared nanocrystals. Concerning the nanocrystals size, the findings indicate that the algorithm delivered accurate predictions for most of the nanocrystals produced through the BWM (Figure 7B(a–d)) and HPH (Figure 7B(e–g)) methods. However, the predicted performance for ASP nanocrystals (Figure 7B(h–k)) fell short, with predicted values being roughly twice as large as the experimentally measured sizes. Regarding PDI predictions, the algorithm also demonstrated effective forecasting for BWM (Figure 8B(a–d)) and HPH (Figure 8B(e–g)) datasets, but showed comparatively poorer performance for ASP (Figure 8B(h–k)). The most likely reasons for this subpar predictive performance were the limited volume of data available for ASP size and PDI datasets used in constructing machine learning models, and the lower data quality stemming from the constraints of the preparation methods. These issues ultimately led to the failure of predictions within the ASP dataset.

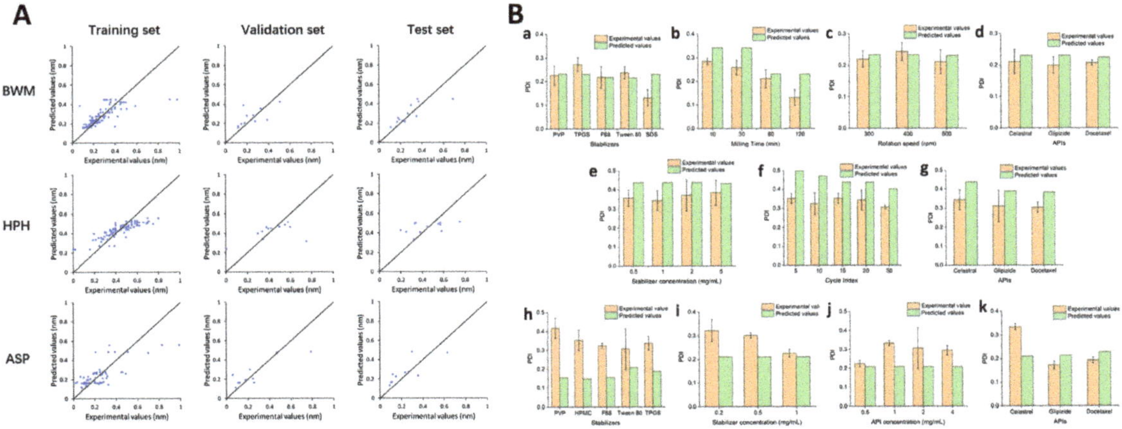

Figure 8. (**A**) Scatter plots comparing the predicted values obtained from the machine learning algorithm with the experimental values for nanocrystal PDI on the training, validation, and test subsets within the BWM, HPH, and ASP size datasets. (**B**) Contrast the predicted values generated by the algorithm with the actual PDI values of nanocrystals prepared by BWM (**a–d**), HPH (**e–g**), and ASP (**h–k**) [105]. **ASP**: antisolvent precipitation; **BWM**: ball wet milling; **HPH**: high-pressure homogenization; **PDI**: polydispersity index.

Overall, the results highlights the potential of using machine learning in nanotechnology manufacturing, providing a promising alternative to traditional, labor-intensive approaches in nanocrystal formulation development [105].

4.4. Digital Twins

Digital twins have emerged as a transformative technology in the pharmaceutical industry, offering a powerful tool for improving drug development processes and product lifecycle management [106]. In the realm of traditional pharmaceuticals, their significance is already well recognized, as digital twins enable the creation of virtual replicas of physical drugs and manufacturing processes, facilitating real-time monitoring, optimization, and quality control [39,40]. However, it is important to highlight the lack of experimental studies on the application of these technologies in the NBCD domain. This is an exciting frontier for innovation and has the potential to significantly advance the development, manufacturing, and quality assurance of these pharmaceutical products.

5. Regulatory Issues

Regulatory agencies, including the FDA, believe that the incorporation of computational methods into the field of pharmaceutics can enhance product quality. When these methods are used, a deeper understanding of the process involved in product design is achieved, aligning with the principles of QbD [7]. In fact, the FDA has been moving towards performance-based regulation, focusing on measurable outcomes rather than prescriptive processes, which aligns well with Pharma 4.0 and its extensive data capabilities [3].

To attain Pharma 4.0, it is essential to embrace cutting-edge manufacturing technologies while simultaneously surmounting regulatory obstacles [12]. For instance, initially, the absence of a well-defined regulatory framework was notable, hindering innovators from integrating digital technologies with traditional processes due to a lack of regulatory precedents. However, more recently, significant strides have been taken in this direction. In particular, the FDA has taken a proactive step by establishing the Digital Health Center of Excellence, aiming to adopt a comprehensive approach to digital health technology [107].

Moreover, filing regulatory applications across different jurisdictions with varying expectations can be burdensome, particularly for emerging manufacturing technologies. Achieving international regulatory convergence could provide clarity and certainty for manufacturers. Besides, the industry may simultaneously comprise companies operating under Pharma 2.0, 3.0, and 4.0 paradigms. Regulating such a diverse landscape requires flexible frameworks to enable the adoption of new technologies without disrupting supply from older technology-based manufacturers [3].

It is important to note that, at present, the FDA has already approved several 3D printed products, which encompass not only drug products—such as Spritam®—but also—and essentially—a diverse range of medical devices that include orthodontic implants, prosthetics, anatomical models, and reaction-wares [108]. In December 2017, the FDA released a set of guidelines titled "Technical Considerations for Additive Manufactured Medical Devices", which provides guidelines covering various aspects, including software and hardware requirements, quality control, and process validation procedures. However, considering the complexity of medicinal products, which often have more demanding requirements than medical devices, separate regulatory considerations are needed. APIs present additional challenges, such as potential incompatibilities and the stability of the active substance during the printing process [109].

Nonetheless, due to the variability of additive manufacturing methods, it is challenging to devise a universal set of guidelines applicable to all 3D printing techniques. The truth is that, given the multitude of factors influencing the quality of computationally designed dosage forms and the safety of their use, the establishment of appropriate regulatory requirements is of utmost importance. However, currently, there are no valid regulations concerning the design, manufacturing process, and quality testing considerations specific to three-dimensional printing in the pharmaceutical industry [110]. Recently, it has been emphasized that 3D printing, as a manufacturing process, does not pose regulatory limitations as long as the final product meets the established requirements. For instance, the previously mentioned approved 3D printed tablet, Spritam®, includes the same excipients that are found in conventional tablets. The only difference lies in the production process. Consequently, it is reasonable to assume that similar quality requirements apply in this case as they do for other orally disintegrating tablets [111].

Overall, as the pharmaceutical industry is transitioning into the Pharma 4.0 era, regulatory agencies are exploring ways to adapt and accommodate the advancements brought by these new technologies [107].

6. Future Prospects

Pharma 4.0 technologies have demonstrated significant promise in the manufacturing of NBCDs. The integration of advanced digital techniques, automation, and data analytics in the pharmaceutical industry has the potential to optimize processes, enhance quality control, enable customization, and improve supply chain efficiency, ultimately leading to improved production and delivery of NBCDS.

However, there is still much potential for further development and some areas where ongoing work and future efforts can be focused. For instance, these technologies can extend to various other NBCDs, such as glatiramer acetate and iron carbohydrate complexes as, to the best of our knowledge, there are no experimental studies available that assess the impact of Pharma 4.0 in these NBCDs. The implementation of digital twins is also expected to assist in simulating and optimizing NBCD manufacturing. By integrating real-time data from sensors and process models, digital twins can enable virtual testing, scenario analysis, and optimization of manufacturing operations to enhance productivity and efficiency. It is important to take into consideration that as the implementation of Pharma 4.0 techniques progresses, regulatory frameworks need to evolve to accommodate the use of advanced technologies in NBCD manufacturing. This includes addressing data security and privacy concerns and establishing guidelines for the validation and qualification of digital systems while ensuring compliance with evolving regulatory requirements.

In the machine learning domain, SVMs and random forests stand out as increasingly promising alternatives to ANNs. Particularly in cases where datasets are limited, ANNs tend to be prone to overfitting due to their complex nature. SVMs, with their remarkable ability to capture intricate relationships within data, and random forests, with their ensemble learning capabilities, offer a more robust and adaptable solution for the challenges unique to NBCDs. These methods, by effectively handling complex NBCD compositions and diverse characteristics, could provide a brighter prospect for the domain, emphasizing precision, reliability, and the capacity to meet quality and safety standards [37,38].

Still in the machine learning domain, experimental studies that employ multiple metrics to quantify the model's performance are surprisingly scarce. This gap in the research landscape highlights the need for a more comprehensive approach to assessing the effectiveness of these models. By incorporating a variety of evaluation metrics, such as accuracy, precision, recall, F1 score, ROC-AUC (receiver operating characteristic–area under the curve), and others tailored to the specific problem, researchers can gain a more nuanced and holistic understanding of their model's performance. This multifaceted evaluation approach is vital in ensuring a more accurate and reliable appraisal, ultimately leading to better-informed decision-making and higher-quality work within the realm of machine learning [112,113].

In addition, it is also important to keep in mind that the implementation of Pharma 4.0 principles and technologies implies a reevaluation and readjustment of economic policies and legal frameworks and the establishment of financial stability to accommodate these emerging techniques. This also calls for a transformation in the academic curriculum to facilitate the acquisition of necessary skills, upskill the workforce, and foster system-wide awareness [6].

Overall, the prospects of Pharma 4.0 in the manufacturing of NBCDs are very promising. The implementation of advanced digital technologies and data-driven approaches can optimize processes, improve quality assurance, enhance customization capabilities, and streamline supply chains, ultimately leading to more efficient and effective NBCD manufacturing.

While the concept of Pharma 4.0 continues to grow and its techniques are slowly applied, there is an ongoing discussion about the potential evolution of the pharmaceutical industry beyond the current Pharma 4.0 framework. In fact, the term Pharma 5.0 has already been mentioned. It represents a possible future stage in which the integration of advanced technologies and data-driven approaches in the pharmaceutical sector goes even further. Hence, the prospects are very ambitious, considering the potential of these tools, but also a challenge, in particular for the regulatory follow-up that will have to be given in this context.

7. Conclusions

Concerning non-biological complex drug manufacturing, Pharma 4.0 techniques such as machine learning, in silico modeling, and 3D printing allow for enhanced overall production efficiency by streamlining operations and reducing production time, ultimately leading to cost savings. Additionally, the increased automation and use of real-time data analytics have improved process monitoring and control, minimized the risk of errors, and ensured a higher level of product quality and consistency.

However, the integration of Pharma 4.0 in the manufacture of NBCDs is still limited, essentially restricted to nanocrystals, liposomes, and polymeric micelles. It would be of great interest to extend the investigation of these techniques to other NBCDs, such as glatiramer acetate and iron carbohydrate complexes, for example. On the other hand, in the realm of machine learning, where extensive research has been conducted, it would be relevant to approach some other algorithms instead of focusing solely on ANN. Another constraint in the machine learning domain is the fact that there is a scarcity of experimental studies that use multiple metrics to gauge the model's performance.

Digital twins seem to be very promising in the field of pharmaceutical industry, but they have not been applied to the domain of NBCDs. However, by integrating real-time data from sensors and process models, digital twins can enable virtual testing, scenario analysis, and optimization of manufacturing operations to enhance productivity and efficiency.

It is also important to acknowledge the challenges associated with the adoption of these technologies, such as the need for skilled personnel capable of operating and maintaining advanced technologies, ensuring data security and privacy, and addressing regulatory concerns regarding the validation and qualification of these novel manufacturing processes.

Overall, it is safe to say that the implementation of Pharma 4.0 technologies in the manufacturing of NBCDs represents a transformative approach and a paradigm shift in the pharmaceutical industry. As we move forward, continuous research and innovation will pave the way for a more sustainable and patient-focused pharmaceutical landscape.

Author Contributions: Conceptualization, F.M.-M.; methodology, V.M. and F.M.-M.; software, V.M. and J.D.; validation, F.M.-M. and F.V.; investigation, V.M. and F.M.-M.; resources, V.M.; data curation, V.M; writing—original draft preparation, V.M., J.D. and F.M.-M.; writing—review and editing, F.M.-M. and F.V.; supervision, F.M.-M. All authors have read and agreed to the published version of the manuscript.

Funding: This research received no external funding.

Institutional Review Board Statement: Not applicable.

Informed Consent Statement: Not applicable.

Data Availability Statement: Data sharing is not applicable to this article.

Conflicts of Interest: The authors declare no conflict of interest.

Abbreviations

ANN	Artificial neural network
AI	Artificial intelligence
API	Active pharmaceutical ingredient
ASP	Antisolvent precipitation
BWM	Ball wet milling
CESS®	Controlled expansion of supercritical solution
CMAs	Critical material attributes
CNS	Central nervous system
CPPs	Critical process parameters
CQAs	Critical quality attributes
3D	Three-dimensional
Dexi	Dexibuprofen
DMT	Disease-modifying treatment
DRZ	Dorzolamide hydrochloride
EAE	Experimental autoimmune encephalomyelitis
EUD	Eudragit
FD	Freeze-dried
FDA	Food and Drug Administration
GA	Glatiramer acetate
GI	Gastrointestinal
hERG	Human ether-a-go-go-related gene
HME	Hot-melt extrusion
HPH	High-pressure homogenization
HPMC	Hydroxypropyl methylcellulose
IOP	Intraocular pressure

ISGS	In situ gelling system
MD	Molecular dynamics
MIMO	Multiple-input–multiple-output
MISO	Multiple-input–single-output
MF	Microfluidic technology
ML	Machine learning
MRE	Mean relative error
MS	Multiple sclerosis
NanoPRX	Nanoformed piroxicam
NN	Neural network
NAP	Naproxen
NBCD	Non-biological complex drug
PEO-PPO-PEO	Poly(ethylene oxide)-Poly(propylene oxide)-Poly(ethylene oxide)
PAL	Palmatine HCL
PAT	Process analytical technology
PDI	Polydispersity index
PVP	Polyvinyl pyrrolidone
QbD	Quality by design
RTD	Room temperature-dried
SDS	Sodium dodecyl sulfate
SVM	Support vector machines
SSE	Semi-solid extrusion
TEER	Transepithelial electrical resistance
TIM	Timolol maleate
TNF-α	Tumor necroses factor-α

References

1. Hariry, R.E.; Barenji, R.V.; Paradkar, A. Towards Pharma 4.0 in clinical trials: A future-orientated perspective. *Drug Discov. Today* **2022**, *27*, 315–325. [CrossRef]
2. Sharma, M.; Sehrawat, R.; Luthra, S.; Daim, T.; Bakry, D. Moving Towards Industry 5.0 in the Pharmaceutical Manufacturing Sector: Challenges and Solutions for Germany. *IEEE Trans. Eng. Manag.* **2022**, 1–18. [CrossRef]
3. Arden, N.S.; Fisher, A.C.; Tyner, K.; Yu, L.X.; Lee, S.L.; Kopcha, M. Industry 4.0 for pharmaceutical manufacturing: Preparing for the smart factories of the future. *Int. J. Pharm.* **2021**, *602*, 120554. [CrossRef] [PubMed]
4. Sharma, D.; Patel, P.; Shah, M. A comprehensive study on Industry 4.0 in the pharmaceutical industry for sustainable development. *Environ. Sci. Pollut. Res.* **2023**, *30*, 90088. [CrossRef] [PubMed]
5. Grangeia, H.B.; Silva, C.; Simões, S.P.; Reis, M.S. Quality by design in pharmaceutical manufacturing: A systematic review of current status, challenges and future perspectives. *Eur. J. Pharm. Biopharm.* **2020**, *147*, 19–37. [CrossRef] [PubMed]
6. Inuwa, H.M.; Ravi Raja, A.; Kumar, A.; Singh, B.; Singh, S. Status of Industry 4.0 applications in healthcare 4.0 and Pharma 4.0. *Mater. Today Proc.* **2022**, *62*, 3593–3598. [CrossRef]
7. Wang, W.; Ye, Z.; Gao, H.; Ouyang, D. Computational pharmaceutics—A new paradigm of drug delivery. *J. Control. Release* **2021**, *338*, 119–136. [CrossRef]
8. Mak, K.K.; Pichika, M.R. Artificial intelligence in drug development: Present status and future prospects. *Drug Discov. Today* **2019**, *24*, 773–780. [CrossRef]
9. Paul, D.; Sanap, G.; Shenoy, S.; Kalyane, D.; Kalia, K.; Tekade, R.K. Artificial intelligence in drug discovery and development. *Drug Discov. Today* **2021**, *26*, 80–93. [CrossRef]
10. Rocco, P.; Musazzi, U.M.; Franzè, S.; Minghetti, P. Copies of nonbiological complex drugs: Generic, hybrid or biosimilar? *Drug Discov. Today* **2019**, *24*, 250–255. [CrossRef]
11. Zagalo, D.M.; Sousa, J.; Simões, S. Quality by design (QbD) approach in marketing authorization procedures of Non-Biological Complex Drugs: A critical evaluation. *Eur. J. Pharm. Biopharm.* **2022**, *178*, 1–24. [CrossRef] [PubMed]
12. Saha, E.; Rathore, P.; Parida, R.; Rana, N.P. The interplay of emerging technologies in pharmaceutical supply chain performance: An empirical investigation for the rise of Pharma 4.0. *Technol. Forecast. Soc. Chang.* **2022**, *181*, 121768. [CrossRef]
13. Ragelle, H.; Rahimian, S.; Guzzi, E.A.; Westenskow, P.D.; Tibbitt, M.W.; Schwach, G.; Langer, R. Additive manufacturing in drug delivery: Innovative drug product design and opportunities for industrial application. *Adv. Drug Deliv. Rev.* **2021**, *178*, 113990. [CrossRef] [PubMed]
14. Muñiz Castro, B.; Elbadawi, M.; Ong, J.J.; Pollard, T.; Song, Z.; Gaisford, S.; Pérez, G.; Basit, A.W.; Cabalar, P.; Goyanes, A. Machine learning predicts 3D printing performance of over 900 drug delivery systems. *J. Control. Release* **2021**, *337*, 530–545. [CrossRef]
15. Kotta, S.; Nair, A.; Alsabeelah, N. Davidopoulou & Ouranidis, 2022. *Curr. Pharm. Des.* **2018**, *24*, 5039–5048. [CrossRef]

16. Jacob, S.; Nair, A.B.; Patel, V.; Shah, J. 3D Printing Technologies: Recent Development and Emerging Applications in Various Drug Delivery Systems. *AAPS PharmSciTech* **2020**, *21*, 220. [CrossRef]
17. Tracy, T.; Wu, L.; Liu, X.; Cheng, S.; Li, X. 3D printing: Innovative solutions for patients and pharmaceutical industry. *Int. J. Pharm.* **2023**, *631*, 122480. [CrossRef]
18. Awad, A.; Yao, A.; Trenfield, S.J.; Goyanes, A.; Gaisford, S.; Basit, A.W. 3D printed tablets (Printlets) with braille and moon patterns for visually impaired patients. *Pharmaceutics* **2020**, *12*, 172. [CrossRef]
19. Awad, A.; Fina, F.; Trenfield, S.J.; Patel, P.; Goyanes, A.; Gaisford, S.; Basit, A.W. 3D printed pellets (Miniprintlets): A novel, multi-drug, controlled release platform technology. *Pharmaceutics* **2019**, *11*, 148. [CrossRef]
20. Melocchi, A.; Uboldi, M.; Briatico-Vangosa, F.; Moutaharrik, S.; Cerea, M.; Foppoli, A.; Maroni, A.; Palugan, L.; Zema, L.; Gazzaniga, A. The chronotopic^{TM} system for pulsatile and colonic delivery of active molecules in the era of precision medicine: Feasibility by 3D printing via fused deposition modeling (fdm). *Pharmaceutics* **2021**, *13*, 759. [CrossRef]
21. Picco, C.J.; Utomo, E.; McClean, A.; Domínguez-Robles, J.; Anjani, Q.K.; Volpe-Zanutto, F.; McKenna, P.E.; Acheson, J.G.; Malinova, D.; Donnelly, R.F.; et al. Development of 3D-printed subcutaneous implants using concentrated polymer/drug solutions. *Int. J. Pharm.* **2023**, *631*, 122477. [CrossRef] [PubMed]
22. Charoenying, T.; Patrojanasophon, P.; Ngawhirunpat, T.; Rojanarata, T.; Akkaramongkolporn, P.; Opanasopit, P. Fabrication of floating capsule-in- 3D-printed devices as gastro-retentive delivery systems of amoxicillin. *J. Drug Deliv. Sci. Technol.* **2020**, *55*, 101393. [CrossRef]
23. Viceconti, M.; Emili, L.; Afshari, P.; Courcelles, E.; Curreli, C.; Famaey, N.; Geris, L.; Horner, M.; Jori, M.C.; Kulesza, A.; et al. Possible Contexts of Use for in Silico Trials Methodologies: A Consensus-Based Review. *IEEE J. Biomed. Health Inform.* **2021**, *25*, 3977–3982. [CrossRef] [PubMed]
24. Brodland, G.W. How computational models can help unlock biological systems. *Semin. Cell Dev. Biol.* **2015**, *47–48*, 62–73. [CrossRef] [PubMed]
25. Seo, Y.; Bang, S.; Son, J.; Kim, D.; Jeong, Y.; Kim, P.; Yang, J.; Eom, J.H.; Choi, N.; Kim, H.N. Brain physiome: A concept bridging in vitro 3D brain models and in silico models for predicting drug toxicity in the brain. *Bioact. Mater.* **2022**, *13*, 135–148. [CrossRef] [PubMed]
26. Hewitt, M.; Ellison, C.M.; Cronin, M.T.D.; Pastor, M.; Steger-Hartmann, T.; Munoz-Muriendas, J.; Pognan, F.; Madden, J.C. Ensuring confidence in predictions: A scheme to assess the scientific validity of in silico models. *Adv. Drug Deliv. Rev.* **2015**, *86*, 101–111. [CrossRef] [PubMed]
27. Ai, N.; Fan, X.; Ekins, S. In silico methods for predicting drug-drug interactions with cytochrome P-450s, transporters and beyond. *Adv. Drug Deliv. Rev.* **2015**, *86*, 46–60. [CrossRef] [PubMed]
28. Montanari, F.; Ecker, G.F. Prediction of drug-ABC-transporter interaction—Recent advances and future challenges. *Adv. Drug Deliv. Rev.* **2015**, *86*, 17–26. [CrossRef]
29. Sung, B. In silico modeling of endocrine organ-on-a-chip systems. *Math. Biosci.* **2022**, *352*, 108900. [CrossRef]
30. Tian, S.; Wang, J.; Li, Y.; Li, D.; Xu, L.; Hou, T. The application of in silico drug-likeness predictions in pharmaceutical research. *Adv. Drug Deliv. Rev.* **2015**, *86*, 2–10. [CrossRef]
31. Villoutreix, B.O.; Taboureau, O. Computational investigations of hERG channel blockers: New insights and current predictive models. *Adv. Drug Deliv. Rev.* **2015**, *86*, 72–82. [CrossRef] [PubMed]
32. Bannigan, P.; Aldeghi, M.; Bao, Z.; Häse, F.; Aspuru-Guzik, A.; Allen, C. Machine learning directed drug formulation development. *Adv. Drug Deliv. Rev.* **2021**, *175*, 113806. [CrossRef] [PubMed]
33. Gupta, R.; Srivastava, D.; Sahu, M.; Tiwari, S.; Ambasta, R.K.; Kumar, P. *Artificial Intelligence to Deep Learning: Machine Intelligence Approach for Drug Discovery*; Springer: Berlin/Heidelberg, Germany, 2021; Volume 25, ISBN 0123456789.
34. Dinh, A.; Miertschin, S.; Young, A.; Mohanty, S.D. A data-driven approach to predicting diabetes and cardiovascular disease with machine learning. *BMC Med. Inform. Decis. Mak.* **2019**, *19*, 211. [CrossRef] [PubMed]
35. Eckhardt, C.M.; Madjarova, S.J.; Williams, R.J.; Ollivier, M.; Karlsson, J.; Pareek, A.; Nwachukwu, B.U. Unsupervised machine learning methods and emerging applications in healthcare. *Knee Surg. Sport. Traumatol. Arthrosc.* **2023**, *31*, 376–381. [CrossRef] [PubMed]
36. Dedeloudi, A.; Weaver, E.; Lamprou, D.A. Machine learning in additive manufacturing & Microfluidics for smarter and safer drug delivery systems. *Int. J. Pharm.* **2023**, *636*, 122818. [CrossRef]
37. Chou, K.C.; Cai, Y.D. Using functional domain composition and support vector machines for prediction of protein subcellular location. *J. Biol. Chem.* **2002**, *277*, 45765–45769. [CrossRef]
38. Cabrera, A.; Bouterse, A.; Nelson, M.; Razzouk, J.; Ramos, O.; Chung, D.; Cheng, W.; Danisa, O. Use of random forest machine learning algorithm to predict short term outcomes following posterior cervical decompression with instrumented fusion. *J. Clin. Neurosci.* **2023**, *107*, 167–171. [CrossRef]
39. Schütt, M.; Stamatopoulos, K.; Batchelor, H.K.; Simmons, M.J.H.; Alexiadis, A. Development of a digital twin of a tablet that mimics a real solid dosage form: Differences in the dissolution profile in conventional mini-USP II and a biorelevant colon model. *Eur. J. Pharm. Sci.* **2022**, *179*, 106310. [CrossRef]
40. Moreno-Benito, M.; Lee, K.T.; Kaydanov, D.; Verrier, H.M.; Blackwood, D.O.; Doshi, P. Digital twin of a continuous direct compression line for drug product and process design using a hybrid flowsheet modelling approach. *Int. J. Pharm.* **2022**, *628*, 122336. [CrossRef]

41. Davidopoulou, C.; Ouranidis, A. Pharma 4.0-Artificially Intelligent Digital Twins for Solidified Nanosuspensions. *Pharmaceutics* **2022**, *14*, 2113. [CrossRef]
42. Schmidt, A.; Helgers, H.; Vetter, F.L.; Juckers, A.; Strube, J. Digital Twin of mRNA-Based SARS-COVID-19 Vaccine Real-Time Release Testing. *Processes* **2021**, *9*, 748. [CrossRef]
43. Sun, Z.; Jiang, J.; Chen, X. Evaluation of Therapeutic Equivalence for the Follow-On Version of Intravenously Administered Non-Biological Complex Drugs. *Clin. Pharmacokinet.* **2020**, *59*, 995–1004. [CrossRef] [PubMed]
44. Klein, K.; Stolk, P.; De Bruin, M.L.; Leufkens, H.G.M.; Crommelin, D.J.A.; De Vlieger, J.S.B. The EU regulatory landscape of non-biological complex drugs (NBCDs) follow-on products: Observations and recommendations. *Eur. J. Pharm. Sci.* **2019**, *133*, 228–235. [CrossRef]
45. Crommelin, D.J.A.; Shah, V.P.; Klebovich, I.; Mcneil, S.E.; Weinstein, V.; Flühmann, B.; Mühlebach, S.; Vlieger, J.S.B. The similarity question for biologicals and non-biological complex drugs. *Eur. J. Pharm. Sci.* **2015**, *76*, 10–17. [CrossRef] [PubMed]
46. Gaspar, R.S.; Silva-Lima, B.; Magro, F.; Alcobia, A.; da Costa, F.L.; Feio, J. Non-biological Complex Drugs (NBCDs): Complex Pharmaceuticals in Need of Individual Robust Clinical Assessment Before Any Therapeutic Equivalence Decision. *Front. Med.* **2020**, *7*, 590527. [CrossRef] [PubMed]
47. Schellekens, H.; Klinger, E.; Mühlebach, S.; Brin, J.F.; Storm, G.; Crommelin, D.J.A. The therapeutic equivalence of complex drugs. *Regul. Toxicol. Pharmacol.* **2011**, *59*, 176–183. [CrossRef] [PubMed]
48. Ghezzi, M.; Pescina, S.; Padula, C.; Santi, P.; Del Favero, E.; Cantù, L.; Nicoli, S. Polymeric micelles in drug delivery: An insight of the techniques for their characterization and assessment in biorelevant conditions. *J. Control. Release* **2021**, *332*, 312–336. [CrossRef] [PubMed]
49. Hwang, D.; Ramsey, J.D.; Kabanov, A.V. Polymeric micelles for the delivery of poorly soluble drugs: From nanoformulation to clinical approval. *Adv. Drug Deliv. Rev.* **2020**, *156*, 80–118. [CrossRef]
50. He, Z.; Wan, X.; Schulz, A.; Bludau, H.; Dobrovolskaia, M.A.; Stern, S.T.; Montgomery, S.A.; Yuan, H.; Li, Z.; Alakhova, D.; et al. A high capacity polymeric micelle of paclitaxel: Implication of high dose drug therapy to safety and in vivo anti-cancer activity. *Biomaterials* **2016**, *101*, 296–309. [CrossRef]
51. Ghosh, B.; Biswas, S. Polymeric micelles in cancer therapy: State of the art. *J. Control. Release* **2021**, *332*, 127–147. [CrossRef]
52. Cagel, M.; Tesan, F.C.; Bernabeu, E.; Salgueiro, M.J.; Zubillaga, M.B.; Moretton, M.A.; Chiappetta, D.A. Polymeric mixed micelles as nanomedicines: Achievements and perspectives. *Eur. J. Pharm. Biopharm.* **2017**, *113*, 211–228. [CrossRef] [PubMed]
53. Ebrahim Attia, A.B.; Ong, Z.Y.; Hedrick, J.L.; Lee, P.P.; Ee, P.L.R.; Hammond, P.T.; Yang, Y.Y. Mixed micelles self-assembled from block copolymers for drug delivery. *Curr. Opin. Colloid Interface Sci.* **2011**, *16*, 182–194. [CrossRef]
54. Guimarães, D.; Cavaco-Paulo, A.; Nogueira, E. Design of liposomes as drug delivery system for therapeutic applications. *Int. J. Pharm.* **2021**, *601*, 120571. [CrossRef] [PubMed]
55. Akbarzadeh, A.; Rezaei-sadabady, R.; Davaran, S.; Joo, S.W.; Zarghami, N. Liposome: Classification, preparation, and applications. *Nanoscale Res. Lett.* **2013**, *22*, 102. [CrossRef] [PubMed]
56. Jensen, G.M.; Hodgson, D.F. Opportunities and challenges in commercial pharmaceutical liposome applications. *Adv. Drug Deliv. Rev.* **2020**, *154–155*, 2–12. [CrossRef] [PubMed]
57. Saraf, S.; Jain, A.; Tiwari, A.; Verma, A.; Panda, P.K.; Jain, S.K. Advances in liposomal drug delivery to cancer: An overview. *J. Drug Deliv. Sci. Technol.* **2020**, *56*, 101549. [CrossRef]
58. Atallah, C.; Viennet, C.; Robin, S.; Ibazizen, S.; Greige-Gerges, H.; Charcosset, C. Effect of cysteamine hydrochloride-loaded liposomes on skin depigmenting and penetration. *Eur. J. Pharm. Sci.* **2022**, *168*, 106082. [CrossRef]
59. Costa, R.; Santos, L. Delivery systems for cosmetics—From manufacturing to the skin of natural antioxidants. *Powder Technol.* **2017**, *322*, 402–416. [CrossRef]
60. Pando, D.; Matos, M.; Gutiérrez, G.; Pazos, C. Formulation of resveratrol entrapped niosomes for topical use. *Colloids Surfaces B Biointerfaces* **2015**, *128*, 398–404. [CrossRef]
61. Chen, S.; Hanning, S.; Falconer, J.; Locke, M.; Wen, J. Recent advances in non-ionic surfactant vesicles (niosomes): Fabrication, characterization, pharmaceutical and cosmetic applications. *Eur. J. Pharm. Biopharm.* **2019**, *144*, 18–39. [CrossRef]
62. Aparajay, P.; Dev, A. Functionalized niosomes as a smart delivery device in cancer and fungal infection. *Eur. J. Pharm. Sci.* **2022**, *168*, 106052. [CrossRef] [PubMed]
63. Chaudhary, H.; Kohli, K.; Kumar, V.K. Nano-transfersomes as a novel carrier for transdermal delivery. *Int. J. Pharm.* **2013**, *454*, 367–380. [CrossRef] [PubMed]
64. Lei, W.; Yu, C.; Lin, H.; Zhou, X. Development of tacrolimus-loaded transfersomes for deeper skin penetration enhancement and therapeutic effect improvement in vivo. *Asian J. Pharm. Sci.* **2013**, *8*, 336–345. [CrossRef]
65. Al Shuwaili, A.H.; Rasool, B.K.A.; Abdulrasool, A.A. Optimization of elastic transfersomes formulations for transdermal delivery of pentoxifylline. *Eur. J. Pharm. Biopharm.* **2016**, *102*, 101–114. [CrossRef] [PubMed]
66. Rocco, P.; Eberini, I.; Musazzi, U.M.; Franzè, S.; Minghetti, P. Glatiramer acetate: A complex drug beyond biologics. *Eur. J. Pharm. Sci.* **2019**, *133*, 8–14. [CrossRef] [PubMed]
67. Weinstock-Guttman, B.; Nair, K.V.; Glajch, J.L.; Ganguly, T.C.; Kantor, D. Two decades of glatiramer acetate: From initial discovery to the current development of generics. *J. Neurol. Sci.* **2017**, *376*, 255–259. [CrossRef] [PubMed]

68. Melamed-Gal, S.; Loupe, P.; Timan, B.; Weinstein, V.; Kolitz, S.; Zhang, J.; Funt, J.; Komlosh, A.; Ashkenazi, N.; Bar-Ilan, O.; et al. Physicochemical, biological, functional and toxicological characterization of the European follow-on glatiramer acetate product as compared with Copaxone. *eNeurologicalSci* **2018**, *12*, 19–30. [CrossRef]
69. Nikravesh, N.; Borchard, G.; Hofmann, H.; Philipp, E.; Flühmann, B.; Wick, P. Factors influencing safety and efficacy of intravenous iron-carbohydrate nanomedicines: From production to clinical practice. *Nanomed. Nanotechnol. Biol. Med.* **2020**, *26*, 102178. [CrossRef]
70. Percy, L.; Mansour, D.; Fraser, I.; Hon, F. Iron deficiency and iron deficiency anaemia in women. *Best Pract. Res. Clin. Obstet. Gynaecol.* **2017**, *40*, 55–67. [CrossRef]
71. Auerbach, M.; Ballard, H. Clinical use of intravenous iron: Administration, efficacy, and safety. *Hematol. Am. Soc. Hematol. Educ. Program* **2010**, *2010*, 338–347. [CrossRef]
72. Zheng, N.; Sun, D.D.; Zou, P.; Jiang, W. Scientific and Regulatory Considerations for Generic Complex Drug Products Containing Nanomaterials. *AAPS J.* **2017**, *19*, 619–631. [CrossRef] [PubMed]
73. Müller, R.H.; Gohla, S.; Keck, C.M. State of the art of nanocrystals—Special features, production, nanotoxicology aspects and intracellular delivery. *Eur. J. Pharm. Biopharm.* **2011**, *78*, 1–9. [CrossRef] [PubMed]
74. Mohammad, I.S.; Hu, H.; Yin, L.; He, W. Drug nanocrystals: Fabrication methods and promising therapeutic applications. *Int. J. Pharm.* **2019**, *562*, 187–202. [CrossRef] [PubMed]
75. Miao, X.; Yang, W.; Feng, T.; Lin, J.; Huang, P. Drug nanocrystals for cancer therapy. *Wiley Interdiscip. Rev. Nanomed. Nanobiotechnol.* **2018**, *10*, e1499. [CrossRef] [PubMed]
76. Lin, Z.; Gao, W.; Hu, H.; Ma, K.; He, B.; Dai, W.; Wang, X.; Wang, J.; Zhang, X.; Zhang, Q. Novel thermo-sensitive hydrogel system with paclitaxel nanocrystals: High drug-loading, sustained drug release and extended local retention guaranteeing better efficacy and lower toxicity. *J. Control. Release* **2014**, *174*, 161–170. [CrossRef] [PubMed]
77. Almeida, A.; Linares, V.; Mora-Castaño, G.; Casas, M.; Caraballo, I.; Sarmento, B. 3D printed systems for colon-specific delivery of camptothecin-loaded chitosan micelles. *Eur. J. Pharm. Biopharm.* **2021**, *167*, 48–56. [CrossRef] [PubMed]
78. Linares, V.; Casas, M.; Caraballo, I. Printfills: 3D printed systems combining fused deposition modeling and injection volume filling. Application to colon-specific drug delivery. *Eur. J. Pharm. Biopharm.* **2019**, *134*, 138–143. [CrossRef]
79. Cisneros, K.; Chowdhury, N.; Coleman, E.; Ferdous, T.; Su, H.; Jennings, J.A.; Bumgardner, J.D.; Fujiwara, T. Long-Term Controlled Release of Simvastatin from Photoprinted Triple-Networked Hydrogels Composed of Modified Chitosan and PLA–PEG Micelles. *Macromol. Biosci.* **2021**, *21*, 2100123. [CrossRef]
80. Sommonte, F.; Weaver, E.; Mathew, E.; Denora, N.; Lamprou, D.A. In-House Innovative "Diamond Shaped" 3D Printed Microfluidic Devices for Lysozyme-Loaded Liposomes. *Pharmaceutics* **2022**, *14*, 2484. [CrossRef]
81. Wang, Z.; Liu, L.; Xiang, S.; Jiang, C.; Wu, W.; Ruan, S.; Du, Q.; Chen, T.; Xue, Y.; Chen, H.; et al. Formulation and Characterization of a 3D-Printed Cryptotanshinone-Loaded Niosomal Hydrogel for Topical Therapy of Acne. *AAPS PharmSciTech* **2020**, *21*, 159. [CrossRef]
82. Groetsch, A.; Stelzl, S.; Nagel, Y.; Kochetkova, T.; Scherrer, N.C.; Ovsianikov, A.; Michler, J.; Pethö, L.; Siqueira, G.; Nyström, G.; et al. Microscale 3D Printing and Tuning of Cellulose Nanocrystals Reinforced Polymer Nanocomposites. *Small* **2023**, *19*, e2202470. [CrossRef] [PubMed]
83. Germini, G.; Peltonen, L. 3D Printing of Drug Nanocrystals for Film Formulations. *Molecules* **2021**, *26*, 3941. [CrossRef] [PubMed]
84. Phan, V.H.G.; Murugesan, M.; Huong, H.; Le, T.T.; Phan, T.H.; Manivasagan, P.; Mathiyalagan, R.; Jang, E.S.; Yang, D.C.; Li, Y.; et al. Cellulose Nanocrystals-Incorporated Thermosensitive Hydrogel for Controlled Release, 3D Printing, and Breast Cancer Treatment Applications. *ACS Appl. Mater. Interfaces* **2022**, *14*, 42812–42826. [CrossRef] [PubMed]
85. Lopez-Vidal, L.; Real, J.P.; Real, D.A.; Camacho, N.; Kogan, M.J.; Paredes, A.J.; Palma, S.D. Nanocrystal-based 3D-printed tablets: Semi-solid extrusion using melting solidification printing process (MESO-PP) for oral administration of poorly soluble drugs. *Int. J. Pharm.* **2022**, *611*, 121311. [CrossRef] [PubMed]
86. Tambe, S.M.; Jain, D.D.; Hasmukh Mehta, C.; Ashwini, T.; Yogendra Nayak, U.; Amin, P.D. Hot-melt extruded in situ gelling systems (MeltDrops Technology): Formulation development, in silico modelling and in vivo studies. *Eur. J. Pharm. Biopharm.* **2023**, *188*, 108–124. [CrossRef] [PubMed]
87. Duran, T.; Costa, A.; Gupta, A.; Xu, X.; Zhang, H.; Burgess, D.; Chaudhuri, B. Coarse-Grained Molecular Dynamics Simulations of Paclitaxel-Loaded Polymeric Micelles. *Mol. Pharm.* **2022**, *19*, 1117–1134. [CrossRef]
88. Bhendale, M.; Singh, J.K. Molecular Insights on Morphology, Composition, and Stability of Mixed Micelles Formed by Ionic Surfactant and Nonionic Block Copolymer in Water Using Coarse-Grained Molecular Dynamics Simulations. *Langmuir* **2023**, *39*, 5031–5040. [CrossRef]
89. Ramajayam, K.K.; Wolfe, A.M.; Motamarry, A.; Yost, J.; Yost, M.J.; Haemmerich, D. Computer Modeling of Drug Delivery with Thermosensitive Liposomes in a Realistic Three-Dimensional Geometry. *Proc. Annu. Int. Conf. IEEE Eng. Med. Biol. Soc. EMBS* **2020**, *2020*, 5021–5024. [CrossRef]
90. Cern, A.; Marcus, D.; Tropsha, A.; Barenholz, Y.; Goldblum, A. New drug candidates for liposomal delivery identified by computer modeling of liposomes' remote loading and leakage. *J. Control. Release* **2017**, *252*, 18–27. [CrossRef]
91. Bunker, A.; Magarkar, A.; Viitala, T. Rational design of liposomal drug delivery systems, a review: Combined experimental and computational studies of lipid membranes, liposomes and their PEGylation. *Biochim. Biophys. Acta—Biomembr.* **2016**, *1858*, 2334–2352. [CrossRef]

92. Pathak, P.; Dhawan, V.; Magarkar, A.; Danne, R.; Govindarajan, S.; Ghosh, S.; Steiniger, F.; Chaudhari, P.; Gopal, V.; Bunker, A.; et al. Design of cholesterol arabinogalactan anchored liposomes for asialoglycoprotein receptor mediated targeting to hepatocellular carcinoma: In silico modeling, in vitro and in vivo evaluation. *Int. J. Pharm.* **2016**, *509*, 149–158. [CrossRef]
93. Wu, X.; Dai, X.; Liao, Y.; Sheng, M.; Shi, X. Investigation on drug entrapment location in liposomes and transfersomes based on molecular dynamics simulation. *J. Mol. Model.* **2021**, *27*, 111. [CrossRef] [PubMed]
94. Jablonka, L.; Ashtikar, M.; Gao, G.; Jung, F.; Thurn, M.; Preuß, A.; Scheglmann, D.; Albrecht, V.; Röder, B.; Wacker, M.G. Advanced in silico modeling explains pharmacokinetics and biodistribution of temoporfin nanocrystals in humans. *J. Control. Release* **2019**, *308*, 57–70. [CrossRef] [PubMed]
95. Ullah, N.; Khan, S.; Ahmed, S.; Govender, T.; Faidah, H.S.; De Matas, M.; Shahid, M.; Minhas, M.U.; Sohail, M.; Khurram, M. Dexibuprofen nanocrystals with improved therapeutic performance: Fabrication, characterization, in silico modeling, and in vivo evaluation. *Int. J. Nanomed.* **2018**, *13*, 1677–1692. [CrossRef] [PubMed]
96. Jones, D.E.; Ghandehari, H.; Facelli, J.C. A review of the applications of data mining and machine learning for the prediction of biomedical properties of nanoparticles. *Comput. Methods Programs Biomed.* **2016**, *132*, 93–103. [CrossRef] [PubMed]
97. Husseini, G.A.; Mjalli, F.S.; Pitt, W.G.; Abdel-Jabbar, N.M. Using ANN and MPC to optimize acoustically assisted Doxorubicin release from micelles. *Proc. IASTED Int. Conf. Model. Simul.* **2009**, *8*, 320–325.
98. Han, R.; Ye, Z.; Zhang, Y.; Cheng, Y.; Zheng, Y.; Ouyang, D. Predicting liposome formulations by the integrated machine learning and molecular modeling approaches. *Asian J. Pharm. Sci.* **2023**, *18*, 100811. [CrossRef] [PubMed]
99. Kashani-Asadi-Jafari, F.; Aftab, A.; Ghaemmaghami, S. A machine learning framework for predicting entrapment efficiency in niosomal particles. *Int. J. Pharm.* **2022**, *627*, 122203. [CrossRef]
100. Subramanian, N.; Yajnik, A.; Murthy, R.S.R. Artificial neural network as an alternative to multiple regression analysis in optimizing formulation parameters of cytarabine liposomes. *AAPS PharmSciTech* **2004**, *5*, E4. [CrossRef]
101. Rebollo, R.; Oyoun, F.; Corvis, Y.; El-Hammadi, M.M.; Saubamea, B.; Andrieux, K.; Mignet, N.; Alhareth, K. Microfluidic Manufacturing of Liposomes: Development and Optimization by Design of Experiment and Machine Learning. *ACS Appl. Mater. Interfaces* **2022**, *14*, 39736–39745. [CrossRef]
102. Baptista, D.; Correia, J.; Pereira, B.; Rocha, M. Evaluating molecular representations in machine learning models for drug response prediction and interpretability. *J. Integr. Bioinform.* **2022**, *19*, 20220006. [CrossRef] [PubMed]
103. Sansare, S.; Duran, T.; Mohammadiarani, H.; Goyal, M.; Yenduri, G.; Costa, A.; Xu, X.; O'Connor, T.; Burgess, D.; Chaudhuri, B. Artificial neural networks in tandem with molecular descriptors as predictive tools for continuous liposome manufacturing. *Int. J. Pharm.* **2021**, *603*, 120713. [CrossRef]
104. Rathore, A.S.; Nikita, S.; Thakur, G.; Mishra, S. Artificial intelligence and machine learning applications in biopharmaceutical manufacturing. *Trends Biotechnol.* **2023**, *41*, 497–510. [CrossRef] [PubMed]
105. He, Y.; Ye, Z.; Liu, X.; Wei, Z.; Qiu, F.; Li, H.F.; Zheng, Y.; Ouyang, D. Can machine learning predict drug nanocrystals? *J. Control. Release* **2020**, *322*, 274–285. [CrossRef] [PubMed]
106. Attaran, M.; Attaran, S.; Celik, B.G. The impact of digital twins on the evolution of intelligent manufacturing and Industry 4.0. *Adv. Comput. Intell.* **2023**, *3*. [CrossRef] [PubMed]
107. Trenfield, S.J.; Awad, A.; McCoubrey, L.E.; Elbadawi, M.; Goyanes, A.; Gaisford, S.; Basit, A.W. Advancing pharmacy and healthcare with virtual digital technologies. *Adv. Drug Deliv. Rev.* **2022**, *182*, 29–39. [CrossRef] [PubMed]
108. Pravin, S.; Sudhir, A. Integration of 3D printing with dosage forms: A new perspective for modern healthcare. *Biomed. Pharmacother.* **2018**, *107*, 146–154. [CrossRef]
109. Bom, S.; Martins, A.M.; Ribeiro, H.M.; Marto, J. Diving into 3D (bio)printing: A revolutionary tool to customize the production of drug and cell-based systems for skin delivery. *Int. J. Pharm.* **2021**, *605*, 120794. [CrossRef]
110. Jamróz, W.; Szafraniec, J.; Kurek, M.; Jachowicz, R. 3D Printing in Pharmaceutical and Medical Applications—Recent Achievements and Challenges. *Pharm. Res.* **2018**, *35*, 176. [CrossRef]
111. Preis, M.; Öblom, H. 3D-Printed Drugs for Children—Are We Ready Yet? *AAPS PharmSciTech* **2017**, *18*, 303–308. [CrossRef]
112. Methods, N.S. Performance Metrics for the Comparative Analysis of Clinical Risk Prediction Models. *Circ. Cardiovasc. Qual. Outcomes* **2021**, *14*, 1076–1086. [CrossRef]
113. Rácz, A.; Bajusz, D.; Héberger, K. Multi-Level Comparison of Machine Learning Classifiers and Their Performance Metrics. *Molecules* **2019**, *24*, 2811. [CrossRef]

MDPI AG
Grosspeteranlage 5
4052 Basel
Switzerland
Tel.: +41 61 683 77 34

Pharmaceutics Editorial Office
E-mail: pharmaceutics@mdpi.com
www.mdpi.com/journal/pharmaceutics

www.ingramcontent.com/pod-product-compliance
Lightning Source LLC
Chambersburg PA
CBHW061621220926
51850CB00005B/563